Library of
Davidson College
VOID

Biology of the Tapeworm *Hymenolepis diminuta*

Academic Press Rapid Manuscript Reproduction

CONTENTS

List of Contributors	ix
Preface	xi
Aspects of the Life History and Systematics of *Hymenolepis diminuta* M. D. B. Burt	1
Structure and Ultrastructure of the Larvae and Metacestodes of *Hymenolepis diminuta* John E. Ubelaker	59
The Morphology, Histology, and Fine Structure of the Adult Stage of the Cyclophyllidean Tapeworm *Hymenolepis diminuta* Richard Dick Lumsden and Robert Specian	157
The Intestine as an Environment for *Hymenolepis diminuta* D. F. Mettrick	281
Development of *Hymenolepis diminuta* in Its Definitive Host Larry S. Roberts	357
The Cultivation of *Hymenolepis* in Vitro William S. Evans	425
Nucleic Acids from Hymenolepids Austin J. MacInnis and Clint Carter	449
Energy Metabolism of Adult *Hymenolepis diminuta* Carmen F. Fioravanti and Howard J. Saz	463
Concepts of Membrane Biology in *Hymenolepis diminuta* Ron B. Podesta	505
Immunity and *Hymenolepis diminuta* C. A. Hopkins	551

Migratory Activity and Related Phenomena in *Hymenolepis diminuta* 615
    Hisao P. Arai

Chemotherapy of Hymenolepiasis 639
    Hugo Van den Bossche

Index *695*

CONTRIBUTORS

Numbers in parentheses indicate the pages on which authors' contributions begin.

Hisao P. Arai (615), Department of Biology, University of Calgary, Calgary, Alberta T2N 1N4, Canada

M. D. B. Burt (1), Department of Biology, University of New Brunswick, Fredericton, New Brunswick E3B 5A3, Canada

Clint Carter (449), Department of Biology, Vanderbilt University, Nashville, Tennessee 37203

William S. Evans (425), Department of Biology, University of Winnipeg, Winnipeg, Manitoba R3B 2E9, Canada

Carmen F. Fioravanti (463), Department of Biological Sciences, Bowling Green State University, Bowling Green, Ohio 43402

C. A. Hopkins (551), Wellcome Laboratories for Experimental Parasitology, University of Glasgow, Glasgow G61 1GH, Scotland

Richard Dick Lumsden (157), Department of Biology, Tulane University, New Orleans, Louisiana 70118

Austin J. MacInnis (449), Department of Biology, University of California, Los Angeles, California 40024

D. F. Mettrick (281), Department of Zoology, University of Toronto, Toronto, Ontario M5S 1A1, Canada

Ron B. Podesta (505), Department of Biology, University of Western Ontario, London, Ontario N6A 5C2, Canada

Larry S. Roberts (357), Department of Biological Sciences, Texas Tech University, Lubbock, Texas 79409

Howard J. Saz (463), University of Notre Dame, Notre Dame, Indiana 46556

Robert Specian (157), Department of Anatomy, Harvard Medical School, Boston, Massachusetts 02115

John E. Ubelaker (59), Department of Biology, Southern Methodist University, Dallas, Texas 75222

Hugo Van den Bossche (639), Laboratory of Comparative Biochemistry, Janssen Pharmaceutica, B-2340 Beerse, Belgium

PREFACE

When Rudolphi first described *Taenia diminuta* in 1819, he could have hardly foreseen that some 160 years later a whole volume would be devoted to considering various aspects of the biology of that particular tapeworm, now renamed *Hymenolepis diminuta*. One of the unique features of this book is that it is the first such volume expressly devoted to consideration of just one species of tapeworm; a parasite, moreover, that has received little or no veterinary or medical attention, i.e., as far as disease and infection are concerned.

One name, whose spirit fills the whole book but is not listed as an author, is that of the late Clark P. Read. In his now classic pamphlet of 1950, Clark Read wrote that "in order to understand the host–parasite relationships of intestinal helminths we must first separately investigate the physiology of the host and of the parasite...resynthesis of the host and parasite physiology will reveal new concepts relative to intestinal parasitism." How true that prediction was is well illustrated in the following contributions.

It is, however, appropriate to reconsider whether we have yet learned the lesson that he expounded in 1963 on the need to bring into parasitology the methodologies and concepts from other disciplines in order to raise the sophistication and quality of experimental studies on helminths to a level acceptable to physiologists, cell biologists, ecologists, biochemists, and members of other disciplines. Clark Read was one of a small number of parasitologists who constantly tried to improve the quality of work in the field of parasitology. It was, and still is, not easy because as Read noted, anyone interested in the physiological and biochemical aspects of parasitism requires a sound grounding in biology as well as training in chemistry, mathematics, and biochemistry; today, one would also have to include biophysics, microbiology, and immunology.

It is disquieting that work on parasitic models in areas such as transport, metabolism, nutrition, ecology, etc. continues to be largely ignored in general review articles on these topics. In addition, many parasitologists seem reluctant to survey the literature in other fields when interpreting their own results. Obviously, we still have inadequate communication with other better developed areas of biology; the complexity of the host–parasite systems demands all ideas and insight be mustered if we are to continue unraveling the intricacies of such associations.

Nonparasitologists may indeed wonder whether the *diminuta*–rat system is the only experimental model that we have. It is not, of course, but it is certainly true that we have a greater understanding of the biology of *H. diminuta* than of practically any other helminth. Therein, we think, lies the challenge of the immediate future. We must be cautious in extrapolating the results from studies on *H. diminuta* to broad generalities for all intestinal parasites or even for all cestodes, until we have a wider range of models on which to base our conclusions. The advances that have been made *H. diminuta* should stimulate others to determine which factors are specific for *H. diminuta* and contribute to its signal success as a pathophysiological agent, as opposed to those features of its biology that are of greater or even widespread generality. We now know the questions that must be asked of other host–parasite systems and, in many instances, we have the methodology and technology to obtain the answers. If this book encourages diversity among future studies in helminth ecology, physiology, immunology, and biochemistry, it will serve its purpose and ensure that parasitology continues along the pathway marked for us by Clark Read and others who have laid the foundations that have resulted in this particular volume.

ASPECTS OF THE LIFE HISTORY AND SYSTEMATICS OF *HYMENOLEPIS DIMINUTA*

M.D.B. Burt

Department of Biology
University of New Brunswick
Fredericton, New Brunswick

I. LIFE HISTORY

Hymenolepis diminuta lives as an adult in a wide variety of rodent hosts but, has also been recorded from other mammals, including man. As well as boasting a large number of definitive hosts, records indicate that this species is almost worldwide in distribution (Table I).

Records of *H. diminuta* from humans are widely scattered in the literature and although it has not been possible to examine every reference, the majority of them are summarised in Table II which shows, when known, the geographical location. Although over 200 cases of human infection have been reported (Turner 1975), records of this worm from man are considered as accidental infections; it is neither considered as a serious health hazard nor of much clinical significance.

Following ingestion by the definitive host, the viable larvae are protected by the outer layers of the cysticercoid during its passage through the stomach. Activation and excystment of the larvae in the definitive host requires, in particular, the presence of bile salts (Rothman 1959). If excysted worms are introduced into the stomach they are destroyed whereas they can establish themselves readily if introduced directly into the small intestine.

Once the young adult *H. diminuta* is established in the definitive host, following ingestion of fully-developed, viable cysticercoid larvae, growth and development are rapid showing an exponential increase in weight for about 10 days (Read 1972). The prepatent period varies from 13 to 21 days and the rate of development and maturation is clearly linked to the size of the infection (Roberts 1961), the nature of the host diet with particular reference to carbohydrates (Mettrick and Munro 1965; Smyth 1969) and the presence of co-parasites (Holmes 1962). Growth of the young adult is most rapid within the first seven days (Roberts 1961), but initially there is a short lag period of about 24h before the growth rate in laboratory rats rises sharply over a 5-day period (Goodchild and Harrison 1961). As the worms mature, they appear to change their site of attachment: 5-day old worms attach within the anterior 39% moiety of the rat gut whereas 7-day old worms are found within the anterior 15% moiety (Cannon and Mettrick 1970). This finding, however, should perhaps be viewed with caution as it appears that worms show a diel migratory pattern within the gut which is related to the host feeding habits (Read and Kilejian 1969; Hopkins 1969, 1970) and which is discussed elsewhere in this volume.

After the formation of each proglottis, its differentiation and maturation is independent of growth or of further proglottis production. However, there does appear to be a relationship between growth rate and shedding of gravid proglottides which maintains a more-or-less constant length of the adult worm at about 70 cm in light infections, although longer worms have been recorded. Worm size in a single host varies not only in relation to the number of worms present, as mentioned previously, but also in relation to the species of definitive host infected (Read and Voge 1954); the average volume of worms recovered from hosts with single-worm infections was found to be greater in rats than in hamsters and albino mice. As is discussed elsewhere, dietary items, such as glucose (Read 1951; Read *et al.* 1958), can affect tapeworm growth.

Gravid proglottides, after breaking away from the strobila, disintegrate within the host intestine and eggs are passed with the host faeces. No further period of embryonation is required, the eggs being infective to a wide variety of intermediate hosts (Table III) immediately upon release from the definitive host. *H. diminuta* has a high biotic potential: an adult worm has been estimated to produce 1149 hexacanths per day (Hager 1941). Although Beck (1951) has shown that egg production can be influenced by the presence of male sex hormones, the appearance of shelled embryos usually occurs about 9 days after proglottis formation (Read 1972). The release of these embryos from hosts typically commences some 17 days after the initial infection (Roberts 1961).

Under natural conditions the life span of adult *H. diminuta* in rats is probably as long as that of the host that harbours it. By artificial passage, from one suitable host to another, however, the worm can live for at least 14 years and, as further pointed out by Read (1972): "there is no reason to believe that it might not live for a much longer period of time".

The egg of *H. diminuta* is atypical of most hymenolepids in that it lacks the characteristic knobs or filaments usually found in association with the embryophore. This is a useful feature in differentiating between *H. diminuta* eggs and those of *H. nana* which are typical. As indicated above, the oncospheres are fully infective when passed by the definitive host and if the stiff outer shell or capsule has not been damaged, they can remain viable for about 6 months (Smyth 1969). If eggs are ingested by a suitable intermediate host, such as an insect living in cereal food, the oncospheres will develop into cysticercoid larvae within the haemocoele of the intermediate host. The feeding insect mechanically ruptures the outer capsule with its mouthparts; the mechanical action of the oncospheral hooks, in conjunction with the penetration glands, affords passage of the oncosphere through the gut wall and into the haemocoele (Read 1972).

A useful account of collection, sterilization and storage techniques of *H. diminuta* "eggs" is provided by Hundley and Berntzen (1969). *In vitro* release of oncospheres was first described by Voge and Berntzen (1961) and later, in further detail, Berntzen and Voge (1965) describe the mechanical rupture of the outer envelope or capsule and the enzymatic digestion of the inner layers thus allowing escape of the hexacanth.

Growth and development of the cysticercoid larva of *H. diminuta* from the hexacanth stage occur in the haemocoele of an intermediate host of which a variety have been implicated in the life cycle (Table III). Penetration of the gut wall is independent of host metamorphosis and the developing larva becomes surrounded by a thin cuticle 2-3 days after entering the haemocoele. Development, which is temperature dependent, can be as early as 5 days at 37°C and as late as 65 days at 15°C (Voge and Turner 1956).

Development of larval *H. diminuta* in *Tribolium* is described by Voge and Heyneman (1957). Whether the scolex develops inside the cystic portion of the cysticercoid or outside, with subsequent invagination, depends on the species. Narihara (1937a) and Rothman (1957) suggest that the scolex of *H. diminuta* and, according to Rothman (1957), that of *H. citelli* develop externally before withdrawing into the cyst. This pattern of development for *H. citelli* is counter to previous findings for this species by Voge (1956), but is similar to findings for *H. exigua* by Alicata and Chang (1939) and *H. cantaniana* by Jones and Alicata (1935). Rothman (1957) notes, however, that in *H. nana* and *H. tenuirostris* scolex development occurs within the cyst. As will be seen elsewhere, in spite of similar manner of development, it is possible to distinguish readily between cysticercoids of *H. diminuta* and *H. citelli*.

II. SYSTEMATIC POSITION AND TAXONOMY

   Order Cyclophyllidea
     Family Hymenolepididae Railliet & Henry, 1909
       Sub-family Hymenolepidinae Perrier, 1897
         Genus *Hymenolepis* Weinland, 1858

Hymenolepis diminuta (Rudolphi, 1819) Blanchard, 1891.

SYNONYMS:

Taenia diminuta Rudolphi, 1819
T. flavopunctata Weinland, 1858; Railliet, 1893
Hymenolepis (Taenia) flavopunctata (Weinland) Weinland, 1858
Hymenolepis flavopunctata (Weinland) Weinland, 1859
Taenia (Hymenolepis) flavopunctata Weinland, 1861
Taenia leptocephala Creplin, 1825; Lutz, 1904
Taenia varesina Parona, 1884
Taenia minima Grassi 1886; Lutz, 1894
Taenia diminuta Zschokke 1899
Hymenolepis diminuta Castellani & Chalmers, 1910
Taenia flavomaculata Leuckart, 1863
Taenia flavopuncta Cobbold, 1864
Taenia flavapuncta Aitken, 1874
Taenia flaviopunctata Vogt, 1878
Taenia flavopunkta Stein, 1882
Taenia flavapunctata Simon, 1897
Taenia ceptocephala Lussana & Romaro
Taenia septocephala Perroncito & Airoldi, 1888
Taenia leptocefala Previtera, 1900
Taenia vererina Huber, 1896
Taenia (Hymenolepis) megaloon von Linstow, 1901
not *Taenia megaloon* Weinland, 1861; Meggitt & Subramanian, 1927
Hymenolepis megaloon (von Linstow) Ransom, 1904
Hymenolepis diminutoides Cholodkovsky, 1913; Meggitt & Subramanian, 1927
Hymenolepis ognewi Skriabin, 1924
Hymenolepis anomala Splendore, 1920; Joyeux & Foley, 1930
Cer. hymenolepis-diminutae (Rudolphi) Railliet, 1892
Cyst. taeniae-diminutae (Rudolphi) Dolly, 1894
Cyst. taenia-flavopunctatae (Weinland) Aitken, 1866

III. INTRA-FAMILIAL RELATIONSHIPS

The genus *Hymenolepis sensu lato* still remains as the largest and probably most confused group of all cestodes. The generic name was coined from two Greek words (*hymen*, membrane and *lepis*, shell) by

Weinland (1858) who, even then, recognized the characteristic membranes and shell surrounding the oncospheres of certain tapeworms as being significantly different to the corresponding structures found in the large *Taenia* species of man. Weinland associates the species he describes as *flavopunctata* with the genus *Hymenolepis*, but causes some taxonomic confusion by further dividing his genus into two subgenera, *Lepidotrias* and *Dilepis*, choosing *Taenia murina* Dujardin, 1845 as the type of the genus *Lepidotrias*. As indicated by both Grassi (1888) and Blanchard (1891), *Taenia diminuta* Rudolphi, 1819 is identical to Weinland's *Lepidotrias flavopunctata* and the involved taxonomy which resulted from the suppresion of *Lepidotrias* to a junior synonym of *Hymenolepis* is discussed in detail by Stiles (1903). The conclusions reached by Stiles are now widely accepted in the establishment of *Hymenolepis diminuta* as the type species of the genus which also contains *Taenia murina* Dujardin, 1845 (not Gmelin, 1789), a junior synonym of *Hymenolepis nana* (von Siebold, 1882).

There have been numerous attempts to find a suitable classification whereby the large and growing number of species can be considered in smaller, and hence, taxonomically, more convenient groups. Thus were erected such genera as: *Echinocotyle* by Blanchard (1891), for those hymenolepids with spiny suckers; *Drepanidotaenia* by Railliet (1892) for those forms from birds with a double crown of hooks. Much of the subsequent work had dealt mainly with avian hymenolepids and contained attempts to split off a growing number of hymenolepid genera from the genus *Hymenolepis* with its type species *H. diminuta*. A major attempt was made by Mayhew (1925) to establish new groupings using, primarily, the arrangement of testes, thus extending the earlier ideas of Cohn (1901, 1904), Clerc (1903) and Fuhrmann (1906). However, his erection of the two new genera *Weinlandia* and *Wardium* and their incorporation along with *Echinorhynchotaenia*, *Hymenofimbria*, *Fimbriaria* and *Hymenolepis* into one sub-family of the family Hymenolepididae, was not generally accepted. It was rejected by Fuhrmann (1932) who foresaw the extent of the resulting subdivision of hymenolepids when he wrote: "Nous maintenons donc le genre *Hymenolepis* sous son ancienne forme avec regret, parce que ce

genre est vraiment trop vaste. Si'on voulait le
subdiviser il faudrait creer, base sur l'anatomie et
la forme et peut-etre aussi le nombre des crochets,
un assez grand nombre de genres".

Hughes (1940), in a general summary of the
genus *Hymenolepis*, lists 328 valid species and later
(Hughes 1941) provides a descriptive key to the
species known at that time. Lopez-Neyra (1942a, b),
in an extensive revision of the genus *Hymenolepis*
Weinland, erects four new genera: *Meggittiella*,
Microsomacanthus, *Sphenacanthus*, and *Hispaniolepis*
and emends the generic diagnoses of *Echinocotyle*,
Drepanidotaenia, *Dicranotaenia* and *Hymenolepis* to
contain most (277) of the species known to him.

Like Mayhew's (1925) earlier scheme, however,
that of Lopez-Neyra has also been more-or-less
rejected by Western authors, although it has been
more widely accepted by Russian authors. The latter,
including Skrjabin and Matevosyan (1942, 1948),
Spasskii (1947, 1948, 1953, 1954), Spasskii and
Spasskaya (1954) and several others, have erected
many new genera which are included in the major work
by Yamaguti (1959) who, himself, erects many new
genera within the Hymenolepididae. In a review of
Volume II of Yamaguti's, *Systema Helminthum*, Baer
(1961) states: "The 20 genera introduced by Yamaguti
to the family Hymenolepididae confound the confusion
that has already been created by the Russian authors
and in no way furthers a clear understanding of this
difficult group".

In a more recent work, Spasskii (1962)
suppresses 19 of the genera listed by Yamaguti (1959)
and accepts 26 genera of tritesticulate cestodes.
As indicated by MacDonald (1969), the fragmentation
and recombination of *Hymenolepis sensu lato* during
the 10 years preceding his work has resulted in the
transfer of several hymenolepid cestodes of waterfowl to as many as four or five different genera.
Although there is a growing acceptance of the
conservative scheme used by Czaplinski (1956) with
reference to anseriform hymenolepids (in which he
accepts seven genera, including *Hymenolepis sensu
lato*, to contain all the tritesticulate species he
deals with), there is still a wide divergence of
opinion regarding the sub-division of this vast

genus as is clear from the recent works of Baer
(1973), Czaplinski (1973) and Matevosyan (1973).

Throughout the taxonomic turbulence referred
to above, *H. diminuta* has been left more-or-less
undisturbed as the type species of the genus. This
position has been maintained even within the genus
Hymenolepis sensu stricto of Yamaguti (1959) who
lists but 13 species, all of which possess either a
rudimentary unarmed rostellum or are lacking a
rostellum altogether, have unarmed suckers, and are
found in rodents. Of the 13 species listed by
Yamaguti, he indicates that one of them (*H.
arvicolina*) is a synonym of *H. horrida* while two
others (*H. megaloon* and *H. ognewi*) and possibly a
third (*H. diminutoides*) are synonyms of *H. diminuta*.
Although *H. citelli* has sometimes been suggested as
a synonym of *H. diminuta*, the available evidence
indicates clearly that they are distinct species, a
distinction well elaborated by Voge (1969). This
effectively reduces the number, accepted by Yamaguti
(1959) as valid, in the genus *Hymenolepis sensu
stricto*, to the following nine species: *H. alpestris*
Baer, 1932; *H. cebidarum* Baer, 1927; *H. citelli*
(McLeod, 1933); *H. diminuta* (Rudolphi, 1819); *H.
horrida* (Linstow, 1900); *H. palmarum* Johri, 1956; *H.
peipingensis* Hsu, 1935; *H. relicta* (Zschokke, 1887);
and *H. scalopi* Schultz, 1939.

TABLE I

Vertebrate hosts and geographical distribution of *Hymenolepis diminuta*.

Hosts	Localities	References
Carnivora		
Canidae		
1. *Canis familiaris*	Japan	Asada (1923) in Ehrenford (1977)
Canis familiaris	Argentina	Rosa & Niec (1959) in Ehrenford (1977)
Canis familiaris	USA	Ehrenford (1977)
Insectivora		
Soricidae		
2. *Neomys fodiens*	Czechoslovakia	Mituch (1964)
3. *Sorex araneus*	Poland	Soltys (1954)
Talpidae		
4. *Scalopus scapanus*	East Pakistan	Hug (1969)
5. *Mogera wogura wogura*	Japan	Shimidsu *et al.* (1951)
Primates		
Cercopithecidae		
6. *Cercopithecus shmidti*	Congo Kinshasa	Gedoelst (1925) in Joyeux & Baer (1929)
Rodentia		
Cricetidae		
7. *Cricetulus migratorius*	USSR	Tokobaev (1960)
8. *Cricetus cricetus*	USSR	Andreiko (1966)
Cricetus cricetus	Romania	Chiriac & Hamar (1966)
9. *Hesperomys pyrrhordinus* (=*Rhipidomys p?*)	Unreported	Baylis (1922)
10. *Mesocricetus auratus*	Experimental	Read (1951)
Mesocricetus auratus	Experimental	Sullivan *et al.* (1977)
11. *Rhipidomys pyrrhorhinus*	Unreported	von Linstow (1878) in Meggitt (1924)
Rhipidomys pyrrhorhinus	Unreported	Ransom (1904) in Meggitt (1924)
Rhipidomys pyrrhorhinus	Unreported	Stiles (1906) in Meggitt (1924)

TABLE I

Vertebrate hosts and geographical distribution of *Hymenolepis diminuta* (cont.)

Hosts		Localities	References
12.	*Sigmodon hispidus*	Unreported	Smith (1908) in Meggitt (1924)
	Sigmodon hispidus	USA	Seidenberg *et al.* (1974)
13.	*Sigmodon hispidus hirsutus*	Venezuela	Diaz-Ungria (1970)
14.	*Zygodontomys brevicauda brevicauda*	Venezuela	Voge & Diaz-Ungria (1958) in Diaz-Ungria (1970)

Echimyidae

15.	*Echimys semivillosus flavidus*	Venezuela	Gallo & Vogelsang (1951)
	Echimys semivillosus flavidus	Venezuela	Flores-Barroeta *et al.* (1958)
	Echimys semivillosus flavidus	Venezuela	Flores-Barroeta & Diaz-Ungria (1958) in Diaz-Ungria (1970)

Gerbillidae

16.	*Meriones hurrianae*	India	Agrawal (1965)
17.	*Meriones shawi shawi*	Algeria	Joyeux & Foley (1930) in Hunkeler (1974)
18.	*Meriones sp.*	Turkey	Kaya (1975)
19.	*Meriones unguiculatus*	Experimental	Vincent *et al.* (1975)
20.	*Tatera indica*	West Pakistan	Buscher (1972)
21.	*Tatera kempi*	Ghana	Paperna *et al.* (1970)

Gliridae

| 22. | *Eliomys quercinus* | Czechoslovakia | Tenora (1965c) |
| 23. | *Glis glis* | Czechoslovakia | Erhardova (1958) |

Microtidae

24.	*Arvicola terrestris*	Czechoslovakia	Erhardova (1958)
25.	*Clethrionomys glareolus*	France	Joyeux & Baer (1936)
	Clethrionomys glareolus	Czechoslovakia	Erhardova (1955) in Erhardova (1958)
	Clethrionomys glareolus	Czechoslovakia	Tenora & Barus (1955) in Erhardova (1958)
	Clethrionomys glareolus	USSR	Sharpilo (1961)
	Clethrionomys glareolus	East Germany	Schmidt (1962)
	Clethrionomys glareolus	Czechoslovakia	Kisielewska (1970a, 1970b)

TABLE I

Vertebrate hosts and geographical distribution of *Hymenolepis diminuta* (cont.)

	Hosts	Localities	References
26.	*Clethrionomys rufocanus*	USSR	Surkov (1972, 1974)
27.	*Ellobius talpinus*	USSR	Zanina & Tokobaev (1962)
28.	*Microtus agrestis*	USA	Moll (1917)
	Microtus agrestis	France	Joyeux & Baer (1936)
	Microtus agrestis	Czechoslovakia	Erhardova (1956) in Erhardova (1958)
	Microtus agrestis	Poland	Soltys (1957)
29.	*Microtus arvalis*	Czechoslovakia	Tenora & Barus (1955) in Erhardova (1958)
	Microtus arvalis	Czechoslovakia	Erhardova (1956) in Erhardova (1958)
	Microtus arvalis	East Germany	Schmidt (1962)
	Microtus arvalis	Romania	Chiriac & Hamar (1966)
	Microtus arvalis	Czechoslovakia	Prokopic (1970)
	Microtus arvalis	Czechoslovakia	Tenora (1972)
30.	*Microtus nivalis mirhanreini*	Czechoslovakia	Erhardova (1955) in Erhardova (1958)
31.	*Microtus gregalis*	USSR	Tokobaev (1960)
32.	*Microtus* sp.	Turkey	Kaya (1975)
33.	*Microtus subterraneus*	Poland	Soltys (1957)
34.	*Pitymys subterraneus*	Czechoslovakia	Erhardova (1955) in Erhardova (1958)
	Pitymys subterraneus	Czechoslovakia	Tenora (1956) in Erhardova (1958)

Muridae

35.	*Acomys cahirinus*	UAR	Rifaat *et al.* (1969)
36.	*Acomys* sp.	Israel	Greenberg (1969)
37.	*Apodemus agrarius*	Poland	Furmaga (1957)
	Apodemus agrarius	Czechoslovakia	Erhardova (1958)
	Apodemus agrarius	East Germany	Schmidt (1962)
	Apodemus agrarius	Czechoslovakia	Tenora (1963, 1965b)
	Apodemus agrarius	Romania	Chiriac & Hamar (1966)
	Apodemus agrarius	Taiwan	Yeh (1970)

TABLE I

Vertebrate hosts and geographical distribution of *Hymenolepis diminuta* (cont.)

Hosts		Localities	References
38.	*Apodemus flavicollis*	France	Joyeux & Baer (1936)
	Apodemus flavicollis	Czechoslovakia	Tenora & Barus (1955) in Erhardova (1958)
	Apodemus flavicollis	Czechoslovakia	Erhardova & Rysavy (1955)
	Apodemus flavicollis	East Germany	Schmidt (1962)
	Apodemus flavicollis	Czechoslovakia	Tenora (1963, 1965a, 1965b)
	Apodemus flavicollis	Czechoslovakia	Prokopic (1970)
	Apodemus flavicollis	Hungary	Tenora & Murai (1972)
	Apodemus flavicollis	Austria	Barus *et al.* (1975)
39.	*Apodemus flavidus*	Czechoslovakia	Tenora (1965b)
40.	*Apodemus microps*	Czechoslovakia	Erhardova (1956) in Erhardova (1958)
	Apodemus microps	Czechoslovakia	Tenora (1963, 1965a, 1965b)
41.	*Apodemus sylvaticus*	France	Joyeux & Baer (1936)
	Apodemus sylvaticus	Poland	Zarnowski (1955)
	Apodemus sylvaticus	Czechoslovakia	Tenora & Barus (1955) in Erhardova (1958)
	Apodemus sylvaticus	Czechoslovakia	Erhardova & Rysavy (1955)
	Apodemus sylvaticus	Poland	Furmaga (1957)
	Apodemus sylvaticus	USSR	Tokobaev (1960)
	Apodemus sylvaticus	Romania	Suciu & Popescu (1962)
	Apodemus sylvaticus	USSR	Tokobaev (1962)
	Apodemus sylvaticus	East Germany	Schmidt (1962)
	Apodemus sylvaticus	Czechoslovakia	Tenora (1963, 1964, 1965a, 1965b)
	Apodemus sylvaticus	France	Mishra & Bercovier (1975)
42.	*Apodemus tauricus*	Romania	Chiriac & Hamar (1966)
43.	*Arvicanthus barbarus pulchellus*	Guinea	Joyeux & Baer (1927) in Hunkeler (1974)
44.	*Arvicanthus niloticus*	Ghana	Paperna *et al.* (1970)
45.	*Bandicota bengalensis*	India	Niphadkar (1977)
	Bandicota bengalensis	East Pakistan	Huq (1969)
46.	*Bandicota indica*	India	Balachandra & Ranade (1978)
47.	*Cricetomys gambianus*	Nigeria	Dipeolu & Ajayi (1976)
48.	*Grammomys surdaster* (=*Thamnomys s.*)	Tanzania	Baylis (1934) in Collins (1972)
49.	*Lemniscomys* sp.	Sudan	Myers *et al.* (1960)

12

TABLE I

Vertebrate hosts and geographical distribution of *Hymenolepis diminuta* (cont.)

Hosts		Localities	References
50.	*Mastomys natalensis*	Rhodesia	Baer (1933)
	Mastomys natalensis	Experimental	Lamler *et al.* (1968)
	Mastomys natalensis	Experimental	Zahner & Texdorf (1968)
	Mastomys natalensis	Ghana	Paperna *et al.* (1970)
51.	*Mastomys* sp.	Central African Republic	Quentin (1964)
52.	*Micromys minutus*	East Germany	Schmidt (1962)
53.	*Mus decumanus* (=*Rattus norvegicus*)	Italy	Grassi (1888)
	Mus decumanus	West Germany	Grassi (1888)
	Mus decumanus	East Germany	Grassi (1888)
	Mus decumanus	Austria	Grassi (1888)
	Mus decumanus	Brazil	Grassi (1888)
	Mus decumanus	Switzerland	Galli-Valerio (1901) in Fuhrmann (1926)
	Mus decumanus	Indochina	Houdemer (1938)
54.	*Mus minutoides*	Ivory Coast	Baer (1972)
	Mus minutoides	Ivory Coast	Hunkeler (1974)
55.	*Mus molossinus*	Japan	Hamajima (1962, 1963)
56.	*Mus musculoides*	Ivory Coast	Baer (1972)
57.	*Mus musculus*	Unreported	Dujardin (1845) in Meggitt (1924)
	Mus musculus	Unreported	Ransom (1904) in Meggitt (1924)
	Mus musculus	Unreported	Stiles (1906) in Meggitt (1924)
	Mus musculus	Romania	Leon (1908, 1924) in Suciu & Popescu (1962)
	Mus musculus	Australia	Johnston (1909, 1918)
	Mus musculus	France	Joyeux & Baer (1936)
	Mus musculus	Somalia	Joyeux *et al.* (1936) in Collins (1972)
	Mus musculus	Canada	Cameron (1949)
	Mus musculus	USSR	Tokobaev (1960)
	Mus musculus	Czechoslovakia	Tenora (1964)
	Mus musculus	UAR	Fahmy *et al.* (1969b)
	Mus musculus	Republic of South Africa	Collins (1972)
	Mus musculus	Afghanistan	Tenora & Kullmann (1970)
	Mus musculus	Turkey	Kaya (1975)
58.	*Mus musculus* var. *gentilis*	Algeria	Joyeux & Foley (1930) in Hunkeler (1974)

TABLE I

Vertebrate hosts and geographical distribution of *Hymenolepis diminuta* (cont.)

Hosts		Localities	References
59.	*Mus musculus domesticus*	East Germany	Schmidt (1962)
60.	*Mus musculus spicilegus*	Romania	Chiriac & Hamar (1966)
61.	*Mus norvegicus* (=*Rattus norvegicus*)	Unreported	Dujardin (1845) in Meggitt (1924)
	Mus norvegicus	Unreported	von Linstow (1878) in Meggitt (1924)
	Mus norvegicus	Unreported	Ransom (1904) in Meggitt (1924)
	Mus norvegicus	Unreported	Stiles (1906) in Meggitt (1924)
	Mus norvegicus	Unreported	Galli-Valerio (1909) in Meggitt (1924)
	Mus norvegicus	Australia	Johnston (1909, 1918) in Meggitt (1924)
	Mus norvegicus	Unreported	Luhe (1910) in Meggitt (1924)
	Mus norvegicus	USA	Moll (1917)
62.	*Mus rattus* (=*Rattus rattus*)	Unreported	Rudolphi (1819) in Meggitt (1924)
	Mus rattus	Unreported	Dujardin (1845) in Meggitt (1924)
	Mus rattus	Italy	Grassi (1888)
	Mus rattus	West Germany	Grassi (1888)
	Mus rattus	East Germany	Grassi (1888)
	Mus rattus	Austria	Grassi (1888)
	Mus rattus	Brazil	Grassi (1888)
	Mus rattus	Unreported	Parona (1901) in Meggitt (1924)
	Mus rattus	Unreported	Leidy (1904) in Meggitt (1924)
	Mus rattus	Unreported	Ransom (1904) in Meggitt (1924)
	Mus rattus	Unreported	Stiles (1906) in Meggitt (1924)
	Mus rattus	Australia	Johnston (1909, 1918) in Meggitt (1924)
	Mus rattus	Switzerland	Galli-Valerio (1909) in Fuhrmann (1926)
	Mus rattus	Hong Kong	Southwell (1922)
	Mus rattus	Switzerland	Fuhrmann (1926)
	Mus rattus	Indochina	Houdemer (1938)
63.	*Mus spicilegus hispanicus*	Spain	Gonzalez Castro (1944)
64.	*Mus sylvaticus* (=*Apodemus sylvaticus*)	Unreported	Dujardin (1845) in Meggitt (1924)
	Mus sylvaticus	Unreported	Ransom (1904) in Meggitt (1924)
	Mus sylvaticus	Unreported	Stiles (1906) in Meggitt (1924)
	Mus sylvaticus	Spain	Gonzalez Castro (1944)
65.	*Mus terraereginae* (=*Rattus terrae-reginae*)	Australia	Johnston (1918) in Meggitt (1924)

TABLE I
Vertebrate hosts and geographical distribution of *Hymenolepis diminuta* (cont.)

Hosts		Localities	References
66.	*Pelomys fallax*	Congo Kinshasa	Southwell & Lake (1939) in Collins (1972)
67.	*Praomys jacksoni*	Tanzania	Baylis (1934) in Collins (1972)
	Praomys jacksoni	Central African Republic	Quentin (1964)
68.	*Praomys (Mastomys) natalensis*	Rhodesia	Baer (1933) in Collins (1972)
	Praomys (Mastomys) natalensis	Republic of South Africa	Collins (1972)
69.	*Nesokia indica*	West Pakistan	Buscher (1972)
	Nesokia indica	Israel	Greenberg (1972)
70.	*Ondatra zibethicus*	USSR	Spasskii *et al.* (1951)
71.	Rat(s)	USA	Moll (1917)
	Rat(s)	UK	Southwell (1922)
	Rat(s)	USA	Riley & Shannon (1922)
	Rat(s)	USA	Chandler (1922)
	Rat(s)	UK	Baylis (1922)
	Rat(s)	Switzerland	Fuhrmann (1926)
	Rat(s)	UAR	Meggitt (1927)
	Rat(s)	Brazil	Hegner *et al.* (1929) in Turner (1975)
	Rat(s)	China	Hsu (1935)
	Rat(s)	USSR	Rusinova (1940)
	Rat(s)	India, Burma	Johri (1950)
	Rat(s)	Venezuela	Gallo & Vogelsang (1951) in Diaz-Ungria (1967)
	Rat(s)	Argentina	Bacigalupo (1951)
	Rat(s)	Spain	Pozo-Lora (1959)
	Rat(s)	Brazil	Amaral Costa (1963, 1964)
	Rat(s)	Venezuela	Mayaudon Tarbes & Gallo (1964) in Diaz-Ungria (1967)
	Rat(s)	Nigeria	Cowper (1969)
	Rat(s)	Brazil	Schmidt *et al.* (1974)
	Rat(s)	Cuba	Rodriquez Balleste *et al.* (1975)
	Rat(s)	Austria	Muller (1976)
	Rat(s)	Japan	Kasai & Kaneko (1977)
	Rat(s)	Malaysia	Sullivan *et al.* (1977)
72.	*Rattus alexandrinus*	France	Joyeux & Baer (1936)
73.	*Rattus coxinga coxinga*	Taiwan	Olsen & Kuntz (1977)

TABLE I

Vertebrate hosts and geographical distribution of *Hymenolepis diminuta* (cont.)

Hosts		Localities	References
74.	*Rattus exulans*	New Zealand	Ford-Robertson & Bull (1966)
	Rattus exulans	New Zealand	Mosby & Wodzicki (1972)
75.	*Rattus flavipectus*	Indochina	Houdemer (1938)
76.	*Rattus leucopus*	New Guinea	Schmidt (1975)
77.	*Rattus losea*	Taiwan	Olsen & Kuntz (1977)
78.	*Rattus norvegicus*	USA	Sturdevant (1907)
	Rattus norvegicus	Romania	Leon (1908, 1924) in Suciu & Popescu (1962)
	Rattus norvegicus	USSR	Podyapolskaya (1924)
	Rattus norvegicus	Burma	Meggitt & Subramanian (1927)
	Rattus norvegicus	Philippine Islands	Tubangui (1931)
	Rattus norvegicus	France	Joyeux & Baer (1936)
	Rattus norvegicus	Indochina	Houdemer (1938)
	Rattus norvegicus	USA	Voge (1952a, 1952b)
	Rattus norvegicus	Tanganyika	Voge (1952b)
	Rattus norvegicus	USA	Voge (1955)
	Rattus norvegicus	Czechoslovakia	Erhardova (1958)
	Rattus norvegicus	Spain	Pozo-Lora (1960)
	Rattus norvegicus	Scotland	Fahmy (1961)
	Rattus norvegicus	France	Dollfus (1961)
	Rattus norvegicus	USSR	Sharpilo (1961)
	Rattus norvegicus	Japan	Takagi *et al.* (1962)
	Rattus norvegicus	USA	Ash (1962)
	Rattus norvegicus	Japan	Sasa *et al.* (1962)
	Rattus norvegicus	Czechoslovakia	Villagiova (1962)
	Rattus norvegicus	Puerto Rico	de Leon (1964)
	Rattus norvegicus	Spain	Guevara-Pozo (1965)
	Rattus norvegicus	USSR	Sinelshchikov (1965)
	Rattus norvegicus	USSR	Semenova & Yarulin (1965)
	Rattus norvegicus	Spain	Anon. (1965)
	Rattus norvegicus	Guyana	Floch *et al.* (1966)
	Rattus norvegicus	Venezuela	Diaz-Ungria (1967)
	Rattus norvegicus	UAR	Rifaat *et al.* (1968)
	Rattus norvegicus	USA	Lichtenfels & Haley (1968)
	Rattus norvegicus	USSR	Mukhin (1967)
	Rattus norvegicus	Japan	Kamiya *et al.* (1968, 1971)

TABLE I

Vertebrate hosts and geographical distribution of *Hymenolepis diminuta* (cont.)

Hosts	Localities	References
Rattus norvegicus	UAR	Fahmy et al. (1969a)
Rattus norvegicus	Venezuela	Diaz-Ungria (1970)
Rattus norvegicus	Taiwan	Yeh (1970)
Rattus norvegicus	UK	Simmons & Walkey (1971)
Rattus norvegicus	Japan	Shogaki et al. (1972)
Rattus norvegicus	Hungary	Tenora & Murai (1972)
Rattus norvegicus	Japan	Hori & Kusui (1972)
Rattus norvegicus	Japan	Hori et al. (1973a)
Rattus norvegicus	Japan	Hori et al. (1974)
Rattus norvegicus	Tunisia	Mishra & Gonzalez (1975)
Rattus norvegicus	France	Mishra & Bercovier (1975)
Rattus norvegicus	India	Niphadkar (1977)
Rattus norvegicus	Taiwan	Olsen & Kuntz (1977)
Rattus norvegicus	Japan	Kasai (1978)
79. *Rattus norvegicus* (white rat)	Switzerland	Fuhrmann (1926)
80. *Rattus norvegicus* (Wistar)	Peru	Caceres & Guillen de Tantalean (1972)
81. *Rattus norvegicus* (white albino)	Cuba	Rodriguez Balleste et al. (1975)
82. *Rattus norvegicus* var. *albinus*	Austria	Muller (1976)
83. *Rattus norvegicus albus*	Japan	Yamaguti (1935)
84. *Rattus norvegicus javanicus*	Java	Holz & Liem Jan Sioe (1965)
85. *Rattus norvegicus norvegicus*	Japan	Yamaguti (1935)
86. *Rattus rattus*	Burma	Meggitt & Subramanian (1927)
Rattus rattus	Egypt	Meggitt (1927)
Rattus rattus	Chile	Nybelin (1929)
Rattus rattus	Republic of South Africa	Baer (1933) in Collins (1972)
Rattus rattus	Rhodesia	Baer (1933) in Collins (1972)
Rattus rattus	Tanzania	Baylis (1934) in Collins (1972)
Rattus rattus	France	Joyeux & Baer (1936)
Rattus rattus	Indochina	Houdemer (1938)
Rattus rattus	Congo Kinshasa	Southwell & Lake (1939) in Collins (1972)
Rattus rattus	Venezuela	Vogelsang & Potenza (1945) in Diaz-Ungria (1967)
Rattus rattus	Venezuela	Vogelsang & Rodriguez (1952)
Rattus rattus	Tanganyika	Voge (1952b)

TABLE I

Vertebrate hosts and geographical distribution of *Hymenolepis diminuta* (cont.)

Hosts	Localities	References
Rattus rattus	Indonesia	Adiwinata (1955)
Rattus rattus	Japan	Sasa *et al.* (1962)
Rattus rattus	Czechoslovakia	Tenora (1964)
Rattus rattus	Central African Republic	Quentin (1964)
Rattus rattus	Ile Europa	Bryogoo (1966)
Rattus rattus	Romania	Chiriac & Hamar (1966)
Rattus rattus	Guyana	Floch *et al.* (1966)
Rattus rattus	East Pakistan	Huq (1969)
Rattus rattus	Taiwan	Yeh (1970)
Rattus rattus	Japan	Kamiya *et al.* (1968)
Rattus rattus	UAR	Rifaat *et al.* (1969)
Rattus rattus	Ghana	Paperna *et al.* (1970)
Rattus rattus	West Pakistan	Buscher & Haley (1971)
Rattus rattus	West Pakistan	Buscher (1972)
Rattus rattus	Japan	Hori & Kusui (1972)
Rattus rattus	Republic of South Africa	Collins (1972)
Rattus rattus	Ivory Coast	Baer (1972)
Rattus rattus	Japan	Hori *et al.* (1973b)
Rattus rattus	Ivory Coast	Hunkeler (1974)
Rattus rattus	Turkey	Kaya (1975)
Rattus rattus	India	Nama & Khichi (1975)
Rattus rattus	India	Nama & Parihar (1976)
Rattus rattus	Taiwan	Olsen & Kuntz (1977)
Rattus rattus	Malaysia	Sullivan *et al.* (1977)
Rattus rattus	India	Balachandra & Ranade (1978)
Rattus rattus	Japan	Kasai (1978)
87. *Rattus rattus* var. *albus*	Hungary	Tenora & Murai (1972)
88. *Rattus rattus alexandrinus*	Unreported	Meggitt & Subramanian (1927)
Rattus rattus alexandrinus	USA	Ash (1962)
89. *Rattus rattus brevicaudatus*	Java	Holz & Liem Jan Sioe (1965)
90. *Rattus rattus diardi*	Java	Holz & Liem Jan Sioe (1965)
91. *Rattus rattus norvegicus*	Vietnam	Nguyen-Van-Ai (1961)

TABLE I

Vertebrate hosts and geographical distribution of *Hymenolepis diminuta* (cont.)

Hosts		Localities	References
92.	*Rattus rattus rattus*	Japan	Yamaguti (1935)
	Rattus rattus rattus	USA	Ash (1962)
	Rattus rattus rattus	Yemen	Kuntz & Myers (1968)
93.	*Rattus rattus rufescens*	India	Nama & Parihar (1976)
	Rattus rattus rufescens	India	Niphadkar (1977)
94.	*Rattus* sp.	India	Patnaik & Acharyo (1970)
95.	*Rattus turcestanicus*	USSR	Tokobaev (1960)
96.	*Steatomys pratensis*	Congo Kinshasa	Southwell & Lake (1939) in Collins (1972)
97.	*Thamnomys surdaster*	Tanzania	Baylis (1934) in Collins (1972)
Sciuridae			
98.	*Citellus citellus*	Yugoslavia	Simitch & Petrovitch (1954)
	Citellus citellus	Czechoslovakia	Erhardova (1958)
	Citellus citellus	Romania	Chiriac & Hamar (1966)
	Citellus citellus	Turkey	Kaya (1975)
99.	*Citellus leucurus*	Experimental	Voge (1952a)

TABLE II

Records of *Hymenolepis diminuta* in *Homo sapiens*

No. cases	Localities	References
1	USA	Weinland (1858)* in Chandler (1922); Weinland (1861)
1	USA	Leidy (1884) in Chandler (1922)
1	Italy	Grassi (1887)
1	USA	Packard (1900) in Chandler (1922)
12	USA	Ransom (1904) in Riley & Shannon (1922)
1	USA	Deaderick (1906) in Riley & Shannon (1922)
1	Philippine Islands	Garrison (1907) in Riley & Shannon (1922)
1	Unreported	Condorelli-Francaviglia (1908) in Riley & Shannon (1922)
1	Brazil	Galli-Valerio (1910) in Riley & Shannon (1922)
1	USA	Nickerson (1911) in Riley & Shannon (1922)
1	West Indies	Noc (1911)
1	Cuba	Garcia Rijo (1911) in Riley & Shannon (1922)
1	West Indies	Leiper (1913a, b, c) in Riley & Shannon (1922)
1	Argentina	Parodi (1915) in Riley & Shannon (1922)
1	Japan	Hoki (1917) in Riley & Shannon (1922)
1	East Africa	Shircore (1917) in Riley & Shannon (1922)
16	Brazil	Gonzaga & Carvahlo (1918) in Riley & Shannon (1922)
1	Venezuela	Cuenca (1919) in Diaz-Ungria (1967)
8	India	Acton (1919) in Riley & Shannon (1922)
1	Belgian Congo	Gedoelst (1920) in Riley & Shannon (1922)
1	USA	Cort (1921) in Riley & Shannon (1922)
1	USA	Hall (1921)
3	USA	Stiles (1921)
2	Nicaragua	Riley & Shannon (1922)
3	USA	Chandler (1922)
1	Philippine Islands	Schwartz & Tubangui (1922) in Tubangui (1931)
23	India	Chandler (1927)
1	Unreported	Momma (1928) in Turner (1975)

20

TABLE II

Records of *Hymenolepis diminuta* in *Homo sapiens*

No. cases	Localities	References
1	USA	Spindler (1929)
8	USA	Keller (1931)
1	Rhodesia	Blackie (1932) in Goldsmid et al. (1976)
1	Canada	Luney (1934)
1	Soviet Union	Seitenok & Kolossov (1936)
?	USA	Sunkes & Seller (1937) in Turton et al. (1975)
?	Italy	Liddo (1938) in Turner (1975)
1	Mexico	Bacigalupo & Aguirre-Pequeno (1938)**
?	Australia	Bearup & Morgan (1939) in Turner (1975)
5	Mexico	Mazzotti & Osorio (1943) in Turner (1975)
1	Argentina	Castex et al. (1951) in Turner (1975)
1	Mexico	Bacigalupo (1951)
32	Brazil	Amaral & Pires (1952) in Amaral Costa (1964)
?	Japan	Dohi (1959)
?	Mexico	Biagi Filizola et al. (1960)
1	Argentina	Rabinovitch & Marcial Crovato (1961) in Turner (1975)
1	Argentina	Marcial Crovato (1961)
5	Peru	Ayulo (1962) in Caceres & Guillen de Tantalean (1972)
?	Turkey	Gokbert & Bayadal (1963)
4	Brazil	Serra (1963a)
?	Brazil	Serra (1963b)
1	Pland	Plotkowiak (1963)
1	Italy	Marzullo & Squadrini (1963)
1	Peru	Ayulo-Robles (1963)
?	India	Chowdhury & Bandyopadhyay (1964)
1	Brazil	Goulart (1964)
1	Poland	Plotkowiak & Zolnowski (1964)
4	Romania	Gherman & Juvara (1964)
1	Guatemala	Aguilar (1964)

TABLE II

Records of *Hymenolepis diminuta* in *Homo sapiens*

No. cases	Localities	References
1	Brazil	Kalil et al. (1965)
?	Unreported	Edelman et al. (1965) in Turner (1975)
?	Surinam	Asin & van Thiel (1965)
1	USA	Ratliff & Donaldson (1965)
?	Unreported	Kihara et al. (1965) in Turton et al. (1975)
1	New Guinea	Vines & Kelly (1966) in McMillan et al. (1971)
1	Iran	Motakef (1968)
?	Easter Island	Meerovitch & Gibbs (1969)
?	India	Abraham et al. (1969)
?	Indonesia	Bintari Rukmono & Talogo (1969)
1	Thailand	Manning et al. (1969)
?	Singapore	Paul & Zaman (1969)
?	Cameron	van Wijk (1969a, b)
?	India	Ahmed & Roy (1970)
6	Indonesia	Cross et al. (1970)
1	Brazil	Lima et al. (1970)
6	New Guinea	McMillan et al. (1971)
?	India	John et al. (1971)
?	Algeria	Sukoli (1971)
5	Iran	Chadirian & Arfaa (1972)
?	Iran	Arfaa (1972)
?	Japan	Kagei et al. (1972)
3	Rhodesia	Goldsmid (1973)
3	Malawi(?)	Goldsmid (1973)
1	Rhodesia	MacDonald & Goldsmid (1973)
?	Indonesia	Clarke et al. (1974)
?	Rhodesia	Goldsmid (1974)
1	England	Turton et al. (1975)

TABLE II

Records of *Hymenolepis diminuta* in *Homo sapiens*

No. cases	Localities	References
?	Zambia	Hira (1975)
3	Poland	Zembrzuski et al. (1975)
1	Rhodesia	Goldsmid et al. (1976)
?	Korea	Moon (1976)
4	Colombia	Newell et al. (1976)
1	Paraguay	Canese & Canese (1976)
1	Japan	Kamegai (1977)
?	Rhodesia	Goldsmid & Flemming (1977)
?	USA	Ruebush et al. (1978)

*First human record of *H. diminuta*; **Transmission of *H. diminuta* of human origin to rats via *Tenebrio molitor*

TABLE III
Hosts of larval *Hymenolepis diminuta*

Hosts	Localities	References
Insecta		
Coleoptera		
1. *Akis spinosa*	Italy	Grassi (1888)
Akis spinosa	Italy	Grassi & Rovelli (1892) in Narihara (1937b)
Akis spinosa	Venezuela	Cuenca (1919) in Diaz-Ungria (1967)
Akis spinosa	France	Joyeux & Baer (1936)
2. *Alphitobus piceus*	Unreported	Anon. (1938) in Dohi (1959)
3. *Alphitophagus bifasciatus*	Unreported	Joyeux & Baer (1937) in Yamaguti (1959)
4. *Ammophorus peruvianus*	Peru	Caceres & Guillen de Tantalean (1972)
5. *Anobium paniceum*	France	Roman (1937)
Anobium paniceum	Unreported	Mendheim (1951)
6. *Anthicus floralis*	Unreported	Joyeux & Baer (1937) in Yamaguti (1959)
7. *Aphodius distinctus*	France	Roman (1937)
Aphodius distinctus	West Germany	Mendheim (1951)
8. *Dermestes peruvianus*	Argentina	Bacigalupo (1929a) in Narihara (1937b)
Dermestes peruvianus	Argentina	Bacigalupo (1935, 1938, 1951)
Dermestes peruvianus	France	Joyeux & Baer (1936)
Dermestes peruvianus	Unreported	Mendheim (1951)
9. *Dermestes* sp.	Peru	Caceres & Guillen de Tantalean (1972)
10. *Dermestes vulpinus*	Argentina	Bacigalupo (1930, 1935, 1938, 1951)
Dermestes vulpinus	Unreported	Mendheim (1951)
11. *Dyscinetus gagates*	Argentina	Bacigalupo (1939)
12. *Epitragus* sp.	Peru	Caceres & Guillen de Tantalean (1972)
13. *Geotrupes sylvaticus*	Unreported	Joyeux (1920) in Narihara (1937b)
Geotrupes sylvaticus	France	Joyeux & Baer (1936)
Geotrupes sylvaticus	Unreported	Mendheim (1951)
14. *Gnathocercus cornutus*	Peru	Caceres & Guillen de Tantalean (1972)
15. *Oryzaephilus surinamensis*	Experimental	Mullee & Voge (1959)
16. *Palembus dermestoides*	Experimental	Chu *et al.* (1977)
17. *Palorus* sp.	Taiwan	Narihara (1937b)
18. *Scaurus striatus*	Italy	Grassi (1888)
Scaurus striatus	Italy	Grassi & Rovelli (1892) in Narihara (1937b)

TABLE III

Hosts of larval *Hymenolepis diminuta* (cont.)

Hosts		Localities	References
	Scaurus striatus	Venezuela	Cuenca (1919) in Diaz-Ungria (1967)
	Scaurus striatus	France	Joyeux & Baer (1936)
	Scaurus striatus	Unreported	Mendheim (1951)
19.	*Sitophilus granaria*	Peru	Caceres & Guillen de Tantalean (1972)
20.	*Sitophilus oryzae*	Peru	Caceres & Guillen de Tantalean (1972)
21.	*Tenebrio molitor*	France	Joyeux (1916)
	Tenebrio molitor	France	Joyeux (1920) in Narihara (1937b)
	Tenebrio molitor	USA	Chandler (1922)
	Tenebrio molitor	Argentina	Bacigalupo (1928)
	Tenebrio molitor	France	Joyeux & Baer (1936)
	Tenebrio molitor	West Germany	Mendheim (1951)
	Tenebrio molitor	Experimental	Houser & Burns (1968)
	Tenebrio molitor	Experimental	Lethbridge (1971b)
	Tenebrio molitor	Experimental	Lackie (1976)
	Tenebrio molitor	Canada	Rau (1979)
22.	*Tenebrio obscurus*	Argentina	Bacigalupo (1928)
	Tenebrio obscurus	France	Joyeux & Baer (1936)
	Tenebrio obscurus	Unreported	Mendheim (1951)
	Tenebrio obscurus	Canada	Rau (1979)
23.	*Tenebrioides mauritanicus*	Peru	Caceres & Guillen de Tantalean (1972)
24.	*Tribolium brevicornis*	Unreported	Mankau (1977)
25.	*Tribolium castaneum*	Unreported	Mendheim (1951)
	Tribolium castaneum	Experimental	Soltice *et al.* (1971)
	Tribolium castaneum	Unreported	Mankau (1977)
26.	*Tribolium confusum*	Experimental	Voge (1952a)
	Tribolium confusum	Experimental	Rothman (1957)
	Tribolium confusum	Experimental	Voge & Heyneman (1957)
	Tribolium confusum	Experimental	Heyneman & Voge (1971)
	Tribolium confusum	Experimental	Lackie (1976)
	Tribolium confusum	Unreported	Mankau (1977)
27.	*Tribolium ferrugineum*	Japan	Narihara (1937b)
	Tribolium ferrugineum	Unreported	Anon. (1922, 1925, 1937) in Narihara (1937b)
28.	*Tribolium navalefabricius*	Unreported	Anon. (1956) in Dohi (1959)
29.	*Ulosonius parvicornus*	Argentina	Bacigalupo (1929b) in Narihara (1937b)
	Ulosonius parvicornus	Argentina	Bacigalupo (1936, 1951)
	Ulosonius parvicornus	Unreported	Mendheim (1951)

TABLE III

Hosts of larval *Hymenolepis diminuta* (cont.)

Hosts	Localities	References
Dermaptera		
30. *Anisolabis annulipes*	Italy	Grassi (1888)
Anisolabis annulipes	Italy	Grassi & Rovelli (1892) in Narihara (1937b)
Anisolabis annulipes	Venezuela	Cuenca (1919) in Diaz-Ungria (1967)
Anisolabis annulipes	USA	Chandler (1922)
Anisolabis annulipes	Argentina	Bacigalupo (1935, 1951)
Anisolabis annulipes	France	Joyeux & Baer (1936)
Anisolabis annulipes	Unreported	Mendheim (1951)
31. *Forficula annulipes*	Italy	Grassi (1888)
Embioptera		
32. *Embia argentina*	Unreported	Mendheim (1951)
33. *Embia (Rhagadochir) argentina*	Argentina	Bacigalupo (1938)
Lepidoptera		
34. *Aglossa didimiata*	Unreported	Mendheim (1951)
Aglossa didimiata	France	Joyeux & Baer (1936)
35. *Aphomia gularis*	Unreported	Mendheim (1951)
36. *Aphomia (Paralipsa) gularis*	Unreported	Anon. (1922, 1925) in Narihara (1937b)
Aphomia (Paralipsa) gularis	France	Joyeux & Baer (1936)
37. *Asopia farinalis*	Venezuela	Cuenca (1919) in Diaz-Ungria (1967)
38. *Ephestia cautella*	Taiwan	Narihara (1937a, b)
39. *Ephestia* sp.	Unreported	Anon (1956) in Dohi (1959)
Ephestia sp.	Unreported	Dohi (1959)
40. *Kakivoria flavofasciata*	Unreported	Anon. (1956) in Dohi (1959)
41. *Pyralis farinalis*	France	Joyeux & Baer (1936)
Pyralis farinalis	Unreported	Mendheim (1951)
42. *Pyralis (Asopia) farinalis*	Italy	Grassi & Rovelli (1892) in Narihara (1937b)
Pyralis (Asopia) farinalis	Unreported	Anon. (1922) in Narihara (1937b)
43. *Tinea granella*	Unreported	Anon. (1922, 1925) in Narihara (1937b)
Tinea granella	France	Joyeux & Baer (1936)
Tinea granella	Unreported	Mendheim (1951)
44. *Tinea pellionella*	Unreported	Anon. (1925) in Narihara (1937b)
Tinea pellionella	France	Joyeux & Baer (1936)
Tinea pellionella	Unreported	Mendheim (1951)

TABLE III

Hosts of larval *Hymenolepis diminuta* (cont.)

Hosts		Localities	References
Orthoptera			
45.	*Blatta orientalis*	Unreported	Mendheim (1951)
46.	*Blatta (periplaneta) orientalis*	USA	Stiles & Hassall (1926) in Narihara (1937b)
47.	*Blatella germanica*	USA	Stiles & Hassall (1926) in Narihara (1937b)
	Blatella germanica	Unreported	Mendheim (1951)
48.	*Gryllus domesticus*	Experimental	Lackie (1976)
49.	*Locusta migratoria*	Experimental	Lackie (1976)
50.	*Locusta pardalina*	Experimental	Lackie (1976)
51.	*Periplaneta americana*	Unreported	Mendheim (1951)
	Periplaneta americana	Experimental	Lackie (1976)
52.	*Periplaneta (Blatta) americana*	USA	Faust (1930) in Narihara (1937b)
53.	*Schistocerca gregaria*	Experimental	Lethbridge (1971b)
	Schistocerca gregaria	Experimental	Lackie (1976)
Siphonaptera			
54.	*Ceratophyllus anisus*	Unreported	Anon. (1936) in Narihara (1937b)
	Ceratophyllus anisus	Japan	Yamada *et al.* (1936)
55.	*Ceratophyllus fasciatus*	UK	Nicoll & Minchin (1911)
	Ceratophyllus fasciatus	Australia	Johnston (1913) in Narihara (1937b)
	Ceratophyllus fasciatus	France	Joyeux (1916)
	Ceratophyllus fasciatus	France	Joyeux (1920)
	Ceratophyllus fasciatus	Japan	Yamada *et al.* (1936)
	Ceratophyllus fasciatus	France	Joyeux & Baer (1936)
	Ceratophyllus fasciatus	Unreported	Mendheim (1951)
56.	*Ceratophyllus wickhami*	Unreported	Oldham (1931) in Narihara (1937b)
	Ceratophyllus wickhami	Unreported	Mendheim (1951)
57.	*Ctenocephalides canis*	France	Joyeux (1916)
	Ctenocephalides canis	France	Joyeux (1920)
	Ctenocephalides canis	Argentina	Bacigalupo (1928)
	Ctenocephalides canis	Unreported	Mendheim (1951)
58.	*Ctenocephalides felis*	UK	Marshall (1967)
59.	*Ctenocephalus canis*	France	Joyeux & Baer (1936)
	Ctenocephalus canis	Unreported	Mendheim (1951)
60.	*Ctenopsyllus regnis*	Unreported	Mendheim (1951)

TABLE III

Hosts of larval *Hymenolepis diminuta* (cont.)

Hosts		Localities	References
61.	*Leptopsylla musculi*	France	Joyeux (1920) in Narihara (1937b)
	Leptopsylla musculi	Japan	Yamada *et al.* (1936)
	Leptopsylla musculi	France	Joyeux & Baer (1936)
62.	*Pulex irritans*	France	Joyeux (1916)
	Pulex irritans	France	Joyeux (1920) in Narihara (1937b)
	Pulex irritans	Argentina	Bacigalupo (1928)
	Pulex irritans	France	Joyeux & Baer (1936)
	Pulex irritans	Unreported	Mendheim (1951)
	Pulex irritans	Peru	Caceres & Guillen de Tantalean (1972)
63.	*Synopsyllus fonquerniei*	Madagascar	Klein (1966)
64.	*Xenopsylla cheopis*	Australia	Johnston (1913) in Narihara (1937b)
	Xenopsylla cheopis	France	Joyeux (1916)
	Xenopsylla cheopis	France	Joyeux (1920) in Narihara (1937b)
	Xenopsylla cheopis	Argentina	Bacigalupo (1928)
	Xenopsylla cheopis	Japan	Yamada *et al.* (1936)
	Xenopsylla cheopis	France	Joyeux & Baer (1936)
	Xenopsylla cheopis	Mexico	Bacigalupo & Aguirre-Pequeno (1938)
	Xenopsylla cheopis	Unreported	Mendheim (1951)
	Xenopsylla cheopis	Peru	Caceres & Guillen de Tantalean (1972)

Diplopoda

65.	*Fontaria virginiensis*	USA	Nickerson (1911)
	Fontaria virginiensis	Unreported	Mendheim (1951)
66.	*Julus* sp.	USA	Nickerson (1911)
	Julus sp.	Unreported	Mendheim (1951)

28

REFERENCES

1. Abraham, T., Saxena, S. N. and Sen, R., *H. diminuta* in human intestine, possible etiologic role in diarrhoea: incidence survey. *Indian Pediat.* 6, 476-482 (1969).
2. Acton, H. W., The incidence and important intestinal entozoa among Indian members of the Mesopotamian Expeditionary Force. *Indian J. Med. Res.* 6, 601-613 (1919).
3. Adiwinata, R. T., List of parasitic worms in mammals and birds of Indonesia. *Hemera Zoa* 62, 229-247 (1955).
4. Agrawal, V. C., *H. diminuta* in *Meriones hurrianae* (Rodentia, Muridae) from India. *J. Zool. Soc. India.* 17, 125-134 (1965).
5. Aguilar, F. J., *H. diminuta* in man, treatment with acridine and salicylamide - Guatemala. *Bol. San. Guatemala.* 34, 167-176 (1964).
6. Ahmed, E. and Roy, S. N., *H. diminuta* in human intestine; possible association with hypovitaminosis A presenting ocular signs. *Indian Pract.* 23, 225-226 (1970).
7. Alicata, J. E. and Chang, E. The life-history of *Hymenolepis exigua*, a cestode of poultry in Hawaii. *J. Parasitol.* 25, 121-127 (1939).
8. Amaral, A. D. F. and Pires, C. D. A. Human cases of *H. diminuta*. *Folia Clin. Biol.* 18, 75-98 (1952).
9. Amaral Costa, C. A., *H. diminuta* in rats from Brazil. *Rev. Cien. Biol.* 1, 81-82 (1963).
10. Amaral Costa, C. A., *H. diminuta* in rats from Belem, Brazil. *Rev. Serv. Espec. Saude Pub., Rio de Janeiro,* 12, 184-187 (1964).
11. Andreiko, A. F., Parasites of hamster (*Cricetus cricetus* L.) in Moldavia. *Parazity Zhivot. i Rasten., Akad. Nauk Moldavsk. SSR. (2),* 97-100 (1966).
12. Anon, *H. diminuta* in *Epimys norvegicus. Rev. Iber. Parasitol.* 25, 447 (1965).
13. Arfaa, F., Status of *H. diminuta* in man in Iran. *Trop. and Geogr. Med.* 24, 353-362 (1972).
14. Asada, J., Studies on *H. diminuta* (Rudolphi) which finds the host in a dog. *Okayama Igakkai Zasshi* 407, 876-890 (1923).
15. Ash, L. R., The helminth parasites of rats in Hawaii and the description of *Capillaria trav-*

erae sp. n. *J. Parasitol. 48*, 66-68 (1962).

16. Asin, H. R. G. and van Thiel, P. H., The detection under field condition of helminthic infections by the Schuffner-Laarman method. *Acta Leidensia 33/34*, 18-26 (1965).
17. Ayulo, V., Cinco casos de infeccion con *H. diminuta*. Libro Res. Jornada Microbiol. y Parasitol. de Trujillo. 57 p. (1962).
18. Ayulo-Robles, V. M., La infeccion humana con *Hymenolepis diminuta* en el Peru. Proc. 7th Internat. Cong. Trop. Med. Malaria (Rio de Janeiro, Sept. 1963) 2, 192 (1963).
19. Bacigalupo, J., Estudio sobre la evolucion biologica de algunos parasitos del genero *Hymenolepis* (Weinland 1858). *Semana Med. No. 35*, 1249-1267 (1928).
20. Bacigalupo, J., El *Dermestes peruvianus* Castelnau en la transmission de la *Hymenolepis diminuta* (Rudolphi). *Semana Med. No. 34*, (1929a).
21. Bacigalupo, J., Un nuevo huesped intermediario de la *Hymenolepis diminuta* (Rudolphi), el *Ulosonia parvicornis* Fairmaire, 1892, *Semana Med. No. 21*, (1929b).
22. Bacigalupo, J., El *Dermestes vulpinus* Fabricius, nuevo huesped intermediario de la *Hymenolepis diminuta*, *Rev. Chilena Hist. Nat. 34*, 13-15 (1930).
23. Bacigalupo, J., El *Anisolabis annulipes* (Lucas) en la transmission de la *Hymenolepis diminuta* y la *Hymenolepis fraterna*. *Rev. Chilena Hist. Nat. 39*, 127-129 (1935).
24. Bacigalupo, J., Nuevo huesped intermediario de la *Hymenolepis diminuta* (Rudolphi 1829), *Embia (Rhagadachir) argentina* Navas. *Rev. Med. Trop. Parasitol., Bacteriol. Clin. Lab. 4*, 45-47 (1938).
25. Bacigalupo, J., El *Dyscinetus gagates* Burm, huesped intermediario de la *Hymenolepis diminuta* (Rudolphi). *Semana Med. 1*, 1318-1319 (1939).
26. Bacigalupo, J., Parasitosis experimental de rata blanca con cepa humana de *Hymenolepis diminuta*. *Rev. Soc. Arg. Bio. 27*, 138-140 (1951).
27. Bacigalupo, J. and Aguirre-Pegueno, E., Un nouveau cas d'*Hymenolepis diminuta* chez l'homme au Mexique. *Bull. Soc. Pathol. Exot. 31*, 502-504 (1938).
28. Baer, J. G., Contribution a l'etude de la faune

helminthologique africaine. *Rev. Suisse Zool.* *40*, 31-84 (1933).
29. Baer, J. G., Review of Yamaguti's *Systema Helminthum.* Vol. II. *Helminthol. Abstracts* *30*, 135-137 (1961).
30. Baer, J. G., Liste critique des parasites (monogenes, cestodes et trematodes) et leur hotes en Republique de Cote d'Ivoire. *Acta Trop. 29*, 341-361 (1972).
31. Baer, J. G., Consideration on the classification of the family Hymenolepididae (Cestoda, Cyclophyllidea). Mater. Internat. Conf. Hymenolepididae. Warszawa, 14-16 September 1973. (B. Bezubik and B. Czaplinski, eds.). Warsaw: Polish Academy Sciences, Parasitological Committee p. 147-153 (1973).
32. Balachandra, D. V. and Ranade, D. R., A preliminary survey of helminth parasites of rats from Poona City. *Indian Vet. J. 55*, 175-176 (1978).
33. Barus, V., Groschaft, J., Sixl, W., and Tenora, F., Note on the helminth fauna of Austria. *Folia Parasitol. 22*, 214 (1975).
34. Baylis, H. A. Observations on certain cestodes of rats, with an account of a new species of *Hymenolepis*. *Parasitology 14*, 1-8 (1922).
35. Baylis, H. A., On a collection of cestodes and nematodes from small mammals in Tanganyika Territory. *Ann. Mag. Nat. Hist., Ser. 10, 13*, 338-353 (1934).
36. Bearup, A. J. and Morgan, E. L., The occurrence of *Hymenolepis diminuta* (Rudolphi 1819) and *Dipylidium caninum* (Linnaeus 1758) as parasites of man in Australia. *Med. J. Australia 1*, 104-106 (1939).
37. Beck, J. W., Effect of diet upon singly established *Hymenolepis diminuta*. *Exp. Parasitol. 1*, 46-59 (1951).
38. Berntzen, A. K. and Voge, M., *In vitro* hatching of oncospheres of four hymenolepidid cestodes. *J. Parasitol. 51*, 225-242 (1965).
39. Biagi Filizola, F., Gonzalez, C., Robledo, C. E., and Martuscelli, Q. A., Frecuencia de parasitosis intestinales en el hospital infantil de Mexico. *Bol. Med. Hosp. Inf. 17*, 857-863 (1960).
40. Bintari Rukmono & Talogo, R. W., Comparative cohort-studies on diarrhea in a selected population. *Madjalah Kedokt. Indonesia 19*, 316-

322 (1969).
41. Blackie, W. K., A helminthological survey of Southern Rhodesia. *Mem. Ser. London Sch. Hyg. Trop. Med. No. 5*, (1932).
42. Blanchard, R., Histoire zoologique et medicale des Teniades du genre *Hymenolepis* Weinland. *Paris* 112 p. (1891).
43. Bryogoo, E. R., Parasites des animaux d'Europe. *Mem. Mus. Nat. Hist., Paris, n.s. 41*, 143-157 (1966).
44. Buscher, H. N., Intestinal helminths of some small mammals collected in West Pakistan. I. Cestodes and trematodes. *Pakistan J. Scient. Res. 24*, 68-71 (1972).
45. Buscher, H. N., and Haley, A. J., Intestinal helminths of *Rattus rattus* from urban and rural areas in the Punjab region of West Pakistan. *Proc. Helminthol. Soc. Wash. 38*, 96-98 (1971).
46. Caceres, I. E. and Guillen de Tantalean, Z., Insectos de Lima relacionados con el cistercoide de *Hymenolepis diminuta* (Rudolphi 1819), (Cestoda: Hymenolepididae). *Rev. Peru. Entomol. 15*, 142-147 (1972).
47. Cameron, T. W. M., Disease carried by house mice. *Can. J. Comp. Med. 13*, 262-266 (1949).
48. Canese, A. and Canese, J., Nuevo hallago en heces de huevos de *Hymenolepis diminuta* (Rudolphi 1819) Blanchard, 189. *Rev. Parag. Microbiol. 11*, 30 (1976).
49. Cannon, C. E. and Mettrick D. F., Changes in the distribution of *Hymenolepis diminuta* (Cestoda: Cyclophyllidea) within the rat intestine during prepatent development. *Can. J. Zool. 48*, 761-769 (1970).
50. Castex, M. R., Wanke, L., Camponovo, L. E., Rechniewski, C., Nuevo caso Argentino de infestacion humana por *Hymenolepis diminuta*. *Prensa Med. Argent. 38*, 1415-1418 (1951).
51. Chadirian, E. and Arfaa, F., Human infection with *Hymenolepis diminuta* in villages of Minab, Southern Iran. *Internat. Parasitol. 2*, 481-482 (1972).
52. Chandler, A. C., Species of *Hymenolepis* as human parasites. *J. Am. Vet. Ass. 78*, 636-639 (1922).
53. Chandler, A. C., The distribution of *Hymenolepis* infections in India, with a discussion of its

epidemiological significance. *Indian J. Med. Res.* 14, 973-994 (1927).

54. Chandler, A. C. "Introduction to Human Parasitology". 4th ed. J. Wiley & Sons, Inc. 655 p. (1930).

55. Chiriac, E. and Hamar, M., Contributions a la connaissance des helminths des petits mammiferes (Rongeurs, Insectivores) de la Roumanie. *Acta Parasitol. Polon.* 14, 61-72 (1966).

56. Chowdhury, A. B. and Bandyopadhyay, A. K., Hymenolepiasis treated with Vistannyl. *Bull. Calcutta School Trop. Med.* 12, 72 (1964).

57. Chu, G. S. T., Palmieri, J. R., and Sullivan, J. T. Beetle-eating: a Malaysia folk medical practice and its public health implications. *Trop. Geogr. Med.* 29, 422-427 (1977).

58. Clarke, M. D., Carney, W. P., Cross, J. H., Hadidjaja, P., Oemijati, S., and Joesoef, A. Schistosomiasis and other human parasitoses of Lake Lindu in Central Sulawesi (Celebes), Indonesia. *Am. J. Trop. Med. Hyg.* 23, 385-392 (1974).

59. Clerc, J. O., Contribution a l'etude de la faune helminthologique de l'Oural. Part III. *Rev. Suisse Zool.* 11, 241-368 (1903).

60. Cohn, L., Zur Anatomie and Systematik der Vogelcestoden. *Nova Acta Leop. Carol. Akad. Nat. Curios.* p. 265-450 (1901).

61. Cohn, L., Helmintologische Mitteilungen, II. *Arch. Naturg. Jena.* 70, 243-248 (1904).

62. Collins, H. M., Cestodes from rodents in the Republic of South Africa. *Onderstepoort J. Vet. Res.* 39, 25-50 (1972).

63. Condorelli-Francaviglia, M., Caso raro di parassitismo, dovuto a contemporanea dimora nell' intestino d'una giovinetta della *Hymenolepis diminuta* (Rud.), dell'*Ascaris lumbricoides* L. e di numerose larve di *Calliphora vomitoria* (L.). *Boll. Soc. Zool. Ital.* 17, 63-78 (1908).

64. Cowper, S. G., Observations on parasites of primates, dogs and some other hosts in Nigeria, mainly in the Ibadan area. *J. West African Sci. Ass.* 13, 39-52 (1969).

65. Cross, J. H., Gunawan, S., Gaba, A., Watten, R. H. and Sulianti, J., Survey for human intestinal and blood parasites in Bojolali, Central Java, Indonesia. *Southeast Asian J. Trop. Med. Pub. Hlth.* 1, 354-360 (1970).

66. Cuenca, H., Sobre un caso de infeccion humana por *Hymenolepis diminuta*. *Centro de Estudiantes de Medicina, Caracas* (1919).
67. Czaplinski, B., Hymenolepididae Fuhrmann, 1907 (Cestoda) parasites of some domestic and wild anseriformes in Poland. *Acta Parasitol. Polon.* 4, 175-373 (1956).
68. Czaplinski, B., The aim and problems of the International Conference devoted to Hymenolepididae. *Mater. Int. Conf. Hymenolepididae* Warszawa 14-36 September 1973 (B. Bezubik & B. Czaplinski, eds.) pp. i-xv. (1973).
69. Deaderick, W. H., *Hymenolepis nana* and *Hymenolepis diminuta* with report of cases. *J. Am. Med. Ass. 47*, 2087-2090 (1906).
70. Diaz-Ungria, C., Parasitologia de los Animales Domesticos en Venezuela. Vol. I. *Ed. Univ., Univ. Zuilia. Consejo de Desarrollo Cient. Hum., Maracaibo, Venezuela* 1097 p. (1970).
71. Dipeolu, O. O. and Ajayi, S. S., Parasites of the African giant rat (*Cricetomys gambianus* Waterhouse) in Ibadan, Nigeria. *E. Afr. Wildl. J. 14*, 85-89 (1976).
72. Dohi, S., (Studies on a new intermediate host of *Hymenoleopis diminuta* referring to human infections.) (Ja). *Tokyo Iji Shinshi 76*, 75-81 (1959).
73. Dollfus, R. P. H., Station experimentale de parasitologie de Richeliu (Indre-et-Loire). Contribution a la fauna parasitaire regionale. Introduction. Chapter I. Liste des parasites par hotes. Chapter II. Liste des parasites par ordre systematique. A. Protozoaires, C. Trematodes, D. Cestodes, H. Hirudinees, I. Oligochaete, J. Linguatulidea, K. Copepodes. *Ann. Parasitol. Hum. Comp. 36*, 174-265, 266-302, 323-324 (1961).
74. Dujardin, F., Histoire naturelle des helminths ou vers intestinaux. *Paris.* 654+15p. (1845).
75. Edelman, M. H., Spingarn, C. L., Nauenberg, W. G. and Gregory, C., *Hymenolepis diminuta* (rat tapeworm) infection in man. *Am. J. Med. 38*, 951-953 (1965).
76. Ehrenford, F. A., True parasitism of dogs by *Hymenolepis diminuta*. *Canine Practice 4*, 31-34 (1977).
77. Erhardova, B., (Helminth fauna of voles and mice of Tatra National Park.). (Sl). *Zool.*

Ent. Listy. 4, 353-366 (1955).
78. Erhardova, B., (Parasitic worms of our murid rodents II.). (Sl) *Csl. Parasitol. 3*, 49-66 (1956).
79. Erhardova, B., (Parasitic worms of rodents in Czechoslovakia.). (Sl) *Csl. Parasitol. 5*, 27-103 (1958).
80. Erhardova, B. and Rysavy, B., (Contribution to the knowledge of parasitic worms of our mice and voles.). (Sl) *Zool. Ent. Listy. 4*, 71-90 (1955).
81. Fahmy, M. A. M., Study on some trematodes and cestodes of rodents. *Vet. Med. J., Giza 7*, 215-229 (1961).
82. Fahmy, M. A. M., Rifaat, M. A. and Arafa, M. S. Helminthic infection of the brown rat, *Rattus norvegicus* (Berkenhout 1769) in U. A. R. *J. Egypt. Publ. Hlth. Assoc. 44*, 147-153 (1969a).
83. Fahmy, M. A. M., Rifaat, M. A., and Arafa, M. S., Helminthic infection of the house mouse, *Mus musculus* (Cretzeschmar 1826) in U. A. R. *J. Egypt. Publ. Hlth. Ass. 44*, 183-187 (1969b).
84. Floch, H. A., Courdurier, J. B. E., and Jacobi, J. C., Sur la menigite a eosinophiles du Pacifique-Sud recherches en Guyana francaise. *Arch. Inst. Pasteur Guyana Franc. et Inini 26*, 1-5 (1966).
85. Flores-Barroeta, L., Hildago, E. and Diaz-Ungria, C., Cestodes de vertebrados, V. *Rev. Iber. Parasitol. 18*, 248-253 (1958).
86. Ford-Robertson, J. de C., and Bull, P. C., Some parasites of the kiore, *Rattus exulans*, on Little Barrier and Hen Islands, New Zealand. *New Zealand J. Sci. 9*, 221-224 (1966).
87. Fuhrmann, O., Cestodes. Catalogue des invertebres de la Suisse. Part 17. *Mus. d'Hist. Nat. Geneve, Geneve.* 149p. (1926).
88. Furmaga, S., (The helminth fauna of field rodents (Rodentia) of the Lublin environment.) (Pl, en). *Acta Parasitol. Polon. 5*, 9-50 (1957).
89. Galli Valerio, B., La collection des parasites du Laboratoire d'Hygiene et de Parasitologie a l'Universite de Lausanne. *Bull. Soc. Vaudoise Sc. Nat. 37*, 343-384 (1901).
90. Galli Valerio, B., Notes de parasitologie et de technique parasitologique. *Centralbl. Bakt., Abt. I, 50*, 538-545 (1909).

91. Gallo, P. and Vogelsang, E. G., Nosografia veterinaria venezolana. *Rev. Med. Vet. Parasitol. 10*, 3-47 (1951).
92. Garcia Rijo, R., *Tenia diminuta*. Actas y Trab. 2. Cong. Med. Nac. (Habana, Feb. 24-28) p. 307 (1911).
93. Garrison, P. E., A preliminary report upon the specific identity of the cestode parasites of man in the Philippine Islands with a description of a new species of *Taenia*. *Philip. J. Sci. 2*, 537-550 (1907).
94. Gedoelst, L., Un cas de parasitation de l'homme par l'*Hymenolepis diminuta* (Rudolphi). *C. R. Soc. Biol. Paris 83*, 190-192 (1920).
95. Gedoelst, L., A propos de l'*Hymenolepis diminuta* (Rud. 1819). *C. R. Soc. Biol. Paris 93*, 1529-1530 (1925).
96. Gherman, I. and Juvara, A., (Considerations on four new cases of hymenolepidosis due to *Hymenolepis diminuta*.) (Ro, ru, fr, en, ge). *Rev. Med. - Chir. Iasi. 68*, 193-196 (1964).
97. Gökbert, C. and Bayadal, K., (Helminthologic survey in school children and indigenous people in Adana-Turkey) (Tr, en). *Türk Hij. Tecrubi Biyol. Derg. 23*, 299-313 (1963).
98. Goldsmid, J. M., A note on the occurrence of *Hymenolepis diminuta* (Rudolphi 1819: Blanchard 1891) (Cestoda) in Rhodesia. *Central African J. Med. 19*, 51-52 (1973).
99. Goldsmid, J. M., The intestinal helminth zoonoses of primates in Rhodesia. *Ann. Soc. Belg. Med. Trop. 54*, 87-101 (1974).
100. Goldsmid, J. M. and Fleming, F., The tapeworm infections of children in Rhodesia. *Central African J. Med. 23*, 7-10 (1977).
101. Goldsmid, J. M., Rogers, S., Parsons, G. S. and Chambers, P. G., The intestinal protozoa and helminths infecting Africans in the Gatooma region of Rhodesia. *Central African J. Med. 22*, 91-95 (1976).
102. Gonzaga, O. and Carvahlo, J., Campanha contra a ancylostomose. Rap. au VIII Congres bresilien de Medicine, Servicio sanitario de Sao Paulo. (1918).
103. Gonzalez Castro, J., Contribucion al estudio del parasitismo por helmintos o sus fases larvarias de diversos Muridos capturados en Granada. *Rev. Iber. Parasitol. 4*, 38-60 (1944).

104. Goodchild, C. G. and Harrison, D. L., The growth of the rat tapeworm, *Hymenolepis diminuta*, during the first five days in the final host. *J. Parasitol.* 47, 819-829 (1961).
105. Goulart, E. G., Enteroparasitos na infancia favelada e nao favela do Estado de Guanabara. *Rev. Brasil. Med.* 21, 359-368 (1964).
106. Grassi, G. B., Bestimmung der vier von Dr. E. Parona in einem kleinen Madchen aus Varese (Lombardei) gefundenen Taenien (*Taenia flavopunctata?* Dr. E. Parona). *Centralbl. Bakt. I Abt.* 1, 9, 257-259 (1887).
107. Grassi, G. B., *Taenia flavopunctata* Wein., *Taenia leptocephala* Creplin, *Taenia diminuta* Rud., *Atti R. Accad. Sc. Torino.* 23, 492-501 (1888).
108. Grassi, G. B. and Rovelli G., Ricerche embriologische sui Cestodi. *Atti Accad. Gioenia Sci. Nat.* 4, 1-109 (1892).
109. Greenberg, Z. Helminths of mammals and birds of Israel. I. Helminths of *Acomys* spp. (Rodentia, Murinae). *Israel J. Zool.* 18, 25-38 (1969).
110. Greenberg, Z., Helminths of birds and mammals from Israel. IV. Helminths from *Nesokia indica* Gray and Hardwicke, 1832 (Rodentia: Muridae). *Israel J. Zool.* 21, 63-70 (1972).
111. Guevara-Pozo, D., Parasitacion de la rata de alcantarilla por *Capillaria hepatica* e *Hydatigera taeniaeformis* en Granada. *Rev. Iber. Parasitol.* 25, 447 (1965).
112. Hager, A., Effects of dietary modification of host rats on the tapeworm, *Hymenolepis diminuta*. *Iowa St. Coll. J. Sci.* 15, 127-154 (1941).
113. Hall, M. C., Society Proceedings. 45th Meeting of the Helminthological Society of Washington. *J. Parasitol.* 7, 186-201 (1921).
114. Hamajima, F., (Studies on the parasites of the Japanese house mouse, *Mus molossinus*. I. Helminth parasites in the mouse living in different environments.) (Ja, en). *Kyushu J. Med. Sci.* 13, 319-323 (1962).
115. Hamajima, F., (Studies on the parasites of the Japanese house mouse, *Mus molossinus*. Helminth parasites of the mouse living in two different environments.) (Ja, en). *Kiseichungaku Zasshi (Jap. J. Parasitol.)* 12, 12-15 (1963).
116. Hegner, R., Root, F. M., Augustine, D. L.,

"Animal Parasitology, with Special Reference to Man and Domesticated Animals." Appleton-Century, New York (1929).

117. Heyneman, D. and Voge, M., Host response of the flour beetle, *Tribolium confusum* to infections with *Hymenolepis diminuta*, *H. microstoma* and *H. citelli* (Cestoda: Hymenolepididae). *J. Parasitol.* 57, 881-886 (1971).

118. Hira, P. R., Human infection with the cestode *Hymenolepis diminuta* (Rudolphi 1819; Blanchard 1891). *Med. J. Malaysia.* 9, 93-95 (1975).

119. Hoki, R., (Report of the finding of the egg of *Hymenolepis diminuta* in men.) (Ja). *Tokyo Iji Shinshi.* No. 2007, 161-168 (1917).

120. Holmes, J. C., Effects of concurrent infections on *Hymenolepis diminuta* (Cestoda) and *Moniliformis dubius* (Acanthocephala). II. Effect on growth. *J. Parasitol.* 48, 87-96 (1962).

121. Holz, J. and Liem Jan Sioe, The parasites of rat in West-Java. *Z. Parasitenkde.* 25, 405-412 (1965).

122. Hopkins, C. A., The influence of dietary methionine on the amino acid pool of *Hymenolepis diminuta* in the rat's intestine. *Parasitology* 59, 407-427 (1969).

123. Hopkins, C. A., Diurnal movement of *Hymenolepis diminuta* in the rat. *Parasitology* 60, 255-271 (1970).

124. Hori, E. and Kusui, Y., (A survey of *Angiostrongylus cantonensis* in the harbor side areas of Tokyo. I. A survey of *Angiostrongylus cantonensis* from house rodents.) (Ja, en). *Kiseichugaku Zasshi (Jap. J. Parasitol.).* 21, 90-95 (1972).

125. Hori, E., Kusui, Y., Matui, A. and Hattori, T., (A survey of *Angiostrongylus cantonensis* in the harbor side areas of Tokyo. II. On the intermediate hosts of *Angiostrongylus cantonensis*.) (Ja, en). *Kiseichugaku Zasshi (Jap. J. Parasitol.)* 22, 209-217 (1973a).

126. Hori, E., Miyamoto, K., Kusui, Y. and Saito, K., (A survey of *Angiostrongylus cantonensis* in Haha-jima, Ogasawara Islands.) (Ja, en). *Kiseichugaku Zasshi (Jap. J. Parasitol.).* 23, 138-142 (1974).

127. Hori, E., Shionaga, S., Wada, Y. and Kusui, Y., (A survey of *Angiostrongylus cantonensis* in the

Chichijima, Ogasawara Islands.) (Ja, en). *Kiseichugaku Zasshi (Jap. J. Parasitol.)* 22, 347-353 (1973b).
128. Houdemer, F. E., Recherches de parasitologie comparee Indochinoise. *Paris.* 235 p. (1938).
129. Houser, B. B. and Burns, W. C., Experimental infection of gnotobiotic *Tenebrio molitor* and white rats with *Hymenolepis diminuta* (Cestoda: Cyclophyllidea). *J. Parasitol.* 54, 69-73 (1968).
130. Hsu, H. T., Contributions a l'etude des Cestodes de Chine. *Rev. Suisse Zool.* 42, 477-570 (1935).
131. Hughes, R. C. The genus *Hymenolepis* Weinland 1858. *Tech. Bull. Oklahoma Agric. Exp. Station No. 8*, 42 p., (1940).
132. Hughes, R. C., A key to the species of tapeworms in *Hymenolepis*. *Trans. Am. Micros. Soc.* 60, 378-414 (1941).
133. Hundley, D. F. and Berntzen, A. K., Collection, sterilization and storage of *Hymenolepis diminuta* eggs. *J. Parasitol.* 55, 1095-1096 (1969).
134. Hunkeler, P., Les Cestodes parasites des petits mammiferes (Ronqeurs et Insectivores) de Cote-d'Ivoire et de Haute-Volta. *Rev. Suisse Zool.* 80, 809-930 (1974).
135. Huq, M. M., A survey of the helminth parasites of roof rats, *Rattus rattus*, digger rats, *Bandicota bengalensis*, and mole *Scalopus scapanus*, in the Mymensingh District, East Pakistan. *Pakistan J. Vet. Sci.* 3, 65-68 (1969).
136. John, T. J., Montgomery, E., Jayabal, P., The prevalence of intestinal parasitism and its relation to diarrhoea in children. *Indian Pediat.* 8, 137-141 (1971).
137. Johnston, T. H., Notes on Australian Entozoa. No. 1. *Rec. Australian Mus.* 7, 329-344 (1909).
138. Johnston, T. H., Notes on some entozoa. *Proc. Roy. Soc. Queensland* 24, 63-91 (1913).
139. Johnston, T. H., Notes on miscellaneous parasites. *Proc. R. Soc. Queensland* 30, 209-218 (1918).
140. Johri, L. N., Report on cestodes collected in India and Burma. *Indian J. Helminthol.* 2, 23-34 (1950).
141. Jones, M. F. and Alicata, J. E., Development

and morphology of the cestode, *Hymenolepis cantaniana*, in coleopteran and avian hosts. *J. Wash. Acad. Sci. 25*, 237-247 (1935).

142. Joyeux, Ch., Sur le cycle evolutif de quelques Cestodes. Note preliminaire. *Bull. Soc. Path. Exot. 9*, 578-583 (1916).
143. Joyeux, Ch., Cycle evolutif de quelques Cestodes. Recherches experimentales. *Bull. Biol. France Belg. Suppl. II*, 1-219 (1920).
144. Joyeux, Ch. and Baer, J. G., Etudes de quelques Cestodes provenant des colonies francaises d'Afrique et de Madagascar. *Ann. Parasitol. Hum. Comp. 5*, 27-36 (1927).
145. Joyeux, Ch. and Baer, J. G., Les cestodes rares de l'homme. *Bull. Soc. Pathol. Exot. 22*, 114-136 (1929).
146. Joyeux, Ch. and Baer, J. G., Faune de France, 30. Cestodes. *Office Centrale de Faunistique, Paris*. 613 p. (1936).
147. Joyeux, Ch. and Baer, J. G., Sur quelques cestodes de Cochinchine. *Bull. Soc. Pathol. Exot. 30*, 872-873 (1937).
148. Joyeux, Ch., Baer, J. G. and Martin, R., Sur quelques cestodes de la Somalie-Nord. *Bull. Soc. Pathol. Exot. 29*, 82-96 (1936).
149. Joyeux, Ch., Baer, J. G. and Martin, R., Sur quelques cestodes de la Somalie-Nord (Deuxieme note). *Bull. Soc. Path. Exot. 30*, 416-423 (1937).
150. Joyeux, Ch. and Foley, H., Les helminthes de *Meriones shawi shawi* Rozet dans le nord de l'Algerie. *Bull. Soc. Zool. Fr. 55*, 353-374 (1930).
151. Kagei, N., Kihata, M. and Igarashi, S., (Observation in transitional aspect of helminthic infection in a rural area, Higashi-Matsuyama City, in Saitama Prefecture.) (Ja, en). *Bull. Inst. Pub. Health, Tokyo. 21*, 1-8 (1972).
152. Kalil, F. A., Basedow, H. J., Telles, C. A. and Monteiro, O., Himenolepiase nana em um educandario de Curitiba. Com adendo sobre "Um caso de Himenolepiase diminuta". *An. Fac. Med. Univ. Parana. 8*, 119-156 (1965).
153. Kamegai, S., (Treatment of a case of human infection by *Hymenolepis diminuta* with Atebrine.) (Ja). *Jap. J. Parasitol. 26*, (Suppl.), 17 (1977).

154. Kamiya, M., Chinzei, H. and Sasa, M., (A survey of helminth parasites of rats in southern Amami, Japan.) (Ja, en). *Kiseichugaku Zasshi (Jap. J. Parasitol.) 17*, 436-444 (1968).
155. Kamiya, M., Yabe, T. and Nakamura, Y., (Helminthic infections of the brown rat, *Rattus norvegicus*, from Kanagawa, Japan.) (Ja, en). *Kiseichugaku Zasshi (Jap. J. Parasitol.) 20*, 490-494 (1971).
156. Kasai, Y., Studies on helminths and protozoan parasites of rats in Sapporo. *Jap. J. Vet. Res. 26*, 31 (1978).
157. Kasai, H. and Kaneko, K., (Parasite fauna of domestic rat in Sapporo.) (Ja). *Jap. J. Parasitol. 26*, (5, Suppl.), 17 (1977).
158. Kaya, F., (Helminthological survey of the intestines of rodents in the districts of Ankara, Konya, Nevsehir and Urfa, Turkey.) (Tu, en). *Ankara Universitesi Tip Fakultesi Mecmuasi 28*, 3-35 (1975).
159. Keller, A. E., Eight cases of human infestation with the rat tapeworm (*Hymenolepis diminuta*). *J. Parasitol. 18*, 108-110 (1931).
160. Kihara, T., Yokohama, H. and Ishii, A., Uber die Resultate von Bandwurmkuren mit Cestocid Bayer 2353 (Yomesan). *Der Landarzt 42*, 1532-1534 (1965).
161. Kisielewska, K., Ecological organization of intestinal helminth groupings in *Clethrionomys glareolus* (Schreb.) (Rodentia). I. Structure and seasonal dynamics of helminth groupings in a host population in the Bialowieza National Park. *Acta Parasitol. Polon. 18*, 121-147 (1970a).
162. Kisielewska, K., Ecological organization of intestinal helminth groupings in *Clethrionomys glareolus* (Schreb.) (Rodentia). IV. Spatial structure of a helminth grouping with the host population. *Acta Parasitol. Polon. 18*, 177-196 (1970b).
163. Klein, J.-M., Donnees ecologiques et biologiques sur *Synopsyllus fonquerniei* Wagner et Roubaud, 1932 (Siphonaptera), puce du rat peridomestiques, dans la region de Tananarive. *Cahiers Office de la Recherche Scientifique et Technique Outre-Mer. Ser. Entomol. Med., Paris 4*, 3-29 (1966).
164. Kuntz, R. E. and Myers, B. J., Helminths of

vertebrates and leeches taken by the U.S. Naval Medical Mission to Yemen, Southwest Arabia. *Can. J. Zool. 46*, 1071-1075 (1968).
165. Lackie, A. M., Evasion of the haemocytic defence reaction of certain insects by larvae of *Hymenolepis diminuta* (Cestoda). *Parasitology 73*, 97-107 (1976).
166. Lamler, G., Zahner, H. and Texdorf, I., Infektionsversuche mit Darmnematoden, Cestoden and Trematoden bei *Mastomys natalensis* (Smith 1834). *Z. Parasitenkde. 31*, 166-202 (1968).
167. Leidy, J., Occurrence of a rare human tapeworm (*Taenia flavopunctata*). *Am. J. Med. Sc.*, n.s. *88*, 110-114 (1884).
168. Leidy, J., Researches in helminthology and parasitology. With a bibliography of his contributions to science arranged and edited by Joseph Leidy Jr. *Smithson. Misc. Collect. 46*, 1-281 (1904).
169. Leiper, R. T., A comment on two recent articles on helminth infections in man. *Brit. Med. J. 2*, 1302 (1913a).
170. Leiper, R. T., Two new genera of helminthes in man. *J. Trop. Med. Hyg. London. 16*, 270 (1913b).
171. Leiper, R. T., Observations on certain helminths of man. *Tr. Soc. Trop. Med. Hyg. 6*, 265-297 (1913c).
172. Leon, D. D. de, Helminth parasites of rats in San Juan, Puerto Rico. *J. Parasitol. 50*, 478-479 (1964).
173. Leon, N., Ein neuer menschlicher Cestode. *Zool. Anz. 33*, 359-362 (1908).
174. Leon, N., "Contribution a l'etude des Parasites Animaux de Roumanie". Bucuresti, (1924).
175. Lethbridge, R. C., The locust as an intermediate host for *Hymenolepis diminuta*. *J. Parasitol. 57*, 445-446 (1971a).
176. Lethbridge, R. C., The hatching of *Hymenolepis diminuta* eggs and penetration of the hexacanth in *Tenebrio molitor* beetles. *Parasitology 62*, 445-456 (1971b).
177. Lichtenfels, J. R. and Haley, A. J., New host records of intestinal nematodes of Maryland rodents and suppression of *Capillaria bonnevillei* Grundmann and Frandsen, 1960 as a synonym of *C. americana* Read, 1949. *Proc.*

Helminthol. Soc. Wash. 35, 206-211 (1968).
178. Liddo, S., *Hymenolepis diminuta* nella provincia di Bari. *Pathologica (Genova) 30*, 436-437 (1938).
179. Lima, D. F., Froes, O. M. and Zingano, A. G., Sobre um caso humano de himenolepidiase diminuta. *Hospital, Rio de Janeiro, 77*, 645-647 (1970).
180. Linstow, O. F. B. von, Compendium der Helminthologie. Ein Verzeichniss der bekannten Helminthen die frei oder in thierischen Korper leben, geordnet nach ihren Wohnthieren, unter Angabe der Organe, in denen sie gefunden sind, und mit Beifung der Litteraturquellen. *Hannover.* 382 p. (1878).
181. Lopez-Neyra, C. R., Division del género *Hymenolepis* Weinland (*s. l.*) en otros mas naturales. *Rev. Ibér. Parasitol. 2*, 46-93 (1942a).
182. Lopez-Neyra, C. R., Division del género *Hymenolepis* Weinland (*s. l.*) en otros mas naturales. *Rev. Ibér. Parasitol. 2*, 113-256 (1942b).
183. Luney, W. F., *Hymenolepis diminuta* (rat tapeworm) in man, with the report of a case. *Can. Med. Assoc. J. 30*, 385-386 (1934).
184. MacDonald, F. and Goldsmid, J. M., Intestinal helminth infections in the Burma Valley area of Rhodesia. *C. Afr. J. Med. 19*, 113-115 (1973).
185. MacDonald, M. E., Catalogue of helminths of waterfowl (Anatidae). *Spec. Scient. Rep. Fish & Wildlife Serv. No. 126*, 692 p. (1969).
186. Mankau, S. K., Sex as a factor in the infection of *Tribolium* spp. by *Hymenolepis diminuta*. *Environ. Entomol. 6*, 233-326 (1977).
187. Manning, G. S. et al., *Fasciolopsis buski* in Thailand, with comments on other intestinal helminths. *J. Med. Ass. Thailand 53*, 425-432 (1969).
188. Marcial Crovato, A., Un nuevo caso de parasitosis por *Hymenolepis diminuta*. Nota previa. *Rev. Ass. Bioquim. Argent. 26*, 3-4 (1961).
189. Marshall, A. G., The cat flea, *Ctenocephalides felis* (Bouche 1835) as an intermediate host for cestodes. *Parasitology 57*, 419-430 (1967).
190. Marzullo, F. and Squadrini, F., Saggi di

funzionalita epatopancreatica in alcune
parassitosi intestinali. *Gior. Mal. Infet.
Parassitar. 15*, 465-467 (1963).
191. Matevosvan, E. M., The status of the genus
Hymenolepis in the system of the cestode family
Hymenolepididae. *Mat. Internat. Conf. on
Hymenolepididae.* Warszawa. 14-16 September
1973. (B. Bezubik & B. Czaplinski, eds.) p.
86-88 (1973).
192. Mayaudon Tarbes, H. and Gallo, P., Algunas
consideraciones sobre las helmintozoonosis en
Venezuela. *Rev. Med. Vet. Parasitol., Maracay,
Year 1963-1964. 20*, 5-21 (1964).
193. Mayhew, R. L., Studies on the avian species of
the cestode family Hymenolepididae. *Illinois
Biol. Monogr. 10*, 1-125 (1925).
194. Mazzotti, L. and Osorio, M. T., Cinco nuevos
casos de infeccion humana por *Hymenolepis
diminuta* en Mexico. *Rev. Inst. Salubr. Enferm.
Trop., Mexico 4*, 49-52 (1943).
195. McMillan, B., Kelly, A. and Walker, J. C.,
Prevalence of *Hymenolepis diminuta* infection
in man in the New Guinea highlands. *Trop.
Geogr. Med. 23*, 390-392 (1971).
196. Meggitt, F. J., "The Cestodes of Mammals".
London 282 pp., (1924).
197. Meggitt, F. J., Report on a collection of
Cestoda, mainly from Egypt. Part II.
Cyclophyllidea: Family Hymenolepididae.
Parasitology 19, 420-448 (1927).
198. Meggitt, F. J. and Subramanian, K., The
tapeworms of rodents of the subfamily Murinae
with special reference to those occurring in
Rangoon. *J. Burma Res. Soc. 17*, 190-237
(1927).
199. Meerovitch, E. and Gibbs, H. C., Intestinal
parasitic infections in the inhabitants of
Easter Island. *Trans. R. Soc. Trop. Med. Hyg.
63*, 370-373 (1969).
200. Mendheim, H. V., Zwischenwirte and
Infektionsmodus beim Rattenbandwurm *Hymenolepis
diminuta* (Rudolphi 1819). *Anz. Schaedlingsk.
24*, 89-91 (1951).
201. Mettrick, D. F. and Munro, H. N., Studies on
the protein metabolism of cestodes. I. Effects
of host dietary constituents on the growth of
Hymenolepis diminuta. Parasitology 5, 453-
466 (1965).

202. Mishra, G. S. and Bercovier, H., Bilan d'une enquete parasitologique chez de micromammiferes sauvage du department de l'Indre (France). *Rec. Met. Vet.* 151, 427-435 (1975).
203. Mishra, G. S. and Gonzalez, J. P., Bilan d'une etude sur les endoparasites du rat, *Rattus norvegicus* Berkenhout, 1769, a Tunis. *Arch. l'Inst. Pasteur Tunis.* 52, 71-87 (1975).
204. Mituch, J., [Contribution on the knowledge of the helminth fauna of the genus *Neomys* (Insectivora) in Slovakia.] (Sl, ru, en). *Studia Helminthol.* 1, 83-100 (1964).
205. Moll, A. M., Animal parasites of rats at Madison, Wisconsin, *J. Parasitol.* 4, 89-90 (1917).
206. Momma, K., On a case of *Hymenolepis diminuta* Rud., 1819. *Ann. Trop. Med. Parasitol.* 22, 1-3 (1928).
207. Moon, J. R., Public health significance of zoonotic tapeworms in Korea. *Internat. J. Zoonoses* 3, 1-18 (1976).
208. Mosby, J. M. and Wodzicki, K., some parasites of the kimoa (*Rattus exulans*) on the Tokelau Islands. *New Zealand J. Sci.* 15, 698-704 (1972).
209. Motakef, M., Report of a case infected with *Hymenolepis diminuta* in Mashad. *J. Mashad School Med.* 10, 472-474 (1968).
210. Mukhin, V. N., [Anomalies in the structure of *Hymenolepis diminuta* (Cestoda) from the intestine of *Rattus norvegicus*.] (Ru.). *Parazitologiya* 1, 324 (1967).
211. Mullee, M. T. and Voge, M., *Oryzaephilus surinamensis* (L)., a new intermediate host for the cestode, *Hymenolepis diminuta*. *J. Parasitol.* 45, 504 (1959).
212. Muller, H., Zur Parasitenfauna der Labortiere. 2. Die Parasitenfauna der weissen Ratte (*Rattus norvegicus* var. *albinus*). *Wiener Tierarzt. Monats.* 63, 31 (1976).
213. Myers, B. J., Wolfgang, R. W. and Kuntz, R. E., Helminth parasites from vertebrates taken in the Sudan (East Africa). *Can. J. Zool.* 38, 833-836 (1960).
214. Nama, H. S. and Khichi, P. S., Studies on cestodes (Hymenolepididae) from *Columba livia* and *Rattus rattus*. *Acta Parasitol. Polon.* 23, 223-228 (1975).

215. Nama, H. S. and Parihar, A., Quantitative and qualitative analysis of helminth fauna in *Rattus rattus rufescens*. *J. Helminthol.* 50, 99-102 (1976).
216. Narihara, N., (Studies on the post-embryonal development of *Hymenolepis diminuta*. Part I. On hatching of the eggs of *Hymenolepis diminuta*.) (Ja, en). *Taiwan Igakkai Zasshi.* 36, 713-729 (1937a).
217. Narihara, N., (Studies on the post-embryonal development of *Hymenolepis diminuta*. Part II. On the development of cysticercoid within the definite intermediate host.) (Ja, en). *Taiwan Igakkai Zasshi.* 36, 732-780 (1937b).
218. Newell, K. W., Dover, A. S., Clemmer, D. I., D'Allessandro, A., Duenas, A., Gracian, M. and LeBlanc, D. R., Diarrheal diseases of infancy in Cali, Colombia: study design and summary report on isolated disease agents. *Bull. Pan Am. Health Org.* 10, 143-155 (1976).
219. Nguyen-Van-Ai., Services pratiques. *Rap. Ann. Fonction Techn. Inst. Pasteur Viet-Nam. 1960*, 115-219 (1961).
220. Nickerson, W. S., An American intermediate host for *Hymenolepis diminuta*. *Science, n.s. (842).* 33, 271 (1911).
221. Nicoll, W. and Minchin, E. A., Two species of cysticercoids from the ratflea (*Ceratophyllus fasciatus*). *Proc. Zool. Soc. London No. 1*, 9-13 (1911).
222. Niphadkar, S. M., Ecological study of helminths of three species of rats in Bombay in relation to veterinary and public health. 1. Incidence. *In: Abst. 1st Nat. Cong. Parasitol., Baroda, 24-26 February 1977. Indian Soc. Parasitol.* p. 45-46 (1977).
223. Noc, F., Les parasites intestinaux a la Martinique. *Bull. Soc. Path. Exot.* 4, 390-395 (1911).
224. Nybelin, O., Saugetier- und Vogelcestoden von Juan Fernandez. *Nat. Hist. Juan Fernandez and Easter Islands* 3, 493-525 (1929).
225. Oldham, J. N., On the arthropod intermediate hosts of *Hymenolepis diminuta* (Rudolphi 1819). *J. Helminthol.* 9, 21-28 (1931).
226. Olsen, O. W. and Kuntz, R. E., Cestodes from *Rattus* Fischer in Taiwan. *Proc. Helminthol. Soc. Wash.* 44, 101-102 (1977).

227. Packard, F. A., *Tenia flavopunctata*, with description of a new specimen. *J. Am. Med. Ass.* 35, 1551-1553 (1900).
228. Paperna, I., Furman, D. P. and Rothstein, N., The parasite fauna of rodents from urban and suburban areas of Accra-Tema, South Ghana. *Rev. Zool. Botan. Africaines* 81, 330-336 (1970).
229. Parodi, S. E., Consideraciones sobre el 1st caso de *Hymenolepis diminuta* observado en la R. Argentina. *Prensa Med. Argent.* 2, 131-132 (1915).
230. Parona, C., Di alcuni cestodi brasiliani raccolti dal Dott. Adolfo Lutz. *Atti. Soc. Ligust. Sci. Nat. Genova.* 12, 3-14 (1901).
231. Patnaik, M. M. and Acharyo, L. N., Notes on the helminth parasites of vertebrates in Baranga Zoo (Orissa). *Indian Vet. J.* 47, 723-730 (1970).
232. Paul, F. M. and Zaman, V., *Hymenolepis diminuta* infestation in a Chinese baby. *J. Singapore Paediat. Soc.* 11, 62-66 (1969).
233. Plotkowiak, J., (Some problems concerning taeniasis in the light of the materials collected on the terrain of Szczecin Province.) (Pl). *Wiadomosci Parazytol.* 9, 547-552 (1963).
234. Plotkowiak, J. and Zolnowski, Z., (A case of infestation by the rat tapeworm *Hymenolepis diminuta*.) (Pl). *Pediatria Polska.* 39, 65-68 (1964).
235. Podyapolskaya, V. L., [Survey of parasitic worm fauna of rats (*Rattus norvegicus*) of Russia.] (Ru). *Vest. Mikrobiol. Epidemiol. Saratov* 3, 280-290 (1924).
236. Pozo-Lora, R., Helmintos de la rata en Cordoba. *An. Univ. Hispalensis.* 19, 55-58 (1959).
237. Pozo-Lora, R., Aportaciones al inventario y ecologia de los helmintos espanoles. Especies encontrados en Cordoba. *Rev. Iber. Parasitol.* 20, 403-410 (1960).
238. Prokopic, J., [A bionomical-faunistic analysis of results of the stationary investigation of cestodes occurring in micromammalia in the vicinity of Klec (South Bohemia).] (De). *Helminthologia (Bratislava).* 11, 201-212 (1970).
239. Quentin, J., Cestodes de rongeurs de Republique Centrafricaine. *Cahiers la Maboke.* 2, 117-140 (1964).

240. Rabinovitch, B. A. and Marcial Crovato, A., Un nuevo caso de parasitosis por *Hymenolepis diminuta*. Prensa Med. Argent. *48*, 2703-2704 (1961).
241. Railliet, A., Notices parasitologiques: *Taenia tenuirostris* Rud. chez l'oie domestique: remarques sur la classification des cestodes parasites des oiseaux. Bull. Soc. Zool. France. *17*, 110-117 (1892).
242. Ransom, B., An account of the tapeworms of the genus *Hymenolepis* parasitic in man, including several new cases of the dwarf tapeworm (*H. nana*) in the United States. U. S. Publ. Health Serv. Hyg. Lab. Bull. *18*, 1-38 (1904).
243. Ratliff, C. R. and Donaldson, L., A human case of *Hymenolepis diminuta* in Alabama. J. Parasitol. *51*, 808 (1965).
244. Rau, M. E., The frequency distribution of *Hymenolepis diminuta* cysticercoids in natural sympatric populations of *Tenebrio molitor* and *T. obscurus*. Int. J. Parasitol. *9*, 85-87 (1979).
245. Read, C. P., *Hymenolepis diminuta* in the Syrian hamster. J. Parasitol. *37*, 324 (1951).
246. Read, C. P., "Animal Parasitism". Prentice-Hall, Inc. Englewood Cliffs, New Jersey. 182 p. (1972).
247. Read, C. P. and Kilejian, A. Z., Circadian migratory behaviour of a cestode symbiote in the rat host. J. Parasitol. *55*, 574-578 (1969).
248. Read, C. P., Schiller, E. L. and Phifer, K., The role of carbohydrates in the biology of cestodes. V. Comparative studies on the effects of host dietary carbohydrates on *Hymenolepis* spp. Exp. Parasitol. *7*, 198-216 (1958).
249. Read, C. P. and Voge, M., The size attained by *Hymenolepis diminuta* in different host species. J. Parasitol. *40*, 88-89 (1954).
250. Rifaat, M. A., Fahmy, M. A. M. and Arafa, M. S., Results of a helminthic survey in a locality highly infected with rats near Cairo, U.A.R. J. Egypt. Publ. Hlth. Ass. *43*, 105-121 (1968).
251. Rifaat, M. A., Mahdi, A. H. and Arafa, M. S., Helminthic infection of the climbing rat, *Rattus rattus* (Linnaeus 1758) in the U.A.R.

J. Egypt Publ. Hlth. Ass. **44**, 119-125 (1969a).
252. Rifaat, M. A., Mahdi, A. H. and Arafa, M. S., Helminthic infection of Cairo spiny mouse, *Acomys cahirinus* (E. Geoffroy, St. Hilaire, 1803) in U.A.R. *J. Egypt. Publ. Hlth. Ass.* **44**, 177-182 (1969b).
253. Riley, W. A. and Shannon, W. R., The rat tapeworm, *Hymenolepis diminuta*, in man. *J. Parasitol.* **8**, 109-117 (1922).
254. Roberts, L. S., The influence of population density on patterns and physiology of growth in *Hymenolepis diminuta* (Cestoda: Cyclophyllidea) in the definitive host. *Exp. Parasitol.* **11**, 332-371 (1961).
255. Rodriguez Balleste, J., Gonzalez de la Torre, P. and Hernandez Minoso, M., Tipos de helmintos encontrados en rats Wistar. *Rev. Cubana Med. Trop.* **27**, 151-157 (1975).
256. Roman, E., Hôtes intermédiaires noveaux d' *Hymenolepis diminuta* (Cestodes Hymenolépididés). *C. R. Soc. Biol. Paris* **126**, 26-28 (1937).
257. Rosa, W. A. and Niec, R., *Hymenolepis diminuta* (Rudolphi 1819) en perro. *Rev. Invest. Ganad., Buenos Aires* **5**, 19-25 (1959).
258. Rothman, A. H., The larval development of *Hymenolepis diminuta* and *Hymenolepis citelli*. *J. Parasitol.* **43**, 643-648 (1957).
259. Rothman, A. H., Studies on the excystment of tapeworms. *Exp. Parasitol.* **8**, 336-364 (1959).
260. Rudolphi, K. A., Entozoorum synopsis cui Accedunt mantissa Duplex et Indices Locupletissimi. *Berolini.* 811 p. (1819).
261. Ruebush, T. K., II., Juranek, D. D., Brodsky, R. E., Diagnoses of intestinal parasites by state and territorial public health laboratories, 1976. *J. Inf. Dis.* **138**, 114-117 (1978).
262. Rusinova, E. A., [On the parasites of rats in the City of Molotov. (With problems in combatting trichinosis).] (Ru). *Trudy Molotov Med. Inst.* **19**, 23-27 (1940).
263. Sasa, M., Tanaka, H., Fukui, W. and Takata, A., Internal parasites of laboratory animals. *In:* "Problems of Laboratory Animal Disease". *(R. G. C. Harris, ed.)* Academic Press, New York. p. 195-214 (1962).
264. Schmidt, G. D., New records of helminths from New Guinea, including descriptions of three

new cestode species, one in the new genus
Wallabicestus n.g. *Tr. Am. Micros. Soc. 94*,
189-196 (1975).
265. Schmidt, R., Untersuchungen uber die
Entoparasitenfauna des Magen-Darmtraktes und
der Leibeshohle von Muriden (Rodentia) der
Umgebung Halles unter besonder Beruksichtigung
der Cestoden und Nematoden. *Wissen. Z. Martin-
Luther Univ., Halle-Wittenberg. 11*, 457-470
(1962).
266. Schmidt, S., da C. Mattos, D., and Alves, E.
L., Incidencia de *Hymenolepis diminuta* em
ratos capturados em Neropolis, Estado de
Goias. (Pt, en). *Rev. Patol. Trop. 3*,
141-142 (1974).
267. Schwartz, B. and Tubangui, M. A., Uncommon
intestinal parasites of man in the Philippine
Islands. *Philip. J. Sci. 20*, 611-618 (1922).
268. Seidenberg, A. J. *et al.*, Helminths of the
cotton rat in southern Virginia, with comments
on the sex ratios of parasitic nematode
populations. *Am. Midl. Nat. 92*, 320-326
(1974).
269. Seitenok, N. and Kolossov, N., (Observations
on the infestations of man with *Hymenolepis
diminuta*.) (Ru). *Med. Parazit. (Moskva). 5*,
811-812 (1936).
270. Semenova, L. F. and Yarulin, G. P., (On the
study of the helminthological fauna of rodents
of Dagestan.) (Ru). *Mater. Nauchn. Konf.
Vsesoyuz. Obshch. Gel'mintol. No. 3*, 221-225
(1965).
271. Serra, R. G., Contribuicao a incidencia de
Hymenolepis diminuta (Rud., 1819) no homem.
Ocorrencia de 4 casos em Sao Paulo. *Rev.
Fac. Farm. Bioquim., Sao Paulo. 1*, 37-42
(1963a).
272. Serra, R. G., Anomalias de *Hymenolepis
diminuta* (Rudolphi, 1819) em exemplares colhidos
no homem. *Rev. Fac. Farm. Bioquim., Sao Paulo.
1*, 43-60 (1963b).
273. Sharpilo, L. D., (On the study of helminth
fauna of rodents in the territory of the
Ukraine.) (Ru). *Trudy Ukrainsk. Respub. Nauch.
Obshch. Parazitol. 1*, 201-206 (1961).
274. Sharpilo, L. D., (On the helminth fauna of
synanthropic rodents in the territory of the
right-bank steppes of Ukranian SSR.) (Ru).

Trudy 4 Nauch. Konf. Parazitol. USSR. pp 286-288 (1963).
275. Shimidsu, S., Horimi, T. and Inagami, H., [Occurrence of *Hymenolepis diminuta* in Japanese mole, *Mogera wogura wogura* (Temminck, 1842).] (Ja). *Eisei Dobutsu. 2*, 62-63 (1951).
276. Shircore, J. O., Notes on the prevalence of intestinal parasites in East Africa. *Tr. Soc. Trop. Med. Hyg. London 10*, 101-108 (1917).
277. Shogaki, Y., Mizuno, S. and Itoh, H., [On *Protospirura muris* (Gmelin), a parasitic nematode of the brown rat in Nagoya City.] (Ja, en). *Kiseichugaku Zasshi (Jap. J. Parasitol.) 21*, 28-38 (1972).
278. Simitch, T. and Petrovitch, Z. L., Ce qu'il advient avec des helminthes du *Citellus citellus* au cours du sommeil hibernal de ce rongeur. *Riv. Parassitol. 15*, 655-662 (1954).
279. Simmons, D. J. C. and Walkey, M., *Capillaria* and *Hymenolepis* in a wild rat: hazards to barrier-maintained laboratory animals. *Lab. Animal. 5*, 49-55 (1971).
280. Sinelshchikov, V. A., (On the helminth fauna of domestic carnivores and rodents in the town of Kishinev.) (Ru). *In: (Parasites of Animals and Plants)*. Kishinev: Kartya Moldovenyaske. No. 1, 61-64 (1965).
281. Skrjabin, K. I. and Matevosyan, E. M., (Types of topographical correlations of sexual glands in cestodes of the family Hymenolepididae and their taxonomic significance.) (Ru). *Dokl. Akad. Nauk SSSR, n.s. 36*, 32-35 (1942).
282. Skrjabin, K. I. and Matevosyan, E. M., (Hymenolepidids of mammals.) (Ru). *Trudy Gel'mintol. Lab., Akad. Nauk SSSR. 1*, 15-92 (1948).
283. Smith, A. J., Synopsis of studies in metazoan parasitology in the McManus Laboratory of Pathology. *Univ. Penn. Med. Bull. 20*, 262-282 (1908).
284. Smyth, J. D., "The Physiology of Cestodes". W. H. Freeman and Co., San Francisco. 279 p. (1969).
285. Soltice, G. E., Arai, H. P. and Scheinberg, E., Host-parasite interactions of *Tribolium confusum* and *Tribolium castaneum* with *Hymenolepis diminuta. Can. J. Zool. 49*, 265-273 (1971).

286. Soltys, A., (Helminthofauna of Soricidae in the Bialowieza National Park.) (Pl, en). *Acta Parasitol. Polon. 1*, 353-402 (1954).
287. Soltys, A., (Studies on parasitic worms of small rodents of National Park in Bialowieza.) (Pl, en). *Acta Parasitol. Polon. 5*, 487-504 (1957).
288. Southwell, T., Cestodes in the collection of the Indian Museum. *Ann. Trop. Med. Parasitol. 16*, 127-152 (1922).
289. Southwell, T. and Lake, F., On a collection of Cestoda from the Belgian Congo. *Ann. Trop. Med. Parasitol. 33*, 63-90 (1939).
290. Spassky, A. A., (On the position of the genus *Echinorhynchotaenia* Fuhrmann, 1909, in the system of cestodes.) (Ru). *Dokl. Akad. Nauk SSSR, n. s. 58*, 513-515 (1947).
291. Spassky, A. A., (*Mathevolepis petrotschenkoi* nov. gen., nov. sp. - a new cestode genus with uterine canals for the production of eggs.) (Ru). *Dokl. Akad. Nauk SSR, n. s. 59*, 1513-1515 (1948).
292. Spasskii, A. A., (On the question of the alteration of generations in cestodes.) (Ru). *Dokl. Akad. Nauk SSSR, n. s. 91*, 445-447 (1953).
293. Spasskii, A. A., (Classification of the hymenolepidids of mammals.) (Ru). *Trudy Gel'-mintol. Lab., Akad. Nauk SSSR. 7*, 120-167 (1954).
294. Spasskii, A. A., Romanova, N. P. and Naidenova, N. V., [New data on the fauna of parasitic worms of the muskrat - *Ondatra zibethica* (L.).] (Ru). *Trudy Gel'mintol. Lab. Akad. Nauk SSR. 5*, 42-52 (1951).
295. Spasskii, A. A. and L. P. Spasskaya, (Systematic structure of the hymenolepidids parasitic in birds.) (Ru). *Trudy Gel'mintol. Lab., Akad. Nauk SSSR. 7*, 55-119 (1954).
296. Spindler, L. A., On the occurrence of the rat tapeworm (*Hymenolepis diminuta*) and dwarf tapeworm (*Hymenolepis nana*) in man in southwest Virginia. *J. Parasitol. 16*, 38-40 (1929).
297. Stiles, C. W., The type species of the cestode genus *Hymenolepis*. *U. S. Publ. Hlth. Serv., Hyg. Lab. Bull. 13*, 19-21 (1903).
298. Stiles, C. W., Society Proceeding. Forty-sixth meeting of the Helminthological Society

of Washington. *J. Parasitol.* 7, 186-188 (1921).
299. Stiles, C. W., Illustrated key to the cestode parasites of man. *Bull. U. S. Publ. Hlth. Serv. Mar. Hosp. Serv.* No. 25, (1906).
300. Stiles, C. W. and Hassall, A., Key-catalogue of the worms reported for man. *U. S. Public Health Serv. Hyg. Lab. Bull.* No. 142, 69-196 (1926).
301. Sturdevant, L. B., Some variations in *Hymenolepis diminuta*. *Univ. Studies, Univ. Nebraska.* 7, 135-148 (1907).
302. Suciu, M. and Popescu, A., (Contribution to the study of intestinal parasites of three species of murines and of *Citellus citellus* in the region of Dobrogea.) (Ro, ru, fr). *Comun. Acad. Repub. Pop. Romine.* 12, 559-564 (1962).
303. Sukolin, G. I., (Allergic skin diseases and intestinal parasites in Algeria.) (Ru). *Vestnik Dermat. Venerol.* 45, 67-70 (1971).
304. Sullivan, J. T., Palmieri, J. R. and Chu, G. S. T., Potential transmission of hymenolepiasis by a practice of Malaysian Chinese folk medicine. *J. Parasitol.* 63, 172 (1977).
305. Sultanov, M. A. and Kabilov, T., (The role of insects in maintaining sources of infection with helminthoses in natural foci in Uzbekistan.) (Ru, uzbek). *Uzbeksk. Biol. Zhurn.* No. 4, 60-63 (1976).
306. Sunkes, E. J. and Sellers, T. F., Tapeworm infestations in the southern United States. *Am. J. Pub. Hlth.* 27, 893-898 (1937).
307. Surkov, V. S., (Distribution of helminths from forest voles of the Sakhalin Island by biotopes.) (Ru, en). *Zool. Zhurn.* 51, 748-750 (1972).
308. Surkov, V. S., (Seasonal dynamics of infestation of forest voles by helminths on Sakhalin Island.) (Ru, en). *Zool. Zhurn.* 53, 184-188 (1974).
309. Takagi, K., Yamaguchi, T. and Suzuki, R., (The helminth parasites of rats captured in an endemic area of clonorchiasis in Tokushima Prefecture.) (Ja). *Shikoku Acta Medica.* 18, 194-197 (1962).
310. Tenora, F., (Review of the parasitic worms in rodents of the genus *Apodemus* in Czecho-

slovakia.) (Sl, en). *Zool. Listy. 12,* 331-336 (1963).
311. Tenora, F., [Report on the parasitic worms found in *Rattus rattus* (L.). living in Czechoslovakia.] (Sl, en). *Zool. Listy. 13,* 88-89 (1964).
312. Tenora, F., Die Helminthenfauna der Kleinnager aus der Untergattung *Sylvaemus* in der C. S. S. R. and ihre Bezeihungen zur Bionomie der Wirte. *Zool. Listy. 14,* 261-272 (1965a).
313. Tenora, F., (Towards the elucidation of the problem of mutual relations among the parasitic helminths in rodents of the genus *Apodemus* in Czechoslovakia.) (Sl, en, ge, ru). *Sborn. Vysoke Zemedelske Brne, Rada D, 1,* 69-75 (1965b).
314. Tenora, F., Supplementary notes on hymenolepidid tapeworms parasitizing glirid dormice in south Slovakian limestone area (Czechoslovakia). *Csk. Parasitol. 12,* 299-303 (1965c).
315. Tenora, F., Notes on the analysis of helminth fauna of the common vole *Microtus arvalis* (Pall.). *Sborn. Vysoke Skoly Zemed. Brne. Rada A. 20,* 655-666 (1972).
316. Tenora, F. and Barus, V., (Cysticercus Taeniae taeniaeformis dangerous parasite of our muskrats.) (Sl). *Sborn. Vysoke Skoly Zemedd. Lesn. Fak. Brne. A. 2,* (1955).
317. Tenora, F. and Kullman, E., (The first findings of cestodes from Rodentia and Lagomorpha from Afghanistan.) (De). *Helminthologia (Bratislava). 11,* 113-126 (1970).
318. Tenora, F. and Murai, E., Recent data on five species of the genus *Hymenolepis* (Weinland, 1858) (Cestoidea, Hymenolepididae) parasitizing rodents in Hungary. *Acta Zool. Acad. Sci. Hungar. 18,* 129-145 (1972).
319. Tokobaev, M. M., (Helminth fauna of rodents of Kirgizia.) (Ru). *Trudy Gel'mintol. Lab., Akad. Nauk SSSR. 10,* 235-247 (1960).
320. Tokobaev, M. M., (Helminth fauna of rodents in the high mountains of Tersk-Ala-Tor, valley of the Chon-Kyzyl-Su River.) (Ru). *Izv. Akad. Nauk Kirgiz. SSR, s. Biol. Nauk 4,* 153-161 (1962).
321. Tubangui, M. A., Worm parasites of the brown rat (*Mus norvegicus*) in the Philippine Islands,

with special reference to those forms that may be transmitted to human beings. *Philip. J. Sci. 46*, 531-591 (1931).
322. Turner, J. A., Other cestode infections. In: Diseases Transmitted from Animals to Man. (W. T. Hubbert, W. F. McCulloch and P. R. Schnurrenberger, eds.) Charles C. Thomas, Springfield, Illinois, p. 708-744 (1975).
323. Turton, J. A., Williamson, J. R. and Harris, W. G., Haematological and immunological responses to the tapeworm *Hymenolepis diminuta* in man. *Tropenmed. Parasitol. 26*, 196-200 (1975).
324. Villagiova, I., (Endoparasites of laboratory rodents.) (Sl). *Csl. Parasitol. 9*, 423-429 (1962).
325. Vincent, A. L., Porter, D. D. and Ash, L. W., Spontaneous lesions and parasites of the Mongolian gerbil, *Meriones unguiculatus*. *Lab. Animal Sci. 25*, 711-722 (1975).
326. Vines, A. P. and Kelly, A., Highlands region survey of intestinal parasites. *Med. J. Aust., 53rd year. 2*, 635-640 (1966).
327. Voge, M., Variability of *Hymenolepis diminuta* in the laboratory rat and in the ground squirrel, *Citellus leucurus*. *J. Parasitol. 38*, 454-456 (1952a).
328. Voge, M., Variation in some unarmed Hymenolepididae (Cestoda). *Univ. Calif. Publ. Zool. 27*, 1-52 (1952b).
329. Voge, M., A list of cestode parasites from California mammals. *Am. Midl. Nat. 54*, 413-417 (1955).
330. Voge, M., Studies on the life history of *Hymenolepis citelli* (McLeod, 1933) (Cestoda: Cyclophyllidea). *J. Parasitol. 42*, 485-490 (1956).
331. Voge, M., Systematics of cestodes - Present and future. In: Problems in Systematics of Parasites (G. D. Schmidt, ed.) University Park Press, Baltimore & Manchester. p. 49-73 (1969).
332. Voge, M. and Bertzen, A. K., *In vitro* hatching of oncospheres of *Hymenolepis diminuta* (Cestoda: Cyclophyllidea). *J. Parasitol. 47*, 813-818 (1961).
333. Voge, M. and Heyneman, D., Development of *Hymenolepis nana* and *Hymenolepis diminuta* (Cestoda: Cyclophyllidea) in the intermediate

host, *Tribolium confusum*. *Univ. Calif. Publ. Zool.* 59, 549-580 (1957).

334. Voge, M. and Turner, J. A., The effect of different temperatures on the development of *Hymenolepis diminuta* in *Tribolium confusum*. *J. Parasitol.* 42 (Supp.), 31 (1956).

335. Vogelsang, E. G. and Potenza, L., Endoparasitos de las ratas silvestres de Caracas. *Pub. Biogen., Caracas.* 3, 21-30 (1945).

336. Vogelsang, E. G. and Rodriguez, C., Ecto y endoparasitos de animales en cautiverio del Jardin zoologico de Maracay. *Rev. Med. Vet. y Parasitol., Caracas.* 11, 311-316 (1952).

337. Weinland, D. F., Human Cestoides. An essay on the tapeworms of man, giving a full account of their nature, organization, and embryonic development; the pathological symptoms they produce, and the remedies which have proved successful in modern practice. To which is added an appendix, containing a catalogue of all species of helminthes hitherto found in man. Metcalf and Co., Cambridge, Massachusetts. 93 p. (1858).

338. Weinland, D. F., Beschreibung zweier neuer Taenioiden aus dem Menschen; Notiz uber die Bandwurmer de Indianer and Neger; Beschreibung einer monstrositat von *Taenia solium* L. und Versuch einer Systematik der Taenien uberhaupt. *Nova Acta Acad. Nat. Curios., Janae* 28, 24 p. (1861).

339. van Wijk, H. B., Infection with *Schistosoma intercalatum* in Mungo Department, Cameroon. *Trop. Geogr. Med.* 21, 362-373 (1969a).

340. van Wijk, H. B., *Schistosoma intercalatum* infection in school children of Loum, Cameroon. *Trop. Geogr. Med.* 21, 375-382 (1969b).

341. Yamada, S., Asada, J. and Miyada, I., [Studies on the life-history of a common rat-tapeworm, *Hymenolepis diminuta* (Rudolphi), especially on the relation between this tapeworm and rat-fleas.] (Ja). *Dobutsu Zasshi.* 48, 437-457 (1936).

342. Yamaguti, S., Studies on the helminth fauna of Japan. Part 7. Cestodes of mammals and snakes. *Jap. J. Zool.* 6, 233-246 (1935).

343. Yamaguti, S., Systema Helminthum. Vol. II. The Cestodes of Vertebrates. Interscience, New York. 806 p. (1959).

344. Yeh, Y. C., A survey on tapeworm infestations in rodents on Taiwan. *J. Taiwan Ass. Animal Husb. Vet. Med. No. 16*, 38-43 (1970).
345. Zahner, H. and Texdorf, I., Uber das Wirt-Parasit-Verhaltnis bei *Mastomys natalensis* (Smith, 1834). *Z. ParasitenKde. 31*, 9-10 (1968).
346. Zanina, Z. L. and Tokobaev, M. M., (Parasitic worms of rodents in the desert regions of Tadzhikistan.) (Ru). *Izv. Akad. Nauk Tadzhikisk. SSR, Otdel. Biol. Nauk. 3*, 70-85 (1962).
347. Zarnowski, E., [Parasitic worms of forest micromammalians (Rodentia and Insectivora) of the environment of Pulawy (district Lublin) I. Cestoda.] (Pl, en). *Acta Parasitol. Polon. 3*, 279-368 (1955).
348. Zembrzuski, K. et al., (Cestodes in the population of Poland in 1973.) (Pl). *Przeglad Epidemiol. 29*, 235-240 (1975).

STRUCTURE AND ULTRASTRUCTURE OF THE LARVAE AND METACESTODES OF *HYMENOLEPIS DIMINUTA*

John E. Ubelaker

Department of Biology
Southern Methodist University
Dallas, Texas

Hymenolepis diminuta is often regarded as a model tapeworm species which is used in many parasitology classes to introduce students to cestode life cycles. The use of this particular species is undoubtedly related to the ease of maintaining both adult and metacestode stages. This cestode, like many others, possesses a basic sequence of development consisting of a monoecious adult which undergoes proglottidation and sexual reproduction in the enteron of rodent definitive hosts. The adult tapeworm produces numerous ova and spermatozoans which upon fertilization form eggs which pass into the uterus and embryonate. Embryogenesis results in a larva, termed a hexacanth larva or oncosphere (Freeman 1973). The six-hooked larva is surrounded by several larval membranes including an outer envelope which is hardened and referred to as a capsule. Probably because of a hardened capsule, the oncosphere is commonly, but erroneously, designated an egg. The larva is passed in the feces of the definitive host and may be found in the gravid proglottids or free in the fecal material. The ingestion of the larva by suitable intermediate hosts results in the release of the oncospheres from the embryonic envelopes, a process of emergence that is incorrectly referred to as hatching. Migration of the oncosphere to a parenteral site is followed by a true metamorphosis which results in reorganization and growth of a metacestode, termed a cysticercoid, while within the intermediate host. The cysticercoid enters the definitive host by ingestion (usually while within the beetle host) and continues its development by approaching sexual maturation in the early proglottids (see Freeman 1973 for review).

The present review concerns only the developmental biology of the fertilized ovum to the formation of the cysticercoid in an insect host. Although much research on these aspects has been accomplished on *H. diminuta*, it has been occasionally necessary to refer to other species which were presumed to be similar in a particular process. The review is largely restricted to *Hymenolepis diminuta* and may not be applicable to other tapeworms. Because of a limitation of space, some aspects of the biology of the larva and metacestode were not covered and some papers concerning the biology of 'eggs', larvae, and metacestodes have not been included. A more general coverage can be found in reviews of cestodes by Freeman (1973), Rybicka (1966a), Slais (1973) and Voge (1967, 1969 and 1973).

I. THE LARVAL STAGES

Although details of development of larval stages leading to the formation of a metacestode are not known for many tapeworms (the exception being some pseudophyllids by Schauinsland 1886, and some taenoids by Janicki 1907, and Spatlich 1925), the contributions of Robert Ogren and Krystyna Rybicka have been illuminating in providing fundamental information on embryonic development of *Hymenolepis diminuta*.

The process of oogenesis has been described by Rybicka (1966b) and by Lumsden and Specian (this volume). The mature ovary contains large primary oocytes which are released into the oviduct. Spermatogenesis has been described at the ultrastructural level by Kelsoe, Ubelaker and Allison (1977) and has been summarized by Rybicka (1966a) and Lumsden and Specian (ibid). Fertilization has not been carefully studied in any cestode. Following complete penetration by a spermatozoan, the oocyte accompanied by a vitelline cell passes through the ootype and enters the uterus.

Hymenolepis diminuta is representative of Cyclophyllidea in that the oocyte becomes associated with a single vitelline cell. The fine structure of vitelline cells has been examined by Swiderski *et al.* (1970). The vitelline cells are ovoid secretory cells of the holocrine type which possess a centrally located nucleus with nucleoli. The cytoplasm is well developed and forms a layer roughly equal to one half the nuclear diameter about the nucleus. The cytoplasm contains ovoid mitochondria with short cristae, numerous free ribosomes, and rough endoplasmic reticulum. Several Golgi zones appear active in packaging numerous large vitelline granules which are distributed throughout the cytoplasm. In other Cyclophyllideans, the vitelline granules coalesce to form one or two large vesicles (see Rybicka 1966a, for review).

Upon entry into the uterus, or possibly just before entry, a membrane appears surrounding the oocyte and vitelline cell. Although many authors refer to this membrane as a capsule, it is uncertain if the membrane perseveres in forming the completed 'shell'. The membrane is apparently secreted in part by the vitelline cell (probably the vitelline granules). The oocyte has been suggested to participate in the formation of the membrane but the nature of the contribution is unknown. Histochemical analysis suggests that the membrane is composed of several polysaccharides and lipoproteins and there is some evidence that the lipoproteins may be derived from secretions of the Mehlis' gland (see discussion by Rybiçka 1966a). The membrane appears to be more than 200 Å in thickness. Both sides of the membrane exhibit finely granulated or flocculated material which increases in thickness during development. The fate of the capsule is not clear. It is generally considered that the capsule is only a protective membrane for the cleaving embryo and it either disintegrates later in development or it persists, becoming incorporated into the 'shell' surrounding the mature oncosphere. Swiderski (1968) presents evidence from an EM study of *Catenotaenia pusilla* that the capsule persists throughout the stages of embryonic development and gives rise to the outer layer of the 'shell'.

The role of the vitelline cell in early development remains unclear. The possible contribution to the capsule has been mentioned above. According to Hedrick and Daugherty (1957), the vitelline cells of *H. diminuta* contain glycogen in contrast to the other tapeworms they examined. Moczon (1975) suggested, on the basis of the patterns of incorporation of ^{14}C-glucose, that while the testes, muscle cell bodies (parenchyma) and vitellaria contain large amounts of glycogen, the oocytes were glycogen free. Release of the vitelline cells resulted in a decrease in glycogen content. Moczon proposed that while the vitelline cell might furnish some energy source for the embryo, it is more likely that this cell does not nourish the embryo but maintains glycogen as its own source of energy.

II. CLEAVAGE

Cleavage has been carefully studied by Rybicka (1966b). Cleavage is initiated after completion of the maturation divisions and entry of the oocyte into the uterus. The first cleavage is total and unequal, resulting in a macromere and a mesomere. The second cleavage is also unequal, the macromere dividing three times to form three micromeres, the mesomere dividing once. Continued divisions serve to increase the numbers of micromeres surrounding the other cells. Eventually, the micromeres and the vitelline cell cytolyze. The cleavage patterns are presented in Figure 1.

The fine structure of macromeres in the cleavage of *H. diminuta* has been studied by Rybicka (1973a). The early macromere (MI) resembles the oocyte (Figure 2). This cell contains clusters of ribonucleoprotein bodies (Rybicka 1967b) concentrated at one pole of the cell. At least two distinct structural kinds of ribonucleoprotein can be distinguished (types A and B). Type A consists of electron dense material appearing as fine granules and fibrils in young cells. Type B appears as spheroid bodies and occurs in older cells. Ribosomes in poly-configurations occur in dense masses. A cytocentrum, composed of centrioles and a 'yolk nucleus' (Golgi bodies and numerous mitochondria) appears at the opposite pole of the cell.

Structure and Ultrastructure of the Larvae and Metacestodes

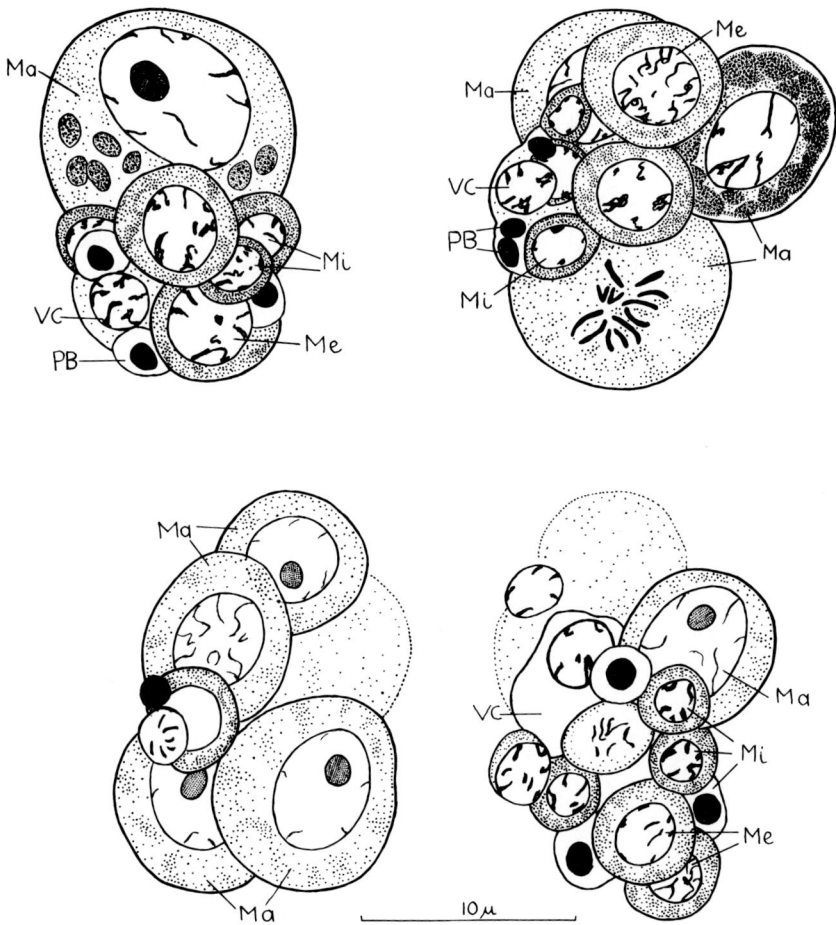

Figure 1. Early cleavage of *Hymenolepis diminuta.* A. One macromere, two mesomeres, vitelline cell and three polar bodies are illustrated. B. Later stage illustrating three micromeres. C, D. Sections of embryo near end of cleavage illustrating pycnosis of micromeres. Ma, macromeres; Me, mesomeres; Mi, micromeres; PB, polar body; VC, vitelline cell. (From Rybicka 1966b).

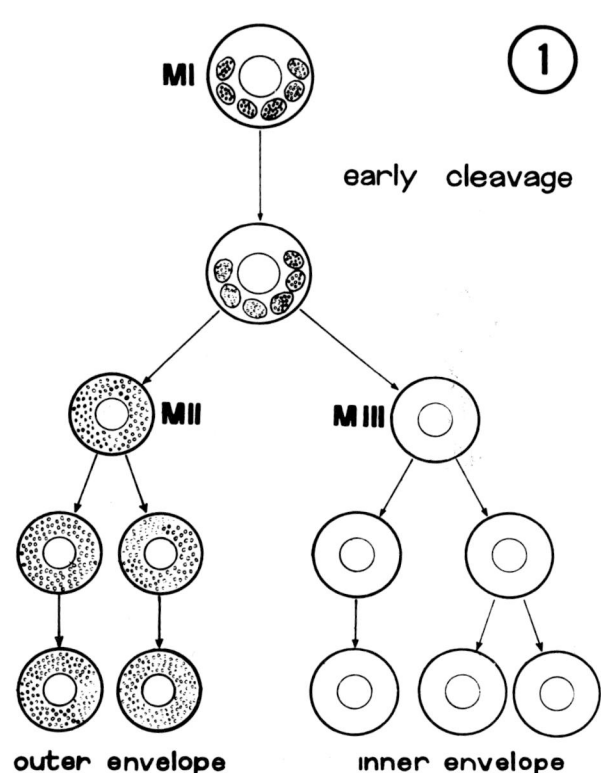

Figure 2. Diagram of macromere division during cleavage. MI, macromere with ribonucleic protein; MII, macromere that will give rise to the outer embryonic envelope; MIII, macromere that will form the inner embryonic envelope. (From Rybicka 1973a).

III. FORMATION OF THE OUTER ENVELOPE

As cells continue to divide, the five macromeres and the vitelline cell separate from the other embryonic cells and form a syncytium surrounding the embryo. The nuclei of this syncytium can be divided into three types (Rybicka 1966b) (Figure 3). The first set of nuclei is small with distinct chromatin. The second set of nuclei (three in number) is larger and has prominent nucleoli with little visible chromatin structure. The third nucleus type is derived from the vitelline cell, which soon degenerates. It is important to note, as mentioned by Rybicka (1972), that the vitelline cell disintegrates before the shell material is produced by the outer envelope. The first set of nuclei moves towards the periphery and forms a cytoplasmic layer that will develop into the outer envelope.

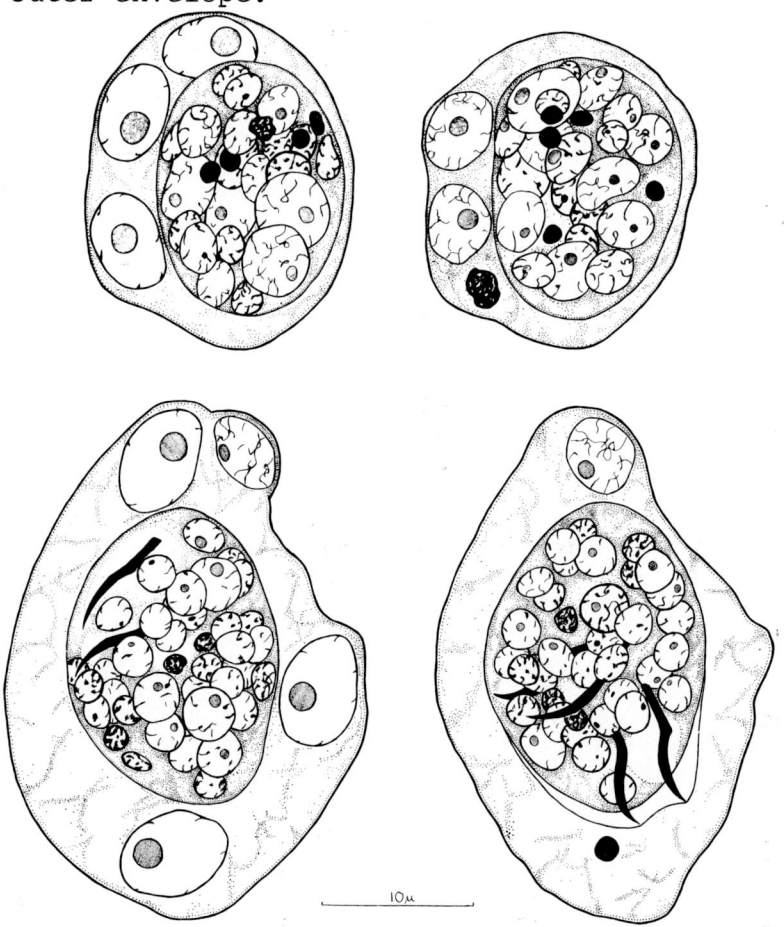

Figure 3. Diagram of sections of preoncosphere. A. Nuclei of inner envelope. B. Nuclei of outer envelope and degenerating nucleus of vitelline cell (Pycnosis evident in micromeres). C, D. Older preoncosphere illustrating movement of some nuclei towards periphery, increase in number of embryonic cells and degeneration of some somatic cells. Oncoblast cells differentiated at this stage. (From Rybicka 1966b).

IV. FORMATION OF THE CAPSULE

Rybicka (1972) described the differentiation of the embryonic envelopes in *Hymenolepis diminuta*. From her work it is clear that the 'shell' is formed in part by at least two cellular types. The first type is the vitelline cell which is responsible for secreting a membranous-like layer (capsule) over the unfertilized ovum and spermatozoan. This membranous-like layer is produced from the secretory granules of the vitelline cells (King and Lumsden 1969). The granules are lost after entering the ootype (Rybicka 1972). As the latter author proposes, the capsule remains around the embryo until 'shell' deposition occurs. Material for the 'shell' is produced by the outer envelope. Rybicka (1973a) demonstrated by electron microscopy that the B type granules, which consist of principally ribonucleoprotein material, are present in the perinuclear cytoplasm of the macromeres composing the outer envelope. Following the fusion of these macromeres into a syncytium, the B type granules disappear and reform at the outer margin of the syncytium below the capsule. The cytoplasm of the outer envelope contains mitochondria, sparse rough endoplasmic reticulum, and few free ribosomes. As development continues, the nuclei of the syncytium degenerate but the nucleoli remain in the cytoplasm surrounded by vesicles and profiles of annulate lamellae.

'Shell' precursor material is apparently synthesized by the outer envelope and secreted into the space below the capsule. As the material polymerizes, it appears to accumulate on the capsule, which increases in size and thickness with these deposits (Figure 4). The random addition of material changes the surface configuration from being smooth, before addition of the 'shell' material, to a rough irregular surface. Following 'shell' production, the dense granules are no longer observed. The outer envelope remains through embryogenesis but consists of a thin, vacuolated layer of cytoplasm. Eventually, the outer envelope disintegrates and in the mature larva only occasionally can remnants of this layer be observed.

It seems reasonable to assume that the 'shell' consists of three components. The first component

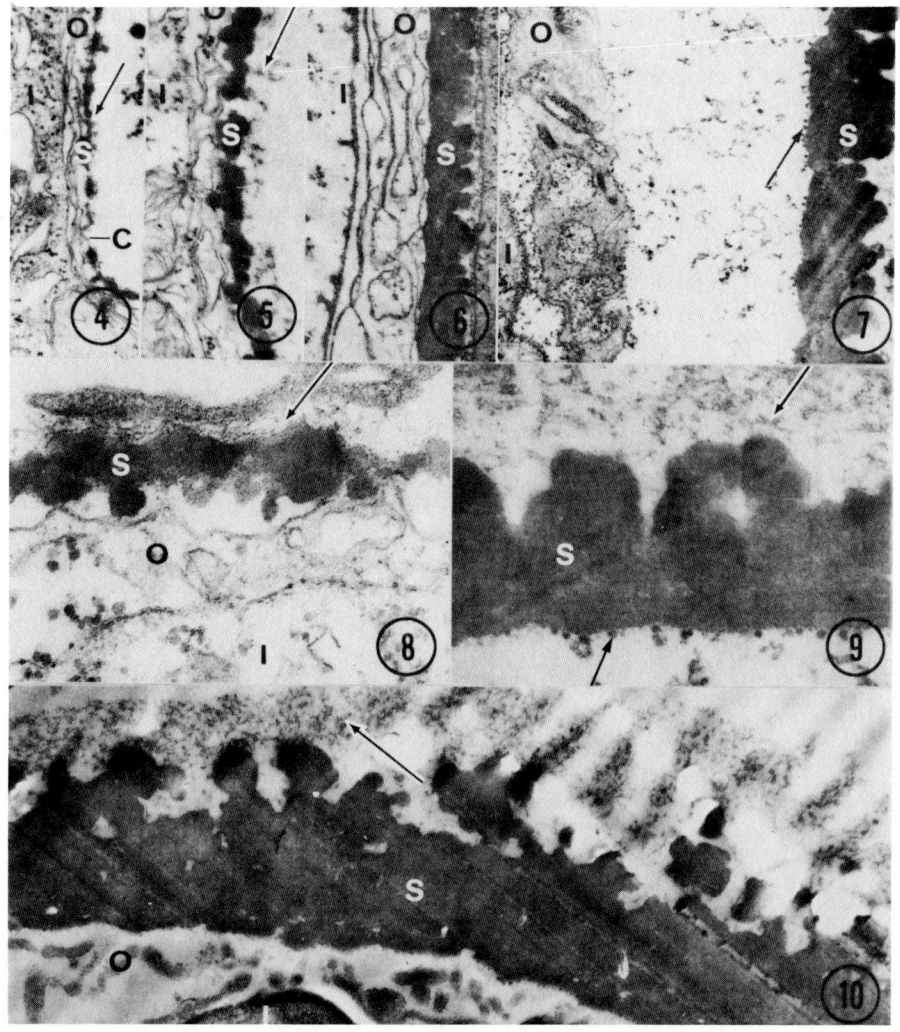

Figure 4. Stages of 'shell' growth in H. diminuta. Early deposits of 'shell' material (white S) in upper left (4, 5, 6) show deposition of material from outer envelope (O) which is deposited against the capsule (C). The appearance of the 'shell' at 7 shows a smooth inner surface and rough outer surface. 'Shell' material appears in vesicles within the outer envelope and probably is released into the space below the 'shell'. Approx. X 22,000. 8, 9 and 10 represent higher magnifications of the 'shell', including the fuzzy coat (white-black arrows). (From Rybicka 1972).

is the membranous-like capsule which forms early in development. This layer often becomes obscured as the 'shell' material is deposited. The capsule may disintegrate (Rybicka 1964), although Swiderski (1968) found that the capsule does persist in *Catenotaenia pusilla* and represents a layer of the so-called 'shell'. The second layer is secreted by the outer envelope. This layer represents the dense and hardened material generally associated with the 'shell'. A third layer, possibly secreted by the uterus, may be formed on the outer surface. Moriyama (1961) reported such a layer secreted by the uterus, based upon the similarity of hematoxylin staining of certain uterine cells and the outer layer of the 'shell'. Ogren and Magill (1962) reported two layers in the 'shell' which contained tyrosine and trytophan. Rybicka (1966a) reported observations by Hoy and Clegg that a similar granular secretion on the outer surface of the capsule by glands in the wall of the uterus of *Moneaia expansa* stained intensely for the presence of keratin. Pence (1970) showed by electron microscopy the presence of a dense layer of finely granular material. Although the relatively high magnifications used by Pence show a smooth surface (Figure 4), mature larvae clearly show an irregular and rough, but not block-like, surface by scanning electron microscopy (Voge 1969).

V. CHEMICAL COMPOSITION OF THE EMBRYONIC ENVELOPES AND 'SHELL'

Contributions to our knowledge of the chemical composition of the embryonic envelopes and 'shell' or capsule have been made by various investigators (Hedrick and Daugherty 1957; Hedrick 1958; Ogren and Magill 1962; Cheng and Dyckman 1964; Rybicka 1967a, b, c). These authors reported the presence of proteins and some lipid-like material in the outer envelope. Ogren and Magill (1962) and Berntzen and Voge (1965) noted that the outer envelope could be partially digested by α-amylase and by trypsin. Using a variety of histochemical techniques, Pence (1970) reported a number of materials in the 'shell' and remnants of the outer envelope. In the mature larva he found basic proteins, some aromatic amino acids, disulphides or sulphydryl radicals, PAS-positive carbohydrates, and acid mucopolysaccharides

TABLE I. *The amino acid composition of the shell material (after Lethbridge 1971b).*

Amino Acid	% of total*	Amino Acid	% of total*
Glycine	2.88	Aspartic acid	4.39
Alanine	2.36	Glutamic acid	8.61
Valine	3.25	Arginine	2.72
Serine	1.38	Lysine	6.99
Threonine	3.53	Proline	8.61
Leucine	1.34	Histidine	17.63
Isoleucine	1.71	Tyrosine	4.99
Cysteic acid	5.97	Phenylalanine	7.19

* Mean of two determinations.

exhibiting a metachromasia. Sudanophilic material was noted in the outer envelope. Pence also found that phenolic substances, phospholipid, RNA and DNA were absent. It is important to note that the outer envelope in a mature larva is generally not intact so the report of the lack of RNA in mature larva should not conflict with the previous report of Rybicka (1967b).

Lethbridge (1971b) also examined the composition of *H. diminuta* mature larvae and amplified the contributions of Pence. He found, histochemically, the presence of protein, tyrosine, tryptophan, and cystine in the capsule, and the absence of arginine, keratin, carbohydrate, acid mucopolysaccharide, and lipid. Some carbohydrates and lipids were found in the remnants of the outer envelope. Catechol tests for the presence of phenolase were negative. He also examined the capsule for amino acid composition and detected 16 amino acids. These amino acids and their relative percentage of occurrence are presented in Table 1.

Moczon (1972) reviewed the literature on the chemical composition of the oncospheral envelopes in *Hymenolepis diminuta*. Based on histochemical data, he concluded that the outer envelope was composed of a protein-polysaccharide complex with the protein component exhibiting properties of soft keratin-like proteins. Moczon also reported the visual observation that oncospheres removed from rat feces are golden brown in color. Although he did not discount coloration from the bile salts he stated that the color change and hardening were "based on enzymic (or spontaneous) oxidation of polyphenols, present in them, to quinones with subsequent formation of so called "quinone tanned protein" that are characteristic for egg shells of some Trematoda and Pseudophyllidea ....". Pence (1970) and Lethbridge (1971b) both indicated the lack of phenol or phenolase in vitellaria and shells of *Hymenolepis diminuta*. The latter author proposed that since electrovalent linkages of S-S bonds were only present in less than 6% of the shell protein, the abundant aromatic and heterocyclic residues (tyrosine, phenylalanine, histidine, and proline) probably form bonds among themselves in adjacent strands of protein via "some highly modified 'autotanning' system ... in which the aromatic and heterocyclic groups are converted to suitable intermediates by oxidative enzymes other than phenolase".

VI.   INNER ENVELOPE AND EMBRYOPHORE

Both the outer and inner envelopes form from the syncytial macromere layer in the preoncosphere. After the two nuclei move toward the periphery, eventually to give rise to the 'shell', the remaining three nuclei remain in place or move toward the inner surface and soon degenerate. Rybicka (1973a) described the changes in this layer that occur at the time of formation of the inner envelope. As the nuclei become irregular in shape and begin to break down, the profiles of annulate lamellae increase in number. Large lipid deposits accumulate and beta-glycogen particles appear in the cytoplasm. Mitochondria enlarge to nearly twice their previous size, the Golgi complex decreases in size, and spheroid membranous bodies appear.

Rybicka (1972) described the morphogenesis of the inner layer based on electron microscopy. She reported that the first noticeable event was the elaboration of numerous membrane bound vesicles containing irregular electron dense material. The vesicles were of various sizes and appeared to fuse into larger ones until they formed an intracellular space within the inner envelope. The intracellular space effectively delaminated a thin cytoplasmic layer lying adjacent to the preoncosphere. This layer subsequently deteriorates. The new plasma membrane of the inner envelope thickens as dense material is deposited against it and this thickened membrane eventually forms the oncospheral membrane. Following formation of this layer, a second series of vesicles appear which, following fusion, delaminate a thin cytoplasmic layer containing the oncospheral membrane.

After delamination of the oncospheral membrane, mitochondria present in the cytoplasm of the inner envelope increase in number. The mitochondria are rougly ovoid with few short cristae. Following mitochondriogenesis, the embryophore begins to form in the outer region of the inner envelope (opposite side from the oncospheral membrane). As presented by Rybicka (1972), the embryophore is not entire, but possesses irregularly occurring holes (Figure 5). As the embryophore becomes thicker it contracts and slowly moves toward the inner surface of the

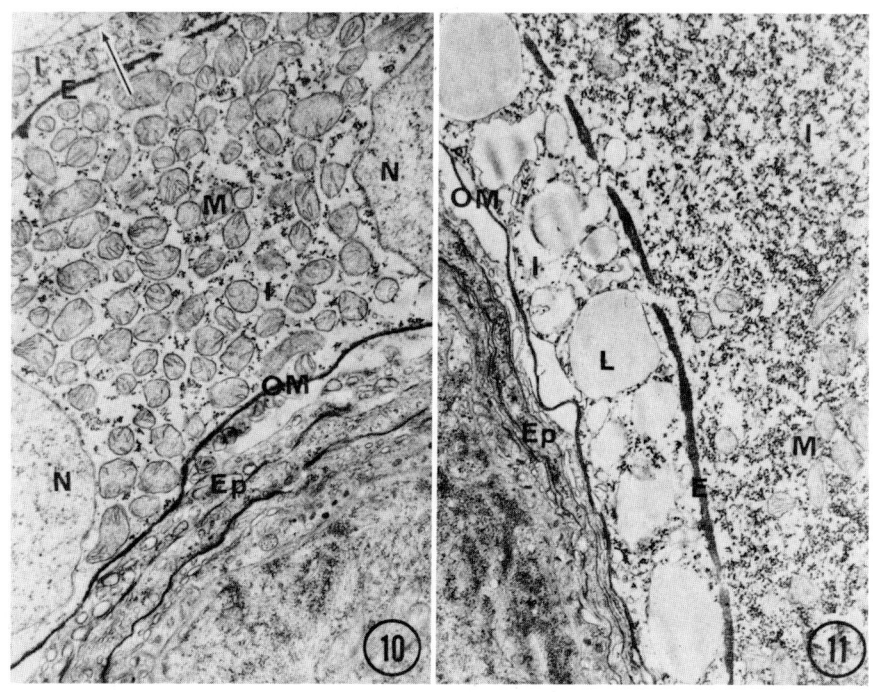

Figure 5. Ultrastructure of the inner envelope of Hymenolepis diminuta. Left photomicrograph showing numerous mitochondria in inner envelope. Embryophore (E), with pores, developing in outer layer of cytoplasm; oncospheral membrane (OM) forming in inner layer of cytoplasm. Note delamination of cytoplasm layer which lies adjacent to epithelium (Ep) of oncosphere. Approx. X 13,100. Right photomicrograph after movement of the embryophore illustrating isolation of lipid droplets. Approx. X 19,600. (From Rybicka 1972).

inner layer, eventually lying close to the oncospheral membrane. Apparently mitochondria are able to pass through these pores and populate the outer layer of cytoplasm. Following contraction of the embryophore, mitochondria are markedly reduced in numbers. According to Rybicka (1972), only cytoplasm and mitochondria are able to pass through the pores during the contraction phase, whereas nuclei and lipid deposits accumulate and eventually form a thin layer between the embryophore and oncospheral membrane. After reaching a site near the inner surface, the embryophore begins increasing in size. The pores become obscured and a single homogeneous electron dense layer forms, reaching approximately 0.7 µ in thickness in the mature larva (Pence 1970) (Figure 6).

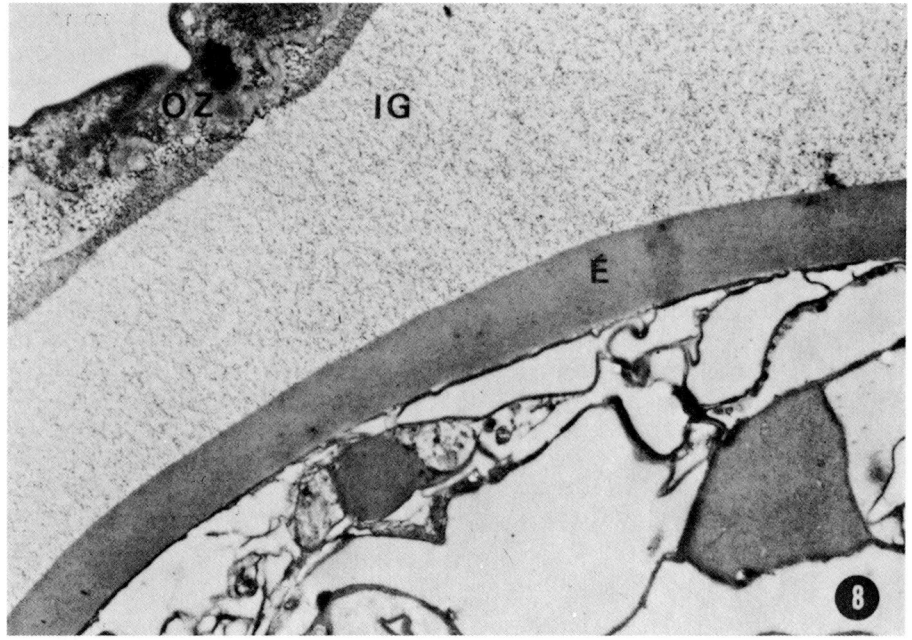

Figure 6. Inner envelope in mature larval stage. Outer zone (OZ) is folded and contains mitochondria (not illustrated). Inner layer (IG) is granular and devoid of organelles. Embryophore (E) is entire and thickened. Cytoplasmic remnants of the lipid filled layer are present. Approx. X 22,400. (From Pence 1970).

The embryophore is generally thicker at the polar regions. The cytoplasmic layer internal to the embryophore eventually becomes distorted and breaks down.

The cytoplasm of the external layer of the inner envelope becomes partitioned into two regions (Fig. 6). The outermost region contains numerous mitochondria and profiles of glycogen. Most of the cytoplasm of this outer layer is probably a remnant of the inner envelope that existed external to the early embryophore prior to its contraction. The inner cytoplasmic layer, which probably results from the contraction of the embryophore, contains no obvious organelles and is represented by a light matrix of irregular granular material (see Fig. 6).

The histochemistry of the inner envelope and embryophore of mature larvae has been studied by various authors. Ogren and Magill (1962) determined that the inner envelope and embryophore were composed of simple proteins containing tyrosine, polysaccharide-bound proteins, mucopolysaccharides, and RNA. Berntzen and Voge (1965) indicated that the inner envelope could be altered by trypsin digestion whereas it was resistant to α-amylase activity (see also reports of Hedrick and Daugherty 1957; Cheng and Dyckman 1964). Rybicka (1967a) reported PAS-resistant material in the inner envelope (cytoplasmic portion) which decreased as the oncosphere reached maturity. Pence (1970) reported the presence of basic proteins, aromatic amino acids, PAS-positive carbohydrates, acid mucopolysaccharides exhibiting a metachromasia, and some phospholipid in the mature larva. A slight reaction for disulphide and sulphydryl radicals was detected. Phenolic substances, general lipids, neutral lipids, RNA and DNA were absent.

Rybicka (1967a) proposed that beta glycogen predominates in the embryonic envelope and reported positive reactions for succinic dehydrogenase and NADH-tetrazolium reductase activites in the inner envelope (1967c). Both observations are correlated with her EM observations (1972) of beta glycogen and dense accumulations of mitochondria in the inner envelope.

Lethbridge (1971b) confirmed previous studies and reported the presence of proteins, tyrosine, -SH groups, cystine, and the absence of arginine, tryptophan, 'keratin', acid mucopolysaccharides and lipids in the cytoplasmic layer. The embryophore was found to be similar in composition, except a doubtful positive reaction was observed for 'keratin'.

Moczon (1972) confirmed the report of Rybicka (1972) that the cytoplasmic region of the inner envelope consists of two regions. The outer layer, referred to as the superficial component, contains basic amino acids and mucopolysaccharides of a weakly acidic nature. The inner component of the envelope contains basic amino acids with a high percentage of histidine and possibly some arginine, serine esterified with phosphoric acid, and acidic mucopolysaccharides. The embryophore was constructed of macromolecules of compact proteins and small quantities of phosphoric acid residues. Keratin was not detected.

The formation of the oncospheral membrane in *H. diminuta* has been described by Rybicka (1972). As detailed above, the membrane forms within the cytoplasm of the inner envelope following the fusion of numerous vesicles which separate the cytoplasm into two layers. Electron dense material is synthesized on the newly formed inner membrane which subsequently develops into a layer of granules forming the oncospheral membrane. Additional plasma membranes may be incorporated into the oncospheral membrane (Figure 7). Following the breakdown of the cytoplasmic layer between this membrane and the embryo and the formation of the embryophore, the oncospheral membrane becomes separated from the inner envelope by the disintegration of the cytoplasm between this membrane and the embryophore (Figure 8). The oncospheral membrane is often difficult to discern in mature larvae, as it adheres closely to the embryophore. It is seen more easily in living material during emergence of the larva.

A diagram of the embryonic envelopes surrounding a late preonocosphere (left side) and a mature oncosphere (right side) is presented in Figure 9.

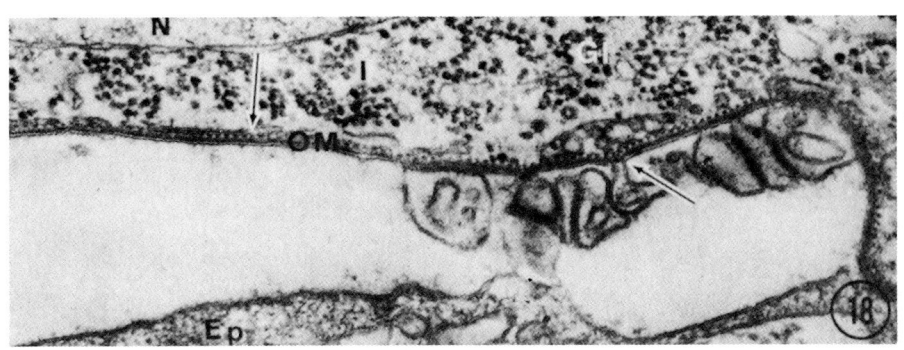

Figure 7. Formation of oncospheral membrane (OM) in the inner envelope, rich in glycogen (G). Note orientation of microtubular elements and membranes (white-black arrows). Approx. X 56,100. (From Rybicka 1972).

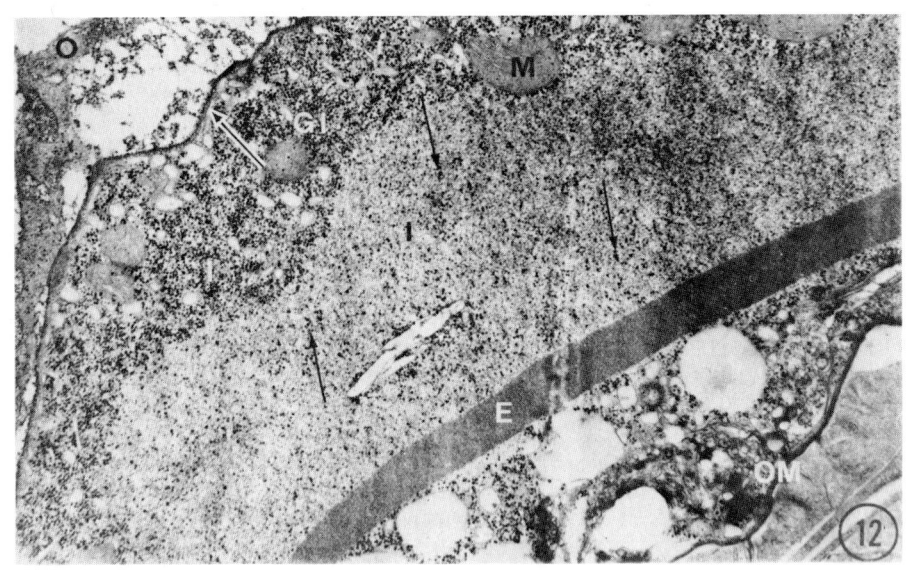

Figure 8. Delamination of oncospheral membrane (OM) illustrating relationship to embryophore (E). Mitochondria (M) and glycogen (G) are present in outer cytoplasmic region. Approx. X 18,900. (From Rybicka 1972).

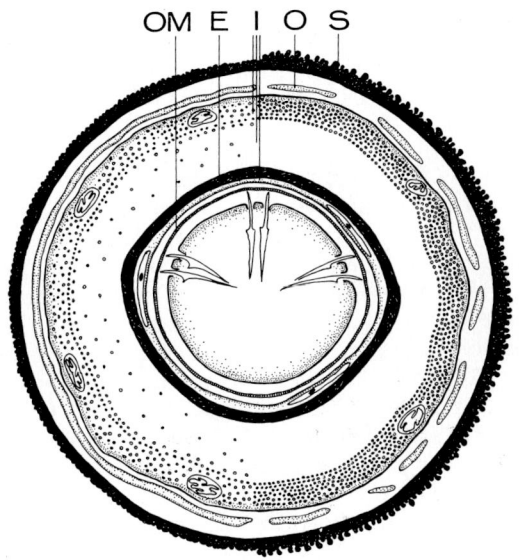

Figure 9. Diagram of early (left) and mature (right) larvae of Hymenolepis diminuta. Symbols are S, 'shell'; O, outer envelope; I, inner envelope showing three cytoplasmic regions: an outer layer, inner layer, and layer internal to the embryophore (E); OM, oncospheral membrane. (From Rybicka 1972).

VII. PREONCOSPHERAL PHASE

The preoncospheral phase can be defined as one of cellular morphogenesis resulting in a fully developed hexacanth larva or oncosphere. Ogren (1868b) proposed that the term preoncosphere be restricted to that period prior to the presence of oncoblasts and the remaining period be referred to as the period of oncosphere differentiation. He further subdivided morphogenesis of the 'embryo' into three major periods to include: morphogenesis of hooks and other structures in the hexacanth; preparation for survival and infectivity, including development of musculature and germinative cells; and reorganization or metamorphosis in the insect hemocoel. While these distinctions are useful in describing morphogenesis of cell lineages, they will not be utilized in this article.

Following early cleavage, the number of embryonic cells increases to approximately 80. Fate maps are not known from cestodes but apparently the oncosphere is formed completely of micromeres, some of which continue to divide and differentiate, while others disintegrate.

Ogren (1968b) observed that, by the time oncoblast cells can first be recognized, the preoncosphere is organized into two regions. The first region, the somatophore or oncophore, contains mostly somatic cells which differentiate rapidly, forming the hooks. The second region, the mesophore, contains some somatic cells and larger embryonic cells referred to as Class I and II cell types (Ogren 1967). Class I cells have distinct chromosomes but little cytoplasm surrounding the nucleus. Class II cells have indistinct chromosomes, prominent nuclei, and more cytoplasm (Figure 10). Ogren (1968a) reported that the Class I cells are germinative cells and are responsible for post-oncosphere development, whereas Class II cells are responsible for development of specialized features of the oncosphere, such as musculature.

During the preoncospheral phase of development, the micromeres that continue to differentiate are responsible for the formation of the Class I and Class II cells, three pairs of hooks, the musculature of the oncosphere, glandular cells, and the surface epithelium.

VIII. HOOK FORMATION

Hook formation has been examined in detail by Ogren (1955, 1957, 1958, 1961a), Rybicka (1966b), and Moczon (1971). In 1961, Ogren distinguished five stages of hook development: (1) early oncoblast initiating hook synthesis, (2) early oncoblast with blade outline completed, (3) late oncoblast synthesizing the shank, (4) late oncoblast with shank completely formed, and (5) degeneration of the oncoblast with completion of the mature hook (see Figure 11 from Moczon 1971). Although Ogren (1955) considered that the hook was formed externally to the oncoblast in *H. nana*, he later (1957, 1958, 1961a) clearly established that the hooks are synthesized within cells. Subsequently, Swiderski (1973) examined on-

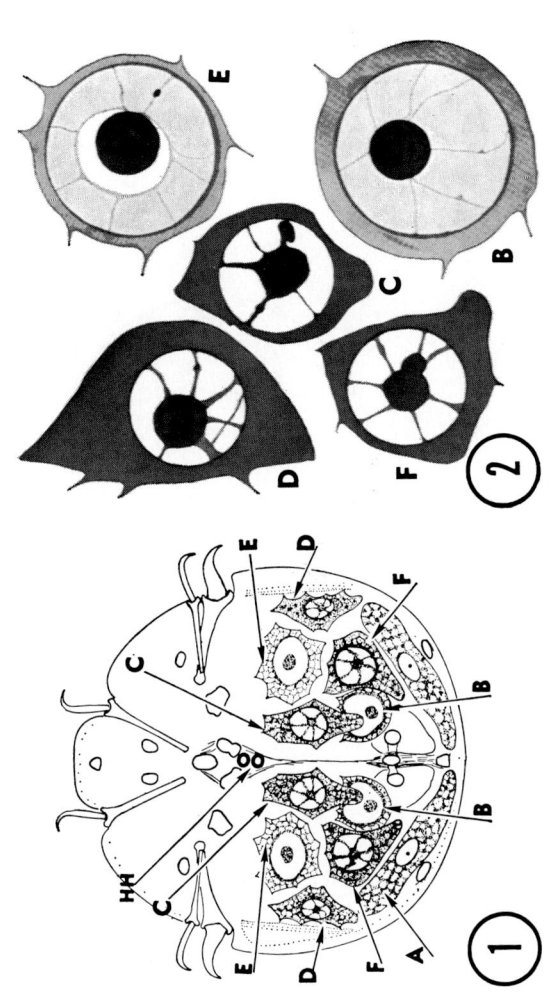

Figure 10. Diagram of invasive oncosphere illustrating Class I (C, D, F) and Class II (B, E) cells. A binucleate epithelial cell is present at HH and glandular cells at A. In *H. citelli*, Collin (1969) identified two nuclei types associated with the musculature which may represent Class I type cells identified by Ogren (1968a). Collin cited a reference by Voge and Johri (1968, Srivastava Commemorative Volume, Izatnagar, U. P. India) describing Type I and Type II nuclei which he thought might correspond to somatic and hook musculature respectively. (From Ogren 1968a).

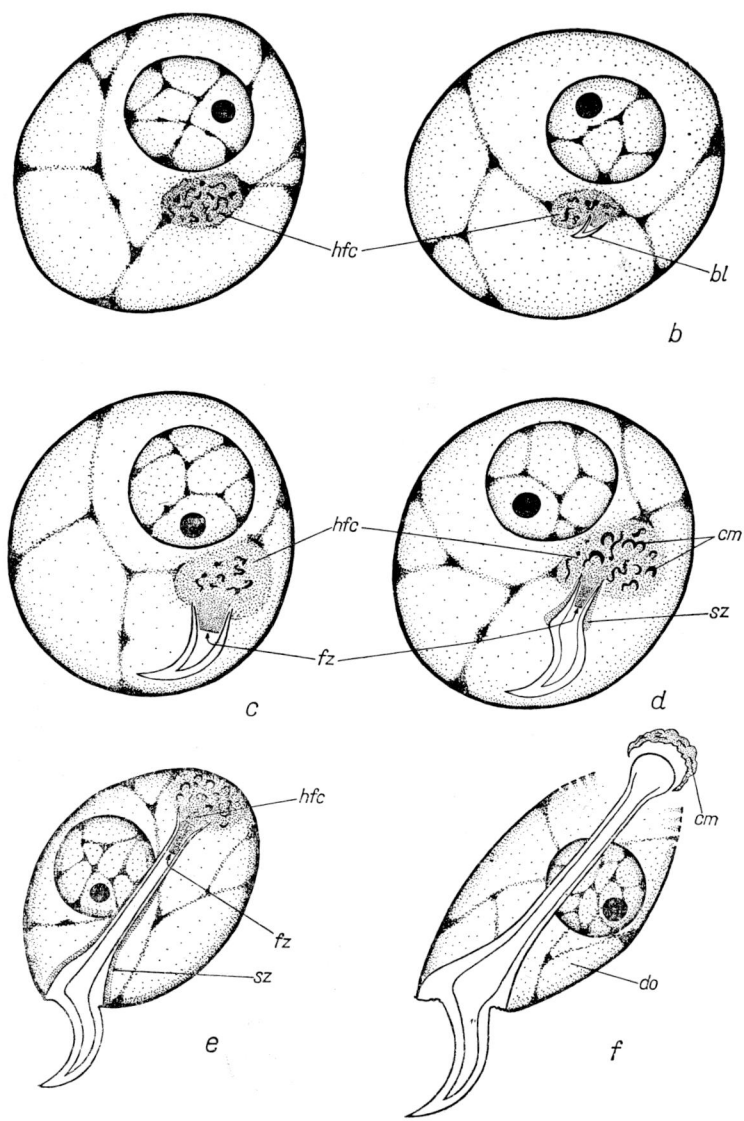

Figure 11. Development of the hooks in oncoblasts of oncospheres (H. diminuta). The hook forming center (a) develops a zone of keratinization (Fz), forming hook (a-d). A second external zone of keratinization (Sz) forms and external layer on the shaft of the hook. Ogren (1968b) referred to the development shown in stages a-c as Stage I (blade formation in oncoblasts) and stages d-f as Stage II (shank formation). (From Moczon 1971).

cospheral hook formation of *Catenotaenia pusilla* by
electron microscopy and found a similar pattern of
formation. In the preoncosphere, certain cells move
into one hemisphere and arrange themselves into three
groups of cells - one medial group and two laterally
located groups of cells. By their positions, each
lateral group consists of a dorsal-lateral and a
ventral-lateral oncoblast. As these cells initiate
differentiation, the nucleus becomes displaced to
one pole. At the opposite pole, a 'hook forming
center' develops. This center consists of numerous
elongate mitochondria with sparse cristae, a dense,
free polyribosome population, and Golgi zones.
Blade formation can be first recognized morphologically with the appearance of a dense granule in the
Golgi complex. With the synthesis of more material
the granule increases in size and elongates into a
blade of the future hook. As it grows, three regions
can be distinguished: an outer dense granular cortex,
an inner fibrous layer, and a central core.

The blade remains within the oncoblast until
the beginning of shank formation. As the shank develops, the blade extends through the unit membrane of
the cells and becomes surrounded by a cellular collar
attached by a septate desmosome. Further development
involves an increase in length of the shank and formation of a guard or collar of the mature hook. As
formation of the hook shank nears completion, somatic cells in the vicinity attach to the base of the
shank and differentiate into a muscular system for
movement of the hooks.

The ultrastructure of mature hooks of *H. diminuta* was first reported by Pence (1970). Three layers
of different densities were observed: an outer granular zone, a middle fibrous layer, and a central core.
This arrangement is also observed in oncosphere hooks
of *H. citelli* (Collin 1968) and *Taenia taeniaeformis*
(Nieland 1968). Other cestodes that have been studied have only two layers, a dense outer cortex and
less dense inner core (*Catenotaenia pusilla* by
Swiderski 1973; *Inermicapsifer madagascariensis* by
Swiderski 1970; *Dipylidium caninum* by Pence 1967).
According to Pence (1970), fibers of the fibrous layer are approximately 30Å in diameter and in composition resemble keratin, although the fiber size is
smaller than normally reported in vertebrate keratin.

The inner core was found to be positive with tests for phospholipids which were not extractable with pyridine and were not reactive with Sudan black B. Moczon (1971) examined the composition of the developing hooks in *H. diminuta* and detected keratin-like protein in the hook forming center which increased during morphogenesis of the hook blade. A second center of keratinization appeared in the area of the collar and subsequently covered the shank of the hook, producing the outer layer. All tests for chitin were negative.

IX. MUSCULATURE

The musculature of the oncosphere can be divided into two groups; somatic and hook musculature (Collin 1968, 1969). According to Ogren (1968a, b), both sets of musculature probably originate from Class II cells that differentiate into myoblasts. The somatic musculature occurs as a series of closely set transverse myofibers that may function in maintaining the shape of the oncosphere (see discussion and photomicrographs presented by Collin 1968 for *H. citelli*). The hook musculature appears to originate from Class II cells which are oriented around the oncoblasts. As the hook completes development, the myoblasts initiate myofilament formation and attach via cytoplasmic connective tissue sheaths to the basal lamina of the oncosphere surface epithelium and to the hooks. Myoblasts undergoing myofilament formation have been observed by Swiderski (1973) in oncospheres of *C. pusilla* (Figure 12). The perinuclear cytoplasm generally resembles that described by Lumsden and Byram (1967) except that the rough endoplasmic reticulum is not well-developed and the large outpockets of sarcoplasm filled with numerous alpha glycogen particles are not yet developed (see discussion by Lumsden and Specian, this volume and Webb 1977).

Ogren (1972) described the musculature of the mature oncosphere. He distinguished three systems: a protraction system which allowed extension of the hooks; an adduction system which returned the hooks to a normal resting position; and a retraction system which pulled the hooks into the body. Schematic views representing the basic musculature for lateral and medial hooks and a composite view are presented in Figures 13 and 14 respectively.

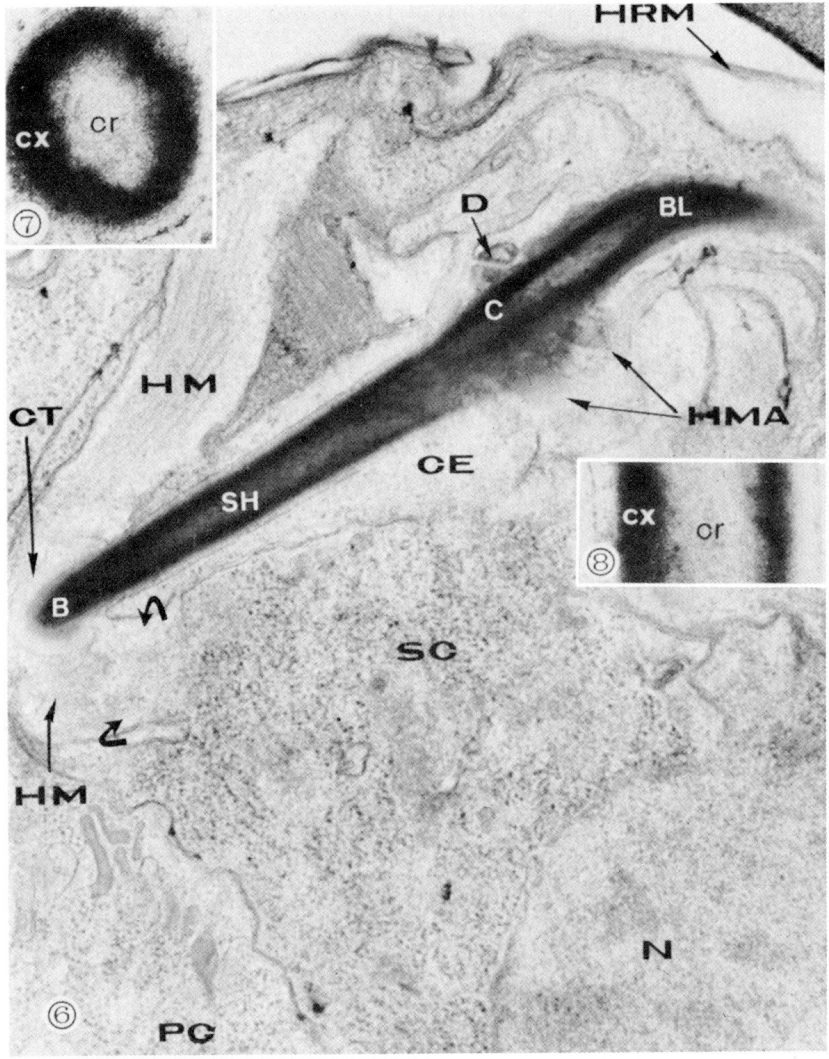

Figure 12. Transmission photomicrograph of mature oncospheral hook shank (B) showing attachment of muscles (HM). The hooks are surrounded by a thin layer of cytoplasm (CE). The sarcoplasmic region of the muscle cell is seen (SC). Approx. X 34,200. (From Swiderski 1973).

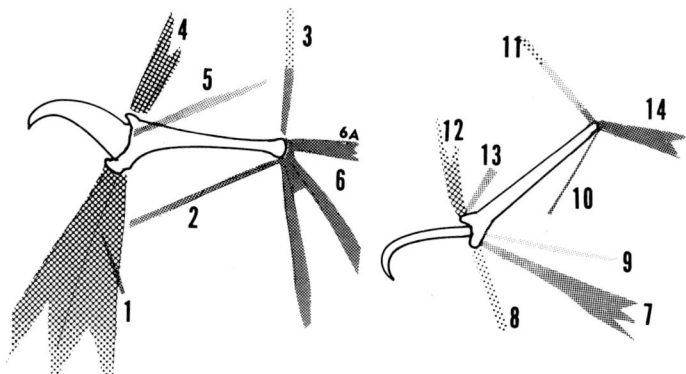

Figure 13. Schematic view of lateral (left) and medial (right) hooks of Hymenolepis diminuta. Protractor (1,7) and adductor (4,5,12,13) muscles insert on the guard, whereas levator (3,11), retractors (6,14), abductors (8,9), and tensors (2,10) insert on the end of shaft. Interhook muscles (6A) are present on lateral hooks. (From Ogren 1972).

X.   PENETRATION GLANDS

Ogren (1968a) reported that some Class II cells in the mesophore develop into secretory cells. These secretory cells develop after the hooks are nearly formed and, in mature oncospheres, are represented by a granular area, first observed by Fülleborn (1922). Reid (1948) considered them to be bilobed unicellular glands, similar to those in oncospheres of *Choanotaenia infundibulum* and termed them "penetration glands'. The cellular nature of these glands was described by Ogren (1955, 1961b), Voge and Heyneman (1957), Rothman (1957) and Moczon (1977c), among others. Pence (1970) and Lethbridge and Gijsbers (1974) described the penetration glands of *H. diminuta* oncospheres as observed by electron microscopy (Figure 15). The glands are represented by a large, U-shaped cell that opens to the surface by cytoplasmic extensions located between the medial and lateral hooks on each side of the body. The cytoplasm is syncytial and represents a secretory cell type. The nuclei are located in the peripheral cytoplasm which contains a few mitochondria and small amounts of rough ER. The majority of the cytoplasm is filled with membrane-bounded secretory bodies and abundant beta glycogen. Two distinct kinds of granules are present and probably represent structural modifications occurring in

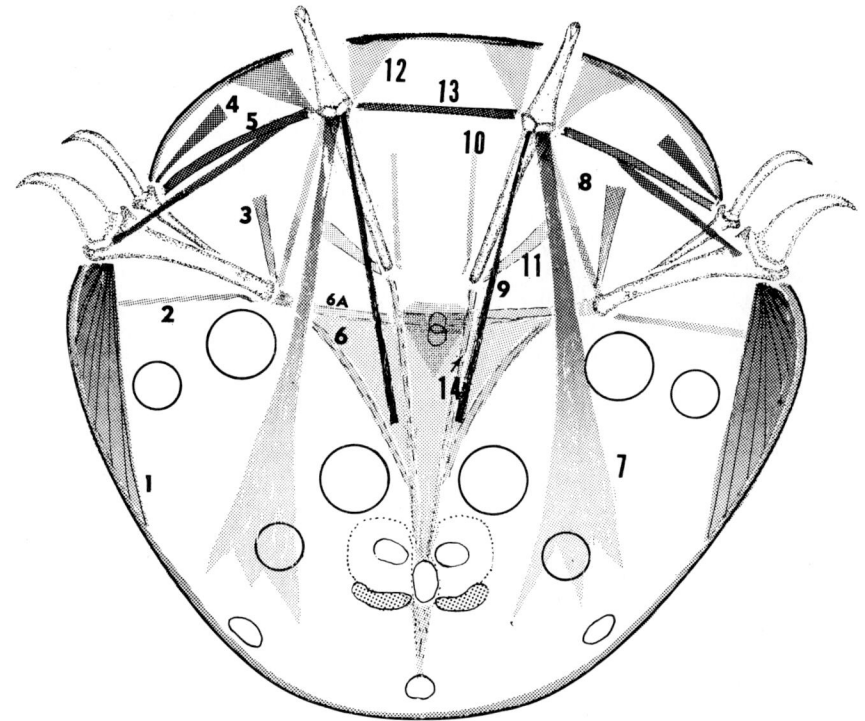

Figure 14. Schematic view of hook musculature of *Hymenolepis diminuta* oncospheres showing relationships of muscles and hooks. Region anterior to the interhook muscle (6A) generally represents the oncophore or mesophore. (From Ogren 1972).

the secretory product prior to secretion. One type of secretory body is sausage-shaped, 0.5 μm by 0.15 μm, and is located basally in the cytoplasm (Figure 16A). The second type of secretory body is large, markedly granular and usually restricted to the apical zone of the cytoplasm (Figure 16B).

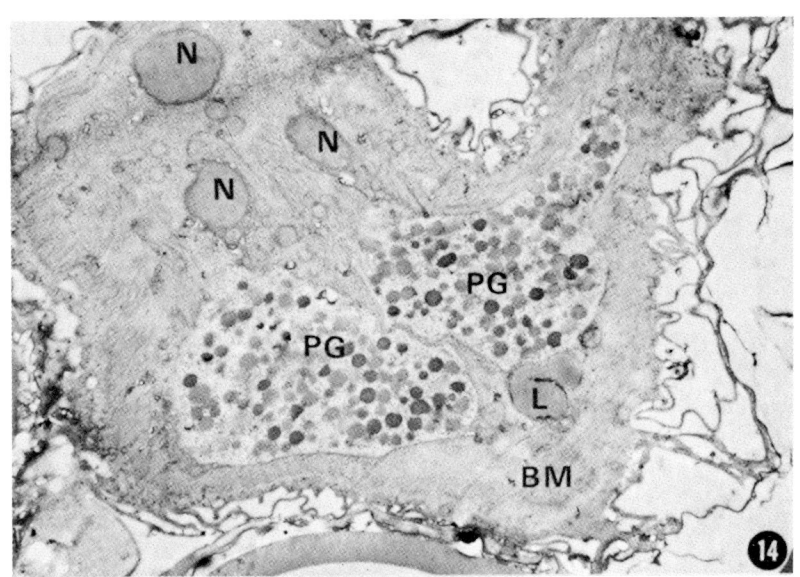

Figure 15. Section of somatophore of oncosphere showing penetration glands. The cytoplasmic connection between the glandular cells (PG) and nuclei are not present in the micrograph. Approx. X 4,800. (From Pence 1970).

XI. EPITHELIUM

Ogren (1968a) showed that, following development of oncoblasts and penetration glands, some Class II cells differentiate to form a binucleate medullary center which he had earlier observed in the mature oncosphere of *H. diminuta* (Ogren 1961b) and in oncospheres of other cestodes (Ogren 1956, 1957 and 1958). The binucleate center contained a large cell with vesicular nuclei and was rich in cytoplasmic RNA. Since this cell was located near the center of the oncosphere and thus, in close contact with the musculature, Ogren considered it to have contractile properties.

The binucleate cell's contribution to the formation of surface epithelium was recognized and described by Rybicka (1973b) in a most important work using techniques of electron microscopy (Figure 17). She reported that the binucleate cell possesses nuclei with large prominent nucleoli and a cytoplasm characterized by abundant free ribosomes, smooth and rough endoplasmic reticulum, Golgi complexes, numerous membrane-bound vesicles, and occasionally, elec-

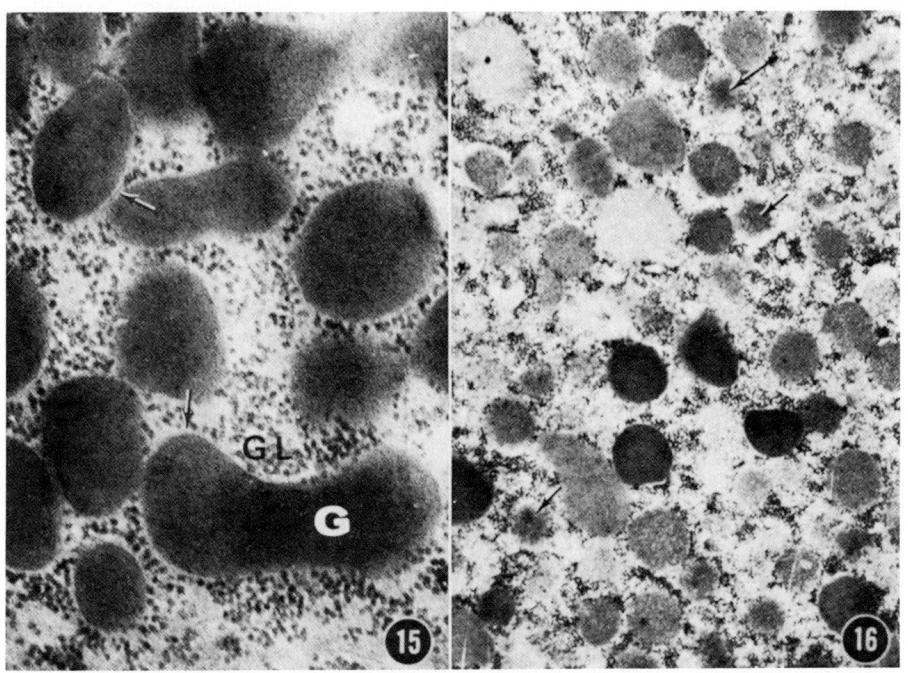

Figure 16. Transmission electron microscopy photomicrograph of penetration gland cells illustrating development in preoncospheres (A) and mature oncospheres (B). Glycogen and secretory granules of variable density and size are evident. Approx. X 51,400 (A) and X 22,850 (B). (From Pence 1970).

tron dense, membrane-bound bodies. This syncytium possessed cytoplasmic 'arms' that extended to the surface of the somatophore, forming a cytoplasmic layer or 'cap' on the surface (Figure 17). The thin layer of cytoplasm spread laterally over the surface of the preoncosphere, eventually investing the preoncosphere in a cytoplasmic layer of syncytial cytoplasm. This architectural arrangement, whereby the cyton occurs below the surface and is connected by cytoplasmic extensions to a surface of 'distal' cytoplasm, is continued throughout the metacestode stage as well as in the adult.

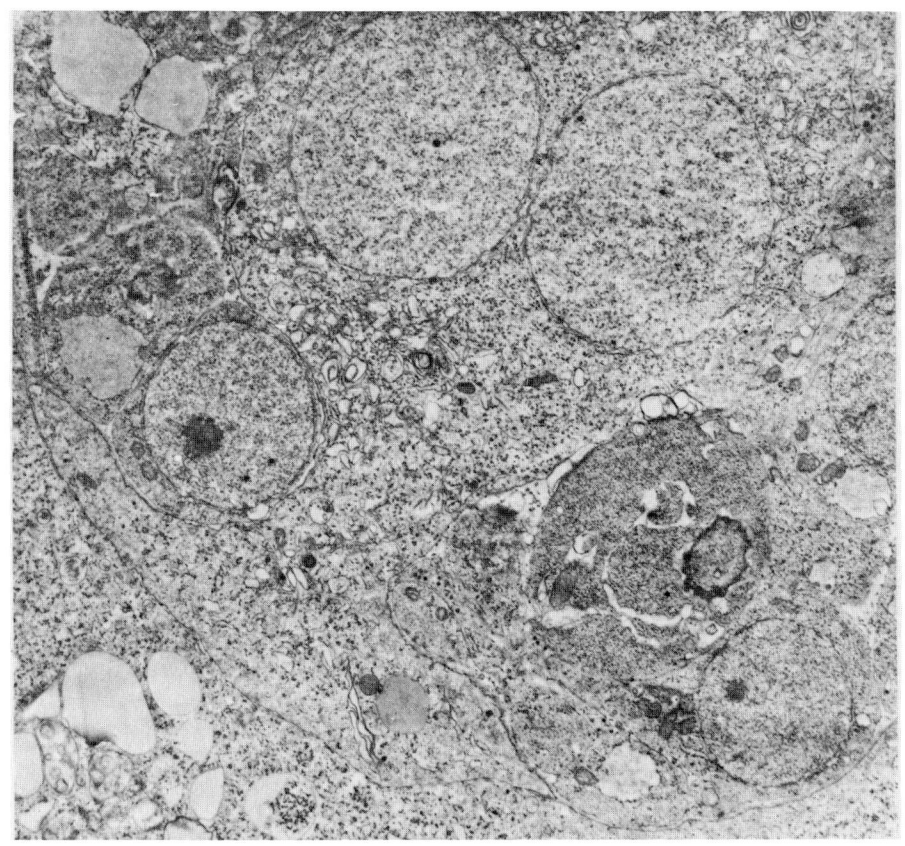

Figure 17. Transmission electron microscopy photomicrograph of binucleate cell showing connection to surface and 'cytoplasmic cap' of epithelium (ep). Approx. X 8,460. (From Rybicka 1973b).

With growth of the distal cytoplasmic layer, small vesicles appear in the cytoplasm and compartmentalize the cytoplasm into three regions, termed basal, intermediate, and peripheral by Rybicka. The outer peripheral zone contains smooth endoplasmic reticulum. The intermediate zone contains dense ribosomes, rough and small ER and Golgi bodies. The basal zone contains numerous membrane-bound dense bodies and mitochondria (Figure 18).

Concurrently with the spreading of the surface cytoplasm over the preoncosphere, the vesicles separating the zones fuse and the outer layers delineate and form long ribbon-like extensions from the surface

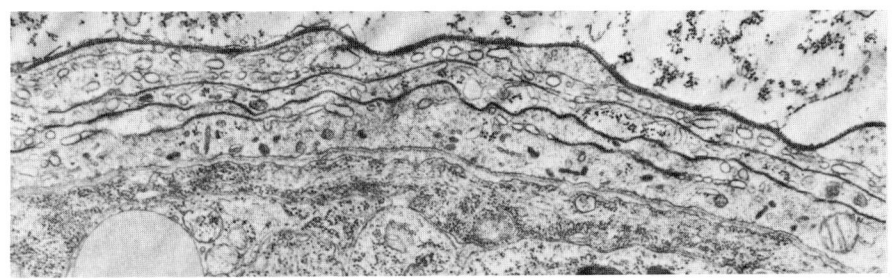

Figure 18. Transmission electron microscopy photomicrograph of epithelium illustrating vesicle fusion and formation of layers. Approx. X 19,800. (From Rybicka 1973b).

(Figure 19). The arms of the epithelial cell extend to the surface by passing between differentiating myoblasts. The external coats (or basal laminae) of both myofibers and epithelium form an interstitial network surrounding the preoncosphere. As the epithelium extends over the preoncosphere, numerous basal plasma membrane invagination form into the surface epithelium (Figure 20).

As illustrated by Collin (1968), the extracellular coat also attaches (or comes into supportive, close contact) to the guard of the hooks, and thus, in mature oncospheres, hooks, musculature, and the surface epithelium are all closely associated and possibly interacting (Figure 21). This would be important in an organism whose larval stage lacked a nervous system.

XII. THE MATURE ONCOSPHERE

The mature oncosphere of *Hymenolepis diminuta* was first figured by Grassi and Rovelli (1892) and this figure has been widely used. Faust (1949)

presented another figure which has also been reproduced. Ogren (1961b) described the mature oncosphere and used photographs to illustrate various salient features, as did Voge and Heyneman (1957) and Rothman (1957). Ogren (1962, 1967), Pence (1970), and Rybicka (1972) also diagrammed the mature oncosphere. A composite diagram is presented in Figure 22.

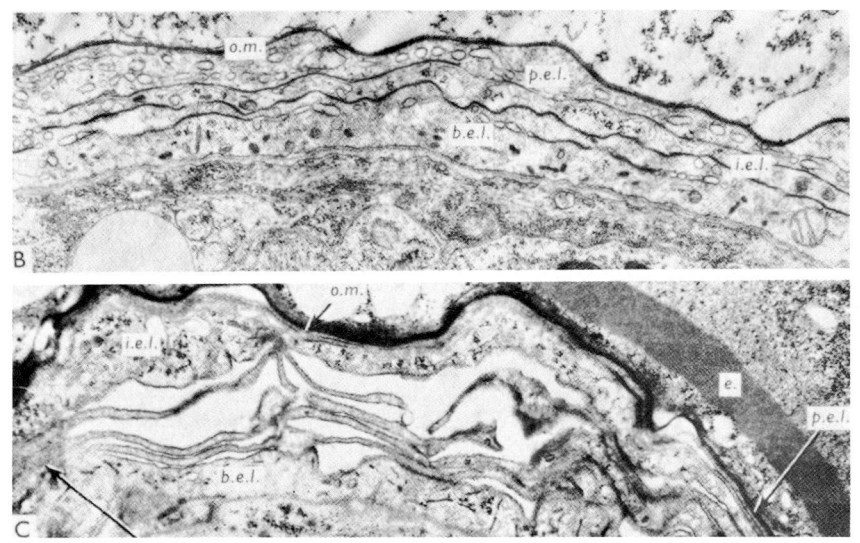

Figure 19. Photomicrograph of separation of syncytial epithelium forming elongate strands of cytoplasm which are continuations of the distal cytoplasm of the tegument (bel). Approx. X 17,750. (From Rybicka 1973b).

Ogren (1961b) presented the orientation of the oncosphere. The mature oncosphere is bilaterally symmetrical and consists of an extensive musculature, three pairs of distinctive hooks, secretory cells, epithelial syncytial cells with perinuclear and distal cytoplasm, and two classes of large embryonic cells. The latter embryonic cells occur in the mesophore and presumably give rise to cells in the metacestode (Figure 23 after Ogren 1967).

Structure and Ultrastructure of the Larvae and Metacestodes

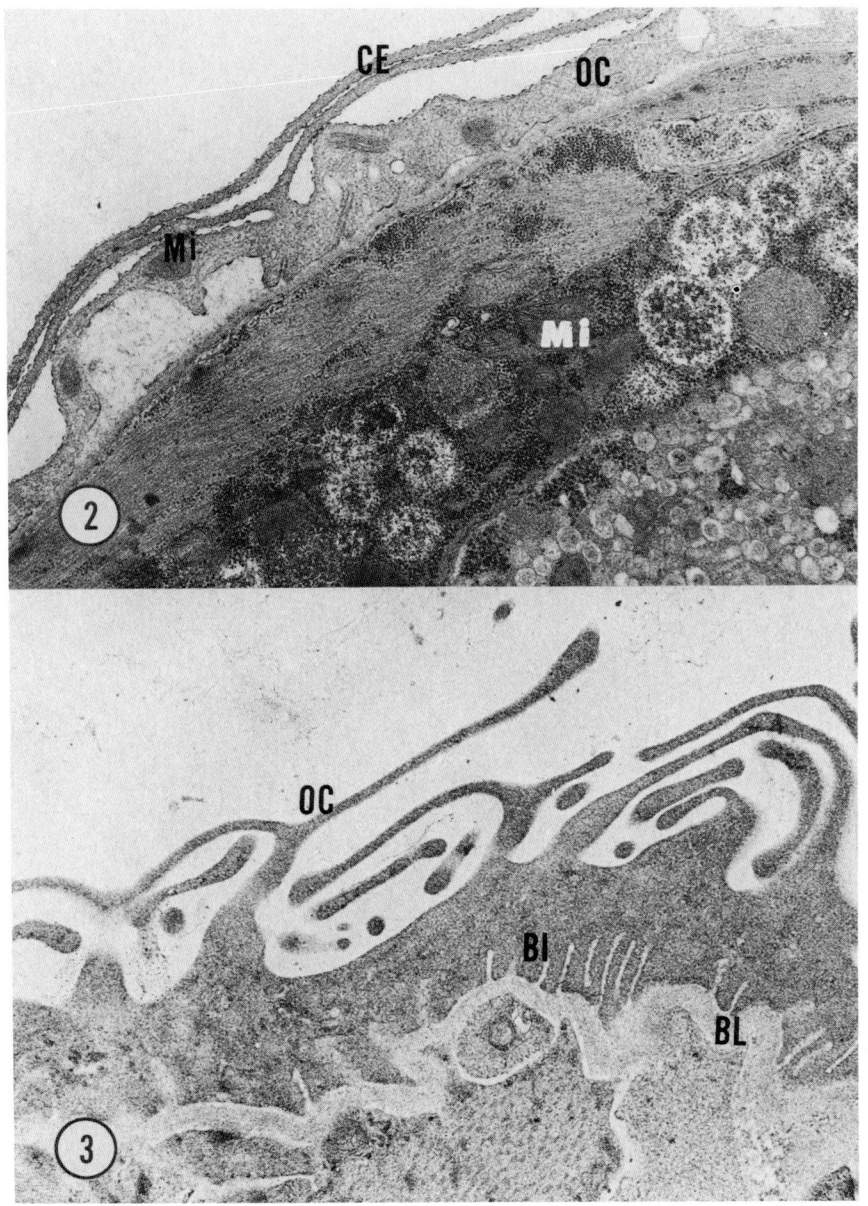

Figure 20. Photomicrograph of distal cytoplasmic layer (H. citelli) showing laminar folds (OC) extending from surface in emergent oncospheres. BI, basal infoldings; BL, basal lamina. Approx. X 35,700. (From Collin 1968).

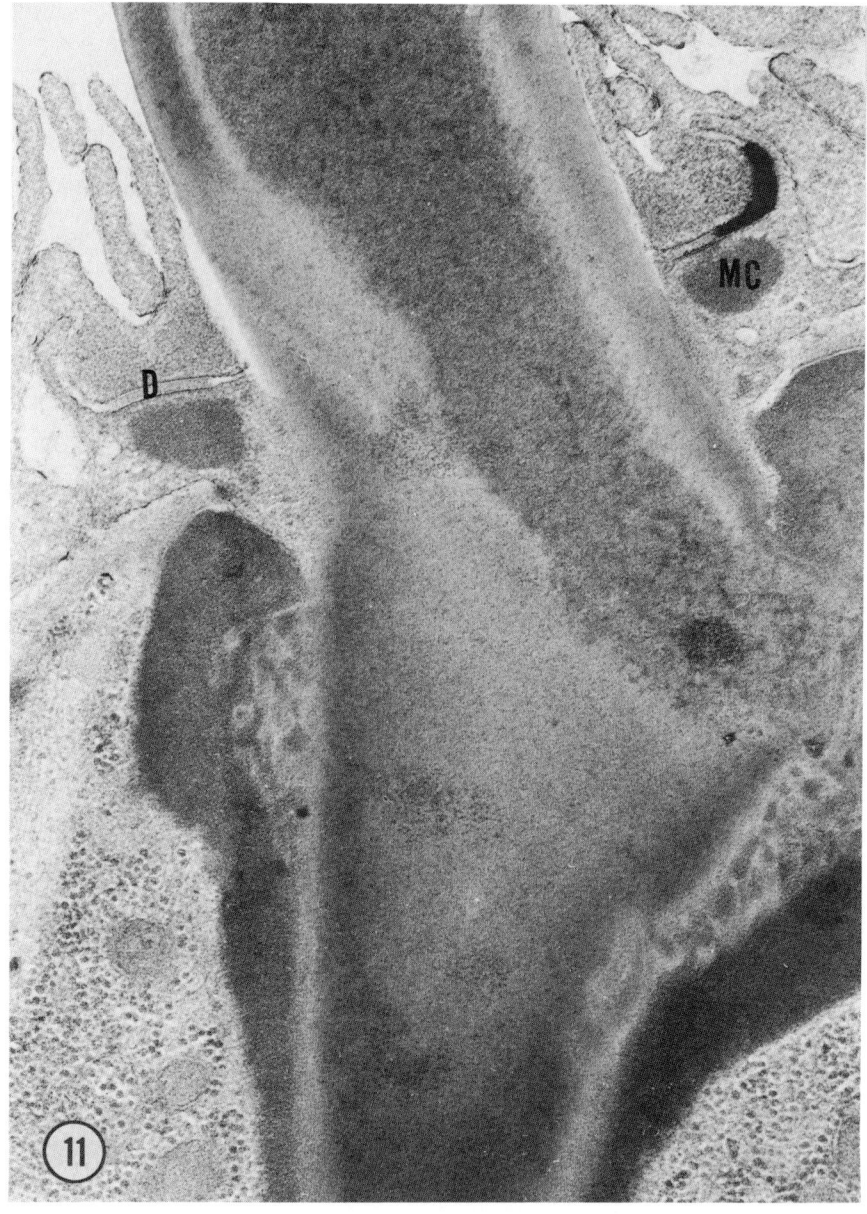

Figure 21. Photomicrograph of hook of H. citelli oncospheres. Distal cytoplasm attaches to external coat of hook by a desmosome (D). Approx. X 43,100. (From Collin 1968).

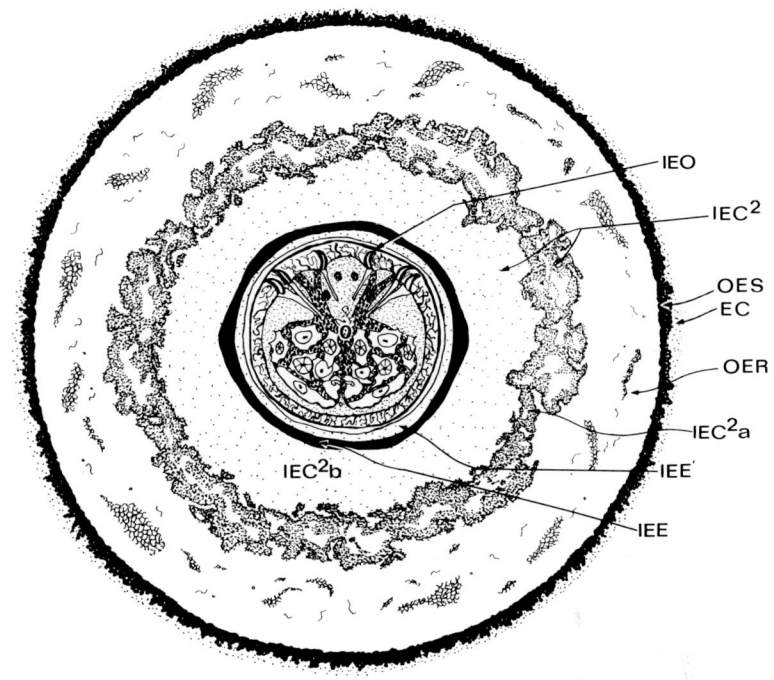

Figure 22. Diagram of oncosphere of Hymenolepis diminuta modified from Pence (1970), Rybicka (1972) and Ogren (1968a). OE, outer envelope derived structures; OES, outer envelope 'shell' which is deposited against the capsule (derived from vitelline gland, see text) obscuring it; OER, outer envelope remnant in various stages of fragmentation. The 'shell' and capsule are covered by a granular material (EC) forming an external coat that may be secreted by the uterus (see text). The inner envelope (IE) forms layers including the inner cytoplasmic layer (IEE^1) and an outer cytoplasmic layer (IEC^2). The outer cytoplasmic layer contains an irregular dense external layer (IEC^2a) and an inner homogeneous lucent layer (IEC^2b). Embryophore (IEE) and oncospheral membrane (IEO) are also present. An oncosphere (O) is present within the embryophore.

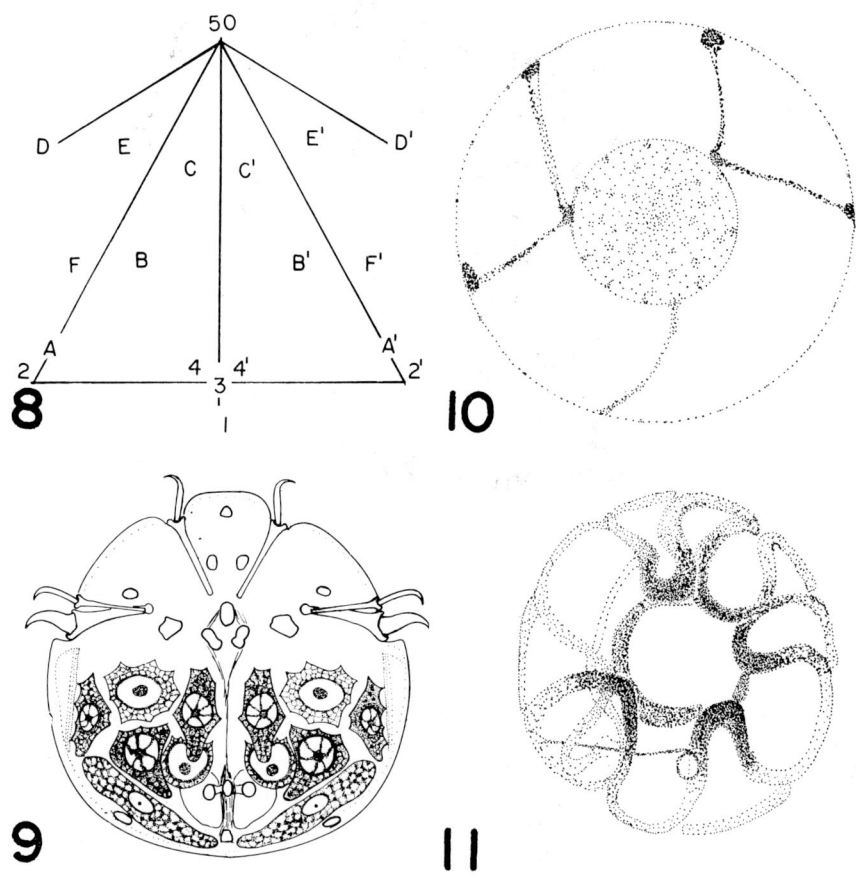

Figure 23. Distribution of cellular patterns in invasive oncospheres. Main axis of cells lie between 3 and 50 (diagram 8). Dorsal view showing cells in diagram 8 presented in diagram 9. Diagram 10 represents class II embryonic cell nuclei. Diagram 11 represents class I embryonic cells. (From Ogren 1967).

As described by Ogren (1961b), each oncosphere has three pairs of hooks which aid in orientation. The two medial hooks are orientated along the longitudinal axis of the body. The blade of these hooks is delicate and sharply curved at the tip. The hooks extend outward from the oncosphere toward the substrate, allowing a distinction between the dorsal surface and the ventral surface of the body, which touches the substrate. The blade of these hooks measures approximately 7 microns long with a shank of 10-11 microns. Similar measurements occur in all hooks. The lateral hooks, located posterior and slightly dorsal to the medial hooks, are arranged with the blades directed toward the mesophore. The anterior-most hook, designated the dorso-lateral hook, is delicate, narrow, and sickle-shaped. The ventral-lateral hook is thicker and, being readily observable, is used for comparison with hooks of other oncospheres (Ogren 1957).

XIII. EMERGENCE AND PENETRATION

Grassi and Rovelli (1892) first reported that emergence of hexacanth larvae (a process often erroneously called hatching) and subsequent development in *H. diminuta* could occur in an insect intermediate host, *Tenebrio molitor*. Although these observations have been documented by nearly every student working with *H. diminuta*, the basic physiological changes that allow emergence and establishment of infection are only rudimentarily understood. In an early study, Isobe (1926) examined intact larvae (oncospheres in embryonic membranes) and observed that establishment of an infection was not a passive phenomenon involving ingestion of the larvae by a correct insect intermediate host, but rather, involved at least two phases: activation of the hexacanth larva and emergence from the larval membranes. Isobe examined intact larvae and observed that activation could be achieved by a variety of drugs and salt concentrations. The presence of distilled or tap water with various salt concentrations, with or without beetle juices, all resulted in stimulating initial activity, particularly hook movements, but generally such activity was not sustained. Reid *et al.* (1951) described the importance of hooks in allowing emergence of the oncosphere from the larval membranes. Careful studies were conducted by Voge and Berntzen (1961) and Berntzen and Voge (1965) on the emergence of oncospheres of several tapeworm species, including *H. diminuta*. These authors clearly established that emergence could only occur following removal of or damage to the 'shell'. They also presented substantial evidence showing that substances present in the beetle were important in the disruption or destruction of the outer and inner envelopes, including the embryophore. Using a variety of media these authors suggested that amylases were important in autolysis of the embryophore and that trypsin dispersed the cytoplasmic region of the inner envelope. Inconsistent results were obtained using saline extracts prepared from *Dermestes vulpinus*, in that the cytoplasmic layer was destroyed but the embryophore was maintained intact. Oncospheres emerged by opening the embryophore with their hooks. Saline preparations of *Tenebrio molitor* were generally not effective in allowing emergence. Emergence was also found to be influenced by temperature. An optimal temperature of 25°C was found to be effective, whereas higher temperatures either decreased the activity or immobilized the oncosphere.

Lethbridge (1971a) confirmed the requirement of breaking the 'shell' in order to initiate emergence of the oncosphere. By analyzing midgut contents of adult and larval *T. molitor*, he showed that nearly 50% of ingested larvae were not damaged (cracked) by the mandibles of the insect. Such larvae passed through the alimentary tract unharmed and were viable when fed to subsequent insects. Approximately 3% of the oncospheres were severely damaged (crushed) and were not able to establish the infection. In roughly 45% of ingested oncospheres, the shell and cytoplasmic region of the outer envelope were ruptured by the mandibles. The cytoplasmic region of the inner envelope subsequently expanded rapidly and expelled the larvae and inner envelope through the opening in the 'shell' into the midgut of the beetle.

The sequence of emergence was diagrammed by Lethbridge (1971a) (Figure 24). Following removal from the 'shell', the cytoplasmic part of the inner envelope disappeared in six minutes, followed by the embryophore in twelve minutes. Observed changes included a loss of refractility and an increase in circumference and elasticity of the embryophore. Although hook movements damaged the embryophore, release from the embryophore was apparently by digestion. Voge and Berntzen (1961) suggested the possibility that lytic secretions produced from the penetration glands might assist emergence. In contrast, Lethbridge (1971a) observed that emergence was essentially due to digestive factors present in the beetle midgut once the 'shell' and outer envelope were broken.

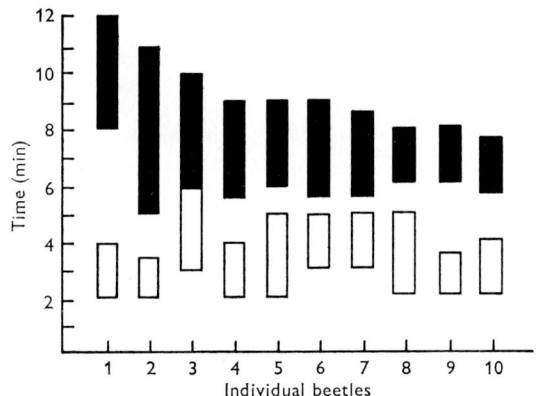

Figure 24. Emergence sequence of Hymenolepis diminuta larvae in Tenebrio molitor adults. The time periods required for digestion of the outer cytoplasmic layer (white) and embryophore (black) of the inner envelope are presented. (From Lethbridge 1971a).

Lethbridge (1971b) observed different roles for each of the embryonic envelopes. He determined that the 'shell' was resistant to hydrolytic enzymes but could be dissolved in hypochlorite. The cytoplasmic region of the outer envelope (called subshell membrane) contained lipid and phospholipid and was unaffected by hypochlorite, many enzymes and histological fixatives, water, and lipid soluble dyes. This layer is important in protecting the hexacanth from external changes that might affect osmotic pressure or pH.

The cytoplasmic layer was shown to consist of a glucosamine-containing mucoprotein. This layer was apparently in a colloidal state that allowed rapid absorption of water upon rupture of the outer envelope. Expansion of this layer is controlled by the concentration of sodium chloride, with swelling inversely related to the salt concentration. Changing salt concentrations allowed swelling or shrinking of this layer and at 1% concentration this layer could be shrunk to its normal size (Figure 25).

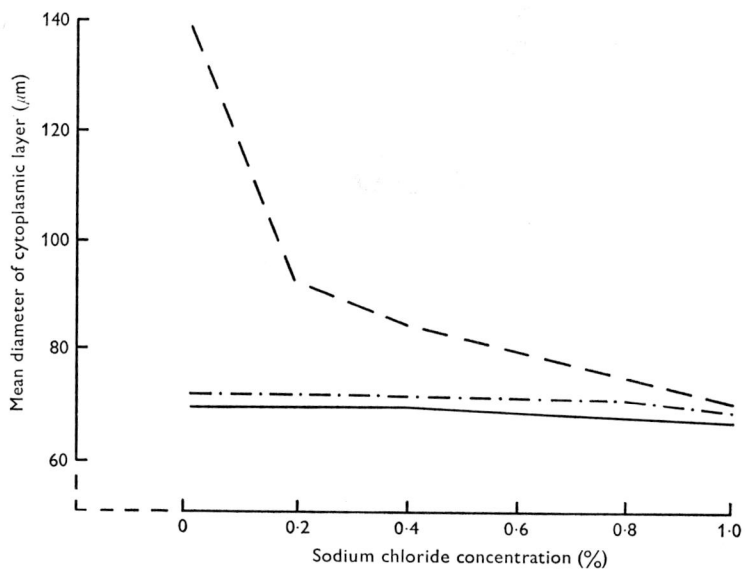

Figure 25. Variation in the diameter of the outer cytoplasmic layer of the inner envelope of H. diminuta larvae after 60 minutes of immersion of intact (-•-•-•-) or mechanically changed (- - - -) or hypochlorite treated (————) larvae. (From Lethbridge 1971b).

Lethbridge (1972) extended the observations by Berntzen and Voge and examined the time required for emergence at different pH concentrations, using saline midgut extracts of *Tenebrio molitor* (one gut/ml) at 25°C (Figure 26). A minimal time of six minutes at pH 6.6 to 6.8 was sufficient to allow dissolution of both layers, with the inner envelope digesting slightly more rapidly than the embryophore. Digestion was inhibited by five minutes incubation of the extracts at 80°C.

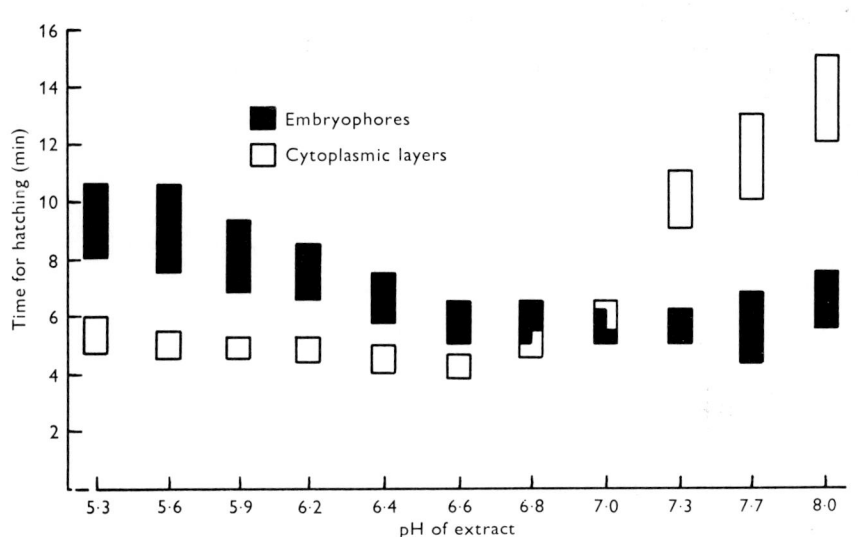

Figure 26. Time periods required for digestion of outer cytoplasmic layer and embryophore of the inner envelope during emergence of H. diminuta larvae in Tenebrio molitor extracts at various pH's. (From Lethbridge 1972).

Storing the extracts for 24 hours at 2°C lengthened the time required for digestion. Dialyzed, aliquots of the stored samples were active in destroying embryophores but did not react against the inner envelope. Concentration of the larval beetle extract generally resulted in rapid digestion (Figure 27).

The elution of beetle midgut extract by electrophoresis and its subsequent effects on emergence of *H. diminuta* was studied by Lethbridge (1972). Four bands were detected. Two bands exhibited intense proteolytic activity and migrated in opposite directions from the origin (Band A moving 10 to 17 mm to the cathode; Band B moving 22 to 26 mm to the anode).

Band A extracts rapidly destroyed the embryophore and slowly dispersed the cytoplasmic material of the inner envelope. Band B digested the cytoplasmic region of the inner envelope and weakened the embryophore, allowing some oncospheres to emerge. Mixtures of eluates prepared from both bands A and B promoted the most efficient emergence. Bands C and D, obtained by electrophoresis, were anodal. Band C was shown to contain amylase and Band D contained no detectable enzymes. Both bands had no effect on digestion of the larval layers.

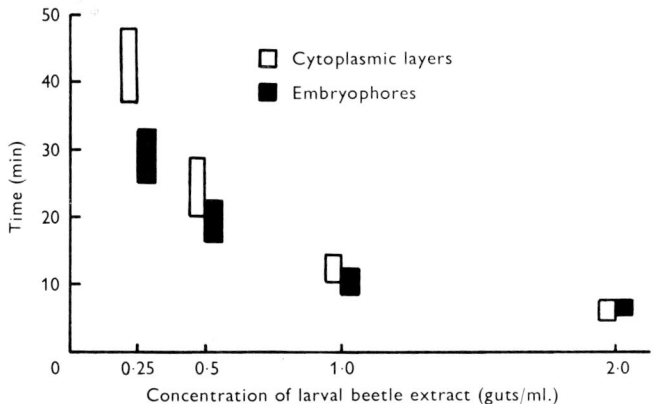

Figure 27. Time periods required for digestion of outer cytoplasmic layer and embryophore of inner envelopes of H. diminuta larvae in varying concentrations of T. molitor extracts at pH 6.8. (From Lethbridge 1972).

The role of amylases was evaluated by incubating 'deshelled' oncospheres with bacterial α-amylase (330 ug/ml; pH 6.8 preparations), human saliva, purified hog amylase, cockroach midgut extract containing amylases, and proteases. Only the cockroach midgut extract digested both layers and allowed emergence. Bacterial α-amylase altered the embryophore, which became elastic and could be punctured by the hooks of the oncosphere, allowing emergence (Lethbridge 1972).

The tryptic activity of larval midgut extracts (*T. molitor*) was found to be equivalent to 17.5 µg/ml of trypsin standard at pH 7.8. Chymotryptic activity of the midgut at pH 6.8 was found to be 30 µg/ml of the chymotrypsin standard. Application of these levels of trypsin and chymotrypsin solutions prepared singly in buffered saline indicated that trypsin sufficiently weakened the embryophore, allowing oncosphere emergence in 60 minutes (Figure 28). The reactions could be inhibited by ovomucoid. Emergence was enhanced by chymotrypsin and 18% of the oncospheres emerged in one hour. In various combinations, emergence was more rapid, but always the embryophore was present and the outer envelope remained unaffected. The embryophore was readily destroyed by the addition of peptidase (5%).

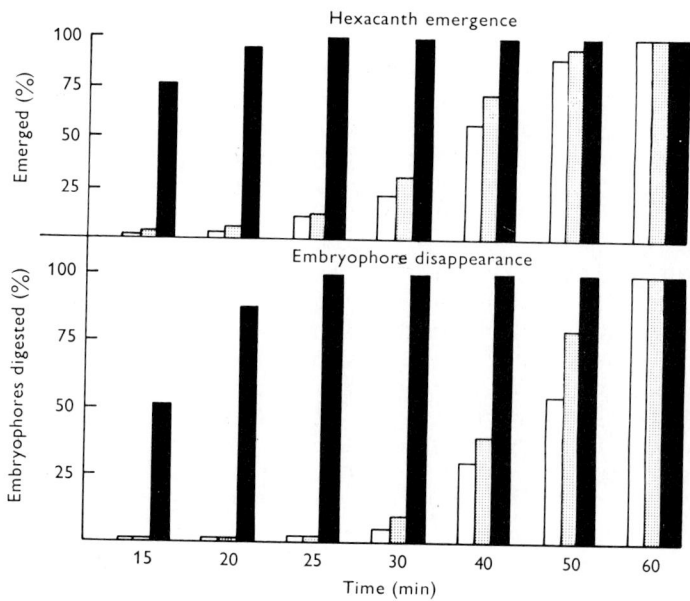

Figure 28. Emergence of oncosphere and disappearance of embryophore in trypsin-chymotrypsin preparations after the addition of 1% (white), 2% (stipple), and 5% (black) peptidase extracts. (From Lethbridge 1972).

Lethbridge (1972) was able to propose a defined medium containing trypsin, chymotrypsin, and peptidase, which digested the embryophore and allowed emergence in times comparable to those obtained in his earlier studies using extracts of the insect gut. Since none of these substances digested the inner envelope, presumably another substance, probably a protease, is involved in *in vivo* emergence, as demonstrated by the fraction separated by electrophoresis of the insect gut extract. As pointed out by Lethbridge, the embryophore appears to be the main barrier to emergence after the outer envelope is broken. The cytoplasmic layer is rapidly dispersed by pepsin, ficin, or papain, whereas the embryophore could be weakened by proteolytic enzymes, but not by amylase.

XIV. PENETRATION OF THE ONCOSPHERE

The ability of oncospheres to penetrate across the intestine of their insect host has been studied by various authors. As early as 1928, Bacigalupo reported differences in susceptibility of larvae versus adults to oncospheres of *H. diminuta*. Voge and Graiwar (1964) found that motile oncospheres emerged in both larvae and adults, but metacestodes occurred primarily in the hemocoels of adult insects. Injection of oncospheres into the body cavity of larval insects resulted in normal metacestode development. Comparing gross histological structure of the intestine, particularly the midgut, Voge and Graiwar suggested that structural differences between the larvae and adults might account for different rates of infection.

The histology of the midgut in larval and adult *T. molitor* is described by Voge and Graiwar (1964) and Lethbridge (1971a). The histology is presented in Figure 29. Essential differences between larval and adult midgut involve a thickened peritrophic membrane in larvae and the presence of crypt-like papillae of columnar cells projecting through the underlying musculature into the body cavity of the adult beetle (Figure 30). It is clear that the muscle bundles do not appear as a sheath but rather as elongate fibers, loosely arrayed. Lethbridge (1971a) found that oncospheres entered the epithelium and within 30 minutes had moved to the muscle layers or to the papillae. Penetration was completed within 45 to 75 minutes. Although Lethbridge reported that the majority of oncospheres penetrated across the papillae, thus avoiding the musculature of the gut, Moczon (1977b) found that oncospheres only rarely utilized the diverticula and that most oncospheres were able to penetrate across the muscular

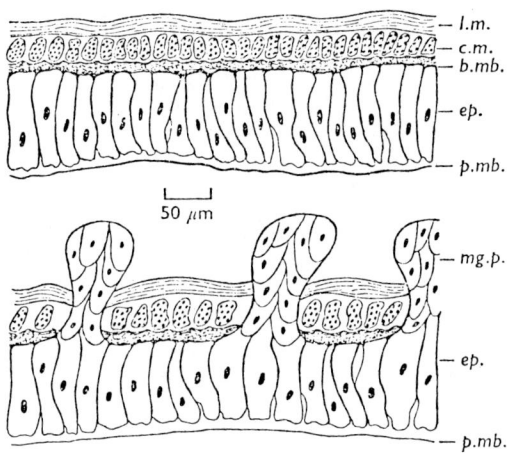

Figure 29. Diagram of longitudinal view of midgut of larval (top) and adult (bottom) Tenebrio molitor. Note the epithelial papillae (mg.p.) which extend into the hemocoel in adult beetles. (From Lethbridge 1971a).

region of the intestine. Lethbridge reported that roughly 45 minutes were necessary for crossing the peritrophic membrane of larval beetles. During the subsequent two hours, oncospheres that had arrived at the musculature were only occasionally able to penetrate. Although rapid larval intestinal emptying times (2 hours) were suggested by Voge and Graiwar (1964) as possibly hindering migration, Lethbridge found it not to be important. Moczon (1977b) suggested that possibly, the chemical composition of the muscles of the adult intestine differs from
that of the larvae and proposed that the oncospheres were able to chemically affect those muscles of the

adult (but not those of the larvae) by secretions of the penetration glands. In view of the observation presented here of the rather loose arrangement of the muscle layers in the wall of the intestine of adult beetles, it might be of interest to examine the musculature of the larval beetles to determine if a similar arrangement is present.

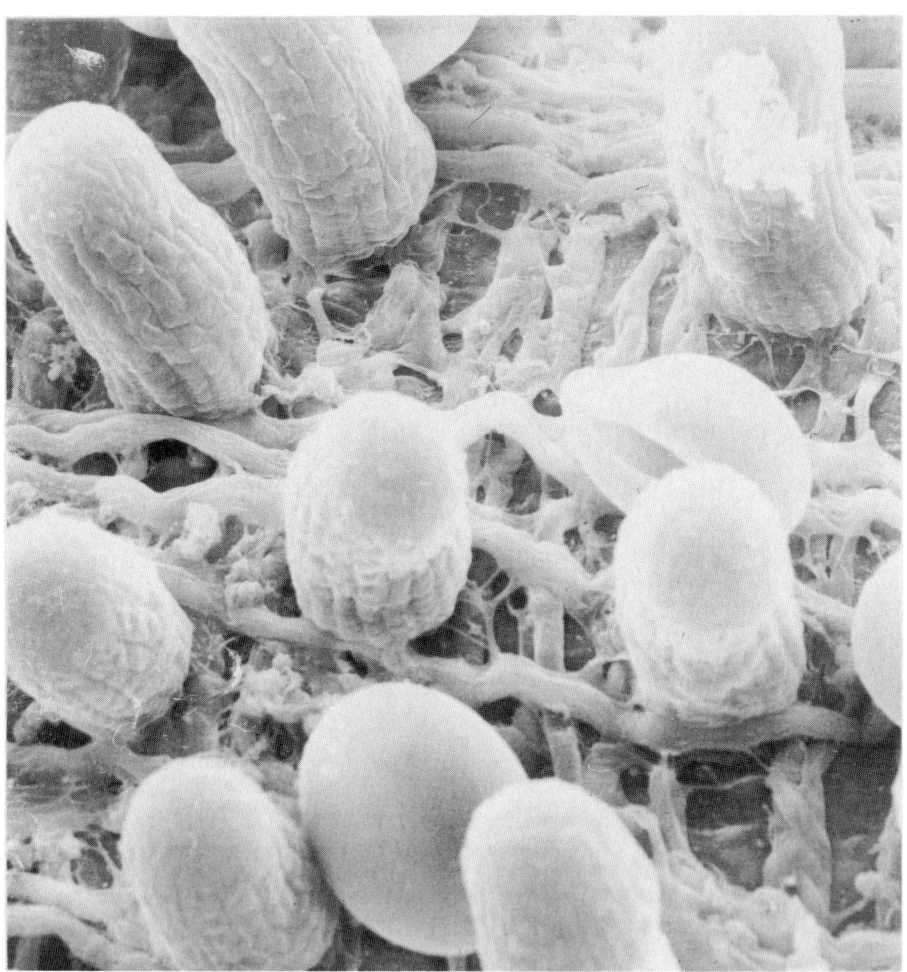

Figure 30. Scanning electron photomicrograph of adult beetle midgut (Tenebrio molitor). Observe the longitudinal and transverse muscle fiber arrangement. X 330.

The initial penetration of *H. diminuta* oncospheres is largely mechanical, due to destruction of the columnar epithelium of the insect gut by movements of the hooks. Moczon (1977b) found that "released from the envelopes, the oncospheres hook into epithelial cells tearing them to pieces in the process and throwing the shreds behind themselves with the hooks". Movements of the oncospheres were first described by Isobe (1926), who noted hook movement of a rapid and slow nature. Reid *et al.* (1951) examined some factors involved in the emergence of *H. diminuta* larvae and related movements of the hooks to this process. Ogren (1969) described fundamental hook movements and the relative times required were reported (Figure 31). Generally, the normal

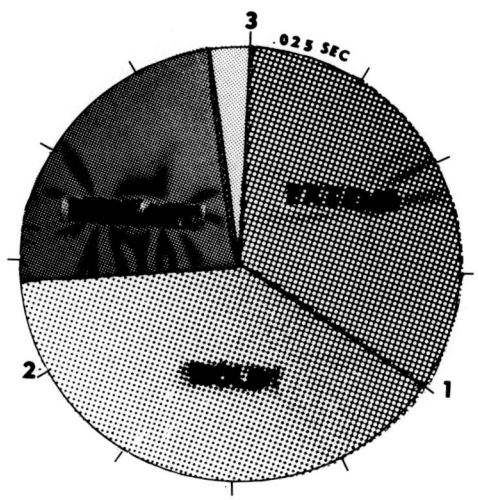

Figure 31. Diagram of time periods required for hook movements of H. diminuta oncospheres during a three second movement cycle. (From Ogren 1969).

rate of movement varied from 15 to 35 extensions per minute. As represented by Ogren, extension of the hooks required approximately 1.0 second; holding, 1.2 seconds; and retraction, 0.7 seconds. During extension, the lateral hooks were extended first, then abducted backward. The medial hooks were extended in a clawinglike motion. Retraction resulted in withdrawing the hooks into the body. According to

Ogren (1969), the following events occurred: "1) lateral hook protraction, 2) anterior enlargement and mid-body constriction, 3) medial hook protraction, 4) holding, 5) retraction, and 6) posterior enlargement". Lethbridge (1971a) confirmed Ogren's observations and determined that extension of the lateral hooks serves to anchor the oncosphere between adjacent epithelial cells. Extension of the medial pair of hooks and their downward rotation allowed forward movement. Movements are greatly influenced by temperature and chemical solutions including neutral red. Since movements are considered a morphological sign of activation, it is apparent that numerous environmental stimuli will serve to activate the oncosphere, especially those involved in removing the 'shell' and outer envelope (Ogren *et al.* 1969).

The chief source of energy for migrating oncospheres appears to be glycogen. Lethbridge (1971a) reported a continued decrease in glycogen content of the hook musculature during penetration. After 3.5 hours of attempted penetration in larval *T. molitor*, levels of glycogen were lower than could be detected histochemically.

The role of the penetration glands remains speculative. Although they were first believed to be functional in providing adhesive properties (see Chen 1934; Reid 1948), assisting the oncosphere in penetration of the host, Silverman and Maneely (1955) demonstrated histochemically that polysaccharide complexes are present in the penetration glands of *Taenia saginata* and *T. pisiformis*. These complexes play an important role in the erosion of the cells of the wall of the intermediate host (Sawada 1961).

The secretory process has been carefully described by Lethbridge and Gijsbers (1974) using neutral red dye which concentrates in the penetration glands. Within 30 minutes of emergence, four blebs appear over the openings of the penetration glands Droplets of secretory substance are released from the surface beginning 15 minutes after emergence. The secretory products are released and replaced by new ones for as long as 135 minutes. Eventually, secretion ceases and little neutral red material remains in the glands (Figure 32).

Expulsion of the secretory material appears to be of the merocrine type. Lethbridge and Gijsbers (1974) believed that the gland opened directly into the peripheral cytoplasmic layer (distal cytoplasm), although this cellular arrangement would be unusual. According to their scheme, secretory products passed into the distal cytoplasm and resulted in localized swellings producing large projections which pinched off the surface (Figure 33).

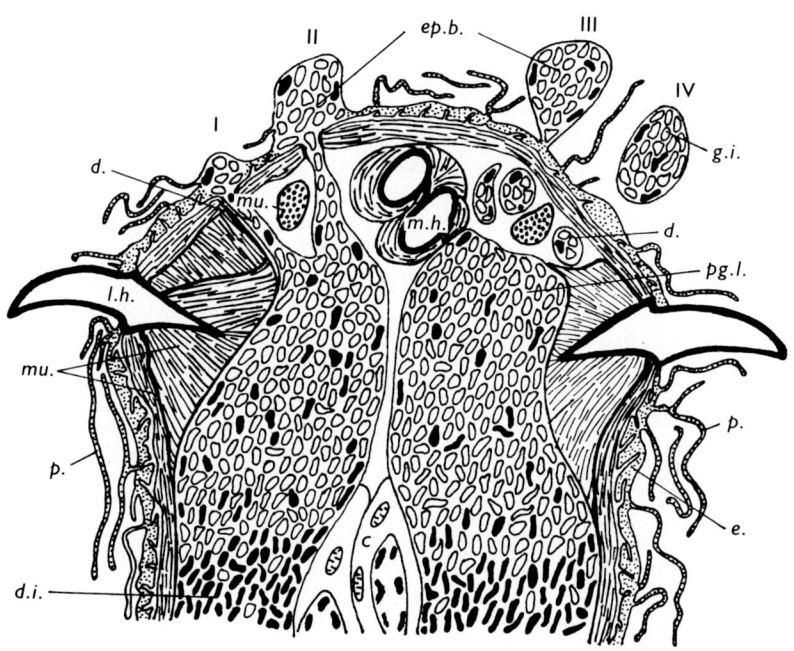

Figure 32. Diagram of mesophore of H. diminuta oncosphere. Penetration glands (pg. 1) extend to surface via ducts (d). The penetration glands appear to open in the distal cytoplasm of the epithelium (tegument) causing blebs to appear on the surface of the oncosphere (see also Collin 1969, Figure 9). If these observations are correct, the penetration glands are epithelial in nature. Their modifications following penetration should be examined. (From Lethbridge and Gijsbers 1974).

The role of penetration gland secretions in invasive organisms has been reviewed by Stirewalt

(1963). Although such secretions are often involved in the lysis of host tissues in many cestode oncospheres, there is conflicting evidence for oncospheres of *H. diminuta*. Lethbridge (1971a) reported a reduction in PAS-positive affinity of midgut connective tissue adjacent to migrating hexacanths, and concluded "On this evidence alone it is not possible to ascribe a lytic function to the secretions of *H. diminuta* hexacanths". Moczon (1977b) described a swelling and breakdown of muscle of adult beetles that are in close contact with the penetration substance. The affected musculature lost its eosin staining ability and became flaccid and gelatinous. He concluded that ".... the muscular tissue of the insect is presumably the true substrate for the penetration enzyme". Moczon showed that the penetration substance apparently had no effect upon human erythrocytes or hemocytes from the beetle. Although Moczon suggested that ".... failure of the oncospheres to penetrate across the wall of the intestine of the insect larva shows that the muscular tissue of this organ is not an appropriate substrate for the penetration enzymes of the oncospheres", no experimental data was presented. Moczon (1977a) found that collagenase and hyaluronidase were not present in the penetration glands, and found that the secretory product was proteinaceous, and that no mucopolysaccharides were detected (1977c).

Houser and Burns (1968) showed that penetration does not appear to be influenced by microorganisms in the insect gut, since normal growth to metacestode occurred in gnotobiotic *Tenebrio molitor*.

XV. METACESTODE DEVELOPMENT

In the life cycle of *Hymenolepis diminuta*, metamorphosis of the invasive oncosphere (larva) occurs in the hemocoel of various insects (Stunkard 1962; Ogren 1968b; Freeman 1973). As first proposed by Rosen (1918) for bothriocephalid cestodes, the metamorphosis of the larva results in the next stage in the life cycle - a metacestode which is infective to the definitive host. The metacestode of *H. diminuta* is commonly referred to as a cysticercoid, a term attributed to Leuckart (Wardle and McLeod 1952).

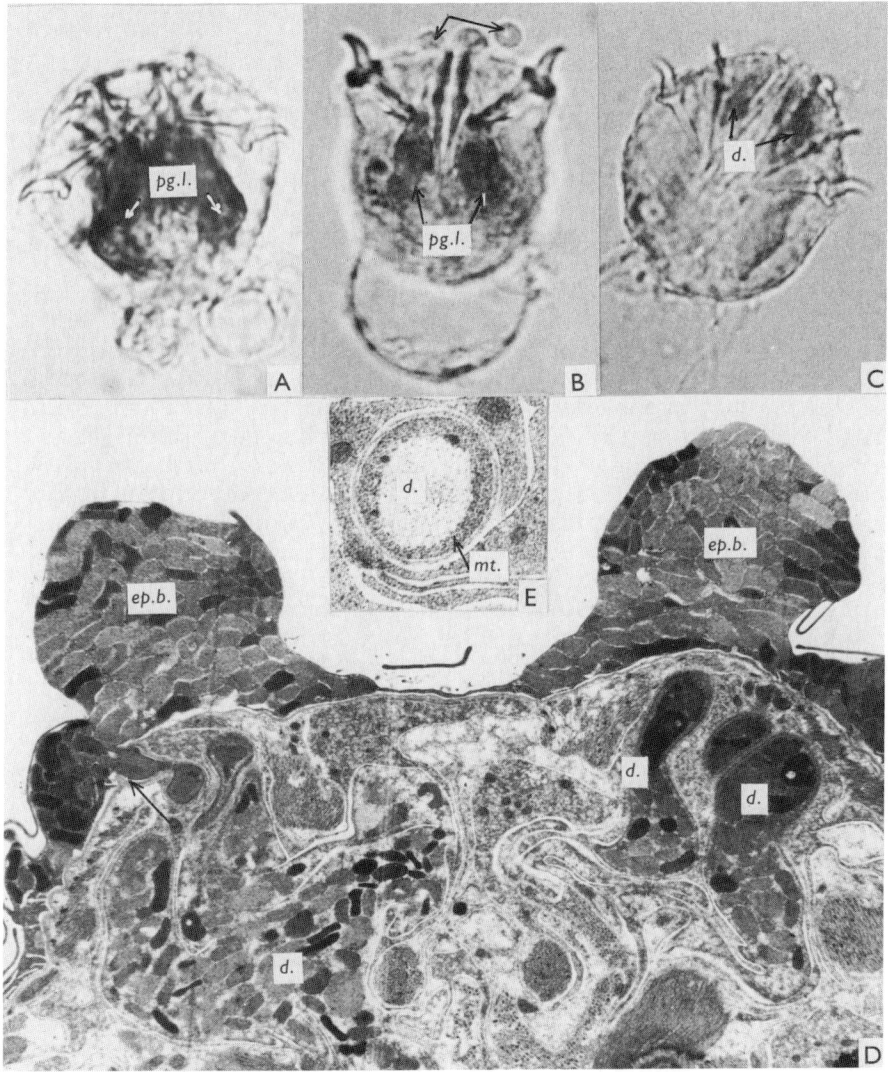

Figure 33. Secretion of penetration gland substance by oncospheres of H. diminuta showing a loss of penetration gland material through time (A, 15 min; B, 75 min; C, 135 min after emergence). Several blebs of penetration gland material appear in D. (From Lethbridge and Gijsbers 1974).

Morphogenesis of the metacestode of *Hymenolepis diminuta* was first observed by Grassi (1887) and Grassi and Rovelli (1892). Their observations established the basic developmental pattern of *H. diminuta*, which has been elaborated on by Joyeux (1920), Rothman (1957), and notably, by Voge and Heyneman (1957). It is clear from these studies that during metamorphosis of the oncosphere there is a reorganization which includes the loss of many larval structures (penetration glands, hook musculature), the assembly of a protonephridial system, a nervous system, specialized metacestode features, and the modification of some structures, such as some musculature of the outer region of the oncosphere and the epithelial surface of the metacestode (including the tegument of the scolex). The oncospheral hooks persist, but appear to be vestigial. A marked change precipitating much discussion is the reported "reversal of polarity" which occurs during metamorphosis. Ogren (1968b) suggests, however, that the reversal may begin before the emergence of the oncosphere into the insect intermediate host. The reversal is morphologically characterized by the rapid and early growth of cells and tissues in the mesophore (end opposite the hooks), resulting in development of a holdfast. An excellent discussion of polarity is presented by Freeman (1973), and I agree with Voge and Heyneman (1957) who conclude that in the development of *H. diminuta* "To speak about polarity and reversal of polarity because of the direction of movement of the relatively undifferentiated oncosphere, as is done by Venard (1938), is meaningless".

The cellular morphological changes of the oncosphere to early metacestode have been examined by Ogren (1962). By careful staining procedures he was able to demonstrate that the infective oncosphere possessed five pairs of cells (termed epidermal glands) located in two groups in the lateral regions of the mesophore (Figure 34). These cells continued through development to form germinative cells of the early oncosphere, which later gave rise to the specialized tissues of the scolex.

Rothman (1957) and Voge and Heyneman (1957) recognized several stages in the normal development of the cysticercoid. The following descriptions of

the stages are based primarily on observations by
the latter authors. The first stage metacestode was
recognized 48 hours after infection of the beetle
intermediate host. The ovoid body, approximately
100 μ in diameter, is covered by an investing cytoplasmic layer, the tegument, which is slightly thicker than in the oncosphere. This cytoplasmic layer
is connected to an underlying nucleated cytoplasm by
cytoplasmic arms extending through the musculature.
This arrangement of the surface architecture is not
changed during morphogenesis of the metacestode.

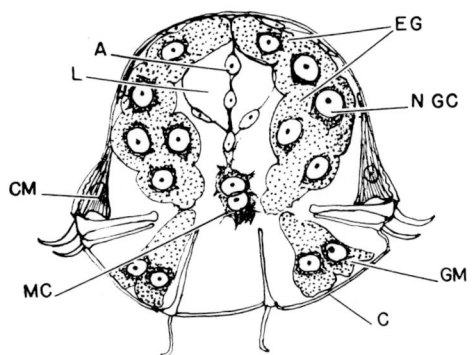

Figure 34. Diagram of infective oncosphere
showing distribution of 5 pairs of germinative cells.
(From Ogren 1962).

Although it is clear that a "primitive lacuna"
develops in the early metacestode, the formation of
this cavity is not well documented. Ogren (1962)
recognized the presence of small vacuolar areas in
the mesophore, which he referred to as lacunae.
Voge and Heyneman (1957) reported that cavity formation always began at the opposite end (somatophore
or oncophore) and was associated with the breakdown
and absorption of the hook musculature. The medial
pair of hooks lose their attachment to the musculature
first and later all hooks become deeply embedded in
the cellular matrix.

The second stage of morphogenesis is characterized by growth and the development of a cavity. By 72 hours the metacestode reaches 180 by 200 μ in size. Collin (1970) found only longitudinal myofibers containing substantial amounts of beta glycogen in similar developmental stages of *H. citelli*. The other cell types observed in this stage are relatively undifferentiated. The majority of cells have large electron opaque nucleoli in electron-lucent nuclei and little cytoplasm. The cytoplasm contains abundant free ribosomes.

The third stage of development occurs between 72 and 120 hours. This stage is characterized by rapid cellular proliferation resulting in growth and elongation of the metacestode. The end containing the oncospheral hooks does not exhibit as much mitotic activity as the prescolex end. The former becomes noticeably smaller and more elongate in comparison to the great increase in size occurring in the mid-region and prescolex end. The growth of this stage is presented by Voge and Heyneman (1957) (Figure 35).

The increase in size is especially evident in the size of the lacuna. This cavity effectively divides the metacestode into three regions termed by Voge and Heyneman (1957) the fore-body, mid-body, and hind-body or cercomer (which contains the hooks).

The division of the metacestode effectively allows each region to continue morphological differentiation almost independently. There is little increase in size. However, cell densities change notably throughout the metacestode. The anterior end contains the greatest density of cells and small lateral projections, representing the differentiation of suckers. At this stage of development there is also an increase in the wall of the lacuna. The increase in size is due to the apparent formation of fibroblastic cells surrounding the lacuna and at least two additional cell types contribute to the outward growth of the wall.

Withdrawal of the presumptive scolex occurs rapidly and represents the fourth stage of development. According to Voge and Heyneman (1957), immediately prior to withdrawal, the metacestode is charact erized by the presence of suckers, a widened midbody, and numerous contractile fibers which occur near the anterior margin of the cavity. These authors suggested that contraction of these fibers, as well as differences in pressure, resulted in waves of contraction and expansion which could be seen over the surface of the metacestode.

As Voge and Heyneman (1957) and others have reported, the primitive lacuna is surrounded early in development by "fibers". Voge (1960c) suggested that the 'spindle-shaped cells' surrounding the lacuna were associated with fiber formation. The ultrastructure of these cells has been described by Allison *et al.* (1972). These authors reported that these cells resemble bipolar epithelial squamous cells consisting of sparse perinuclear cytoplasm, containing ribosomes, large lipid droplets, mitochondria, and small amounts of rough endoplasmic reticulum. Extending from the perinuclear cytoplasm are slender cytoplasmic strands that form a dense layer around the lacunae (Figure 36).

Scolex retraction has been carefully studied in *Hymenolepis microstoma*. In this species retraction is a rapid process which is completed in 30 to 60 seconds. The relationship of various regions of the metacestode during retraction has been presented by Caley (1974) (Figure 37).

As Voge and Heyneman first noted, the retraction of the scolex is accompanied by rhythmical muscular contractions that extend from the presumptive scolex to the posterior end of the body. If analogies can be drawn from *H. microstoma*, the muscles occur as both longitudinal and transverse fibers. The transverse fibers are more numerous in the anterior regions of the body than around the lacuna. According to Caley, the muscle cells are similar to the type described by Lumsden and Byram (1967) and Webb (1977) (see Lumsden and Specian, this volume). The unstriated muscles of the metacestode lie immediately below the tegument and are bound by hemi-desmosomes to the basal lamina of the epidermis. The relationship of muscle fibers in the metacestode of *H. microstoma* before and after scolex retraction is presented in Figure 38. Caley observed that at 25°C the contractions lasted from 3 to 5 seconds and gradually increased until tetanus was achieved. Contractions of the scolex forced it to become squeezed into the mid-body, compressing the fluid filled primitive lacuna and causing the lacuna to become cup-shaped. The lacuna eventually is constricted and the pressure in the lacuna, as well as large circular muscles, maintain the anterior canal. Withdrawal of the scolex

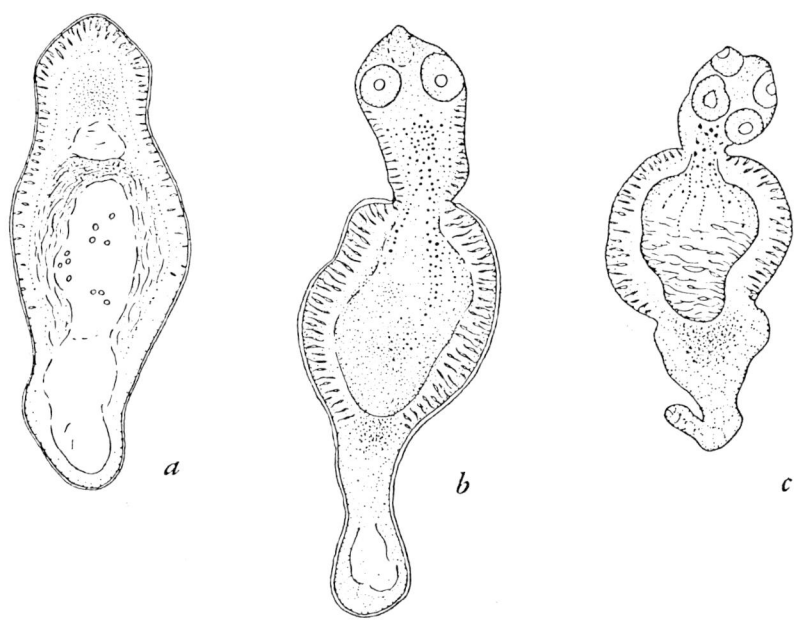

Figure 35. Diagram of the third stage of development illustrating the early form of the cysticercoid (a) showing three body divisions, extension of the primitive lacuna with surrounding cells. Late stage 3 (b) showing outlines of suckers and apical organ and later stage 3 (c) at beginning of withdrawal. (From Voge and Heyneman 1957).

into the lacuna does not result in determination of infectivity. Voge and Heyneman (1957), utilizing feeding tests in rats, demonstrated that the metacestode is not infective at this stage.

The last stage of development (Stage 5) has been described by Voge and Heyneman (1957). During this stage at least two important histological changes

Structure and Ultrastructure of the Larvae and Metacestodes 115

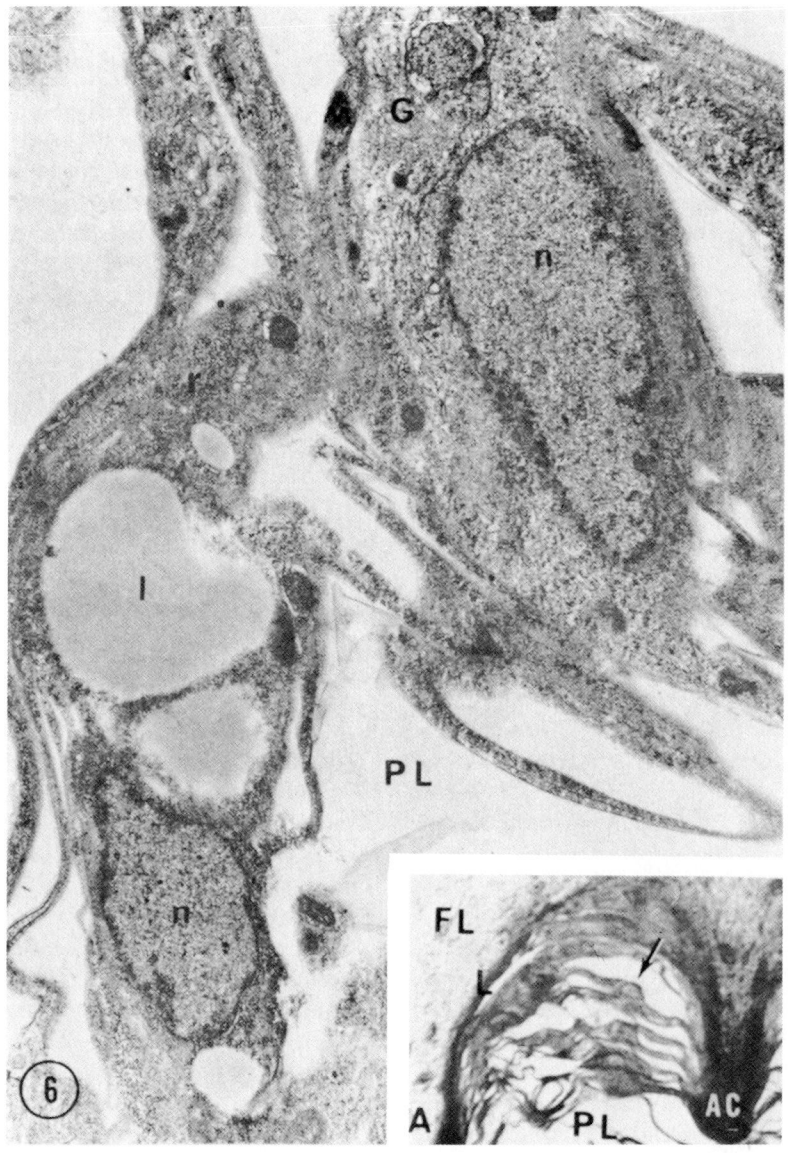

Figure 36. Bipolar squamous epithelial cells that surround the lacuna (inset). Approx. X 2500. Electron photomicrograph illustrates their elongate nature. Approx. X 16,000. (From Allison et al. 1972).

occur. The first change, the completion of a mitochondrial border on the surface tegument of the immature worm, is completed rapidly after withdrawal. The second change represents histogenesis of the wall of the capsule. Initial observations of the histology of the wall are presented by Voge and Heyneman (1957). Voge (1960b) accurately described the fully developed cysticercoid and described the histogenesis of the cysticercoid (1960c). Her data were substantiated and extended by Ubelaker *et al.*

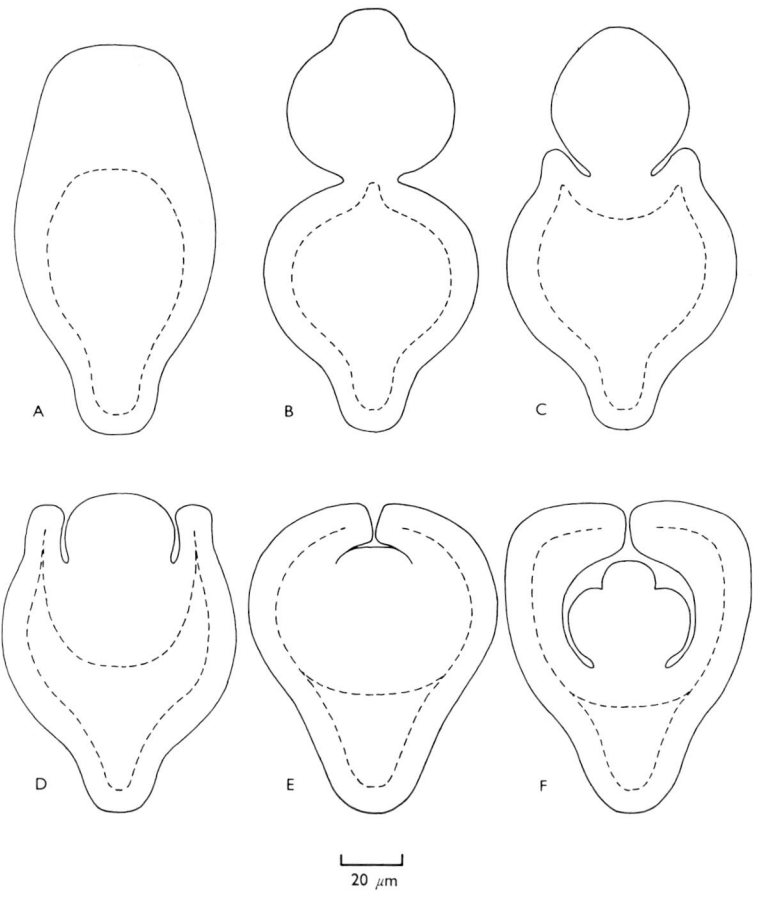

Figure 37. Diagram of retraction of scolex of H. microstoma. Note the cytoplasmic continuity from the scolex to the outer wall of the metacestode. (From Caley 1974).

(1970a). The relationship of the outer layers of the capsule wall of the metacestode is shown in Figure 39. As can be seen in this light photomicrograph, the outer cytoplasmic layer appears as a

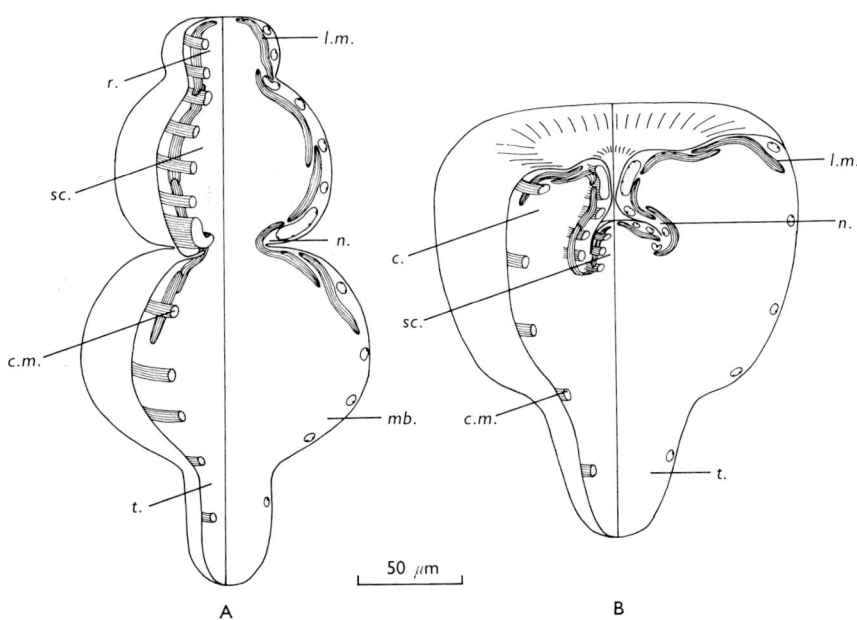

Figure 38. The musculature of the metacestode of Hymenolepis microstoma. The general distribution of circular (c.m.) and longitudinal (l.m.) muscles before (A) and after (B) withdrawal of the scolex. (From Caley 1974).

dense cytoplasmic fringe. By electron microscopy the wall of the cysticercoid (often referred to as the cyst wall or capsule) is a continuation of the cellular architecture observed first in the oncosphere (Figure 40). The outer cytoplasmic layer is continuous with a perinuclear cytoplasm lying below the musculature and basement membrane. This cellular type was described by Bogitsh (1969) as type II cells. It should be emphasized that this cell type is present during the early development of the metacestode and that the distal cytoplasm of this layer apparently

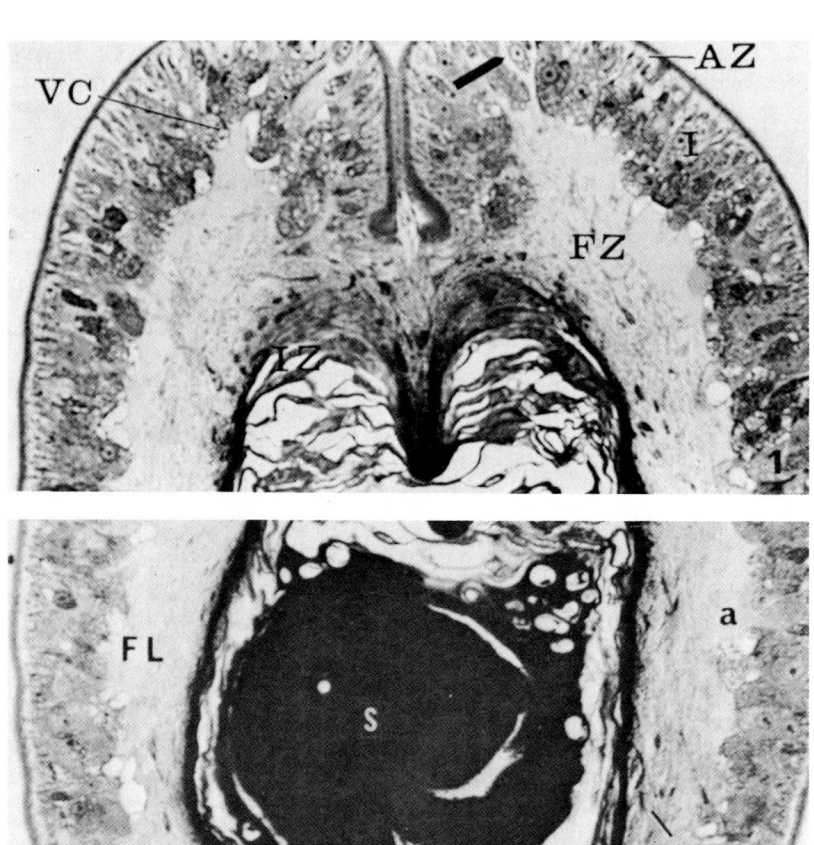

Figure 39. The arrangement of cells in the outer wall of the metacestode (often called 'capsule' or 'cyst') at 8 days of age. The 'hairy layer' is not formed at this stage. The intermediate layer of the wall (FL) is evident and the outer layer (which will form the 'hairy layer') contains numerous cellular types. Anterior canal (A) remains open throughout development. Approx. X 1050. (From Ubelaker et al. 1970a, (top), and Allison et al. 1972 (bottom)).

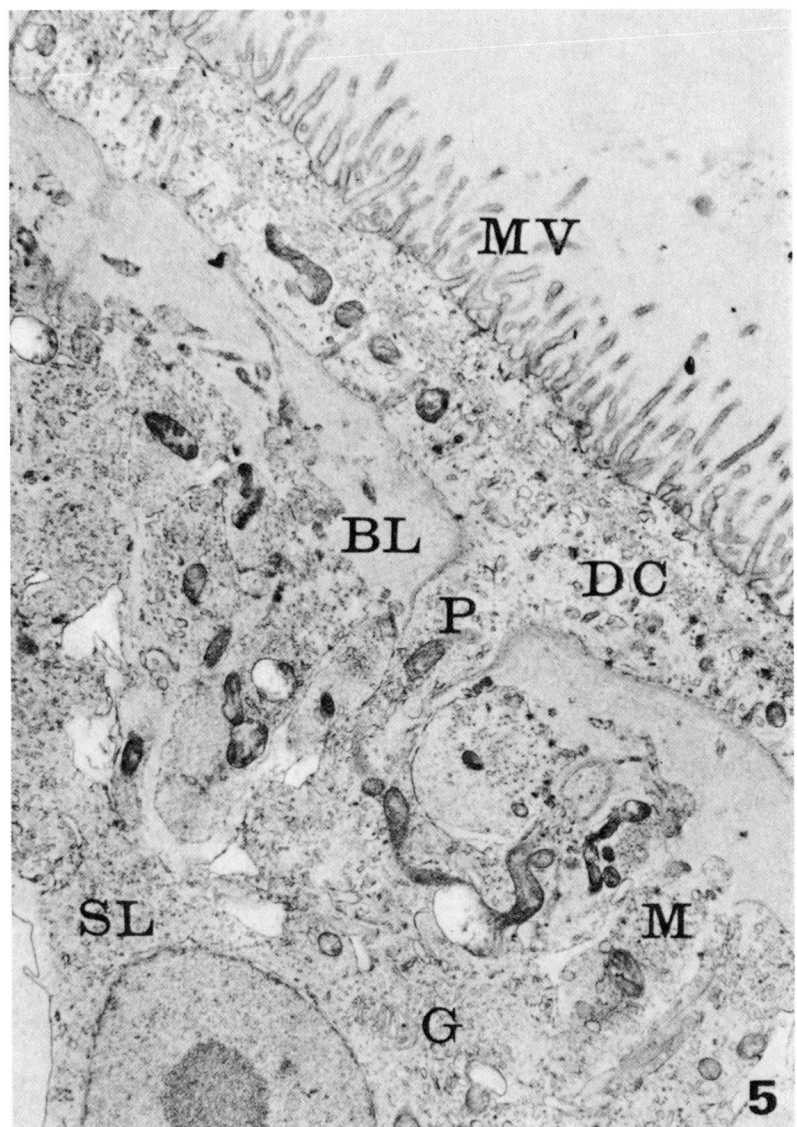

Figure 40. Longitudinal view of outer margin of H. diminuta metacestode. Numerous branched microvilli are present (MV). BL, basal lamina; P, arm of epithelial cell which connects the perinuclear cytoplasm (SL) with surface distal cytoplasm (DC). Approx. X 16,000 (From Ubelaker et al. 1970a).

forms an uninterrupted sheath covering the entire organism, including the developing prescolex. This sheath continues to develop for a short time after withdrawal of the scolex and modifies the scolex surface by the formation of microtriches. As seen in Figure 40, the major alteration of the distal layer following withdrawal of the scolex is a continued thickening of the distal cytoplasm and greater elaboration of the basement layer, particularly the basal lamina component.

A second cellular type observed in the wall of the cysticercoid is a secretory cell characterized by dilated cisternae of granular endoplasmic reticulum. This cell was reported by Bogitsh (1969) as Type 1 cells. The cell was described in detail by Ubelaker et al. (1970a)(Figure 41). The cell has a vesiculated appearance with the highly distended cisternae of rough endoplasmic reticulum. The cisternae are more distended in the peripheral regions of the cell as compared to the perinuclear region.

Bogitsh (1969) found that this cell contains acid phosphatase activity, as demonstrated by a lead salt method. The activity was detected in the product formed in the cisternae. As both Bogitsh and Ubelaker et al. reported, this cell is apparently important in the synthesis of microtubules for the production of bundles of circular fibers located at the base of the peripheral layer.

The inner fibrous region of the wall of the cysticercoid is composed of an active connective tissue cell. This cell type (designated Type A by Allison et al. 1972) contains numerous elongate cytoplasmic products within an amorphous extracellular ground substance filled with fibrillar elements (Figure 42). The cytoplasm of this cell contains mitochondria with numerous cristae, granular endoplasmic reticulum with distended cisternae, and free ribosomes and Golgi elements. This layer of the wall of the cysticercoid lies adjacent to the fibrous layer surrounding the primitive lacuna.

The wall of the cysticercoid of H. diminuta changes dynamically after eight days, with substantial growth occurring in the distal cytoplasm of the surface epithelium. The distal cytoplasm at this

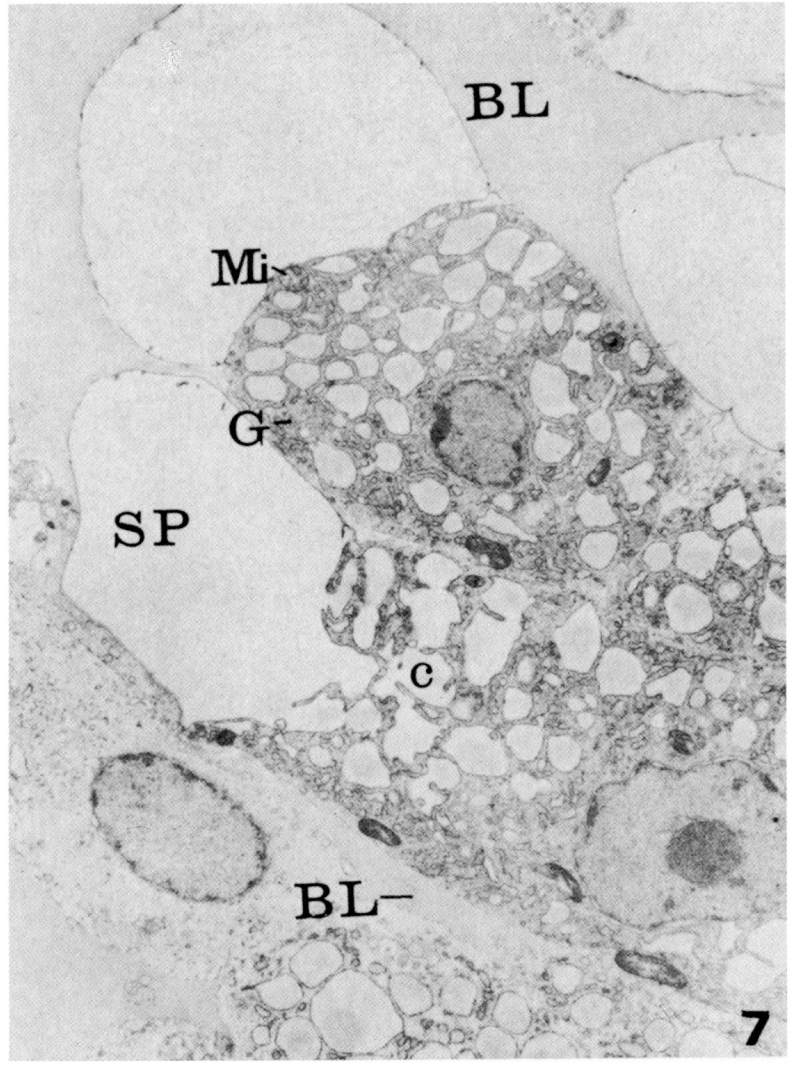

Figure 41. Secretory cells in outer layer of metacestode wall. Early stages of secretion; cells releasing a product (SP) that eventually gives rise to circular fibrils. (From Ubelaker et al. 1970a).

stage of development is clearly arranged into two layers (Figure 43). The outer layer contains a dense network of filaments suggestive of a terminal web whereas the inner component is less dense and contains mitochondria. After the 8th day of development the inner component begins a rapid growth phase and increases greatly in thickness. In addition to many clear vesicles, elongate fibrils are produced which extend through the basement membrane into the distal cytoplasm. The fibrils frequently become grouped together to form bundles. As development continues more bundles form and they represent the 'hairy processes' described by Voge (1960b).

The greatly enlarged distal cytoplasm is presented in Figure 44. Although the dense region of outer cytoplasm is thicker, the inner component has greatly increased. The cytoplasm contains numerous electron-lucent vesicles, membranes, and elongate fibrils.

This cytoplasmic layer is elaborated by the type II cells described by Bogitsh (1969). These cells are still located below the basal lamina and muscles in the vicinity of the type I cells described. The type II cells appear active in producing the electron-lucent vesicles which form large assemblages in the peripheral regions of the cytoplasm, extending into the cytoplasmic arms which connect to the distal cytoplasm. The cytoplasm is filled with ribosomes with small amounts of rough endoplasmic reticulum (Figure 45).

Following the elaboration of the distal cytoplasm, cell type I continues to produce fibrils until the space around the muscles forms a dense fibrillar zone. When this fibrillar zone is completely developed it appears to form bundles of fibrils closely packed together. The fibrils appear to intertwine and do not show any periodicity (Figure 46). The nature of the fibrils is unknown. It seems likely that this arrangement of fibrils was misinterpreted by Voge (1960c) as representing cells of the peripheral layer which she believes gave rise to the hairy layer.

Following development of the outer layer of cytoplasm in the wall of the cysticercoid, many of

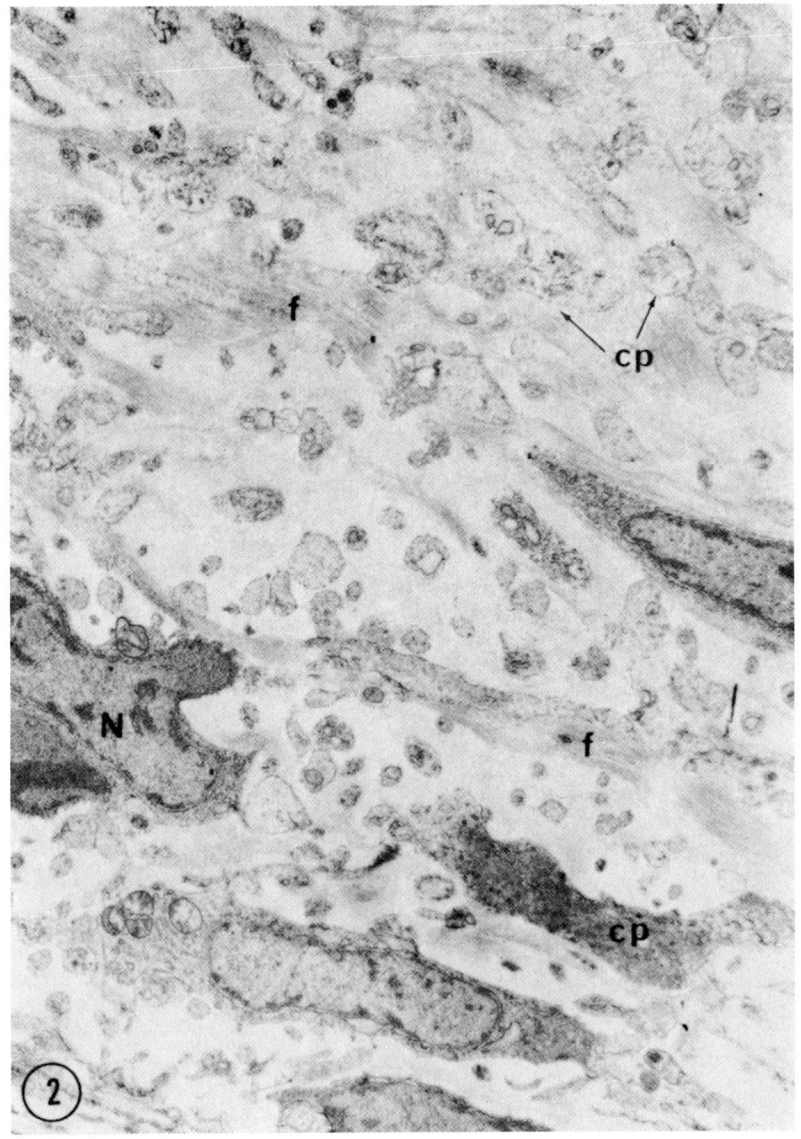

Figure 42. Fibroblastic cells in the inner region of the metacestode wall. Cytoplasmic processes (CP) and extracellular fibrils (EF) are extensive. Approx. X 16,400. (From Allison et al. 1972).

the fibrils join together to form thick fibers which show a clear periodicity (Figure 47). As described by Bogitsh (1969), these fibers have a cross-striation pattern with wide bands of 350 Å alternating with narrow bands of 175 Å. The fibers show a resemblance to collagen fibrils.

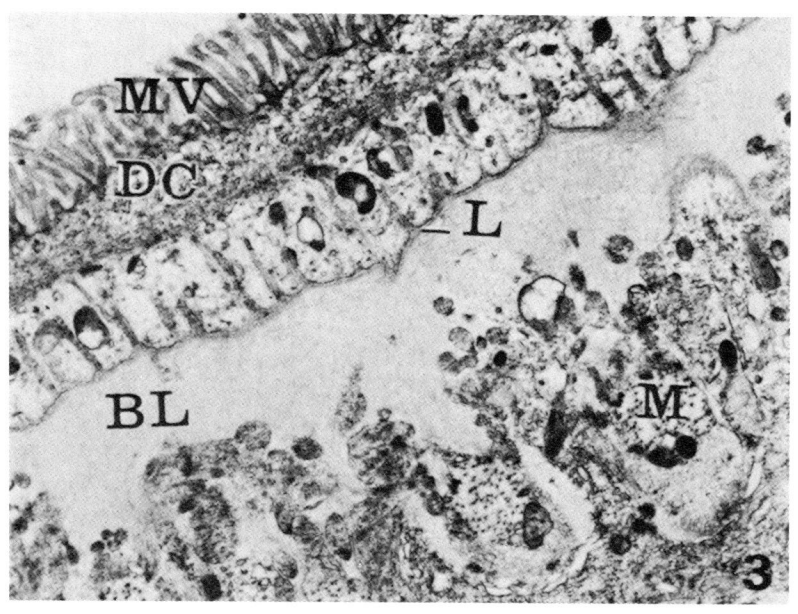

Figure 43. Distal cytoplasm of metacestode wall at 8 days of age. Note microvilli (MV) and distal cytoplasm (DC) divided into an outer dense layer and an inner less dense layer. Approx. X 17,000. (From Ubelaker et al. 1970a).

The inner layer of the cysticercoid wall is filled with an active connective tissue cell which also produces fibrillar elements and is much more dense at maturity than at day 8 (Figure 48; compare with Figure 47). The fibrillar elements appear similar in size and composition to the fibrillar elements produced by the type I cell except in this layer the fibrillar elements are grouped together into strands which are interwoven.

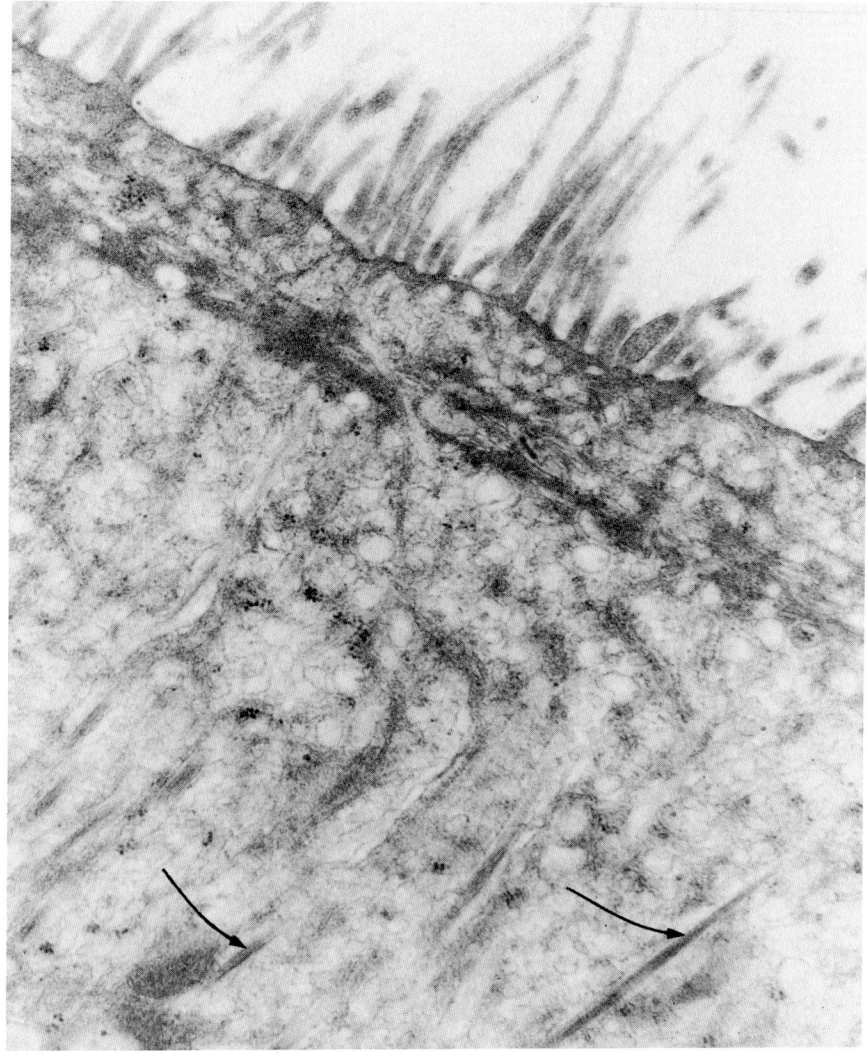

Figure 44. Metacestode wall of 18 day old metacestode of H. diminuta. Distal cytoplasm is more extensive. Two regions are still present but dense fibrils appear in the inner layer (arrows). X 18,000.

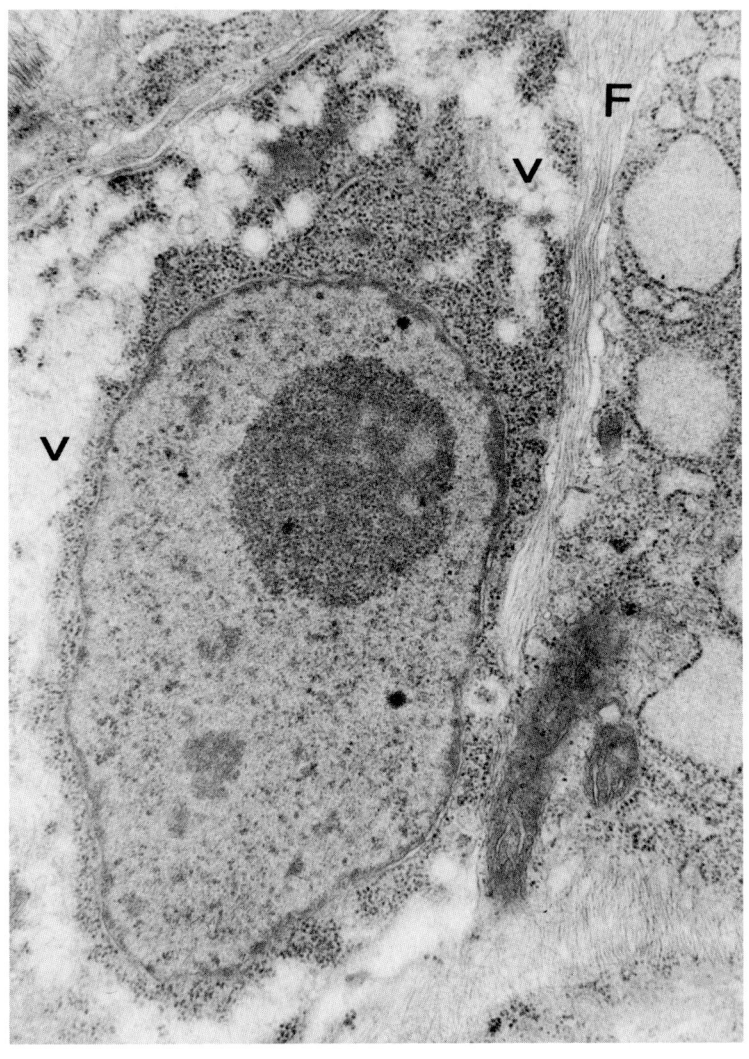

Figure 45. Perinuclear cytoplasm of 18 day old tegumental cell. Nucleus and nucleoli prominent. Nuclear membrane with dense irregular chromatin. Cytoplasm next to nucleus dense with ribosomes, with sparse rough endoplasmic reticulum. Periphery of cell dense with electron lucent vesicles (V) which extend into cytoplasmic arms and distal cytoplasm (see Figure 44). Note fibrils (F) produced by secretory cells (Figure 41). X 33,000.

There are no studies concerned with the development of the excretory system in *H. diminuta*. Goodchild and Harrison (1961) and Freeman and Webb (cited in Freeman 1973) reported that a terminal vesicle and pore may develop at the juncture of the fore-body and mid-body. Excretory canals do extend through the wall of the metacestode and flame cells are frequently encountered (Figure 49). The excretory canals are probably the tubular system mentioned by Voge (1960c).

The surface epithelium of *H. diminuta* is uniform in structure during the first 5 days of metacestode development. Collin (1968) clearly demonstrated by electron microscopy that the surface of newly emerged oncospheres of *H. citelli* possessed an outer covering epithelia containing numerous lamella-like folds that extended from the surface cytoplasm. Collin (1970) extended his observations to the postembryonic stages. Examination of the surface features during the first five days of development in the beetle intermediate host indicated that the entire surface of the metacestode was covered by folds which gradually became smaller and fewer in number. The lamellar-like nature of the surface folds which are evident in the emerged oncosphere disappear and/or become transformed into microvilli. Numerous host cells were observed on the surface. The cells contained microvilli which apparently joined or interdigitated with the microvilli of the metacestode. Since many of the insect hemocytes were apparently cytolyzed, Collin concluded that the beetle hemocytes were not capable of encapsulating the metacestode. Ubelaker *et al.* (1970a) demonstrated by electron microscopy the presence of branched microvilli on the outer capsule wall of mature cysticercoids of *H. diminuta*. Branching of the microvilli occurred at various levels but was most frequently observed near the base. These authors also observed hemocytes in various stages of decay. Numerous vesicles, which appeared to arise from the microvilli, were seen in the vicinity of the cytolyzing hemocytes. The authors proposed the possibility of a secretory function of the surface epithelia, which might suggest a defensive mechanism on the part of the metacestode. Evidence that beetles respond to the presence of *H. diminuta* metacestodes has been provided by Soltice *et al.* (1971), who showed

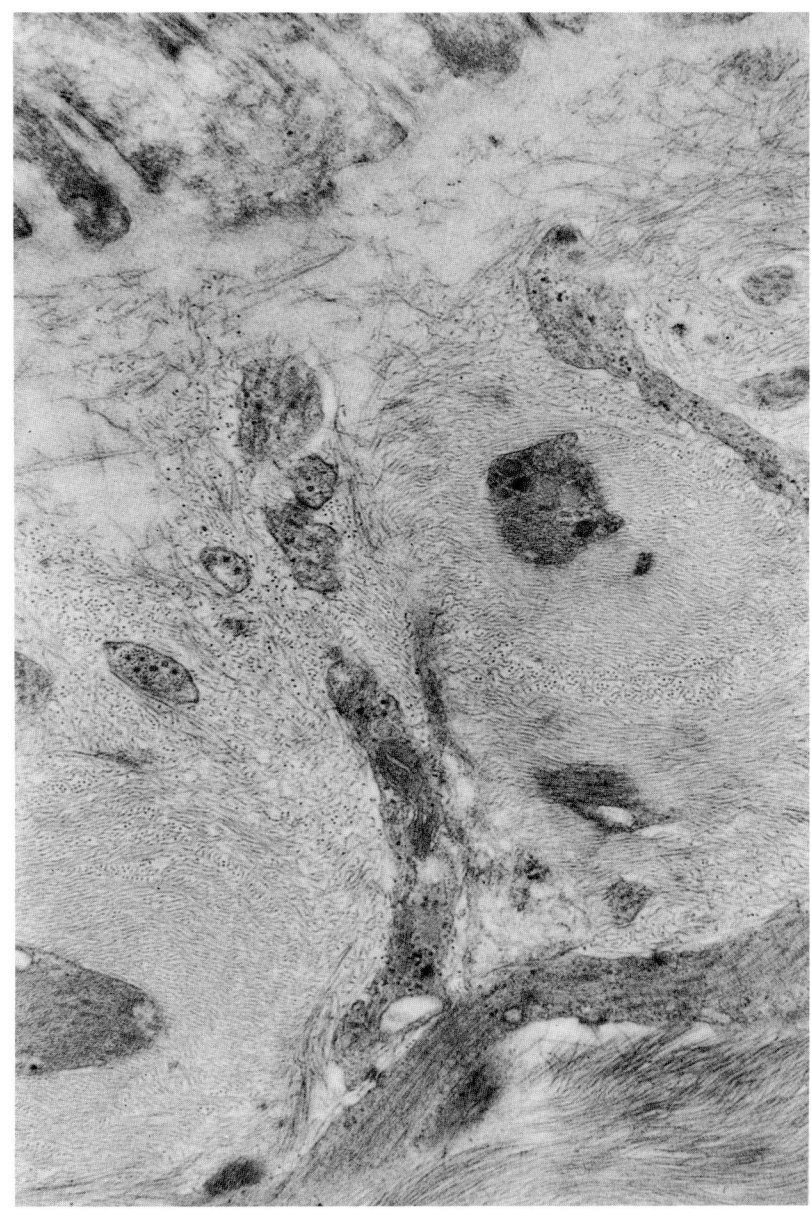

Figure 46. Low magnification of outer wall of metacestode (23 days of age). DC, distal cytoplasm; B, basal lamina; M, muscles; F, fibrils produced by secretory cells. X 14,000.

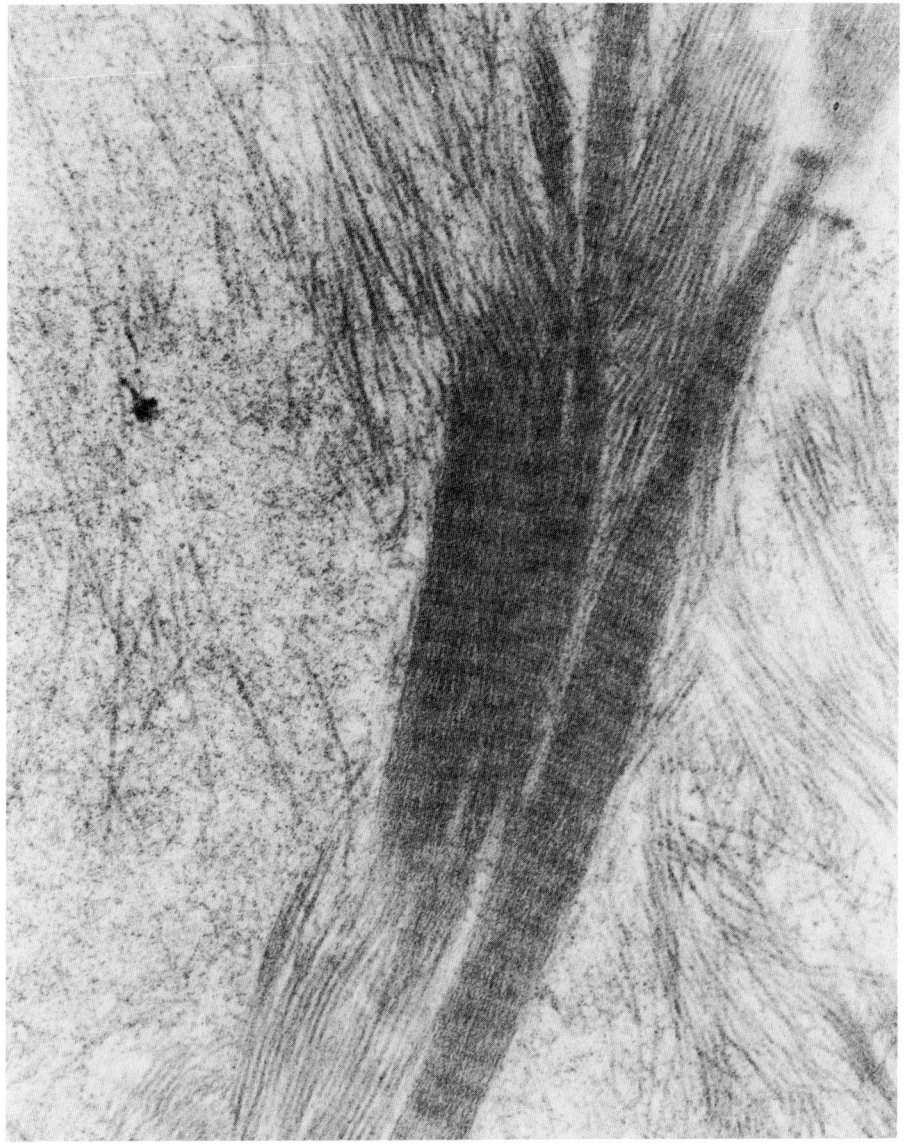

Figure 47. High magnification of fibrils (arrows) collected together in bundles in distal cytoplasm. Note the periodicity. These bundles probably comprise the 'hairy layer' of Voge, 1960a. X 72,800.

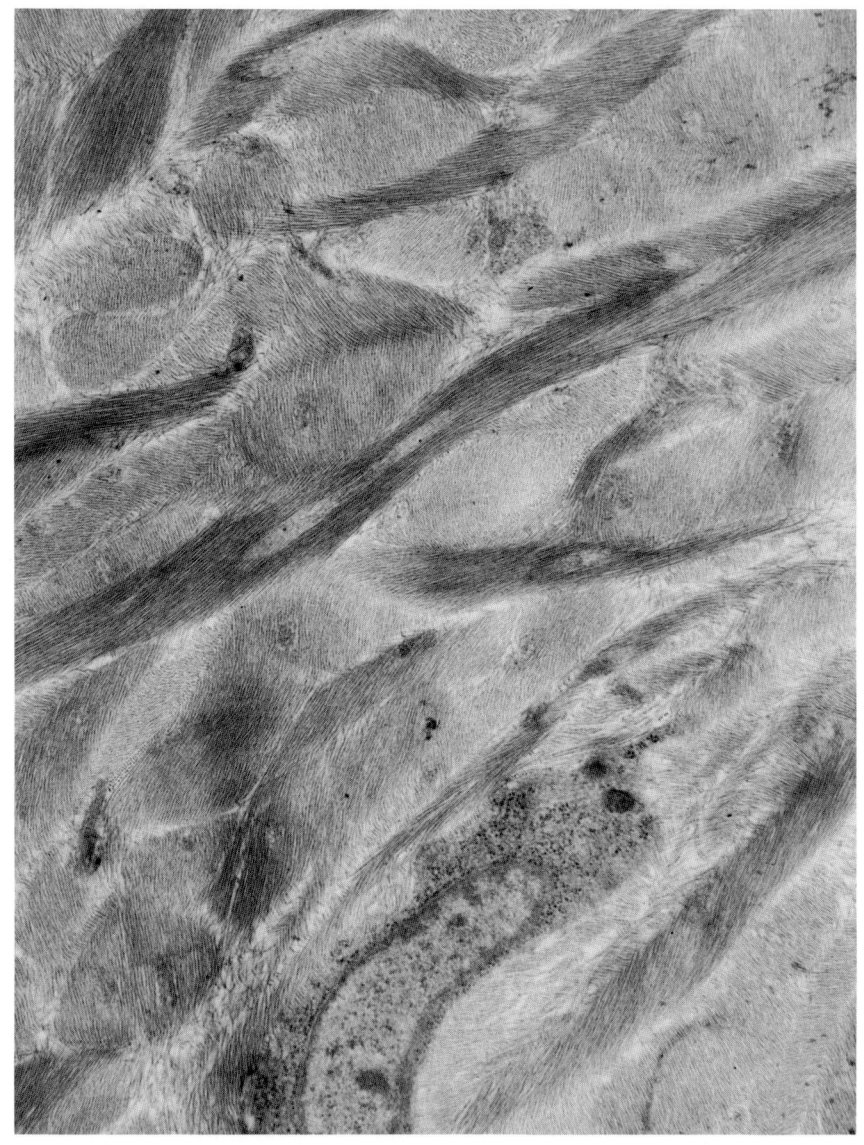

Figure 48. Transmission electron microscopy photomicrograph of inner layer of mature metacestode wall. As observed here, the strands are inter-woven with few cell bodies apparent. N, nucleus of cell body; C, cytoplasm of cell; F, fibrillar region of cell. X 36,900.

that infected beetles have a higher respiratory rate than non-infected ones. MacDonald and Wilson (1964) and Dunkley and Mettrick (1971) showed that mortality was higher in heavily infected beetles than in lightly infected ones. Heyneman and Voge (1971) compared the responses of *Tribolium confusum* infected with *H. citelli*, *H. microstoma*, and *H. diminuta*. Hemocytes were observed on the surfaces of all metacestodes early in the infection but only *H. citelli* oncospheres became encapsulated (although temporarily). Heyneman and Voge suggested that the "…. disappearance of the host cells, as seen under the light microscope …. suggests the possibility that the microvillar layer interfaces with or destroys the host cells".

The evasion of the hemocytic defense reaction of certain insects by metacestodes of *H. diminuta* was elegantly studied by Lackie (1976). Utilizing sterile culture techniques, she removed metacestodes from the body cavity and placed them on a monolayer of hemocytes in tissue culture. After four hours, significant differences could not be detected between hemocytes exposed or not exposed to the metacestodes. Further experimentation indicated that latex beads injected into the body cavity of infected beetles are rapidly covered by a layer of hemocytes 2 hours after implantation, whereas, the metacestode surface remains relatively clean of hemocytes or debris, which might be expected to occur if damage to the hemocytes was occurring. Lackie concluded that lysis of hemocytes on the parasite's surface is probably due to some action of the parasite, but probably not directly as a protective measure. Lackie suggested that perhaps some product of the digestive or excretory process released at the parasite's surface may be responsible. Identification of this material requires further investigation.

At present, the available evidence suggests that, prior to withdrawal, the entire surface epithelium of the metacestode is covered by a branched microvillar border which resists hemocyte action. Voge and Heyneman (1957) clearly demonstrated that withdrawal of the scolex occurs at 5 to 6 days after infection of beetles maintained at 30°C. Although the rudiments of suckers are evident, it is not clear if the tegument itself had begun to transform into the microtriches that characterize the adult tegument

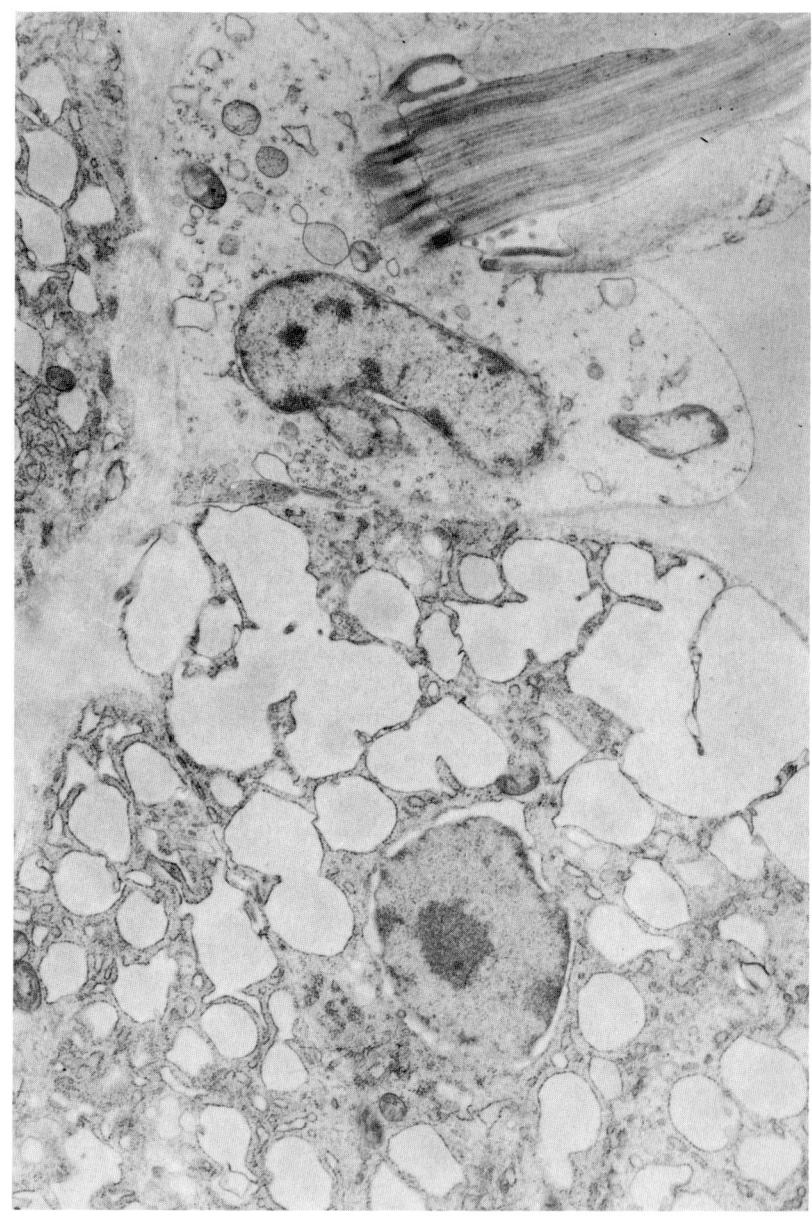

Figure 49. Protonephridium in wall of metacestode. N, nucleus; C, cytoplasm; arrow points to cilia. The protonephridium is located adjacent to three secretory cells in outer wall. X 18,000.

Structure and Ultrastructure of the Larvae and Metacestodes

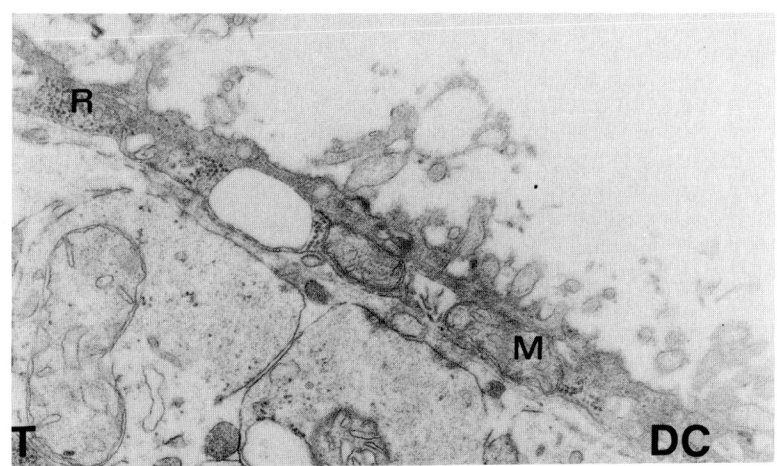

Figure 50. Surface of scolex prior to withdrawal illustrating distal cytoplasm (DC) which is rich in mitochondria (M), and dense populations of ribosomes (R). Ribosomes also appear in the tegumental cell body (T). X 31,200.

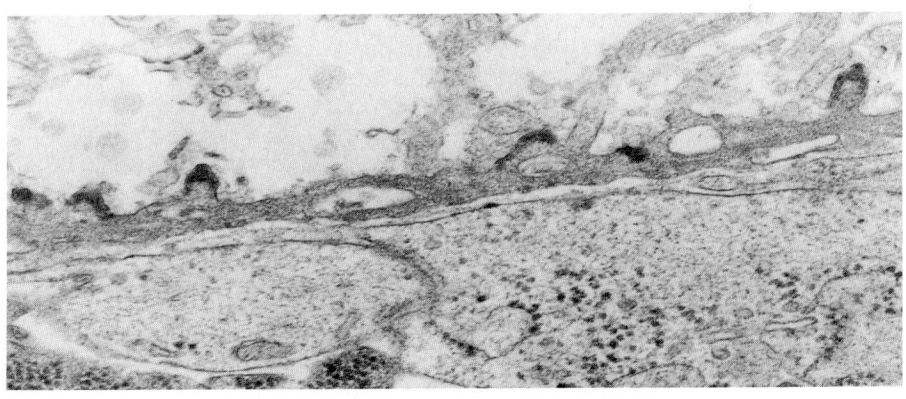

Figure 51. Accumulation of electron dense material at surface membrane forming multilaminate base plates. The lack of microvilli at these sites, but the presence of debris, suggests that sloughing of the microvilli may occur. X 44,550.

(see discussion of microtriches by Lumsden and Specian, this volume).

To determine if withdrawal of the scolex is required for microtriches to develop, experiments were conducted in my laboratory. Infected beetles were maintained at 22°C, which delayed withdrawal of the prescolex until day 7 or 8. Although infections varied from light to heavy, there was considerable variation in withdrawal of the scolex. Examination of the scolex surface before microtrichal formation revealed a structure similar to that described by Collin (1970) for *H. citelli*. Prior to a morphological change in the surface features, numerous ribosomes, singly and in clusters, were observed to occur in the cytons of the epithelium lying below the surface and then to accumulate in the distal cytoplasm (Figure 50). Following the appearance of ribosomes, an electron dense granular material appears below the surface membrane but does not extend into the microvilli which are often observed in the same field (Figure 51). There is some evidence that the microvilli are sloughed from the surface but no conclusion could be drawn from the static photomicrographs. Multilaminate baseplates are formed first and additional granular materials appear to be synthesized, forming the shaft of the microtrich (Figure 52). The synthesis of the dense material occurs below the surface of the plasma membrane. This observation is in contrast to the mechanism of microtrich formation described for a pseudophyllidean, *Spirometra mansonoides*. This species was carefully studied by Lumsden *et al.* (1974), who suggested that synthesis of the shaft material occurred at some distance from the microtrich and was transported there in vesicles. From our study, we found that microtrich formation begins at the apical end and extends posteriorly to the suckers. Before withdrawal, the metacestode may have branched microvilli covering all free surfaces except the anterior end of the prescolex where microtriches are developing. Following withdrawal, the surfaces that are withdrawn into the cavity (primitive lacuna) continue to form microtriches in a posterior wave. The surfaces of the metacestode, including the lining of the anterior canal, maintain the branched microvilli. The shafts of microtriches present on the scolex grow extremely long (see Cooper *et al.* 1975).

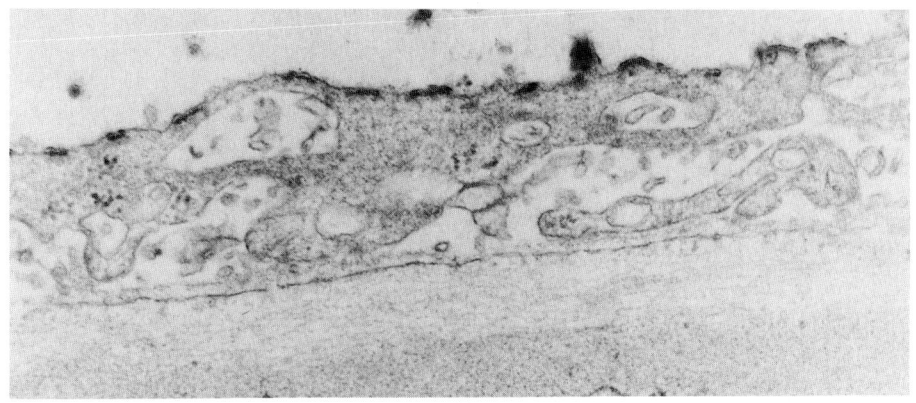

Figure 52. Scolex tegument as base plates form. X 35,000.

XVI. CHEMICAL COMPOSITION

Since the report of Prescott and Voge (1959) indicating the synthesis of RNA in the wall of the cysticercoid, several investigators have reported on the chemical composition and the biosynthetic activities of the cysticercoid. The results of these studies are presented below.

A. *Proteins*. Goodchild and Wells (1957) reported sixteen amino acids in 48 hour hydrolysates from cysticercoids of *H. diminuta* (20 days old). Three amino acids, methionine, arginine, and threonine, were absent in the 48 hour hydrolysates. However, both methionine and arginine were demonstrated in 36 hour hydrolysates.

Baron (1971) demonstrated proteins in all tissues of cysticercoids of *Raillientina cesticellus*. Areas of protein concentration of either tyrosine or tryptophan, or both, included the distal cytoplasm of the capsule, nuclei of the intermediate layer, and nuclei of the scolex. Reflexed tissue (lining of the cysticercoid cavity) around the scolex also possessed proteins but were less reactive with the stain. The globules present in abundance in the distal cytoplasm were shown to be proteinaceous, containing

TABLE 2. Effect of various compounds at a concentration of 8.0mM on the uptake of 0.4mM AIB in cysticercoids of Hymenolepis diminuta. Values listed are means of 4 determinations. Significance of inhibition was determined by t-test at 5% level (after Armes and Coates 1971).

Compound	Inhibition (%)	Compound	Inhibition (%)
Glucose	0	L-Alanine	92.5
Galactose	0	L-Aspartic acid	28.0
Fructose	0	Cycloleucine	87.7
Lactose	0	L-Histidine	37.9
Adenine	0	L-Leucine	68.8
Uracil	0	L-Lysine	0
Sodium acetate	0	L-Arginine	0
Sodium stearate	0	L-Methionine	91.1
Sodium lactate	0	L-Tryptophan	41.7
Betaine	0	L-Valine	48.5
Sarcosine	0	D-Alanine	85.9
		D-Methionine	80.8
		D-Valine	61.0

particularly tyrosine. Protein, probably in association with muco-substances (hyaluronic acid) forms the ground substance of most cells and functions hydrodynamically to control turgescence and physiologically to control random diffusion of large molecules. Although it is also known that the protein content of the 'cuticle' of young plerocercoids decreases with age (Morris and Finnegan 1968), no information is available for cysticercoids of *H. diminuta*.

Arme and Coates (1971) found α-aminoisobutyric acid (AIB) labeled with ^{14}C was taken up linearly with time for 10 minutes at a specific site. Millimolar alanine and aspartic acid competitively inhibited the uptake, but arginine had no effect. These authors (1973) expanded their observations and reported the uptake was saturable with a K_t of 0.27 nM and a V_{max} of 1.78 nmoles/100 cysticercoids/2 minutes and was pH dependent. Compounds that inhibited or did not inhibit AIB uptake are presented in Table 2. The authors could not determine if the scolex, wall of the metacestode, or both were important in absorption of the AIB.

B. *Enzymatic activity*. Heyneman and Voge (1960), Bogitsh and Nunnally (1966) and Bogitsh (1967) reported the presence of succinic dehydrogenase activity in several species of *Hymenolepis*, including *H. diminuta*. The scolex inner fibrous layer and cells in the cercomer showed high concentrations of activity. Temperature influenced the intensity of the enzymatic activity during development. Temperatures above 37°C inhibited enzyme activity in developing *H. diminuta* but not in *H. nana*.

Lactate dehydrogenase activity was detected in larvae and cysticercoids of *H. diminuta* by Walkey and Fairbairn (1973). These authors observed that the enzyme kinetics in these forms are distinctly different from the kinetics of lactate dehydrogenase in the adult. Carter and Fairbairn (1975) reported two isozymes of pyruvate kinase in oncospheres and cysticercoids of *H. diminuta*, whereas three additional ones were present in the juvenile worms and adult worms. The isozymes were found to be activated by fructose-1,6-P_2, but were not inhibited by alanine which is consistent with a fermentative function. These authors suggested that the probable function is to control the specific composition of lactic, acetic, and succinic acid mixtures that are secreted (excreted) at different stages of development. As suggested by Fairbairn (1970), the presence of specific different isozymes in the larval and metacestode stages provides evidence for adaptive control of metabolism (Carter and Fairbairn 1975).

Bogitsh (1967) presented evidence for the presence of nonspecific acid phosphatase activity of pH 5.0 in the intermediate cell layer and tail parenchyma of the capsules of both *H. diminuta* and *H. microstoma*. At the cellular level, Bogitsh (1969) demonstrated activity in smooth membrane-bound vesicles in the cytoplasm of Type I cells and in apparently degenerating cytoplasm in larger vesicles and he found a similar distribution for aryl sulfatase. Phosphatase activity was also detected in the tegument of the scolex. Highest activity occurred at pH 6 and persisted through pH 9.0. Bogitsh postulated a role for these enzymes in excystation.

Adenosine phosphatase was reported by Bogitsh (1967) in the musculature of the scolex and in the circular fibers of the capsule wall. A diffuse reaction of LDH, SDH and MDH activity was observed in the intermediate cell layer of the capsule. Additionally, NADH-NBT reductase activity was present in the tegument and parenchyma of the scolex and intermediate cell layer of the capsule. These mitochondrial enzymes indicate the presence of active mitochondria. Based on histochemical evidence, Bogitsh suggested the presence of mitochondria in the tegument (distal cytoplasm) of the scolex of the metacestode, in contrast to the scolex of the adult tapeworm. The presence of these mitochondria in the tegument of the metacestode scolex has been confirmed by ultrastructural observations (Allison *et al.* 1972).

Cholinesterase activity was detected in the larval tegument and nerves of the scolex. According to Bogitsh (1967), cholinesterase as well as the above stated phosphatase activity may indicate membrane transport in the metacestode, a function subsequently lost in the adult.

Moczon (1973b) found nine specific or nonspecific phosphatases in oncospheres and cysticercoids

TABLE 3.

Distribution of phosphatases in oncospheres and cysticercoids of *Hymenolepis diminuta* (after Moczon 1973b).

No. of test	Enzyme and author of the method	pH of the incubating method	Intensities of the histochemical reactions					
			oncosphere	cercomere	cysticercoid			scolex
					outer envelope	fibrous zone	inner envelope	
1	Nonspecific alkaline phosphatase (α-Naphthyl phosphate – Fast Red TR)	10.0	–	–	–	–	±	++
2	Nonspecific acid phosphatase (α-Naphthyl phosphate – Fast Blue)	5.0	–	++	++	+	+++	+++
3	ATP-ase (Mg^{2+}) (Wachstein and Meisel 1957)	7.2	+++	++	+++	–	+++	+++
4	ATP (Ca^{2+}) (Padykula and Herman 1955)	9.4	+++	++	+++	–	+++	+++
5	5 – Nucleotidase (Wachstein and Meisel 1957)	7.2	–	–	+	–	–	–
6	Nucleoside diphosphatase (Lazarus and Burden 1962)	7.2	+	±	+	–	+	+
7	Glucose-6-phosphatase (Allen 1961)	5.5	–	–	–	–	–	–
8	Thiamine pyrophosphatase (Novikoff and Goldfischer 1961)	7.2	–	+	–	–	±	±
9	Fructose-1, 6-diphosphatase (Brolin *et al.* 1968)	7.4	–	–	–	–	–	–

of *H. diminuta* (Table 3). Oncospheres were found to possess only three phosphatases, whereas cysticercoids possessed seven. The lack of alkaline phosphatase in the tegument of the wall of the cysticercoid and the presence of this enzyme in the tegument of the scolex suggested to Moczon that only the scolex was active in absorption.

Moczon (1973a) surveyed twenty-one additional enzymes from oncospheres and cysticercoids of *H. diminuta*. The activities of these enzymes and their distribution are presented in Table 4. Based on these findings and the report of Soltice *et al.* (1971) that cysticercoids of *H. diminuta* have an intensive oxygen consumption, Moczon concluded that cysticercoids probably have an aerobic metabolism, possibly a tricarboxylic acid cycle and cytochrome system. The presence of two enzymes of the pentose cycle also suggests an anerobic path of glucose metabolism. The nitrogen metabolism of cysticercoids differed from the oncospheres in regards to the source of excretory nitrogen, this source being L-glutamate in cysticercoids and L-methionine and probably other D- or L-amino acids in the oncospheres. The distribution of some enzymic activities in tissues of cysticercoids of *H. diminuta* was illustrated by Moczon and is presented in Figure 53.

C. *Polysaccharides*. The only polysaccharide identified in cysticercoids of *H. diminuta* is glycogen, and this compound has been observed in the cercomer, scolex musculature, and tegument of the scolex (Heyneman and Voge 1957). The amount of glycogen increased during development and growth of the cysticercoid. Glycogen was reduced in cysticercoids developing at suboptimal temperatures and older cysticercoids (90 days) did not show changes in the distribution or amount of this polysaccharide. Bogitsh and Nunnally (1966) and Moczon (1977d) have confirmed the observations of Heyneman and Voge.

By electron microscopy, Collin (1970) reported the presence of beta-glycogen in myofibers and both alpha-and beta-glycogen in cells lining the central cavity of cysticercoids of a related cestode *H. citelli* at 3 days of age.

TABLE 4

Activities of some enzymes (oxidoreductases) in oncospheres and cysticercoids of *Hymenolepis diminuta* (after Moczon 1973a).

No. of test	Enzyme	Intensities of histochemical reactions					
		oncosphere	cysticercoid				
			cercomere	outer envelope	fibrous zone	inner envelope	scolex
1.	Isocitrate: NAD oxidoreductase	-	-	-	-	+|+	+
2.	Isocitrate: NADP oxidoreductase	+++	+	+	-	+|+	+|+
3.	Succinate dehydrogenase	++	+++	+	s	+++	+++
4.	L-Malate: NAD oxidoreductase	++	+	+|+	s	+++	+++
5.	NADH: tetrazolium oxidoreductase (NADH diaphorase)	+++	++	++	s	++	++
6.	NADPH: tetrazolium oxidoreductase (NADPH diaph.)	++	+|+	+	s	+	+
7.	NADH: tetrazolium oxidored. ⎱ as soluble "menad-	++	+++	+++	-	+++	+++
8.	NADPH: tetrazolium oxidored. ⎰ ione reductases"	+|+	-	+|+	s	+	++
9.	NADPH: NAD transhydrogenase	+|+	+|+	+|+|+	|+	+++	+++
10.	Cytochrome oxidase	s	+	+	s	+++	+++
11.	Glycerol-3-phosphate dehydrogenase	++	+	+|+|+	-	++	++
12.	L-Lactate: NAD oxidoreductase	+	+	+|-	s	+	+
13.	Glucose-6-phosphate: NADP oxidoreductase	++	-	-	-	++	+++
14.	as above but with NAD instead of NADP	+|+	-	+|-	s	+++	++
15.	6-Phosphogluconate: NADP oxidoreductase	-	++	+|+|-	s	+++	+++
16.	L-Glutamate: NAD oxidoreductase	-	+|-	-	-	+++	+++
17.	L-Glutamate: NADP oxidoreductase	+++	-	-	-	++	++
18.	L-Methionine: oxygen oxidoreductase	-	-	-	-	-	-
19.	3-Hydroxybutyrate: NAD oxidoreductase	-	-	-	-	-	-
20.	Alcohol: NAD oxioreductase	-	-	-	-	-	-
21.	Choline: tetrazolium oxidoreductase	-	-	-	-	-	-
22.	Peroxidase	+	+	+	-	+	++

The intensities of histochemical reactions with the use of TNBT as an electron acceptor were read and evaluated after preparations were incubated for 45 minutes in appropriate media at 35°C.

Key: +++ high intensity; ++ moderate intensity; + low intensity; and s scarcely perceptible intensity; - no reaction.

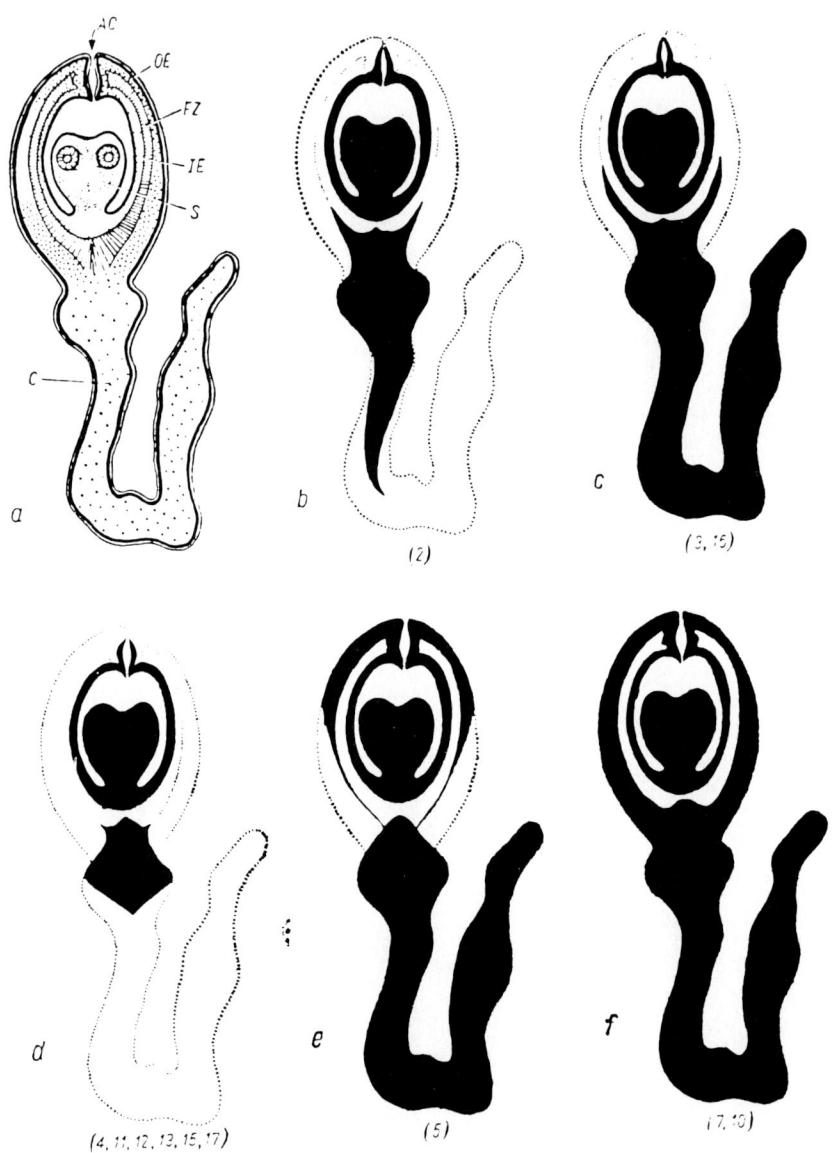

Figure 53. Schematic diagrams of selected enzymatic activities in the cysticercoid of *H. diminuta*. Black areas represent moderate to high activity; clear areas represent absence of or low activity. The morphology of the mature cysticercoid of *H. diminuta* is presented at a. Note the open anterior canal (AC). The remnant of the primitive lacuna is not shown. It is located between the reflexed region of the scolex (S) and the fibrous zone (FZ). (After Moczon 1973a).

Graham and Berntzen (1970) suggested the uptake of glucose by metacestodes by examining *in vitro* cultures of *H. diminuta*. Subsequently, Arme, Middleton and Scott (1973) reported the absorption of glucose and sodium acetate by metacestodes of *H. diminuta*. Two minute incubations in glucose concentrations between 0.2 and 3.0 mM resulted in a nonlinear uptake of the compound with respect to concentration. K_t values of 1.54 mM and a V_{max} of 6.6×10^{-4} μmoles/100 cysticercoids/2 minutes were obtained. Galactose was found to be a competitive inhibitor and its K_i as an inhibitor of glucose uptake was 1.19 mM. Uptake of glucose was not inhibited by fructose, fatty acids, or amino acids. Sodium acetate was observed to be absorbed nonlinearly with respect to concentrations between 0.2 and 3.0 mM but linearly in concentrations between 5 and 20 mM, which suggested a diffusion component at high concentrations. A diffusion rate of 0.6×10^{-4} μmoles/100 cysticercoids/2 minutes was calculated. Acetate uptake was inhibited with short-chain fatty acids. A long-chain fatty acid, sodium stearate, showed no inhibition. Sodium butyrate and sodium propionate were competitive inhibitors of acetate uptake. The results indicate kinetically distinct transport loci for the absorption of α-aminoisobutyric acid, glucose, and sodium acetate. Moczon (1977e) reported the localization of the phosphorylase system and of amylo-(1, 4-1, 6)-transglucosidase in the scolex, inner envelope, and cercomer of the metacestode of *H. diminuta*. The ratio of alpha- to beta-phosphorylases was reported to be controlled by cAMP-dependent protein kinase, phosphorylase b kinase, and protein phosphatase. Moczon (1977f) reported glycogen synthetase activity in the scolex, 'inner envelope', cercomer, and musculature of the wall of the metacestode.

D. *Lipids*. Voge (1960a) demonstrated the presence of lipid-like substances in the peripheral tissue layer, the wall and the cavity of the lacuna, and scolex. Cerebroside and cholesterol positive reactions were also observed.

XVII. EXTERNAL FACTORS INFLUENCING DEVELOPMENT

It is commonly observed by students that exposure of oncospheres to beetle hosts results in a seemingly random distribution of cysticercoids in the beetle population. Some beetles apparently contain only a few metacestodes, while others contain numerous specimens and the metacestodes usually exhibit variation in their development.

A major parameter of infection and subsequent development is temperature. Voge and Turner (1956) reported that the most favorable temperature for development of the metacestodes of *H. diminuta* was 30°C, whereby mature metacestodes were obtained in eight days. Decreasing temperatures had the effect of lengthening the time of development (23 days at 20°C), whereas increasing temperatures increased the abnormalities in the metacestodes (Voge and Heyneman 1958). These results have been confirmed by many investigators including Soltice *et al.* (1971) and Dunkley and Mettrick (1971). Voge (1959a) found that the higher temperature of 38.5°C at days 3 and 5 of development produced two general effects: failure of scolex withdrawal and lack of infectivity. She also reported that abnormalities, apparently due to the high temperature stresses, could be markedly reduced by changing the diet of the adult or larval beetles to pure sugars instead of whole wheat flour (1959b), and that the length of temperature stress was important (1961). High ambient temperatures sustained shorter than 24 hours only delayed growth and maturation, whereas similar stress of 48 hour duration interfered with differentiation - enhancing or inhibiting normal histogenesis, and thus producing abnormal metacestodes. Soltice *et al.* (1971) proposed that the effect of temperature on the intensity of infection was probably related to the activity of enzymes involved in digesting the embryonic envelopes or to those enzymes involved in activation and penetration of the oncosphere. Dunkley and Mettrick (1971) suggested that increased feeding activity, allowing the intake of more food and thus more oncospheres, was the most important factor regulated by temperature that influenced infections in beetles.

Sex of the intermediate host is rarely recorded. Kelly *et al.* (1967) reported that the sex of an intermediate host *Tribolium confusum* influenced infectivity. In beetles less than five weeks old, females had a higher percentage of infection than males. Beetles older than 23 weeks had a higher percentage of infection in male beetles than in females. Soltice *et al.* (1971) found no differences in the percentage of infection in *T. confusum* or *T. castaneum* males or females, but reported that development of the metacestode was more rapid in the female of each species (although age differences could not be discounted).

Starvation of beetles prior to feeding is generally practiced by most investigators to insure a heavy infection. While Kelly *et al.* (1967) found prior starvation of *T. confusum* did not influence infectivity, Dunkley and Mettrick (1971) reported that a minimum period of four days starvation was required to cause significant increases in metacestodes recovered per beetle. These latter authors concluded ".... that the number of cysticercoids recovered per beetle was directly related to the amount of feeding carried out by the beetles".

Crowding effects in heavily infected beetles have been noted (Voge and Turner 1956; Voge and Heyneman 1957; MacDonald and Wilson 1964; Dunkley and Mettrick 1971). Cysticercoids in heavily infected beetles are generally smaller in size, with shorter cercomers, compared with those from light infections. However, crowding appears to have no effect on infectivity of the cysticercoids to their definitive hosts.

Kelly *et al.* (1967) found that age of the intermediate host *Tribolium confusum* influenced the incidence and size of metacestodes of *H. diminuta*. Older females had a significantly smaller burden and prevalence of cysticercoids than young or middle-aged females. Among males, those of middle-age were shown to have a higher incidence than young or old beetles. Dunkley and Mettrick (1971) confirmed these observations and showed an increase in the average number of cysticercoids established per beetle as the age of the beetles increased.

The length of time beetles fed on oncospheres was found by Dunkley and Mettrick (1971) to have the greatest influence on the establishment of an infec-

tion in beetles. These authors suggested that "....
the four significant factors affecting the number of
mature cysticercoids established per beetle may all
be explained in terms of food intake by the beetles".

Several substances are known to interfere with
development of metacestodes of *H. diminuta*. Evans
and Novak (1976) fed infected beetles on mixtures of
flour containing 0.005 to 20 grams of mebendazole
(Telmin: methyl-5-benzoyl benzimidazole-2-carbamate).
At 0.1 gram/10 gram flour, a retarding effect on
development was observed. One gram or higher concentrations were lethal to some, but not all, cysticercoids.

Mettrick and Parnell (1967) found lethal effects
upon metacestodes in *Tribolium confusum* which had
walked for one to three hours on filter paper dampen-
ed in a chemosterilant triethylene-thiophoramide.
They found a 100% mortality when exposure of beetles
to this drug occurred at least two days before, and
three days after, initiation of infection.

REFERENCES

1. Allison, V. F., Ubelaker, J. E. and Cooper, N. B., The fine structure of the cysticercoid of *Hymenolepis diminuta*. The inner wall of the capsule. *Z. Parasitenk.* *39*, 137-147 (1972).
2. Arme, C. and Coates, A., Active transport of an amino acid by cysticercoid larvae of *Hymenolepis diminuta*. *J. Parasitol.* *57*, 1369-1370 (1971).
3. Arme, C. and Coates, A., *Hymenolepis diminuta*: Active transport of α-aminoisobutyric acid by cysticercoid larvae. *Int. J. Parasitol.* *3*, 533-560 (1973).
4. Arme, C., Middleton, A. and Scott, J. P., Absorption of glucose and sodium acetate by cysticercoid larvae of *Hymenolepis diminuta*. *J. Parasitol.* *59*, 214 (1973).
5. Bacigalupo, J., Estudio sobre la evolución biólogica de algunos parásitos del genéro *Hymenolepis* (Weinland 1958). *Semana Médica* *35*, 1249-1267 (1928).
6. Baron, J. P., On the histology, histochemistry and ultrastructure of the cysticercoid of

Raillietina cesticillus (Molin 1958) Fuhrmann 1920 (Cestoda, Cyclophyllidea). *Parasitology 62*, 233-245 (1971).

7. Berntzen, A. K. and Voge, M., In vitro hatching oncospheres of four hymenolepidid cestodes. *J. Parasitol. 51*, 235-242 (1965).

8. Bogitsh, B. J., Histochemical localization of some enzymes in cysticercoids of two species of *Hymenolepis*. *Exp. Parasitol. 21*, 373-379 (1967).

9. Bogitsh, G. J., Fine structural localization of acid phosphatase and aryl sulfatase activities in the intermediate layer of *Hymenolepis diminuta* cystercoids. *Trans. Am. Micros. Soc. 88*, 411-419 (1969).

10. Bogitsh, B. J. and Nunnally, D. A., Histochemistry of *Hymenolepis microstoma* (Cestoda: Hymenolepididae) II. Regional distribution of succinic dehydrogenase. *Parasitology 56*, 55-61 (1966).

11. Caley, J., The functional significance of scolex retraction and subsequent cyst formation in the cysticercoid larva of *Hymenolepis microstoma*. *Parasitology 68*, 207-227 (1974).

12. Carter, C. E. and Fairbairn, D., Multienzymic nature of pyruvate kinase during development of *Hymenolepis diminuta* (Cestoda). *J. Exp. Zool. 194*, 439-488 (1975).

13. Chen, H. T., Reactions of *Ctenocephalides felis* to *Dipylidium caninum*. *Z. Parasitenk. 6*, 603-637 (1934).

14. Cheng, T. C. and Dyckman, E., Sites of glycogen deposition in *Hymenolepis diminuta* during the growth phase in the rat host. *Z. Parasitenk. 24*, 27-48 (1964).

15. Collin, W. K., Electron microscope studies of the muscle and hook systems of hatched oncospheres of *Hymenolepis citelli* McLeod 1933 (Cestoda: Cyclophyllidea). *J. Parasitol. 54*, 47-88 (1968).

16. Collin, W. K., The cellular organization of hatched oncospheres of *Hymenolepis citelli* (Cestoda, Cyclophyllidea). *J. Parasitol. 55*, 149-166 (1969).

17. Collin, W. K., Electron microscopy of post-embryonic stages of the tapeworm *Hymenolepis citelli*. *J. Parasitol. 56*, 1159-1170 (1970).

18. Cooper, N. B., Allison, V. F. and Ubelaker, J. E., The fine structure of the cysticercoid of *Hymenolepis diminuta*. III. The scolex. Z.

Parasitenk. 46, 229-239 (1975)
19. Dunkley, L. C. and Mettrick, D. F., Factors affecting the susceptibility of the beetle *Tribolium confusum* to infection by *Hymenolepis diminuta*. *J. N. Y. Entomol. Soc. 79*, 133-138 (1971).
20. Evans, W. S. and Novak, M., The effect of mebendazole on the development of *Hymenolepis diminuta* in *Tribolium confusum*. *Can. J. Zool. 54*, 1079-1083 (1976).
21. Fairbairn, D., Biochemical adaptation and loss of genetic capacity in helminth parasites. *Biol. Rev. 45*, 29-72 (1970).
22. Faust, E. C., "Human Helminthology". Lea and Febiger, Philadelphia. (1949).
23. Freeman, R. S., Ontogeny of cestodes and its bearing on their phylogeny and systematics. *Advances in Parasitology (B. Dawes, ed.) 11*, 481-557 (1973).
24. Fulleborn, F., Ueber *Hymenolepis diminuta* (Rud.) 1819. *Arch. Schiffs-u. Tropen. Hyg. 26*, 193-202 (1922).
25. Goodchild, C. G. and Harrison, D. L., The growth of the rat tapeworm, *Hymenolepis diminuta*, during the first five days in the final host. *J. Parasitol. 47*, 819-829 (1961).
26. Goodchild, C. G. and Wells, O. C., Amino acids in larval and adult tapeworms *(Hymenolepis diminuta)* and in the tissues of their rat and beetle hosts. *Exp. Parasitol. 6*, 575-585 (1957).
27. Graham, J. J. and Berntzen, A. K., The monoxenic cultivation of cysticercoids with rat fibroblasts. *J. Parasitol. 56*, 1184-1188 (1970).
28. Grassi, G. B., Entwicklungsgeschichte der *Taenia nana*. *Zentrbl. Bakt. Abt. 1. 2*, 94-95 (1887)
29. Grassi, G. B. and Rovelli, G., Ricerche embriologiche sui cestodi. *Atti Accad. Gioenia, Catania. Sec. Nat. 4*, 1-108 (1892).
30. Hedrick, R. M., Comparative histochemical studies on cestodes. II. The distribution of fat substances in *Hymenolepis diminuta* and *Raillietina cesticillus*. *J. Parasitol. 44*, 75-84 (1958).
31. Hedrick, R. M. and Daugherty, J. W., Comparative histochemical studies on cestodes. I. The distribution of glycogen in *Hymenolepis diminuta* and *Railietina cesticillus*. *J. Parasitol. 43*,

497-504 (1957).
32. Heyneman, D. and Voge, M., Glycogen distribution in cysticercoids of three hymenolepidid cestodes. *J. Parasitol.* *43*, 527-531 (1957).
33. Heyneman, D. and Voge, M., Succinic dehydrogenase activity in cysticercoids of *Hymenolepis* (Cestoda: Hymenolepididae) measured by the tetrazolium technique. *Exp. Parasitol.* *9*, 14-17 (1960).
34. Heyneman, D. and Voge, M., Host response of the flour beetle, *Tribolium confusum*, to infections with *Hymenolepis diminuta*, *H. microstoma* and *H. citelli* (Cestoda: Hymenolepididae). *J. Parasitol.* *57*, 881-886 (1971).
35. Houser, B. B. and Burns, W. C., Experimental infection of gnotobiotic *Tenebrio molitor* and white rats with *Hymenolepis diminuta* (Cestoda: Cyclophyllidea). *J. Parasitol.* *54*, 69-73 (1968).
36. Isobe, M., The significance, physiochemical conditions, and pharmacological studies on the movement of the hexacanth embryo. *Acta. Sch. Med. Univ. Kioto 8*, 519 (1926).
37. Janicki, C., Ueber die Embryonalentwicklung von *Taenia serrata* Goeze. *Ztschr. f. Wissenschaftliche Zoologie 87*, 685-724 (1907).
38. Joyeux, C., Cycle evolutif de quelques cestodes. *Bull. Biol. France et Belgique* Suppl. II, 1-219 (1920).
39. Kelly, R. J., O'Brien, D. M. and Katz, F. F., The incidence and burden of *Hymenolepis diminuta* as a function of the age of the intermediate host *Tribolium confusum*. *J. N. Y. Entomol. Soc. 75*, 19-23 (1967).
40. Kelsoe, G. H., Ubelaker, J. E. and Allison, V. F., The fine structure of spermatogenesis in *Hymenolepis diminuta* (Cestoda) with a description of the mature spermatozoan. *Z. Parasitenk. 54*, 175-187 (1977).
41. King, J. W. and Lumsden, R. D., Cytological aspect of lipid assimilation by cestodes. Incorporation of linoleic acid into the parenchyma and eggs of *Hymenolepis diminuta*. *J. Parasitol. 55*, 250-260 (1969).
42. Lackie, A. M. Evasion of the haemocytic defence reaction of certain insects by larvae of *Hymenolepis diminuta* (Cestoda). *Parasitology 73*, 97-107 (1976).
43. Lethbridge, R. C., The hatching of *Hymenolepis*

diminuta eggs and penetration of hexacanths in *Tenebrio molitor* beetles. Parasitology 62, 445-456 (1971a).
44. Lethbridge, R. C., The chemical compositions and some properties of the egg layers in *Hymenolepis diminuta* eggs. Parasitology 63, 275-288 (1971b).
45. Lethbridge, R. C., *In vitro* hatching of *Hymenolepis diminuta* eggs in *Tenebrio molitor* extracts and in defined enzyme preparations. Parasitology 64, 389-400 (1972).
46. Lethbridge, R. C. and Gijsbers, M. F., Penetration gland secretion by hexacanths of *Hymenolepis diminuta*. Parasitology 68, 303-311 (1974).
47. Lumsden, R. D. and Byram, J. III., The ultrastructure of cestode muscle. J. Parasitol. 53, 326-342 (1967).
48. Lumsden, R. D., Oaks, J. A. and Mueller, J. F., Brush border development in the tegument of the tapeworm, *Spirometra mansonoides*. J. Parasitol. 60, 209-226 (1974).
49. MacDonald, I. G. and Wilson, P. A. G., Host-parasite relations of the cysticercoid of *Hymenolepis diminuta*. Parasitology 54, 7 p. (1964).
50. Mettrick, D. F. and Parnell, J. R., Exposure of *Tribolium confusum* to thio-TERA, and its effects upon development of *Hymenolepis diminuta* cysticercoids. Exp. Parasitol. 20, 17-26 (1967).
51. Moczon, T., Histochemical study of the development of embryonic hooks in *Hymenolepis diminuta*. Acta Parasitol. Polon. 19, 269-274 (1971).
52. Moczon, T., Histochemistry of oncospheral envelopes of *Hymenolepis diminuta* (Rudolphi 1819) (Cestoda, Hymenolepididae) Acta Parasitol. Polon. 20, 517-531 (1972).
53. Moczon, T., Histochemical studies on the enzymes of *Hymenolepis diminuta* (Rud. 1819) (Cestoda). I. Some oxidoreductases in oncospheres and cysticercoids. Acta Parasitol. Polon. 21, 85-97 (1973a).
54. Moczon, T., Histochemical studies on the enzymes of *Hymenolepis diminuta* (Rud. 1819) (Cestoda). II. Non-specific and specific phosphatases in oncospheres and cysticercoids. Acta Parasitol. Polon. 21, 99-106 (1973b).
55. Moczon, T., Glycogen distribution and accumulation of radioactive compounds in tissues of

mature specimens of *Hymenolepis diminuta* (Cestoda) after incubation in glucose $-^{14}C$ 1-6. *Acta Parasitol. Polon.* 23, 135-145 (1975).

56. Moczon, T., Negative results of biochemical tests for collagenase and hyaluronidase activities in extracts of *Hymenolepis diminuta* (Cestoda) oncospheres and *Nippostrongylus muris* (Nematoda) invasive larvae, *Bull. l'Acad. Polon. Sci.* 25, 479-481 (1977a).

57. Moczon, T., Penetration of *Hymenolepis diminuta* oncospheres across the intestinal tissues of *Tenebrio molitor* beetles. *Bull. l'Acad. Polon. Sci.* 25, 531-535 (1977b).

58. Moczon, T., Penetration glands of oncospheres of *Hymenolepis diminuta* (Cestoda). Histochemical studies. *Bull. l'Acad. Polon. Sci.* 25, 619-622 (1977c).

59. Moczon, T., Glycogen distribution and accumulation of radioactive compounds in oncospheres and cysticercoids of *Hymenolepis diminuta* (Cestoda) after incubation in glucose $-^{14}C_{1-6}$. *Acta Parasitol. Polon.* 24, 269-274 (1977d).

60. Moczon, T., Histochemical studies on the enzymes of *Hymenolepis diminuta* (Rud. 1819) (Cestoda). VI. Some enzymes of the synthesis and phosphorolytic degradation of glycogen in oncospheres and cysticercoids. *Acta Parasitol. Polon.* 24, 275-282 (1977e).

61. Moczon, T., Histochemical studies on the enzymes of *Hymenolepis diminuta* (Rud. 1819) (Cestoda). VIII. Enzymes of the synthesis and hydrolytic degradation of glycogen in three developmental stages. *Acta Parasitol. Polon.* 25, 45-53 (1977f).

62. Moriyama, S., Studies on the structure and embryonal development of the ova of Tetrabothridiata. F. On the structure and embryonal development of the ova of *Hymenolepis diminuta* (Rudolphi 1819) Blanchard, 1891. *Jap. J. Parasitol.* 10, 272-278 (1961).

63. Morris, G. P. and Finnegan, C. V., Studies of the differentiating plerocercoid cuticle of *Schistocephalus solidus*. I. The histochemical analysis of cuticle development. *Can. J. Zool.* 46, 115-121 (1968).

64. Nieland, M. L., Electron microscope observations on the egg of *Taenia taeniaeformis*. *J. Parasitol.*

54, 957-969 (1968).
65. Ogren, R. E., Development and morphology of glandular regions in oncospheres of *Hymenolepis nana*. *Proc. Pa. Acad. Sci.* 29, 258-364 (1955).
66. Ogren, R. E., Development and morphology of the oncosphere of *Mesocestoides corti*, a tapeworm of mammals. *J. Parasitol.* 42, 414-428 (1956).
67. Ogren, R. E., Morphology and development of oncospheres of the cestode *Oochoristica symmetrica* Baylis, 1927. *J. Parasitol.* 43, 505-520 (1957).
68. Ogren, R. E., The hexacanth embryo of a dilepidid tapeworm. I. The development of hooks and contractile parenchyma. *J. Parasitol.* 44, 477-483 (1958).
69. Ogren, R. E., Observations on hook development in the oncoblasts of hexacanth embryos from *Hymenolepis diminuta*, a tapeworm of mammals (Cestoda: Cyclophyllidea). *Proc. Pa. Acad. Sci.* 35, 23-31 (1961a).
70. Ogren, R. E., The mature oncosphere of *Hymenolepis diminuta*. *J. Parasitol.* 47, 197-204 (1961b).
71. Ogren, R. E., Continuity of morphology from oncosphere to early cysticercoid in the development of *Hymenolepis diminuta* (Cestoda: Cyclophyllidea). *Exp. Parasitol.* 12, 1-6 (1962).
72. Ogren, R. E., The cellular pattern in invasive oncospheres of *Hymenolepis diminuta* as revealed by an enzyme-acetic acid-orcein method. *Trans. Am. Micros. Soc.* 86, 250-260 (1967).
73. Ogren, R. E., Characteristics for two classes of embryonic cells in oncospheres of *Hymenolepis diminuta* stained for cytoplasmic substances. *Trans. Am. Micros. Soc.* 87, 82-92 (1968a).
74. Ogren, R. E., The basic cellular pattern for undifferentiated oncospheres of *Hymenolepis diminuta*. *Trans. Am. Micros. Soc.* 87, 448-463 (1968b).
75. Ogren, R. E., Oncosphere movement: an interesting feature of invasive embryos from the tapeworm *Hymenolepis diminuta*. *Proc. Pa. Acad. Sci.* 43, 238-248 (1969).
76. Ogren, R. E., Basic hook musculature in invasive oncospheres of the tapeworm, *Hymenolepis diminuta* *J. Parasitol.* 58, 240-243 (1972).
77. Ogren, R. E. and Magill, R. M., Demonstration of protein in the protective envelopes and embryonic muscle in oncospheres of *Hymenolepis diminuta*, a

tapeworm of mammals. *Proc. Pa. Acad. Sci. 36*, 160-167 (1962).
78. Ogren, R. E., Ogren, J. J. and Skarnulis, J., Effects of salt and neutral red solutions on movements of invasive oncospheres from the tapeworm *Hymenolepis diminuta. Proc. Pa. Acad. Sci. 43*, 56-60 (1969).
79. Pence, D. B., The fine structure and histochemistry of infective eggs of *Dipylidium caninum. J. Parasitol. 53*, 1041-1054 (1967).
80. Pence, D. B., Electron microscope and histochemical studies on the egg of *Hymenolepis diminuta. J. Parasitol. 56*, 84-97 (1970).
81. Prescott, D. M. and Voge, M., Autoradiographic study of the synthesis of ribonucleic acids in cysticercoids of *Hymenolepis diminuta. J. Parasitol. 45*, 587-790 (1959).
82. Reid, W. M., Penetration glands in cyclophyllidean oncospheres. *Trans. Am. Micro. Soc. 67*, 177-182 (1948).
83. Reid, W. M., Allaman, L. and Fitch, F., Some factors involved in the hatching of *Hymenolepis diminuta* oncospheres (abstract). *J. Parasitol. 37*, (5-2), 24 (1951).
84. Rosen, F., Recherches sur le developpement des cestodes. I. Le cycle evolutif des Bothriocephales. Etude sur l'origine des Cestodes et leurs etats larvaines. *Bull. Soc. Neuchatel. Sci. Nat. 43*, 241-300 (1918).
85. Rothman, A. H., The larval development of *Hymenolepis diminuta* and *H. citelli. J. Parasitol. 43*, 641-648 (1957).
86. Rybicka, K., Embryonic development of *Moniezia expansa* (Rud: 1810) (Cyclophyllidea, Anoplocephalidae) *Acta Parasitol. Polon. 12*, 313-330 (1964).
87. Rybicka, K., Embryogenesis in cestodes. *Advances in Parasitology (B. Dawes, ed.) 4*, 107-186 (1966a).
88. Rybicka, K., Embryogenesis in *Hymenolepis diminuta*. I. Morphogenesis. *Exp. Parasitol. 19*, 366-379 (1966b).
89. Rybicka, K., Embryogenesis in *Hymenolepis diminuta*. II. Glycogen distribution in the embryos. *Exp. Parasitol. 20*, 98-105 (1967a).
90. Rybicka, K., Embryogenesis in *Hymenolepis*. III. Distribution of ribonucleic acid. *Exp. Parasitol. 20*, 177-185 (1967b).
91. Rybicka, K., Embryogenesis in *Hymenolepis*

diminuta. IV. Distribution of succinic dehydrogenase, reduced form of nicotinamide-adenine dinucleotide oxido-reductase, and cytochrome oxidae. *Exp. Parasitol. 20*, 255-262 (1967c).
92. Rybicka, K., Ultrastructure of embryonic envelopes and their differentiation in *Hymenolepis diminuta* (Cestoda). *J. Parasitol. 58*, 849-863 (1972)
93. Rybicka, K., Ultrastructure of macromeres in the cleavage of *Hymenolepis diminuta* (Cestoda). *Trans. Am. Micros. Soc. 92*, 241-255 (1973a).
94. Rybicka, K., Ultrastructure of the embryonic syncytial epithelium in a cestode *Hymenolepis diminuta*. *Parasitology 66*, 9-18 (1973b).
95. Sawada, I., Penetration glands in the oncosphere of *Raillietina cesticillus*. *Exp. Parasitol. 11*, 141-146 (1961).
96. Schauinsland, H. H., Die embryonale Entwicklung der Bothriocephalen. *Jenaische Ztschr. Naturw. 19*, 520-572 (1886).
97. Silverman, P. H. and Maneely, R. B., Studies on the biology of some tapeworms of the genus *Taenia*. III. The role of the secreting gland of the hexacatnh embryo in the penetration of the intestinal mucosa of the intermediate host, and some of its histochemical reactions. *Ann. Trop. Med. Parasitol. 49*, 326-330 (1955).
98. Slais, J., Functional morphology of cestode larvae. *Advances in Parasitology (B. Dawes, ed.) 11*, 395-380 (1973).
99. Soltice, G. W., Arai, H. P. and Scheinberg, E., Host-parasite interactions of *Tribolium confusum* and *T. castaneum* with *Hymenolepis diminuta*. *Can. J. Zool. 49*, 265-275 (1971).
100. Spatlich, W., Die Furchung und die Embryonalhullenbildung des Eies von *Diorchis inflata*. Rud. *Zool. Jahrb. Abt. Anat. 47*, 101-112 (1925).
101. Stirewalt, M. A., Chemical histology of secretions of larval helminths. *Ann. N. Y. Acad. Sci. 113*, 36-53 (1963).
102. Stunkard, H. W., The organization, ontogeny, and orientation of the Cestoda. *Quart. Rev. Biol. 37*, 23-34 (1962).
103. Swiderski, Z., Electron microscopy of embryonic envelope formation by the cestode *Catenotaenia pusilla*. *Exp. Parasitol. 23*, 104-113 (1968).
104. Swiderski, Z., Electron microscopy of embryonal hook formation by the cestode *Inermicapsifer*

madagascariensis (Cyclophyllidea, Davaineidae). *Proc. Sec. Int. Cong. Parasitol. Wash. D. C.*, pp. 337-338 (1970).
105. Swiderski, Z., Electron microscopy and histochemistry of oncospheral hook formation by the cestode *Catenotaenia pusilla*. *Int. J. Parasitol. 3*, 27-33 (1973).
106. Swiderski, Z., Huggel, H. and Schönenberger, N., Comparative fine structure of vitelline cells in cyclophyllidean cestodes. *Septième Cong. Int. Micros. Electron.*, *Grenoble*, pp. 825-826 (1970).
107. Ubelaker, J. E., Cooper, N. B. and Allison, V. F., The fine structure of the cysticercoid of *Hymenolepis diminuta*, I. The outer wall of the capsule. *Z. Parasitenk. 34*, 258-270 (1970a).
108. Ubelaker, J. E., Cooper, N. B. and Allison, V. F., Possible defensive mechanism of *Hymenolepis diminuta* cysticercoids to hemocytes of the beetle *Tribolium confusum*. *J. Invert. Pathol. 16*, 310-312 (1970b).
109. Voge, M., Sensitivity of developing *Hymenolepis diminuta* larvae to high temperature stress. *J. Parasitol. 45*, 175-181 (1959a).
110. Voge, M., Temperature stress and development of *Hymenolepis diminuta* in *Tribolium confusum* on different diets. *J. Parasitol. 45*, 591-596 (1959b).
111. Voge, M., Fat distribution in cysticercoids of the cestode *Hymenolepis diminuta*. *Proc. Helminthol. Soc. Wash. 27*, 1-4 (1960a).
112. Voge, M., Studies in cysticercoid histology. I. Observations on the fully developed cysticercoid of *Hymenolepis diminuta* (Cestoda: Cyclophyllidea). *Proc. Helminthol. Soc. Wash. 27*, 32-36 (1960b).
113. Voge, M., Studies in cysticercoid histology. IV. Observations on histogenesis in the cysticercoid of *Hymenolepis diminuta* (Cestoda: Cyclophyllidea). *J. Parasitol. 46*, 717-725 (1960c).
114. Voge, M., Effect of high temperature stress on histogenesis in the cysticercoid of *Hymenolepis diminuta* (Cestoda: Cyclophyllidea). *J. Parasitol. 47*, 189-195 (1961).
115. Voge, M., The post-embryonic developmental stages of cestodes. *Advances in Parasitology (B. Dawes, ed.) 5*, 247-297 (1967).
116. Voge, M., Systematics of cestodes--present and

future. *In* "Problems in Systematics of Parasites" (G. D. Schmidt, ed), pp. 49-72. Univ. Park Press. Baltimore. (1969).
117. Voge, M., The post-embryonic developmental stages of cestodes. *Advances in Parasitology (B. Dawes, ed.) 11*, 707-730 (1973).
118. Voge, M. and Berntzen, A. K., *In vitro* hatching of oncospheres of *Hymenolepis diminuta* (Cestoda: Cyclophyllidea). *J. Parasitol. 47*, 813-818 (1961).
119. Voge, M. and Graiwer, M., Development of oncospheres of *Hymenolepis diminuta* hatched *in vitro*, in the larvae of *Tenebrio molitor*. *J. Parasitol. 50*, 267-270 (1964).
120. Voge, M. and Heyneman, D., Development of *Hymenolepis nana* and *Hymenolepis diminuta* (Cestoda: Hymenolepididae) in the intermediate host *Tribolium confusum*. *Univ. Calif. Publ. Zool. 59*, 549-580 (1957).
121. Voge, M. and Heyneman, D., Effect of high temperature on the larval development of *Hymenolepis diminuta* (Cestoda: Cyclophyllidea). *J. Parasitol. 44*, 249-260 (1958).
122. Voge, M. and Turner, J. A., Effect of temperature on larval development of the cestode *Hymenolepis diminuta*. *Exp. Parasitol. 5*, 580-586 (1956).
123. Walkey, M. and Fairbairn, D., L(+)-lactate dehydrogenase from *Hymenolepis diminuta* (Cestoda). *J. Exp. Zool. 183*, 365-374 (1973).
124. Wardle, R. A. and McLeod, J. A., "The Zoology of Tapeworms". Univ. of Minnesota Press, Minneapolis. (1952).
125. Webb, R. A., The organization and fine structure of the muscles of the scolex of the cysticercoid of *Hymenolepis microstoma*. *J. Morphol. 154*, 339-356 (1977).

THE MORPHOLOGY, HISTOLOGY, AND FINE STRUCTURE OF THE ADULT STAGE OF THE CYCLOPHYLLIDEAN TAPEWORM *Hymenolepis diminuta*

Richard Dick Lumsden

Department of Biology,
Tulane University,
New Orleans, Louisiana

Robert Specian

Department of Anatomy,
Harvard University School of Medicine,
Boston, Mass.

I. INTRODUCTION

The first description of the tapeworm known today as *Hymenolepis diminuta* was published by Rudolphi in 1819. Rudolphi followed the Linnaen tradition whereby all adult tapeworms were assigned to a single genus, *Taenia*, and, as this was a relatively small tapeworm, Rudolphi named it *Taenia diminuta*. In 1858, Weinland published an account of some tapeworm specimens passed by an infant in Boston, Massachusetts. Believing these worms to be previously unknown to science, he erected a new genus and species to accommodate them, *Hymenolepis flavopunctata*. The generic name emphasizes the presence of transparent "membranes" surrounding the embryos, which among other features, Weinland believed, distinguished these tapeworms from those described up to that time. Grassi, in 1888, and Blanchard, in 1891, nonetheless concluded that *H.*

flavopunctata was, in fact, the same species described earlier by Rudolphi, i.e., *Taenia diminuta*. The morphology of these worms, of which Blanchard gave a particularly detailed account, clearly warranted their separation from the genus *Taenia*, so now this and some 300 additional species since described bear the generic taxon *Hymenolepis*.

The foregoing is not intended to reiterate the taxonomy and systematics of *H. diminuta*, more authoritatively reviewed elsewhere in this volume, but to emphasize that *H. diminuta* has been a subject of study for a long time. Indeed, owing in no small measure to the relative ease with which its life cycle can be maintained in the laboratory, *H. diminuta* has become a model for investigating not only tapeworm morphology, but embryology, biochemistry, and physiology was well. The result is that for no other cestode do we have better correlation between information about structure and information about function.

The first systematic studies of tapeworm metabolism were carried out by Dr. Clark Read during the late 1940's and early 1950's, and were based primarily on *H. diminuta*. It was during this period that other biologists, with the aid of electron microscopes, were making significant progress in correlating subcellular structure with function, as exemplified by the contributions of Drs. George Palade, Keith Porter, and Albert Claude. Most of these studies were being conducted on vertebrate cells and tissues. Read, while not an electron microscopist himself, readily appreciated the potential value of fine structural information on helminth parasites, and was not bashful about soliciting the collaboration of colleagues skilled in the technique. It is not improbable that, with Read's persuasion, the first examination of tapeworms by electron microscopy was inflicted on *H. diminuta*. In any event, the first (to our knowledge) published electron micrograph of tapeworm tissue appeared in an article by Read (1955) which reviewed aspects of intestinal physiology related to host-parasite relationships. This image, provided Read by his colleagues Dr. Fred Bang and Mrs. Illse Vellisto, was of the body surface of *H. diminuta* and revealed a structure superficially not unlike that of the host mucosa; at least, it was so interpreted at that time.

It was not very long thereafter that Read and his students turned their attention to the absorptive properties of tapeworms, articulated the concept of the host-parasite interface, and defined, with *H. diminuta* as the primary model, many of the intricate molecular interactions between symbionts and their hosts (the progress of this and other aspects of Read's research has been reviewed by Stewart *et al.* 1976). Meanwhile, investigations into the fine structure of tapeworms and other parasites blossomed. The electron microscope provided images of cytoarchitecture which in many instances drastically revised concepts of fifty or more years standing, and opened the way for correlations between morphology and physiology never before possible.

It is neither to unduly credit the electron microscope nor to hold it accountable for any missteps in our progress to knowledge about tapeworm biology that we note here its impact on the discipline of parasitology as a whole. We would take this opportunity to recognize Read as one of the first parasitologists to bring to bear the new approaches and concepts which set the pattern of investigations in parasitology that have prevailed during this half of the 20th century. As Dr. Aurel Foster remarked nearly two decades ago, parasitologists have profited immeasureably from the application of ".... ultramicroscopy, tracer methods .... tissue cultivation techniques ...." etc. (Foster 1960; Lumsden 1976), perhaps no better documented than in the literature on *H. diminuta* published since 1950.

The first detailed account of *H. diminuta* ultrastructure was presented by Dr. Alvin Rothman (a student of Read's) at the national meetings of the American Society of Parasitologists in 1959. Rothman's principal subject was the tegument (then called the cuticle), a topic since addressed by at least half the current total of EM-based papers on cestodes. The preponderance of literature on the tegument stems from (1) the importance of the body surface to the physiology of these organisms; and (2) at the EM-level, the tegument is the most readily located, identified, and otherwise interpreted organ system. Many years ago, Young (1935) remarked that, in tapeworms, ".... the true relations of various cellular elements (e.g., muscle and connective tissue fibrils, nerves and excretory tubules) are difficult to distinguish, and easily distorted by fixatives, producing puzzling artifacts". Twenty five years later, electron microscopists were saying the same thing. To be sure, early interpretations of tapeworm fine structure were hampered by many misconceptions and much ambiguous terminology perpetuated from light microscopy-based descriptions, and the difficulty with which faithful preservation of tapeworm cell structure could be obtained with the fixatives and embedments used by the majority of the electron microscopists of the 1950's and early 1960's. Even today, there are aspects of tapeworm cytoarchitecture which remain, disconcertingly, enigmatic. We would agree, at the onset of this review on the microanatomy and fine structure of *H. diminuta*, that "Tapeworms are unfavorable objects for histological study" (Wardle and McCleod 1952), but only in the technical sense, and to the extent that phylogenetically higher organisms, or those much lower, have preoccupied the attention of most modern-day cell biologists.

We acknowledge that many biologists would condemn not only the lifestyle of tapeworms but also their structure as being hopelessly degenerate. Certainly, tapeworm histology differs, in some cases remarkably so, from what one is accustomed to seeing in most other kinds of animals. But to regard tapeworm structure as degenerate is, to the present authors, highly inappropriate. Rather, in our judgement, tapeworms are uniquely well specialized for meeting the demands of what Allee *et al.* (1949) recognized as the world's third habitat (after the aquatic and terrestrial) - other living organisms. In the course of evolution, tapeworms have merely exaggerated certain features and diminished others in adapting most successfully to a lifestyle which exemplifies the ultimate welfare state.

II. THE GENERAL BODY PLAN

Anatomically, the body of adult *H. diminuta* is divisible into three components. Anteriormost is the *scolex*, followed by the *neck*, from which the segmented *strobila* arises. The scolex contains the

principal co-ordinative neural elements (the major
ganglia, commissures, etc.) and mounts four muscular
suckers which provide for attachment of the worm to
its host's intestinal mucosa (Fig. 1). At the apex
of the scolex is an unarmed (hookless) rostellum, a
dome-shaped, protrusible organ consisting of a muscular capsule surrounding some prominent, apparently
glandular cells. The neck contains the germinative
anlagen, a mass of mitotically active cells from
which the somatic and reproductive tissues of the
strobilar proglottids differentiate. In sexually
mature worms, the craspedote strobila may consist of
several hundred proglottids, with those occupying
roughly the posterior two-thirds of the strobila
containing differentiated reproductive organs. Like
most tapeworms, *H. diminuta* is hermaphroditic.
Sexual maturation of the proglottids is protandrous,
the organs of the male system developing before
those of the female system. The posteriormost
proglottids are gravid and apolytic - i.e., the
terminal proglottids, filled with shelled embryos,
detach from the strobila (Fig. 2), after which they
disintegrate and release the eggs.

For more than a hundred years, zoologists have
debated the question of whether the tapeworm is an
individual or a colony. In our opinion, the preponderance of evidence, reviewed by Stunkard (1962),
is compelling in favor of the monozootic view.
Except for a repetition of reproductive organs in
successive proglottids, the tissues manifest organic
unity. As Stunkard (1962) remarked, ".... in turbellarians, nemertines, and annelids, ... serial
repetition of gonads is accepted as a sexual phenomenon within an individual rather than colony formation, and application of the same reasoning would
seem to apply to the cestode".

As for tapeworms generally, there is no trace of
a mouth or alimentary tract - *H. diminuta* is truly a
"gutless wonder". The only lumenal organs which are
patent to the external environment are the posterior
ends of the excretory canals and those of the terminal male genitalia. Internally, the body is for
the most part a solid mass of somatic and reproductive tissue held together by a rather loose excelsior
of reticular connective tissue fibrils. There is no
body cavity, and the only channelized fluid is that
sequestered within the canals and tubules of the
excretory system.

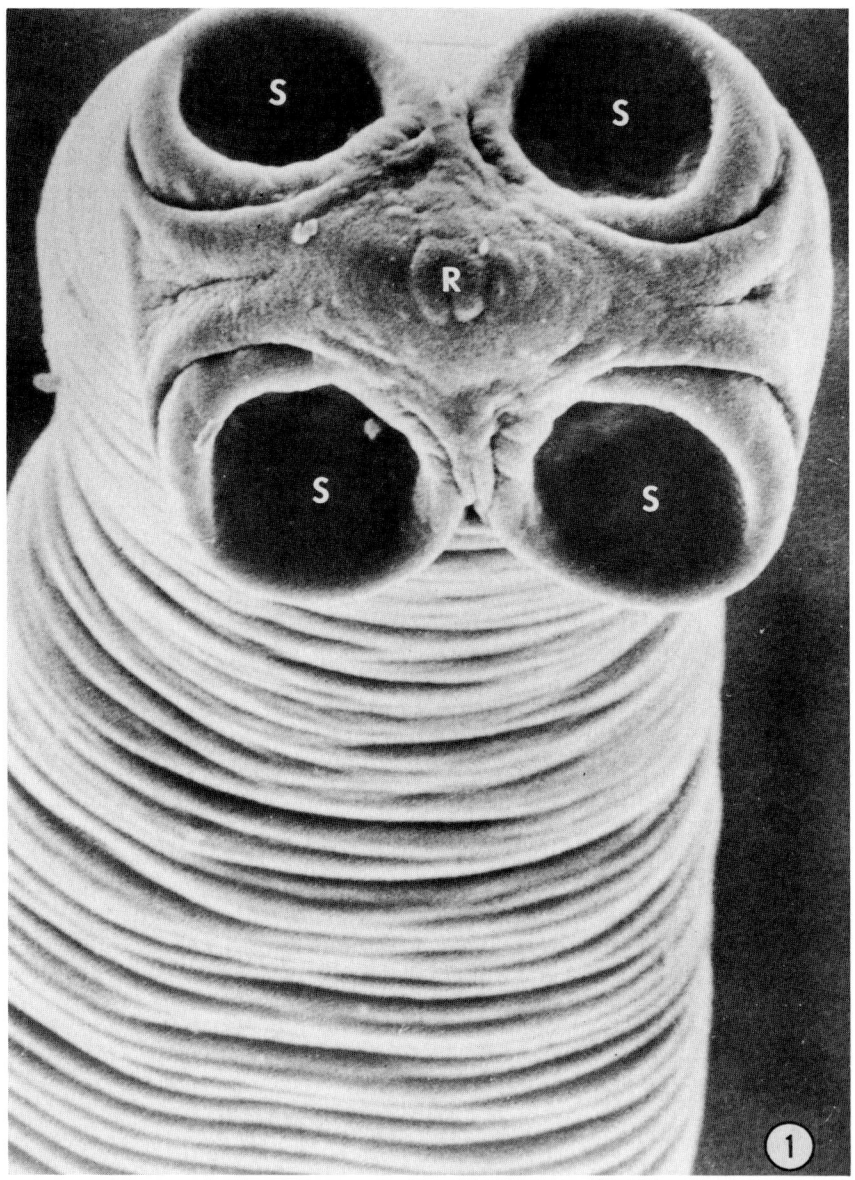

Fig. 1. En face scanning electron micrograph of scolex of Hymenolepis diminuta showing relationship of apical rostellum (R) to bilateral suckers (S). (From Ubelaker et al. 1973). X435.

The Morphology, Histology, and Fine Structure of the Adult Stage 163

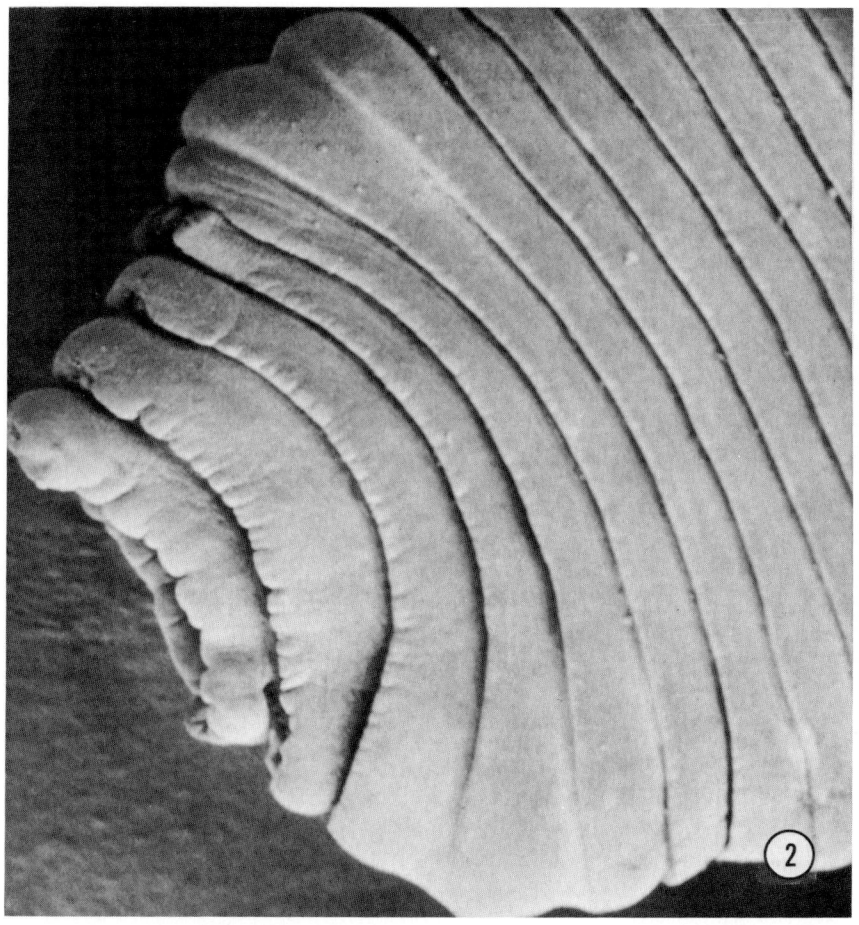

Fig. 2. Scanning electron micrograph of terminal prolottids, revealing topographical features associated with apolysis. X45.

As viewed in section, a proglottid can be divided roughly into two zones - the cortex and the medulla (Fig. 3). The cortex consists principally the tegument, superficial musculature, some nerve fibers, and terminal elements (i.e., flame cells and associated ducts) of the excretory system (Fig. 4). The medulla is set off by a zone of longitudinal muscle fibers and contains the major excretory canals and nerve trunks, germinal tissue and/or reproductive organs (Fig. 5). Though the strobila of *H. diminuta* is externally segmented, or divisible into a number of discrete proglottids (Fig. 6), the tegument, major longitudinal muscles, the excretory canals, and nerve cords are continuous from one proglottid to the next over the entire length of the worm (Fig. 7).

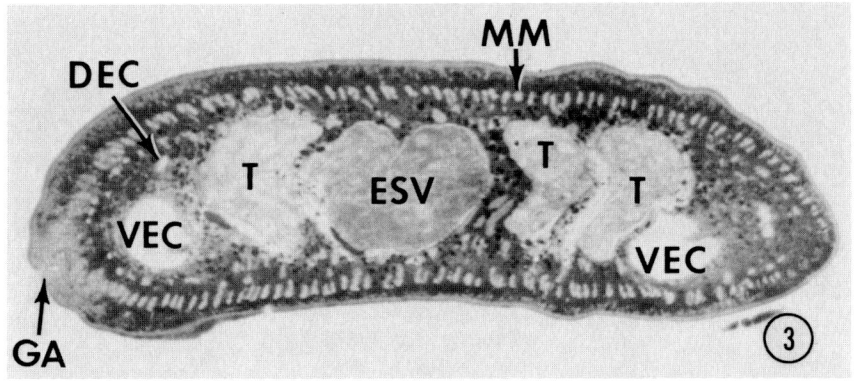

Fig. 3. Cross section through mature proglottid. Medullary muscles (MM) separate cortex from medullary region of proglottid. Cortical region contains tegument and superficial musculature, as well as genital atrium (GA). Apparent within medullary region are male reproductive organs - the testes (T) and the external seminal vesicle (ESV) filled with mature spermatozoa. Lateral margins occupied by dorsal (DEC) and ventral (VEC) excretory canals. Plastic section stained with acid fuchsin-azure II. X40.

Most of the volume between the tegument and germinal/reproductive organs is occupied by the so-called parenchyma. Once thought to be comprised of a discrete cell type (see, e.g., Lumsden 1965a, 1966a), it now appears that the majority of the "parenchymal cells", at least in *H. diminuta*, are in reality the non-contractile regions of muscle cells, containing the nuclei, large amounts of glycogen, and, frequently, lipid droplets. The intercellular space is occupied by a connective tissue of very fine and loosely packed fibrils.

The greatest concentration of nerve tissue in the proglottids is found in a pair of laterally placed cords which parallel the longitudinal body axis. Fine fibers extend from these cords, especially toward the body surface as components of sensory receptors. Others serve to innervate the musculature and reproductive organs. Cross-commissures connect the lateral cords at the intersection of individual proglottids.

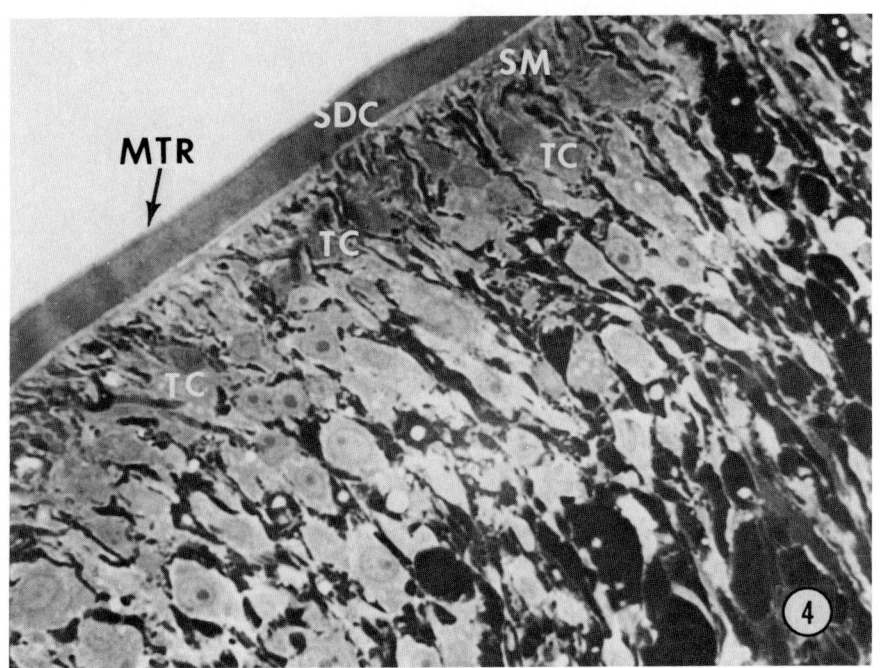

Fig. 4. Cross section through cortical region of immature proglottid. Syncytial distal cytoplasm (SDC) with microtriches (MTR) lining the free surface. Tegumental cytons (TC) beneath superficial musculature (SM) support syncytial layer. Interspersed dark areas are concentrations of glycogen within cortical myocytons, which have been stained with the PAS reaction. Plastic section stained with PAS and methylene blue-azure II. (From Lumsden 1966b). X1050.

The excretory system consists of paired dorsolaterally - and ventrolaterally - positioned canals, which drain a system of fine, branching tubules. Each of these tubules terminates, ultimately, in a ciliated flame cell. In that adult *H. diminuta* behaves in media of changing salinity like an osmometer, it seems inappropriate to refer to this system as "osmoregulatory", as is often done in descriptions of tapeworm microanatomy.

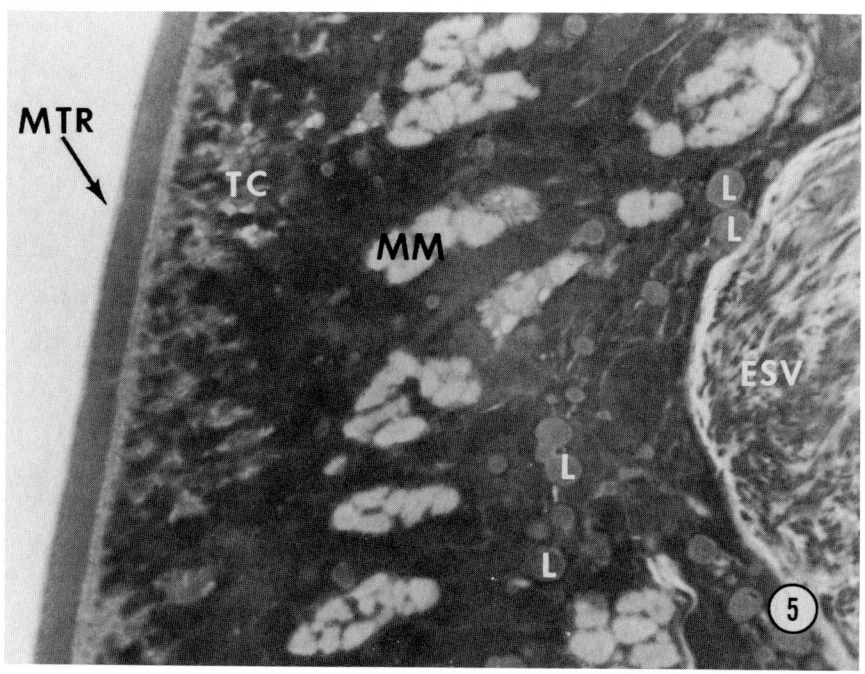

Fig. 5. Cross section through mature proglottid. Medullary muscles (MM) separate cortex from medulla. Tegument with syncytial surface layer extended as microtriches (MTR) supported by basal tegumentary cytons (TC). Abundant lipid distributed throughout "parenchyma" of medullary region. Portion of external seminal vesicle (ESV) shown in medullary region of proglottid. Plastic section stained with acid fuchsin-azure II. X800.

At the risk of oversimplification, the body plan of *H. diminuta*, at least of the strobila, may be analogized as a gut turned inside-out; the body covering, both structurally and functionally, is more like that of an absorptive mucosa than an epidermis. While the skin of most organisms serves as insulation from the environment, that of *H. diminuta* and other tapeworms promotes nearly all forms of chemical interchange between the environ-

The Morphology, Histology, and Fine Structure of the Adult Stage

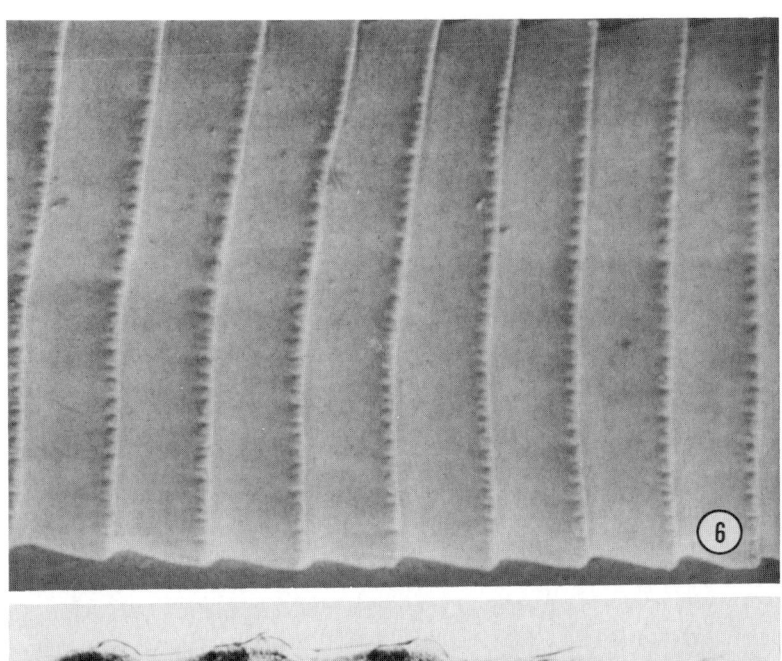

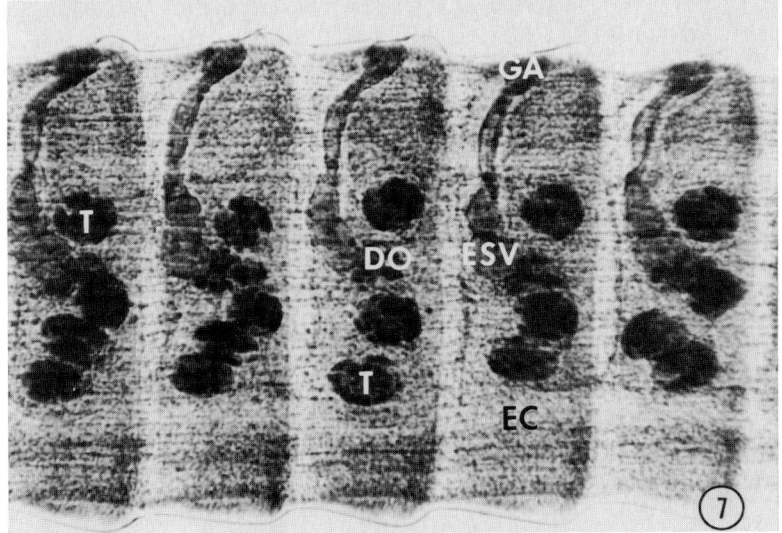

Fig. 6. Scanning electron micrograph of topographical features of mature proglottids. X40.

Fig. 7. Mature proglottids revealing orientation of medullary testes (T), external seminal vesicle (ESV) and developing ovary (DO). Excretory canals (EC) extend through proglottids. Sperm duct (SD) terminates within lateral genital atrium (GA). Whole mount stained with paracarmine. X35.

ment and the internal tissues, especially the absorption of nutrients. The concept that adult parasites eat not merely to live but to reproduce is abundantly manifested in the structural organization of these tapeworms, where the nutrient assimilating tissue (the tegument) and nutrient-storing tissue (the "parenchyma") surround the reproductive organs. Structural development for other functions, e.g., locomotion, sensory reception, osmoregulation, etc., has in these tapeworms been subordinated to the development of an anatomy which can most efficiently capitalize on an environment rich in already digested foodstuffs to meet the demands of growth and reproduction.

Among the more unusual features of tapeworm histology is the prevalence of syncytial tissue organization - in the skin, or tegument, the musculature/parenchyma, and the ducts of the excretory and reproductive systems. A syncytium is a multinucleated mass of protoplasm which forms by fusion of mononucleated cells. In this latter feature, a syncytium differs from a plasmodium, which develops by repeated nuclear divisions in the absence of cytokinesis. Syncytial tissues are not often encountered in higher animals, the principal ones in mammals, for example, being striated muscle and the syncytiotrophoblast. Syncytial organization permits rapid and/or sustained growth without restructuring of previously differentiated tissue. It also provides efficient transfer of substances throughout a large tissue volume. Thus, syncytial tissue organization is clearly an advantage to tapeworms, the majority of which grow continually by budding (strobilization) and none of which have an alimentary tract, circulatory system, or body cavity.

Plasmodial structure is, not surprisingly, incurred in the germinative tissues, at least insofar as spermatogenesis is concerned. This situation, as noted by Bloom and Fawcett (1975), is ".... probably responsible for the synchrony of development of large numbers of germ cells".

As unorthodox as tapeworm histology may seem otherwise, these worms do not violate the fundamental "neuron doctrine", insofar as their nerve cells appear to be distinctive in structure and function and are not in cytoplasmic continuity with themselves or other cytological elements. In this respect, tapeworms evidence at least a modicum of "conventional" epithelial histology, with which Angevine (1975) would credit the nervous systems of metazoans as a whole.

Besides the already emphasized syncytial nature of many tapeworm tissues, their cytological elements are intercoupled with one another, principally via nexus-type junctions, to an uncommon degree. In addition to the expected associations of this type between neurons, neurons and muscle cells, etc., there is in tapeworms such as *H. diminuta* an abundance of such junctional complexes between, e.g., tegument and muscle elements, individual muscle cells, "parenchymal" and excretory elements, and so on. Surprisingly, perhaps adhesive junctions of the desmosomal variety (i.e., zonula adherens, septate desmosomes, etc.) are rarely encountered. In *H. diminuta*, we have seen septate desmosomes only at the attachment of sensory dendrites (sensilla) and tegument; we have not been able to identify to our satisfaction the classic zonula adherens in any of the tissues, though "half desmosomes" are represented at the interface of tegument and muscle elements with connective tissue. It is worth noting here that the nexus ("close" or "gap") type junction has been identified functionally in other organisms with electrical coupling (reviewed by Bloom and Fawcett 1975), and in the context of tapeworm tissue/cell interaction, this is undoubtedly of paramount physiological significance.

We will return to a consideration of these features of the tapeworm body plan at the conclusion of this chapter, where an attempt will be made to weave the thread of morphology into the tapestry of these most fascinating organisms' overall biology. Meanwhile, as antecedent to the following sections, we would identify the following general principles regarding tapeworm histology, cytology, and fine structure:

(1) Tapeworms, as exemplified by *H. diminuta*, exhibit a remarkable degree of conservatism with respect to the number of morphologically different somatic cell types.

(2) With the exceptions of the reproductive organs and the scolex, regional differentiation of tissue structure is essentially non-existent.

(3) Albeit, cells of closely similar appearance in the electron microscope may be otherwise quite diverse in their specific functions.

(4) At the ultrastructural level, the cells of *H. diminuta* and other tapeworms are not unlike those of other organisms - i.e., in the kinds of organelles present, the essential substructure of these organelles, etc., they do not diverge remarkably from the pattern established for eukaryotic cells found everywhere else in the animal kingdom.

(5) Albeit, the manner in which the cytological elements of tapeworms interact are, in many respects, unique.

(6) The closest parallel to the histological organization of tapeworms is that of trematodes.

III. THE TEGUMENT

A. *Structure*

The "skin" of *H. diminuta* and other tapeworms was originally described as consisting of a cuticle, produced by secretions from either the parenchyma (Pratt 1909) or specialized subcuticular cells (Blochmann 1896). This interpretation proved to be an erroneous one when, in the 1960's, studies employing the electron microscope were directed to the tapeworm body surface. Among the early reports on its fine structure were those of Threadgold (1962), on *Dipylidium caninum*, Rothman (1963), on *H. diminuta*, Beguin (1966a), on *Caryophyllaeus laticeps*, and Lumsden (1966b), on *H. diminuta*, *Lacistorhynchus tenuis*, and *Calliobothrium verticillatum*. These and other studies (reviewed by Lumsden 1975a, 1975b) revealed the "cuticle" to be, in reality, part of a cytoplasmic syncytium, demarcated at its free and basal surfaces by a plasma membrane, and continuous with nucleated cell bodies (the "subcuticular cells" of (Blochmann 1896) lying in the cortical parenchyma (Fig. 8). The tapeworm body covering is now most commonly referred to as the tegument.

The tegument consists of two principal zones - the most superficial (comprising what was formerly termed the cuticle) is frequently called the "distal cytoplasm", to differentiate it from the underlying, nucleus-containing cell bodies (tegumentary cytons or perikarya). Connecting the distal cytoplasm and cell bodies are tendrillar internuncial processes which extend through the layers of the superficial muscle fibers and perforate the basement layer of connective tissue supporting the distal cytoplasm. Cytoplasmic bridges are also present between the individual perikarya.

The terms "distal cytoplasm", tegumentary cytons, perikarya, etc., have been widely used since the earliest electron microscope level descriptions of the tapeworm body surface. Nonetheless, a less cumbersome terminology is that coined much earlier by Westblad (1940) for the syncytial epidermis of other flatworms - the *epicytium* and *ectocytium*, respectively. However, since the newer terms are now the most familiar to students of tapeworm fine structure, we will continue to employ "distal cytoplasm", etc., in this review.

The free surface of the tegument is covered by digitiform projections (Fig. 11), for which Rothman (1963) coined the term *microtriches* (G. *thrix (trich-)*, hair). Tapering to a conical apex, these microtriches have a maximum diameter of approximately 0.14 μm, and a maximum length of about 0.9 μm. Within the distal tip of each microthrix is a dense accumulation of fibrils, set off from the remainder of the shaft by a multilaminate baseplate (Fig. 9). The core of each microthrix contains a number of longitudinally oriented, fine (ca. 5 nm diameter) filaments, resembling the actin components of microvilli (e.g., Ishikawa *et al.* 1969) (Fig. 10). Indeed, in most aspects of their structure and in that they are arranged to form what amounts to a "brush border", the microtriches are more reminiscent of microvilli than "microhairs" (as the term microthrix connotes). Estimates of the surface area amplification provided adult *H. diminuta* by these projections range from a factor of 3-fold (Berger and Mettrick 1971) to 16-fold (Rothman 1963).

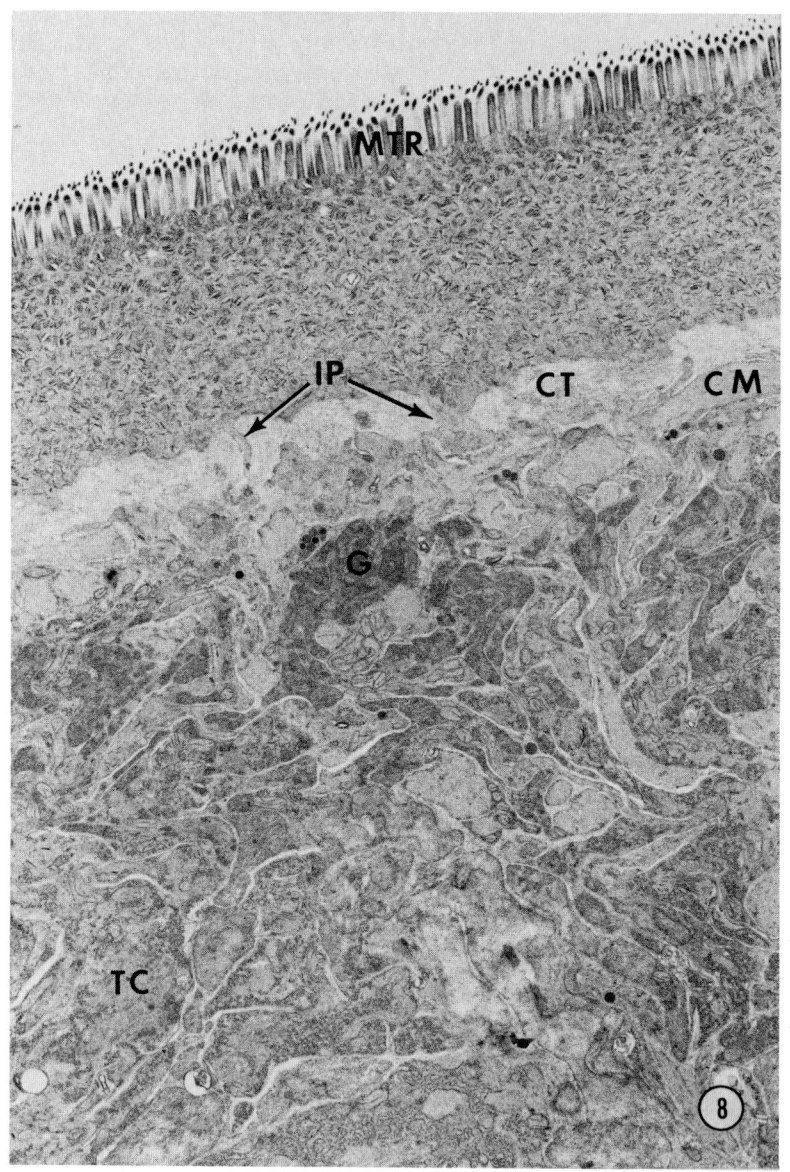

Fig. 8. Longitudinal section through immature proglottid showing nature of tegumentary cortical region. Basal tegumentary cytons (TC) surrounded by glycogen (G) filled processes of cortical myocytons. Internuncial processes (IP) from tegumentary cytons

The Morphology, Histology, and Fine Structure of the Adult Stage

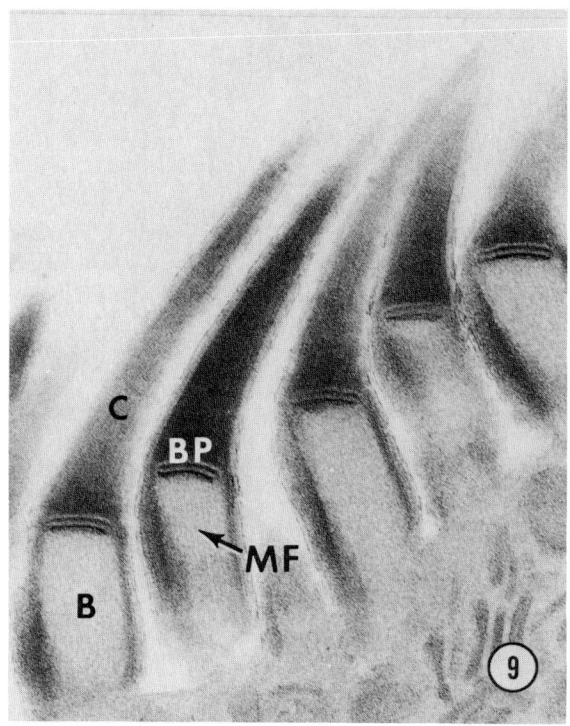

Fig. 9. Sagittal section of tegumental microtriches. Electron opaque cap (C) separated from the base (B) by multilaminar baseplate (BP). Microfilaments (MF) regularly arranged within base. Tegumental plasmalemma extends over entire length of each microthrix. X71,000.

In chemically preserved, plastic embedded and thin sectioned material, the free surface plasma membrane appears by electron microscopy to be trilaminate, measuring about 12 nm in thickness. The outermost leaflet is somewhat thicker than the inner leaflet, reflecting the presence of a surface layer of carbohydrate-containing macromolecules, the

---

extend through longitudinal (LM) and circular (CM) muscles, as well as connective tissue (CT) layer (= basement lamina) before joining syncytial distal cytoplasm (SDC). Microtriches (MTR) line free surface of syncytial layer. X5900.

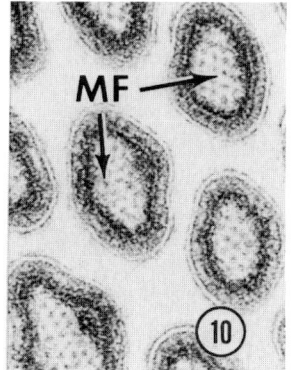

Fig. 10. Cross section through bases of tegumental microtriches revealing orderly array of microfilaments (MF) surrounded by accumulation of electron dense material. X120,000.

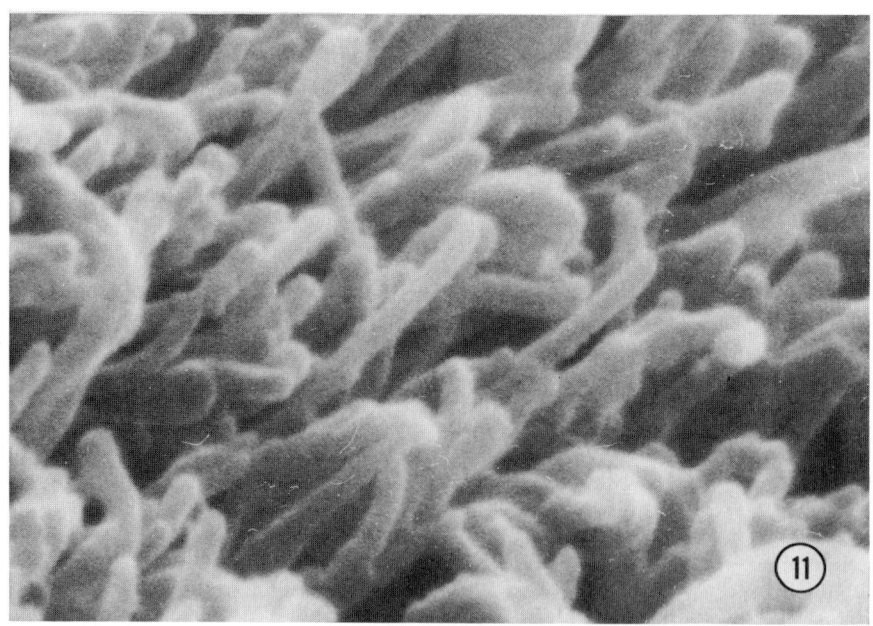

Fig. 11. Scanning electron micrograph of scolex microtriches. (From Ubelaker et al. 1973). X75,500.

glycocalyx which is best demonstrated cytochemically (Lumsden et al. 1970; Lumsden 1975a, b). Employing the technique of freeze-fracturing/etching to study the surface membrane of *Taenia crassiceps*, Belton (1977) obtained images of internal particulate substructure, suggestive of a membrane more along the lines of a "fluid-mosaic" (Singer and Nicolson 1972) than of a "unit" (Robertson 1959) construction. The same is true of the tegument plasma membrane of *H. diminuta* (Lumsden, unpublished observations).

The membrane delimiting the basal surface of the distal cytoplasm measures about 8 nm in thickness. Infoldings of this membrane have been observed, often in the form of tubules (Threadgold and Read 1970a). Hemidesmosomes are present, serving to anchor the membrane to an underlying layer of connective tissue, identified in the early descriptions of tapeworm microanatomy as the "cuticular basement membrane". This structure has two components resolvable by electron microscopy: (1) a dense, felt-like layer approximately 50 nm thick adjacent to the basal plasma membrane of the distal cytoplasm; and (2) a layer about 1.5 µm thick of fibrils, each about 12 nm in diameter, which extends to the level of the superficial musculature (Figs. 8, 12, 13 and 14). As not to confuse this extracytoplasmic component with membranes that are part of cells, it is preferable to use the term basement (or basal) *lamina*. This type of supportive structure is ubiquitously associated with epithelial tissues (see, e.g., Bloom and Fawcett 1975). Fibrils from the tegumentary basement lamina extend from its proximal surface to merge with those of the interstitial parenchymal ground substance. The fine structure of this connective tissue is detailed in a following section.

The distal cytoplasm is rather dense, and filled with flattened, discoidal membranous inclusions measuring about 140 x 15 nm (Figs. 8 and 13). The majority of these have an opaque, carbohydrate-rich matrix, surrounded by a membrane about 10 nm thick. These bodies are elaborated by the Golgi complexes of the tegumentary cytons, and are delivered to the distal cytoplasm via the internuncial processes. Concentrated in the basal third of the distal cytoplasm are numerous mitochondria. These mitochondria are small (about 300 x 200 nm)

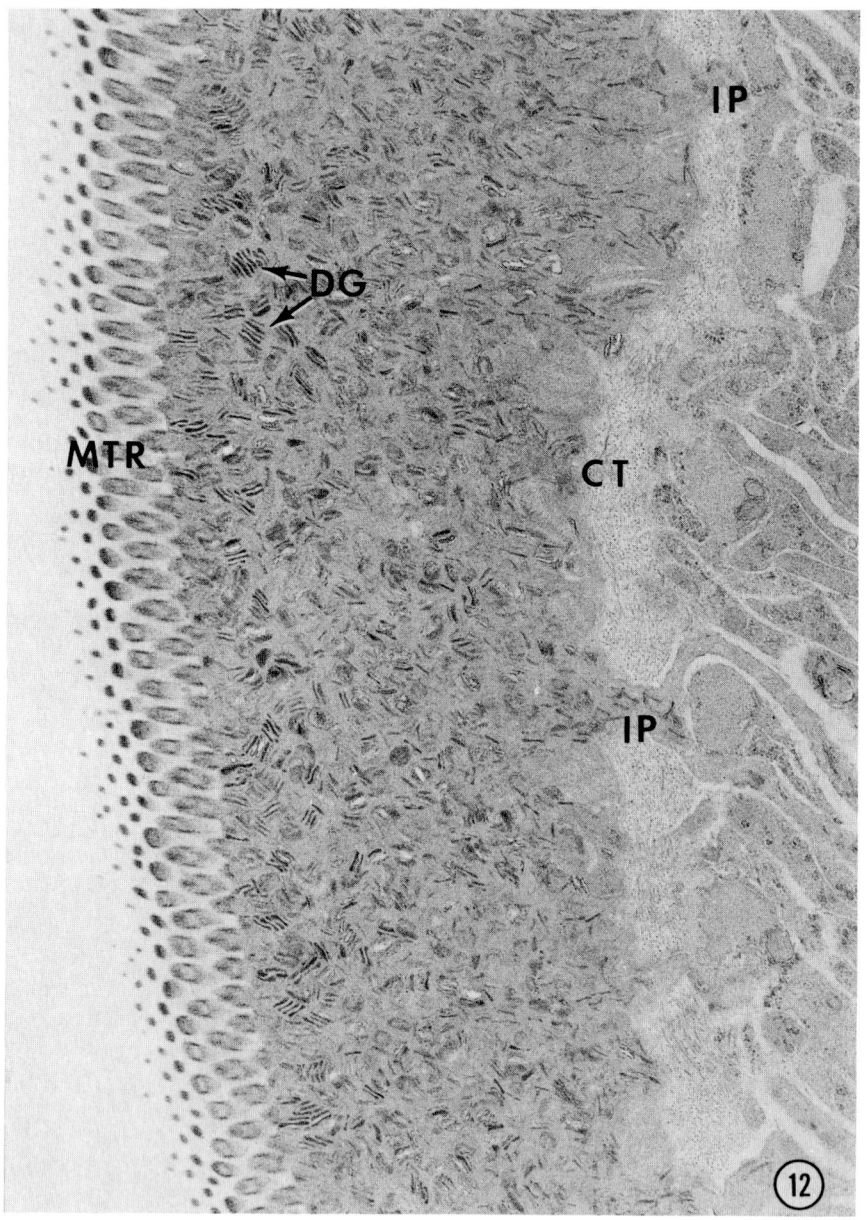

Fig. 12. Longitudinal section through immature proglottid. Microtriches (MTR) line free surface. Numerous discoidal granules (DG) occupy distal cytoplasm. Internuncial processes (IP) extend through connective tissue (CT) layer, arising from submuscular tegumentary cytons. X11,500.

and contain only a few very short cristae (Fig. 13). Early accounts of "cuticular pore canals" may be attributed to the investigators' failure to correctly interpret these structures as neural elements.

The tegumentary cytons are flask-like to fusiform in shape, with the long axis perpendicular to the basal surface of the distal cytoplasm. Each contains a prominent, generally round nucleus. The perinuclear cytoplasm is filled with free ribosomes, contains prominent Golgi bodies, and cisternae of granular endoplasmic reticulum. The majority of these cisternae are closely approximated to the plasma membrane. One or more tendrillar internuncial processes extend from the perinuclear cytoplasm toward the surface, where the plasmalemma of each internuncial process becomes continuous with the basal plasmalemma of the distal cytoplasm and intracytoplasmic continuity is established. The internuncial processes contain microtubules, paralleling the long axis, and, occasionally, granules of the type found in the distal cytoplasm and Golgi zones of the tegumentary cytons (Fig. 14).

Interdispersed between the tegumentary cytons are glycogen-rich extensions of muscle/parenchymal cells (glycogen is not present in the tegumentary cytons or distal cytoplasm). The fine structure of these elements and their relationship to the myofibrils which form the superficial body musculature is described in a following section on the muscle system. Gap junctions occur between muscle and tegument cell bodies (Fig. 22)

Also present are dendritic neurosensory processes, which originate with cell bodies in the lateral nerve cords and extend through the distal cytoplasm to the free surface. The terminus of these processes is cylindrical to bulb-shaped, bears a projecting cilium, contains numerous clear and opaque spherical vesicles and mitochondria, and is joined to the plasmalemma of the distal cytoplasm by a septate desmosome. From their structure, which is like that of known chemoreceptors in other organisms, it has been suggested that these tegumentary nerve processes, termed sensilla, serve chemo - and/or tactosensory functions in *H. diminuta* and other tapeworms (see e.g., Morseth 1967; Webb and Davey

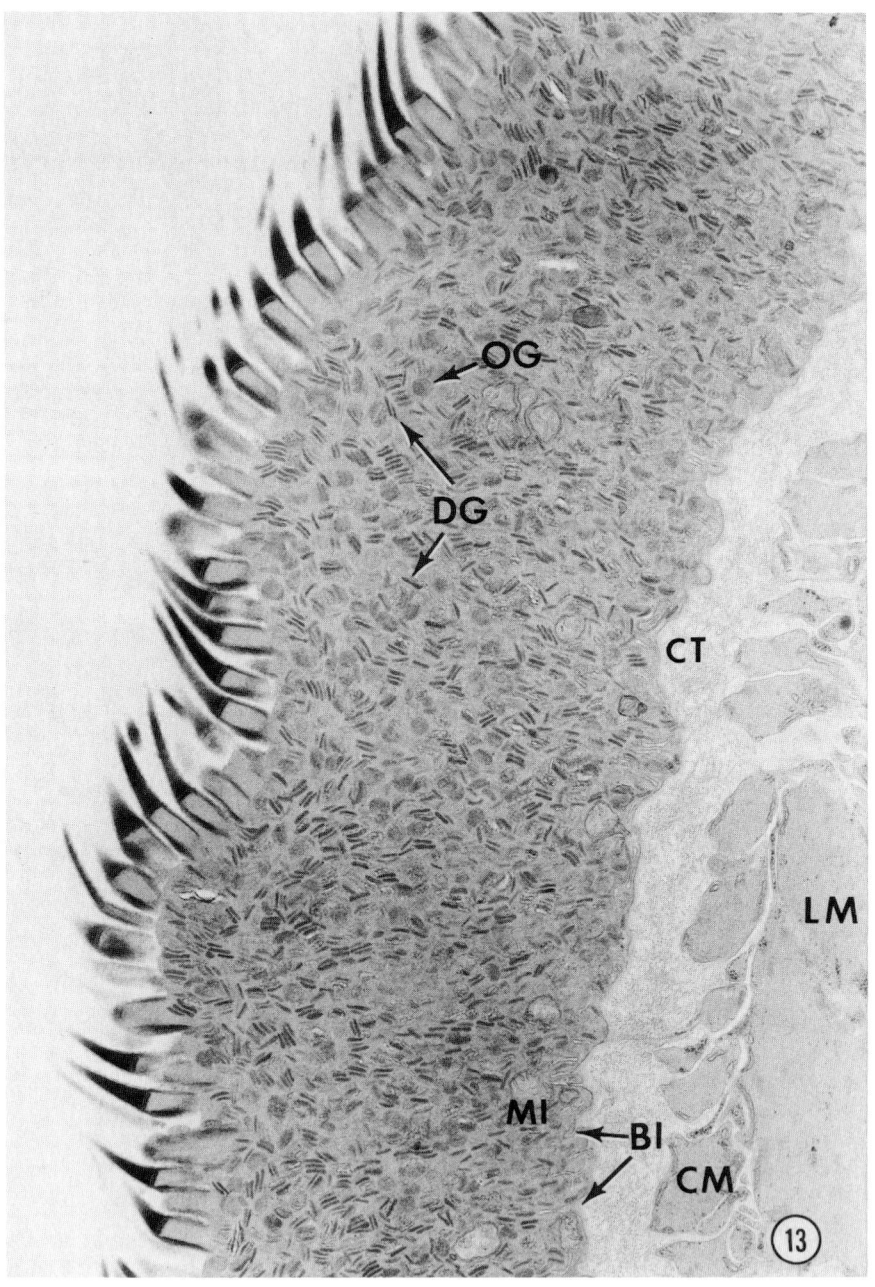

Fig. 13. Longitudinal section through scolex tegument. Microtriches stouter than on strobilar tegument. Syncytial cytoplasm filled with mixed population of discoidal granules (DG) and ovoid granules (OG) from rostellar tegument. Mitochondria (MI)

1974; Cooper et al. 1975). Further commentary on the tegumentary sensilla is to be found elsewhere in this chapter (see Nervous System).

The foregoing account applies generally to the strobilar tegument, and the same cytoarchitecture applies, for the most part, to the tegument covering the neck and scolex as well. Details which apply specifically to the tegument of the scolex are provided in a following section of this chapter.

B. *Functional Correlates*

A major function of the tegument, at least that of the strobila, is absorption. The physiology of this process, addressed in other chapters of this book and elsewhere reviewed by Pappas and Read (1975), is clearly served by the fine structure encountered particularly in the distal cytoplasm. The analogy with more conventional absorptive epithelia, e.g., the vertebrate intestinal mucosa, was emphatically conveyed by Beguin (1966b) (Figs. 14 and 15), and has since been stressed by many other authors. The tegumentary cytons represent a region of high biosynthetic activity, notably the synthesis of peptides (Lumsden 1966c) and glycoproteins (Oaks and Lumsden 1971). These products are involved at least in part with the maintenance of what appears to be a highly dynamic surface (Oaks and Lumsden 1971).

The tegument, by virtue of its sensilla, is also materially involved in sensory reception (see sections on nervous system and scolex). Given the sodium transport functions of the tegument, the nexus-type junctions (Fig. 22) between the tegument and muscle cell bodies is noteworthy.

---

apparent in basal third of cytoplasm. Infoldings (BI) of basal plasma membrane also present. CT, connective tissue; CM and LM, circular and longitudinal muscle, respectively. X19,000.

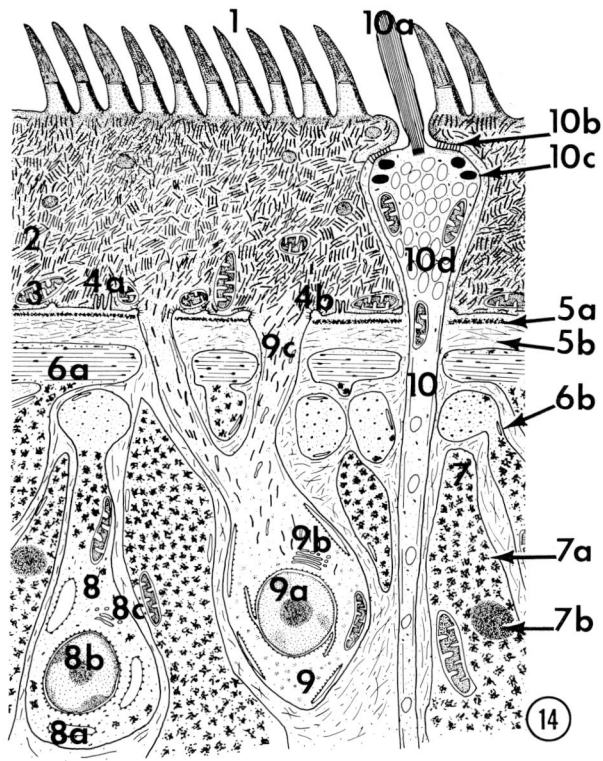

Fig. 14. Diagram of tegument of H. diminuta. 1. Brush border of microtriches; 2. Dense granules of distal cytoplasm; 3. Mitochondria of distal cytoplasm; 4a. Infoldings of basal plasma membrane of distal cytoplasm; 4b. Hemidesmosomes; 5a. Felt-like layer of basement lamina; 5b. Fibrillar layer of basement lamina; 6a. Contractile elements of superficial musculature; 6b. Agranular endoplasmic reticulum forming dyadic complex with sarcolemma; 7. Process of medullary myocyton; 7a. Alpha-glycogen particles; 7b. Lipid; 8. Cortical myocyton; 8a. Dilated cisternae of granular endoplasmic reticulum; 8b. Myocyton nucleus; 8c. Myocyton Golgi; 8d. Beta-glycogen particles; 9. Tegumentary cyton; 9a. Nucleus; 9b. Golgi of tegumentary cyton; 9c. Internuncial

The Morphology, Histology, and Fine Structure of the Adult Stage 181

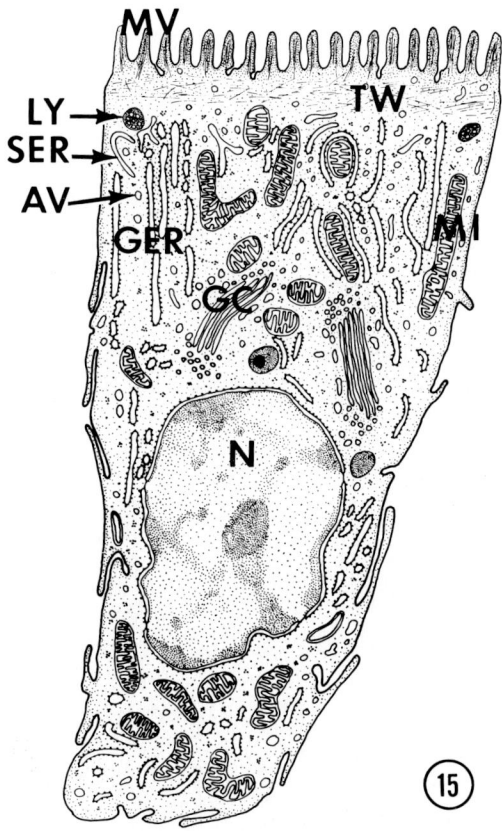

Fig. 15. Diagram of columnar epithelial cell from mammalian small intestine, for purposes of comparison with cestode tegument. Apical vesicles (AV), ectoplasm (EC), endoplasm (EN), Golgi complex (GC), granular endoplasm reticulum (GER), lysosomes (LY), brush border of microvilli (MV), mitochondria (MI), nucleus (N), smooth endoplasmic reticulum (SER), terminal web (TW). (After Lentz 1971).

---

process connecting tegumentary cyton with distal cytoplasm; 10. Sensory nerve process; 10a. Cilium; 10b. Septate desmosome; 10c. Electron dense collar; 10d. Large lucent vesicles; EC. Ectoplasm; EN. Endoplasm.

C. *Histogenesis*

It must be appreciated that tegument growth is a continual process in adult *H. diminuta*, as new proglottids are formed in the neck region and subsequently increase in volume and surface area as they undergo maturation. Protein synthesis occurs continuously in the tegumentary cytons (Lumsden 1966c), and most of this protein is exported to the distal cytoplasm where it contributes to the expansion of matrix, membrane, etc. The relative number of tegumentary cytons per unit area does not differ appreciably between the neck and maturing proglottids. Thus, with the growth of the proglottids, especially circumferentially, the number of tegumentary cytons must increase either by multiplication *in situ* or through the addition of new cells from nontegumentary sites of proliferation.

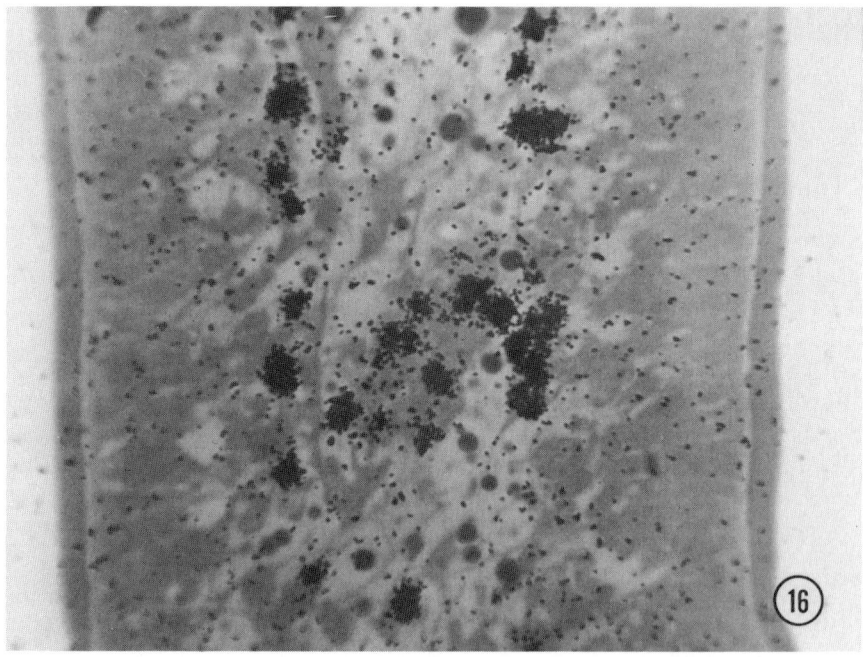

Fig. 16. Autoradiograph of neck region following incubation in ^3H-thymidine. Dense accumulation of exposed silver grains found over mitotically active germinal cells. X200.

Prenant (1922) recognized the existence of two primordial cell types in the medullary zone of immature *H. diminuta* proglottids, which he referred to as "cellules fixes", which supposedly gave rise to the majority of somatic tissues, and gametogenic "cellules libres". If this were true, however, one would expect a certain mobility of the "cellules fixes" during differentiation. Precedent for the role of cellular migration in the growth of the cestode tegument and other tissues can be found in the observations recorded by Douglas (1961) on morphogenic movements of tissue progenitors in some nematotaeniid tapeworms. Douglas (1961) concluded that, in addition to histogenesis of the reproductive structures, ".... nearly all the cellular components of mature and gravid proglottids appear to be derived from a single streak of cells located immediately posterior to the scolex - the primary anlage". Bolla and Roberts (1971) concluded that in adult *H. diminuta* these germinal cells are the only somatic ones which divide, and so act as stem cells for strobilar development of the mature worm.

In the embryonic development of *H. diminuta* oncospheres, both zones of the tegument (distal cytoplasm and tegumentary cytons) differentiate from a single cell type (Rybicka 1973), though postembryonic growth involves fusion with the distal cytoplasm of cells which migrate into the cortex from germinative centers in the medulla (Lumsden 1965b; Bentley 1973). As determined by pulse labeling with ^{3}H-thymidine and autoradiography, tegumentary cytons in growing proglottids do not undergo division. Replication is a function of a pool of undifferentiated cells which, in the neck and anterior proglottids are located principally in the germinal anlage (see Bolla and Roberts 1971). The pattern of ^{3}H-thymidine incorporation in worms after two hours incubation with the radioactive nucleoside is shown in Fig. 16; no labeling of the tegument cyton nuclei is evident, though cells of the germinal anlagen and peripheral medulla incorporate the DNA precursor. However, in worms allowed to assimilate ^{3}H-thymidine for two hours, then cultured *in vitro* or returned to the host intestine for 40-60 hours, labeled cyton nuclei are detected (Fig. 17). Tegument growth in other cestodes occurs by the same process, as demonstrated for *Taenia crassiceps* by Bentley (1973) and for *Diphyllobothrium latum* by Wikgren and Knuts (1970). It is a mechanism employed ubiquitously by syncytial tissues, as exemplified by the mammalian trophoblast. Individual cells of the inner layer, the cytotrophoblast, are mitotically active; daughter cells contribute to the

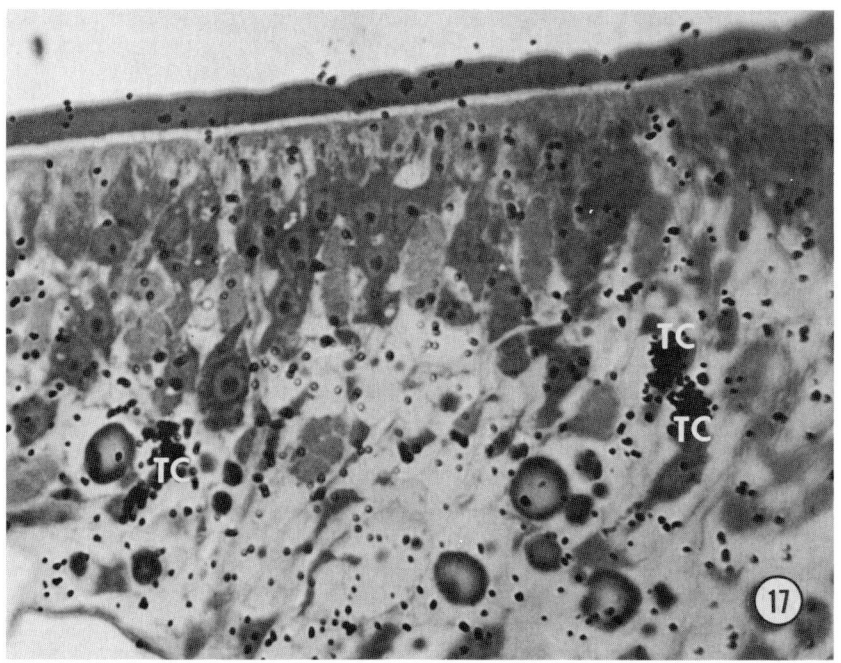

Fig. 17. Autoradiograph of neck region following incubation in ^3H-thymidine. Migration of developing tegumentary cytons (TC) to cortical region of proglottid proliferation marked by localization of exposed silver grains. X700.

increasing mass of the outer syncytiotrophoblast by fusing with and becoming part of the syncytium (see Bloom and Fawcett 1975).

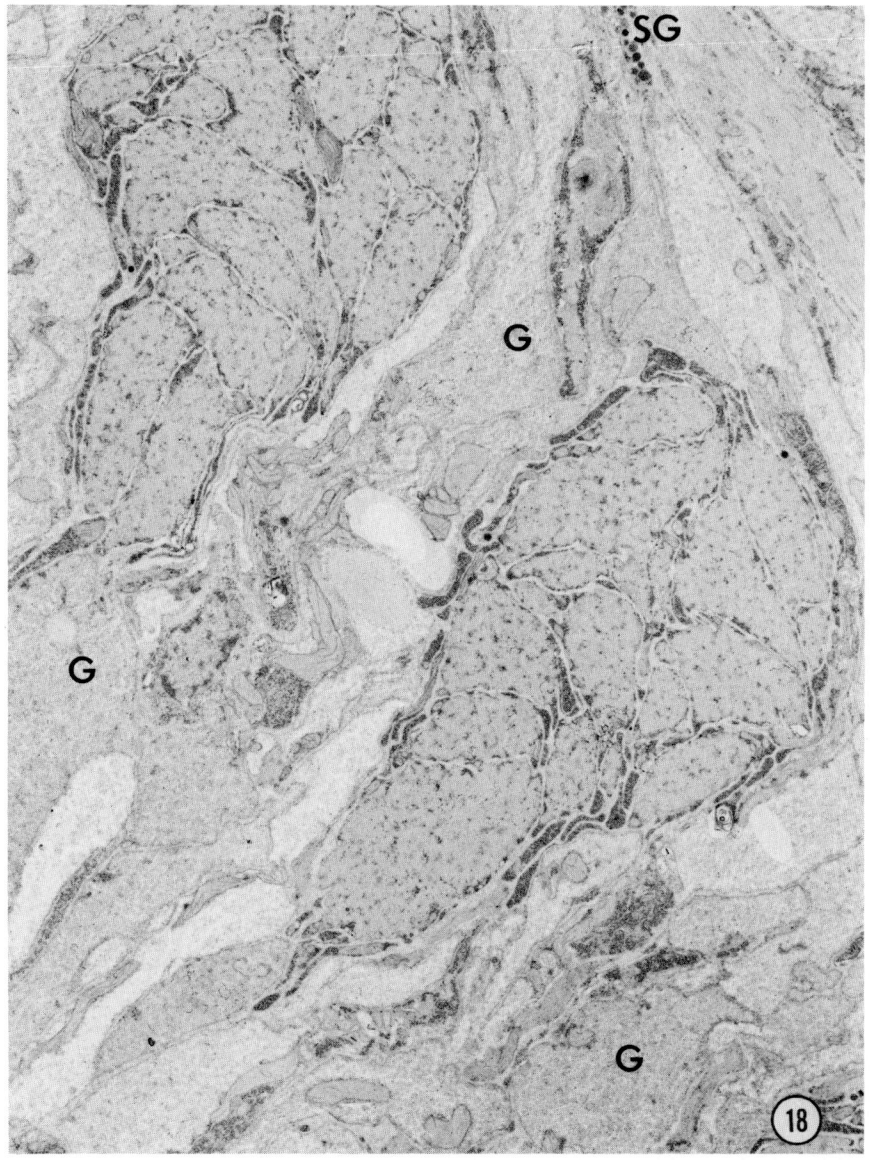

Fig. 18. Cross section through medullary muscles within neck region. Contractile elements are grouped into fascicles, with the glycogen (G) filled processes of the medullary myocytons occupying surrounding area. Secretory granules (SC) of endocrine cell interspersed with muscle tissue. (Micrograph courtesy of Dr. F. M. Gress). X5,500.

IV. MUSCLE

The major musculature of adult *H. diminuta* consists of the longitudinal medullary fibers, cortical transverse fibers, subtegumentary longitudinal and circular fibers, the suckers, rostellum, and the contractile elements associated with the terminal genitalia.

A given muscle cell consists of two major components: (1) the contractile myofibril, containing the actin and myosin myofibrils; and (2) what we would here term the myocyton, the non-contractile, nucleus-containing cytoplasm. The myocytons are typically positioned lateral to and often at some distance from the myofibrils, with cytoplasmic continuity established via tendrillar processes (Fig. 26). In the classical descriptions of the early 1900's, the myocytons were frequently mistaken for neural elements - e.g., the "neuromuscular" cells of Young (1908). Part of the confusion was due to the fact that metal impregnation methods used to identify neural elements in higher organisms also stain at least some of the muscle cell bodies of tapeworm.

A. *Fine Structure of the Myofibril*

Anatomically, the myofibrils are often grouped into fasicles, in which the sufaces of the individual myofibrils are very closely approximated (Fig. 18). Within and surrounding a fasicle, the myofibrils are bound together by connective tissue.

Lacking intact Z-discs, there is no division of the myofibril into sarcomeres. While both thick (myosin) and thin (actin) myofilaments are present, their distribution is not ordered to the extent that there is a clear demarcation into A and I bands. Tapeworm muscles are, accordingly, said to be of the non-striated or "smooth" variety (Lumsden and Byram 1967).

Each muscle cell unit typically contains but one myofibril (those of the suckers and some in the strobilar musculature are branched). The myofibril

The Morphology, Histology, and Fine Structure of the Adult Stage

is invested with a plasma membrane (or sarcolemma) which is continuous with the surface membrane of its associated myocytons. Nothing approximating the transverse sarcolemmal invaginations (T-tubules)

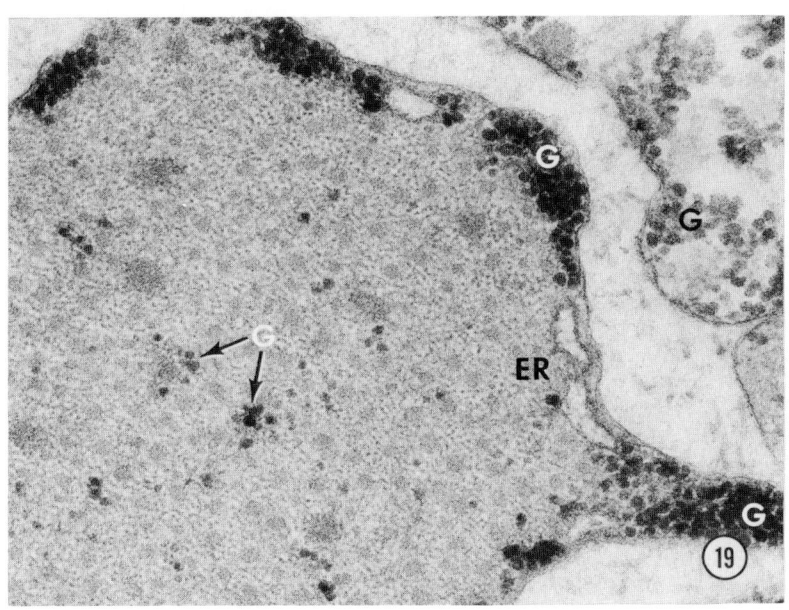

Fig. 19. Higher magnification of fibrillar portion of muscle cell. Peripheral regions of cell occupied by distended cisternae of endoplasmic reticulum (ER) and beta-glycogen (G) particles. Betaglycogen also interspersed with thick and thin filaments. CT, connective tissue. X79,000.

present in vertebrate striated and many kinds of higher invertebrate muscle cells has been observed for any muscle cell type in *H. diminuta*. Cisternae of agranular endoplasmic (sarcoplasmic) reticulum are, however, consistently distributed along the periphery of the myofibril, in close proximity to the sarcolemma; the intervening space between the two membrane systems may be as little as 20 nm or less (Fig. 19). This approximates the intermembrane distances observed in the triads (T-tubule/paired SER cisternae complexes) of striated fibers of other organisms.

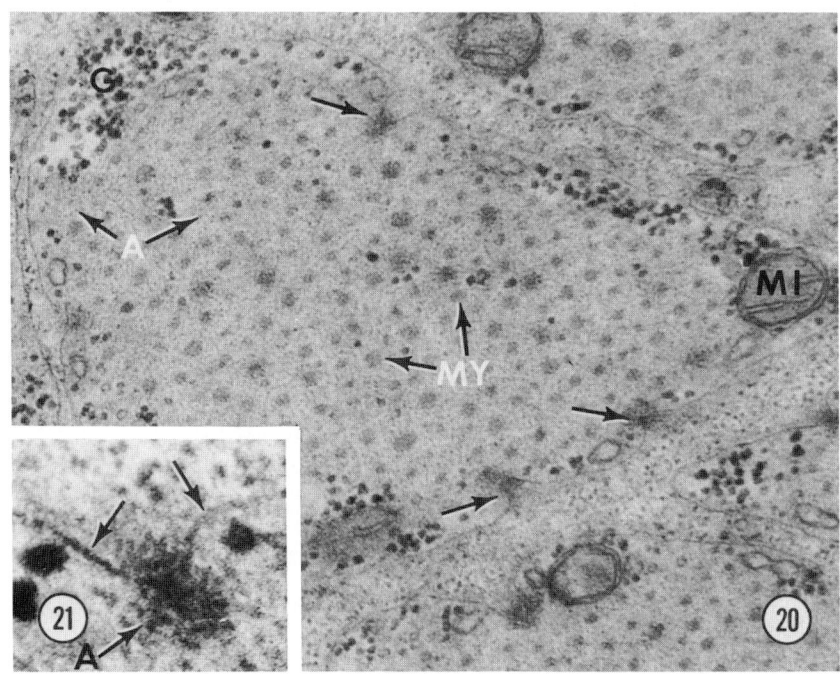

Fig. 20. Cross section through portion of medullary muscle bundle. Dense bodies (arrows) associated with infoldings of sarcolemma. Beta-glycogen (G) and mitochondria (MI) located in peripheral cytoplasm. Central cytoplasm filled with cross-sectioned thick (MY) and thin (A) filaments. (From Lumsden and Byram 1967). X60,000.

Fig. 21. Higher magnification of dense body showing relationship with sarcolemma (arrows). Structures at A are cross-sectioned thin filaments. (From Lumsden and Byram 1967). X198,000.

The myofibrilar cytoplasm is filled with myofilaments, of which there are two size classes - one with an average diameter of 5 nm, the other with a maximum diameter of approximately 30 nm. The myofilaments are oriented parallel or slightly oblique to the longitudinal axis of the myofibril. The 30 nm filaments are thickest in the middle and taper toward both ends. Thus, in shape, they resemble known myosin type myofilaments. However, the myosin filaments of striated vertebrate muscle have a maximum diameter of only 10 nm. The 5 nm myofilaments are presumably composed of actin. Each thick filament is surrounded by an orbital array of up to 12 or more thin filaments (Fig. 20), a ratio of thin:thick filaments considerably higher than is encountered in striated myofibrils (6:1), but much lower than that for vertebrate smooth muscle. The thin filaments are attached to small dense bodies which, at the periphery of the myofibril, anchor the filaments to the sarcolemma (Figs. 20 and 21). The structure of these dense bodies where they interface with the connective tissue, is not unlike a half-desmosome. The afilamentous cytoplasm between the cell surface and myofilaments contains cisternae of agranular endoplasmic (sarcoplasmic) reticulum (noted in the preceding paragraph), occasional microtubules, mitochondria, and numerous glycogen particles.

Junctional complexes, including some described (perhaps erroneously) as desmosomes, have been noted between muscle cells (Threadgold and Read 1970b). From our own observations, these junctions appear more like the "gap" ("close") or nexus variety (Figs. 22 and 23). Interestingly, gap junctions are also observed between muscle and tegument (Fig. 22), as well as between muscle and an associated endocrine cell type (Figs. 24, 43 and 48; see following section on scolex).

B. *Functional Correlates*

While little is known about the physiology of tapeworm muscle contraction, it seems safe to assume that a two filament (actin-myosin) sliding mechanism (as per the Huxley model) obtains for these muscle cells as it has for all other invertebrate and vertebrate systems studied to date. The dense bodies appear to have a cohesive function; their occurrence at nodal points where thin filaments appear to be bound together laterally and where they are attached to the sarcolemma is consistent with this view. Interaction of the thin filaments with the thick would exert tension against the cell surface at the many points of dense body insertion. Body movements would result with the transmission of this force to the surrounding connective tissue (see following section).

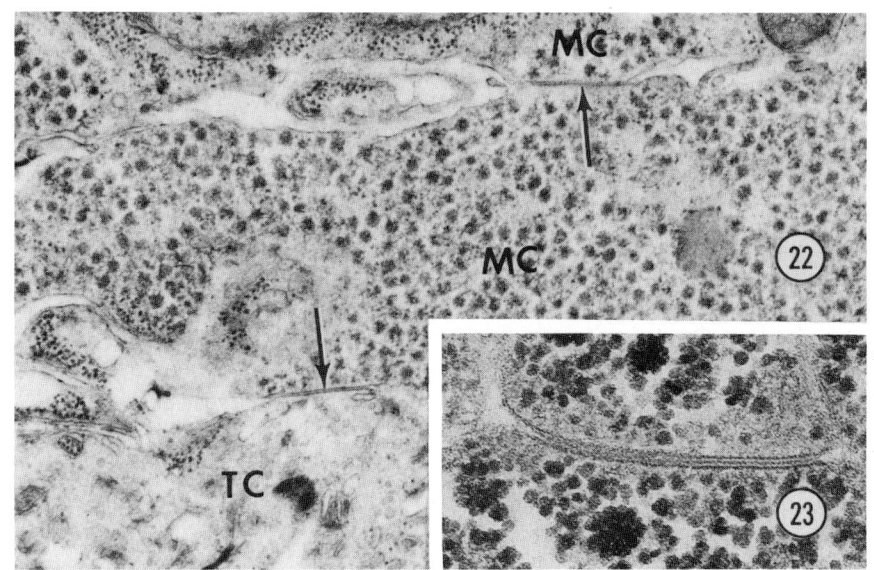

Fig. 22. Adjacent medullary myocytons (MC) and tegumentary cyton (TC) joined by gap junctions (arrows). X28,000.

Fig. 23. Higher magnification of junction joining adjacent myocytons. X82,000.

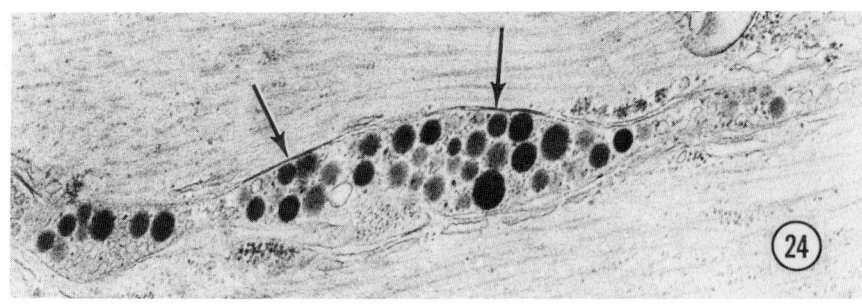

Fig. 24. Endocrine cell process within acetabular musculature. Junctions (arrows) connect secretory cell process with sarcolemma surrounding contractile fibers. X38,000.

Calcium is a ubiquitous requirement for the activation of actin-myosin contractile system, and though its role in tapeworm muscle remains to be established, it would be surprising if this system proved to be calcium insensitive. In a wide variety of invertebrate and vertebrate muscles, calcium, during the resting (relaxed) state, is sequestered within the sarcoplasmic reticulum. Excitation induces a flow of calcium from the sarcoplasmic reticulum into the cytoplasm where binding to myofilaments results in ATP hydrolysis, actin-myosin crosslinkages, and contraction. In muscles with a paucity of agranular ER (e.g., vertebrate smooth muscle), it has been suggested that the plasmalemma mediates cytoplasmic calcium concentration relative to an extracellular pool. Given the modest development of the agranular ER in the muscle of *H. diminuta*, but its consistent proximity to the sarcolemma, either or both mechanisms for regulating calcium concentrations may be operable. The dyadic (sarcolemma/single SER cisterna complex) may have the effect of reducing membrane impedance to ion flow, facilitating cell-to-cell conductivity of excitatory stimuli, and accommodating intracellular movement of contraction-activating substances (e.g., calcium), as is the case in many other kinds of muscle cells.

The myofibrilar fine structure of adult *H. diminuta* conforms to that of slow-contracting fibers in other organisms, and, certainly, the observed movements of these worms are anything but fast. A major role of muscle contraction in these worms, especially of the longitudinal musculature, must be to resist expulsion, by maintaining a state of body tonus against the peristaltic movements of the host intestine. For this purpose, the anatomical distribution and fine structure of the myofibrils are well-suited. Smooth muscles generally are able to sustain contraction for long periods with a relatively modest expenditure of energy. There is evidence, reviewed elsewhere in this volume that adult *H. diminuta* locomote, as their migrations up and down the host gut would testify. Equally, muscular contractions would be expected to play a significant role in excretion, reproduction, and cephalic adhesion, as noted more specifically elsewhere in this chapter.

C. *Neuromuscular Interactions*

The most richly innervated muscles appear to be those in the scolex, especially the suckers (see Wilson and Schiller 1969), the neck, and those of the terminal male genitalia. In specimens of adult *H. diminuta* stained for acetylcholine esterase activity, Wilson and Schiller (1969) also described "numerous" nerve fibers along the main longitudinal trunks of the strobila which led into the marginal, longitudinal musculature. They identified the termini of these nerve fibers as "motor end plates". However, in thin sections examined by electron microscopy, morphologically identifiable myoneural junctions are very infrequently encountered within the strobila. Where such have been observed, they consist at most of slight concavity of the muscle cell surface which accommodates the axon, analogous to but by no means as definitive as the synaptic troughs associated with, the motor end plates of vertebrate skeletal muscle. Oftentimes, the axon merely passes close to the muscle cell, with little or no modification of muscle cell topography. The myoneural junction is otherwise marked by a close parallarity of the muscle cell and axonal membranes, which are separated by space of 20 nm or less. Small, spherical vesicles are usually accumulated in the axonal cytoplasm at these junctions; the majority are electron-lucent, while some are dense-cored. Occasionally, tendrillar processes from the contractile portion of a muscle cell will extend into the neuropile of an adjacent ganglion or nerve cord, thus establishing neuromuscular communication. In *H. diminuta*, this is most often observed in association with the medullary muscles, and the transverse and oblique muscles of the scolex. While the exception in *H. diminuta*, this form of neuromuscular interaction is commonplace in many other lower invertebrate groups (see Bullock and Horridge 1965 for review).

As we describe elsewhere in detail (see Nervous System and Scolex), there is associated with the sucker musculature, in particular, a cell type, possibly endocrine, which may serve as a long-acting modulator of muscle activity. This element is characterized by the presence of large, spherical, electron dense granules (which at the light microscope level stain with paraldehyde fuchsin), (Figs.

24, 43 and 48). The secretory activity of these cells may, in turn, be regulated by neurosecretory elements and/or conventional neurons.

It does not seem to us hazardous to presume that at the motor end plates previously described, the vesicles accumulated in the axonal cytoplasm contain neurotransmitter substances. Most commonly, the one contained within the electron-lucent variety is acetylcholine. Wilson and Schiller (1969) found that certain anti-acetylcholinesterase compounds stimulate muscle activity in *H. diminuta*, while cholinomimetic drugs are inhibitory. These observations led Wilson and Schiller (1969) to conclude that acetylcholine functions as an inhibitory neurotransmitter, and that a second, stimulatory motor neurotransmitter must be present. The subsequent identification of 5-hydroxytryptamine (Lee *et al.* 1978) within at least certain neurons of *H. diminuta* suggests this substance as the possible neurotransmitter effecting muscle contraction.

In higher organisms, especially vertebrates, cholinergic myoneural junctions are frequently excitatory; binding of acetylcholine to the sarcolemma increases sodium permeability, resulting in depolarization. In mammalian cardiac muscle, however, acetylcholine inhibits the generation of action potentials, by increasing potassium, rather than sodium, conduction (the resting potential is accordingly shifted closer to the potassium equilibrium value, which is more negative than the normal resting potential). In some cases, inhibition by acetylcholine is effected by an increase in chloride permeability of the muscle cell.

It is of interest that the great majority of the "motor end plates" so far identified histochemically in *H. diminuta* are cholinergic; 5-hydroxytryptamine has so far been localized only in the cirrus sphinter musculature (Wilson and Schiller 1969; Lee *et al.* 1978). If, indeed, acetylcholine in these tapeworms is an inhibitory neurotransmitter (see also Tomosky-Sykes *et al.* 1977) and the majority of neuromuscular junctions prove to be cholinergic, it follows that muscle excitation must be accomplished by an alternate mechanism to direct innervation.

The apparent paucity of the traditional kinds of neuromuscular interactions in the strobila makes it likely that the excitation of a given tapeworm muscle cell need not require direct innervation, but the stimuli may be passed from one muscle cell to another, or self-generated. At least the rhythmic contractions of the longitudinal strobilar muscles appear to be independent of direct neural control. Rietschel (1935) found that cutting the longitudinal body nerve cords had no effect on this muscular activity. Moreover, when a proglottid was compressed, the waves of contraction were interrupted at that level but resumed distally; when the pressure was released, contractions passed over the formerly compressed area as before. Among the local stimuli known to initiate contraction in smooth muscle fibers generally is stretch, to which the longitudinal body musculature, especially, would most appropriately be receptive.

Junctional complexes resembling the nexus or gap junction have been reported between adjacent muscle cells in *H. diminuta* (Threadgold and Read 1970b). As seen in Figures 22 and 23, the plasma membranes of adjacent cells are closely apposed, with an intervening space of about 15 nm or, often, much less. The nexus is believed to be the principal, if not only, type of junction that mediates direct electrical coupling between cells. Invertebrate smooth muscle, gap junctions allow the contraction of a group of muscles from a single nerve impulse, with the separate cells acting in concert, without extensive innervation. A similar mechanism is envisioned for smooth muscle in *H. diminuta*.

D. *Fine Structure of the Myocyton*

The most readily identified myocytons in the *H. diminuta* strobila are those associated with the superficial circular and longitudinally directed myofibrils underlying the distal cytoplasm and basement lamina of the tegument. These are interdispersed among the tegumentary perikarya, and may be confused for them. The myocytons are distinguished by a more electron transparent cytoplasmic ground substance, frequently dilated cisternae of granular endoplasmic reticulum, and glycogen granules, usually concentrated in the cytoplasm proximal to the myofibril. Glycogen is not found in the tegumentary perikarya. The perinuclear cytoplasm of the myocyton contains an abundance of free ribosomes and a highly vesicular Golgi apparatus. Mitochondria are inconspicuous (Fig. 26).

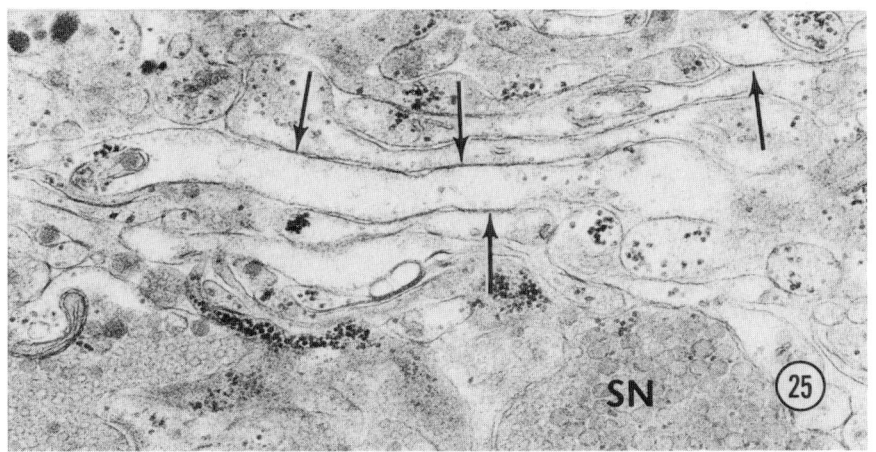

Fig. 25. Cross section through lateral nerve cord within neck region. Junctions (arrows) join adjacent neurites, not at terminals, but along length of nerve processes. Sensory neurite (SN) filled with large lucent vesicles also apparent. X38,500.

In the medullary parenchyma, the chief cytological element encountered is a large cytoplasmic body, typically filled with glycogen granules and containing prominent lipid droplets (Fig. 28). In comparison with most other *H. diminuta* cell types, mitochondria here are relatively large and abundant. The perinuclear cytoplasm is filled with free ribosomes and contains occasional, flattened profiles of granular endoplasmic reticulum. Golgi complexes are inconspicuous. The glycogen and lipid deposits occupy the cytoplasm peripheral to the nucleus-containing region. This glycogen-rich cytoplasm is highly attenuated, with elongate, branching processes extending out from the cell center. It is now apparent that many of these processes merge at their distal extremities with myofibrils, as first argued by Reissig and Colucci (1968). It therefore seems reasonable to regard these medullary "parenchymal cells" as myocytons. It appears that in some cases a given myofibril may have associated with it more than one myocyton. Since two or more myocytons may thus be cytoplasmically interconected, the musculo-parenchymal tissue can be considered syncytial, at least to an extent. Myocytons are also associated with one another by nexus or "gap" junctions (Threadgold and Read 1970b).

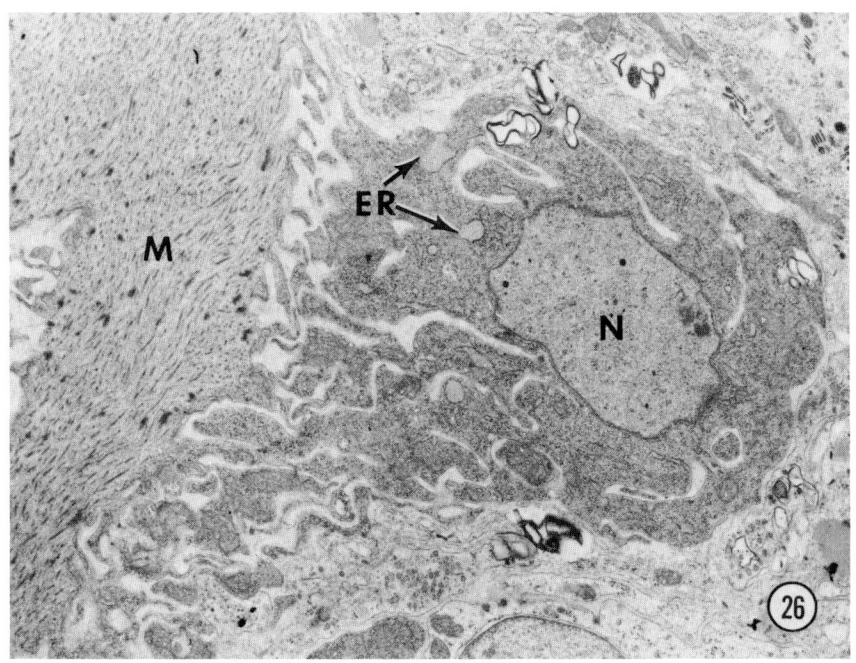

Fig. 26. Cortical myocyton characterized by prominent nucleus (N), distended cisternae of endoplasmic reticulum (ER) and numerous ribosomes; glycogen not prominent. Tendrillar processes join perinuclear region to contractile elements. X8,000.

The organization of the tapeworm parenchyma has long been a puzzle to helminthologists. In the classical accounts of the late 1800's and early 1900's, it was often described as highly vacuolar. This appearance may be attributed to fixatives and embedments which failed to preserve glycogen, severe shrinkage and separation of elements during microtechnical processing, or to stains which failed to tincture polysaccharide. The disagreement in this literature as to whether the major amount of "parenchymal space" is intra - or intercellular was resolved in favor of the former by electron microscopy (e.g., Lumsden 1965a, 1966a; Lumsden and Byram 1967). The greatest amount of the parenchymal volume is clearly cytoplasmic, with the cytological units separated by ordinarily relatively narrow interstitial spaces occupied by connective tissue.

E. *Functional Correlates of Myocyton Fine Structure*

As reviewed elsewhere in this book, energy metabolism in adult *H. diminuta* is predicated on the

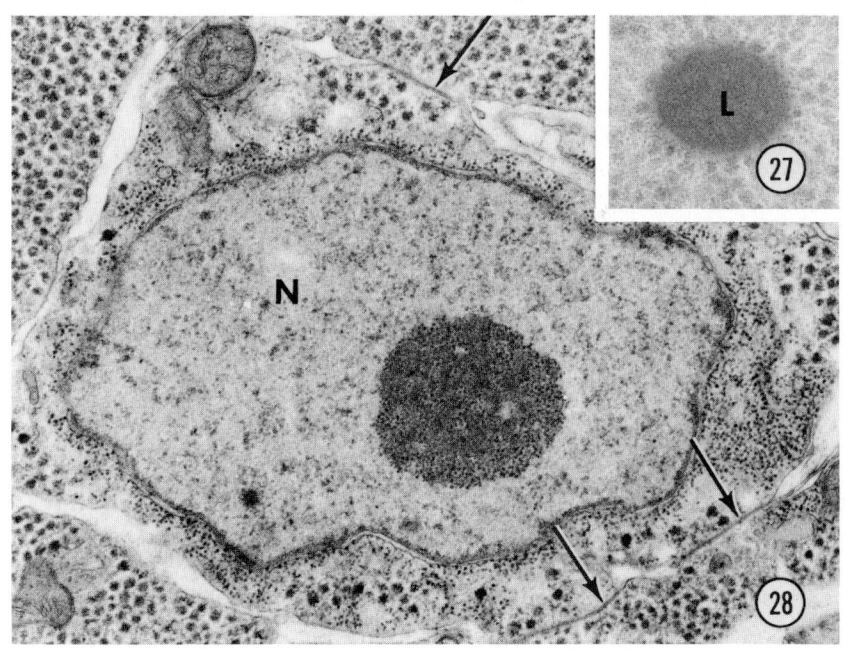

Fig. 27. *Peripheral cytoplasm of medullary myocyton containing lipid (L) surrounded by alpha-glycogen rosettes. X30,000.*

Fig. 28. *Medullary myocyton characterized by nucleus (N) with prominent nucleolus. Perinuclear cytoplasm filled with free ribosomes, peripheral*

anaerobic oxidation of glucose. A principal function of the musculature, at least of the medullary parenchymal myocytons, is glycogen storage. "Parenchymal" glycogen, which may constitute as much as half the dry weight of these worms, is readily degraded to glucose, especially under conditions which deprive the worms of exogenous supplies of this hexose sugar. Likewise, much of the glucose absorbed from the host intestine is initially incorporated into glycogen (Colucci et al. 1966), the principal site of this glycogen synthetic activity being the musculature (Lumsden 1965a). The musculoparenchyma is also the principal site of lipid storage (Fig. 27). Fatty acids, absorbed from the environment, are esterified with glycerol and deposited as microscopically visible droplets in the medullary myocytons (Lumsden and Harrington 1966). Some of this lipid is subsequently transferred to the eggs (King and Lumsden 1969). Though suggested many years ago that tapeworm lipids might be derived from the worm's prodigious carbohydrate metabolism (von Brand 1952), there is no evidence that the high lipid content of *H. diminuta* is related to the formation of metabolic waste products (Ginger and Fairbairn 1966a, 1966b), nor do such lipids contribute materially to the worm's energy metabolism.

For reasons presented in the following section, the muscle cells (myocytons) are the most likely candidates, to date, for the origin of tapeworm connective tissue.

F. *Histogenesis*

Reissig and Colucci's (1968) interpretation of the structural relationship of "parenchymal cells" to "muscle fibers" is an analysis in which we concur. However, there yet remain some unanswered questions. The myocytons prevalent in the cortical region differ structurally in certain respects from those prevalent in the medullary region. It is not unlikely, however, that both originate from a common myoblast precursor,

mitochondria and abundant alpha-glycogen. Cell junctions (arrows) join adjacent myocytons. X28,000.

with the medullary type of myocyton simply becoming more specialized for glycogen storage, etc. On the other hand, there is the possibility of two distinct cell lines - the myofibril-forming myoblast, from which all muscle units are initially derived, and another which secondarily merges with myofibrils after they are differentiated. Gough (1911) described the histogenesis of parenchymal muscle in *Avitellina centripunctata* as originating with spindle shaped myoblasts which elaborated the contractile fibers. According to Gough (1911), as the tubular cavity of the fiber fills peripherally with "muscle substance" (presumably myofilaments), the nuclei of the axial myoblasts "disappear", while nuclei of the differentiated fiber come to lie lateral to it. In embryos of *H. citelli*, Collin (1970) could distinguish between what he suggested were "parenchymal cell" precursors, as such, and myoblasts, *sensu stricto*. Additional studies on the development of the tapeworm musculo-parenchymal tissue are clearly in order.

V.   THE CONNECTIVE TISSUE

Traditionally, the connective tissue of metazoans is described as consisting of (1) a matrix of extracellular fibrous proteins and polysaccharides, and (2) the fiber and ground substance producing cells. By these standards, the connective tissue of *H. diminuta* and other tapeworms is rather ill-defined. Not infrequently, the interstitial spaces appear vacant. In many instances, there is reason to believe that this is the result of extraction during microtechnical preparation, but even in specimens which otherwise satisfy the criteria for faithful preservation, connective tissue elements are oftentimes inconspicuous. The structural components of tapeworm connective tissue recognizable in electron micrographs are exceedingly fine (ca. 10 nm diameter) fibrils, loosely dispersed in optically empty space. These fibrils are most frequently encountered in proximity to muscle cells, where their orientation tends to parallel the longitudinal axis of the myofibrils. Extracellular connective tissue fibrils are most densely concentrated in the basement lamina lying between the distal cytoplasm of the tegument and circular superficial musculature. A distinctive fibrogenic cell type has not, to date, been indentified.

A. *The Nature of Animal Connective Tissues*

Among the ubiquitous fibrous components of the connective tissue of vertebrates and higher invertebrates is collagen. Collagen and related fibrous connective tissue proteins are most dependably identified and distinguished from one another by their amino acid composition, but collagen, in particular, is usually recognizable as well by its morphological hallmarks. Typically, collagen fibrils are transversely striated, with a periodic spacing of 60-70 nm. In cross section, they appear solid, and have a diameter of 20-100 nm. Smaller diameter, non-banded fibrils encountered extracellularly in connective tissues have been associated with the early stages in collagen formation, or with the presence of elastic connective tissues. As described by Greenlee *et al.* (1966) and others, vertebrate elastic tissue has two components: (1) microfibrils, having a diameter of about 10 nm, in cross section appearing tubular, and in longitudinal section appearing beaded; and (2) an abundant amorphous component composed of the protein elastin. A variant of elastic connective termed oxytalan has been described by Fullmer (1958), Fullmer and Lillie (1958) Fullmer *et al.* (1974), Cotta-Pereira *et al.* (1976) and others in a variety of vertebrate connective tissues - skin, tendons, peridontal membranes, etc. The microfilaments of oxytalan are identical in structure to those of elastic connective tissue, *sensu strictu*, (see Carmichael and Fullmer 1966, and Greenlee *et al.* 1966) but oxytalan is lacking in the amorphous elastin component. Accordingly, oxytalan does not stain with the usual procedures employed for the demonstration of elastic connective tissue, such as orcein, resorcinol fuchsin, aldehyde fuchsin, orcinol new fuchsin, or Verhoff's hematoxylin (see, e.g. Pearse 1968), and is resistant to removal by elastase. However, following peracetic acid oxidation, oxytalan-type elastic connective tissue stains with orcein, resorcinol and aldehyde fuchsin, and is removed by elastase.

In vertebrates and many of the higher invertebrates, the extracellular components of both collagenic and elastic connective tissues are elaborated by fibroblasts, which are recognized as such by their usually fusiform shape, abundant granular endoplasmic reticulum, and prominent Golgi apparatus (see, e.g., Porter 1964). In vertebrates, cells of non-fibroblastic origin with the potential for collagen and elastic connective tissue sythesis include smooth muscle (Ross 1973, 1974; Ross and Klebakoff 1971).

B. *The Classification of Tapeworm Connective Tissue - Fine Structural and Functional Properties*

Data on the molecular structure and chemical composition of the fibrous extracellular components of *H. diminuta* are as yet insufficient to classify them as collagen, elastic connective tissue, etc. Collagen-type proteins have been identified from a variety of lower invertebrates, including nematodes, acanthocephalans, and at least one digenetic trematode - *Fasciola hepatica* (see, e.g., Gross 1963; Nordwig and Hayduk 1969; Josse and Harrington 1964; Fujimoto 1968; Cain 1970). However, as they appear in electron microscope images, the elements of the connective tissue of *H. diminuta* and other cestodes more closely resemble those of oxytalan than collagen: (1) the microfibrils do not materially exceed 10 nm in diameter; (2) in fortuitous cross sections, they appear to have a hollow core; and (3) in longitudinal section, a finely beaded substructure with a periodicity of less than 5 nm can be resolved (Fig. 30). Moreover, by its staining properties, the tegumentary basement lamina of the trematode *Schistosoma mansoni* has been identified as an oxytalan-type connective tissue (Kohn *et al.* 1979). This tissue in *S. mansoni* is identical in its fine structure to the connective tissue of *H. diminuta*.

Indeed, logic favors an identification of tapeworm connective tissue as being of an elastic, rather than collagen, type. Tapeworms are highly resistant to permanent deformation imposed by stretch. The ease with which the strobila can be extended and the ready return to original shape and dimensions when a moderate stretching force is removed can most logically be attributed to the physiology and anatomical arrangement of the musculature (see preceding section) and the physical properties of its surrounding connective tissue. Collagen fibers, while flexible to a degree, offer great resistance to a pulling force. On the other hand, elastic connective tissue stretches easily and retains its resiliency even when extended to as much as 150% of its original length.

In addition to the functions of mechanical support and providing cohesion, tapeworm connective tissue undoubtedly plays a significant role in the exchange of metabolites with the other tissues that it surrounds and permeates. While acoelomate flatworms are often thought of as being internally "solid", the extracellular fluid space of tapeworms, as represented by the parenchymal interstitium, is considerable. Its generally "loose" consistency would facilitate the circulation of inorganic ions, dissolved gases (e.g., carbon dioxide), nutrients, and metabolic wastes, as is the case for the highly hydrated loose connective tissues of other organisms.

Morphologically distinguishable binding sites between the connective tissue and cellular elements are most apparent in the tegument and musculature. The former include the hemidesmosome-like structures along the basal plasmalemma of the distal cytoplasmic component. The sites of muscle tissue interaction with connective tissue include the dense bodies associated with the sarcolemma of the myofibrils.

C. *Histogenesis*

A discrete connective tissue fiber-forming cell has yet to be identified in *H. diminuta* or other tapeworms. The somatic cell type whose fine structure is most compatible with connective tissue protein synthesis and export to the extracellular space is muscle, specifically the myocytons thereof. Besides containing numerous ribosomes and a relatively well developed granular endoplasmic reticulum, vesicles containing fine fibrils have been observed in the cytoplasm of tapeworm parenchymal myocytons (e.g., Lumsden 1966c); in their structure, these fibril-containing vesicles are not unlike those elaborated by fibroblasts (see Ross 1968; Porter 1964; Goldberg and Green 1964) which deliver the precursors of collagen, etc., to the intercellular matrix in the connective tissues of other organisms.

Occasionally encountered in *H. diminuta* are cells of the type illustrated in Fig. 29; these, which may represent a type of myocyton or be a

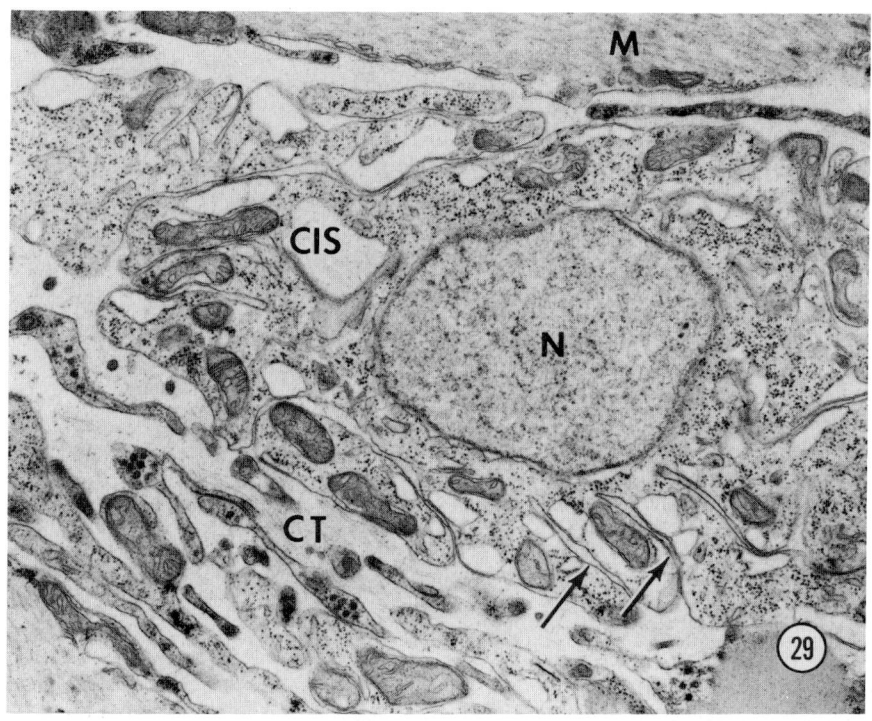

Fig. 29. *Possible fibrogenis cell. Perinuclear region characterized by numerous free ribosomes and peripherally located mitochondria. Distended cisternae (CIS) containing fine fibrillar matrix located throughout peripheral cytoplasm. Infoldings (arrows) of surrounding extraxcellular connective tissue (CT) apparent. M, myofibril. X25,000.*

derivative thereof, are notable in the abundance of ribosomes and large vacuoles, the latter apparently derived from the endoplasmic reticulum. These vacuoles contain a flocculent, finely fibrillar matrix, and are frequently positioned in close proximity to deep invaginations of the cell surface, the extracellular space of which contains oxytalan-like microfibrils. This cell type differs from the typical medullary myocyton in lacking significant amounts of glycogen and lipid. Additional support for the hypothesis that tapeworm connective tissue is produced by myocytons is that in vertebrates,

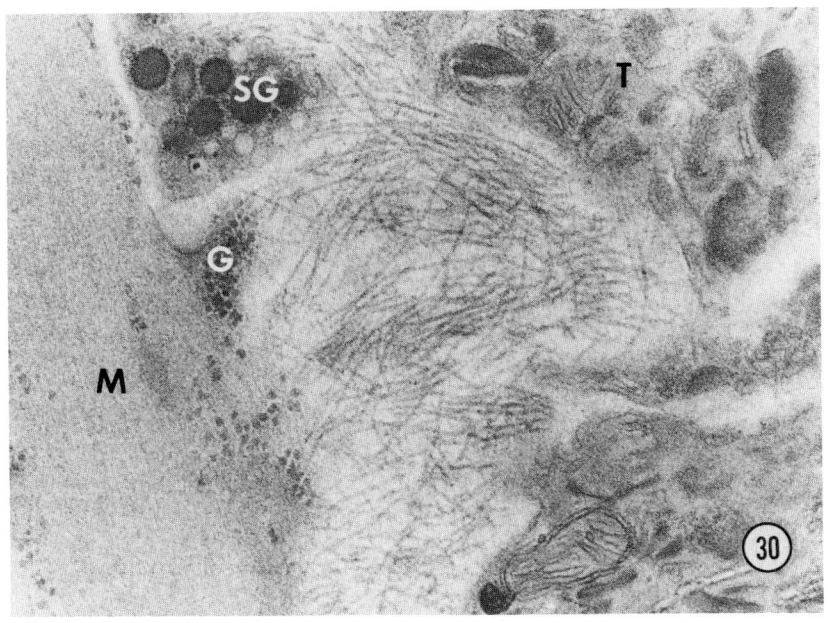

Fig. 30. Connective tissue fibrils from basement lamina between tegumental distal cytoplasm (T) and superficial circular muscles (M). Process containing secretory granules (SG) is from endocrine cell. X49,000.

smooth muscle cells have the potential for synthesizing both collagen and elastic connective tissue fibers (Ross 1973, 1974; Ross and Klebakoff 1971).

VI. THE EXCRETORY (PROTONEPHRIDIAL) SYSTEM

The term "protonephridia" has been generously applied by several authors to the fluid-filled system of ducts which pervades the parenchyma of tapeworms.

The term connotes at least functional analogies with the nephrons of higher organisms, though until recently, the functions attributed to tapeworm protonephridia have been based more on speculations derived from comparative anatomy and fine structure than on hard data from physiological investigations. Nephrons, *sensu stricto*, serve primarily to remove metabolic wastes from the body fluids. In addition to their excretory function, true kidneys have a conservative function, where electrolytes and other physiologically valuable substances are resorbed from the filtrate. In the process, nephrons often play a critical role in homeostasis, especially as regards the osmotic constancy of the body fluids. The mechanisms by which these functions are accomplished include selective filtration, secretion, and absorption. Indications that such mechanisms are operative for tapeworm "protonephridia" remain largely circumstantial. Of the major nephridial functions, only that of excretion is unambiguously supported by direct evidence to date. Therefore, we preferentially use here the term "excretory system", though other functions may eventually be demonstrated. We would also point out that the tegument is undoubtedly also a major route of efflux for a variety of organic and inorganic substances, including those which would classify as metabolic wastes.

A. *Canals and Collecting Ducts*

The microanatomy of the excretory system in adult *H. diminuta*, other cestodes, and related flatworms, has been reviewed by Wilson and Webster (1974). For *H. diminuta*, it consists of three major components: (1) the four longitudinal collecting canals (two dorsolateral, two ventrolateral); (2) a network of capillary-like tubules; and (3) the flame cells. The ventral canals are distinguished from the dorsal canals by their much larger diameter (Fig. 3). Near the posterior end of each proglottid, and in the scolex, at the base of the rostellum, the ventral canals are joined by a transverse vessel. The dorsal and ventral canals are united in the scolex at the base of the rostellum, their confluence marked by bulb-like swellings (Fig. 46). From these swellings, four smaller-caliber canals extend anteriorly into the rostellum, where they are united by a ring-like vessel at base of the rostellar anterior canal (an invagination of tegument at the apex of the scolex). In the first terminal proglottid formed, the dorsal and ventral canals merge to form a common bladder which opens to the outside via a median, posterior pore. When this proglottid is shed, the four canals open independently to the exterior. The capillary connecting tubules arise from the longitudinal canals and transverse vessels and form a branching array which extends into the cortical parenchyma. Each of these tubules terminates, ultimately, at a flame cell, the junction of the tubule and flame cell being referred to as the terminal protonephridial "organ". From calculations based on radioassay measurements of injected ^{14}C inulin, Webster (1971) approximated the average fluid volume of the protonephridial canal system to be on the order of 20-40 µl. Fluid, propelled by ciliary movement of the flame cells, is drained from the capillary tubules into the major collecting canals. According to Wardle and McLeod (1952), Stunkard (1962) and others, fluid is circulated, for the most part, anteriorly in the dorsal canals and posteriorly in the ventral canals. According to Webster (1971), however, fluid flows, in the protonephridial canals of *H. diminuta*, primarily from anterior to posterior, promoted by peristaltic contractions of the body musculature, with a mean fluid output rate of some 3.4 µl/minute.

The walls of the collecting canals and tubules are syncytial. Associated with the major longitudinal canals are nucleated cytons which extend laterally into the surrounding parenchyma. Nuclei of the capillary tubules lie within the periductal cytoplasm (Fig. 31). The lumenal surface of the canals and tubules is covered with short, clavate microvilli (Figs. 31 and 32). The adlumenal surface is smooth (i.e., devoid of infoldings etc.,) and surrounded by the loose connective tissue of the parenchymal interstitium (see preceding section). Junctional complexes between "parenchymal" cells and excretory ducts have been reported by Threadgold and Read (1970b). The ductal cytoplasm contains microfilaments, the majority of which are arranged in a layer just beneath the lumenal border, occasional mitochondria, and a sparse population of electronlucent vesicles. The pericanalicular cytons contain a modestly developed granular endoplasmic reticulum, mitochondria, and vesicles. Golgi complexes are inconspicuous. Glycogen granules and lipid droplets are absent.

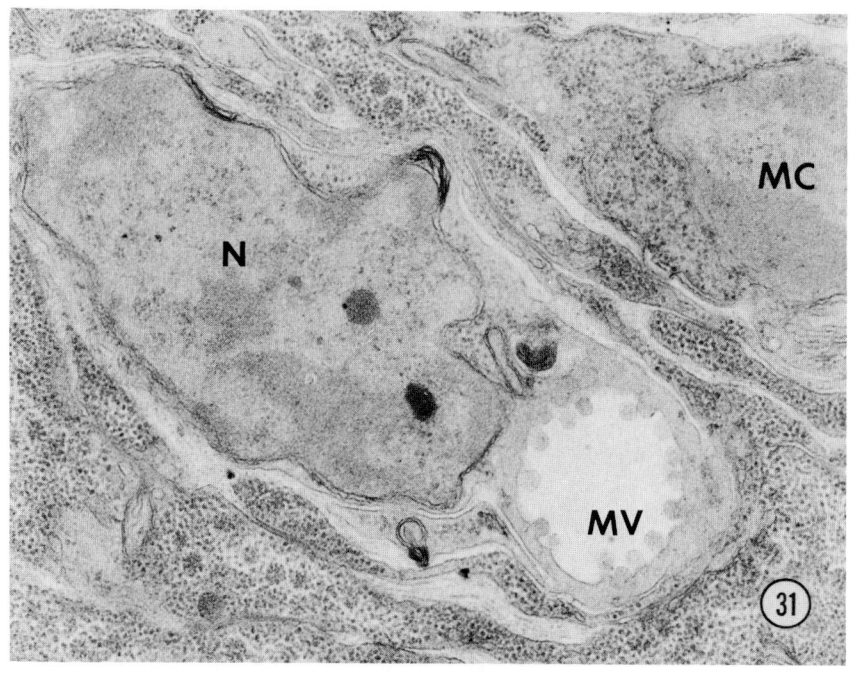

Fig. 31. Collecting duct of excretory system. Nucleus (N) directly adjacent to syncytial cytoplasm of duct. Ductal cytoplasm extended as short clavate microvilli (MV) at free surface. Carbohydrate-storing myocytons (MC) surround duct. X43,900

In its syncytial nature, the ductal system of H. diminuta differs from that of planarians (see Pedersen 1961; Wetzel 1962; McKanna 1968), where the tubules and canals are formed by discrete cells joined by desmosomes.

B. Flame Cells

Flame cells are cup-shaped, the concave surface facing the capillary tubule lumen (Fig. 33). This

surface bears the "flame", consisting of a tuft of
50 or more closely apposed cilia (Fig. 34). Each
cilium contains an axoneme of nine doublet peripheral
microtubules surrounding a pair of central singlet
microtubules (Figs. 35 and 36); the axoneme

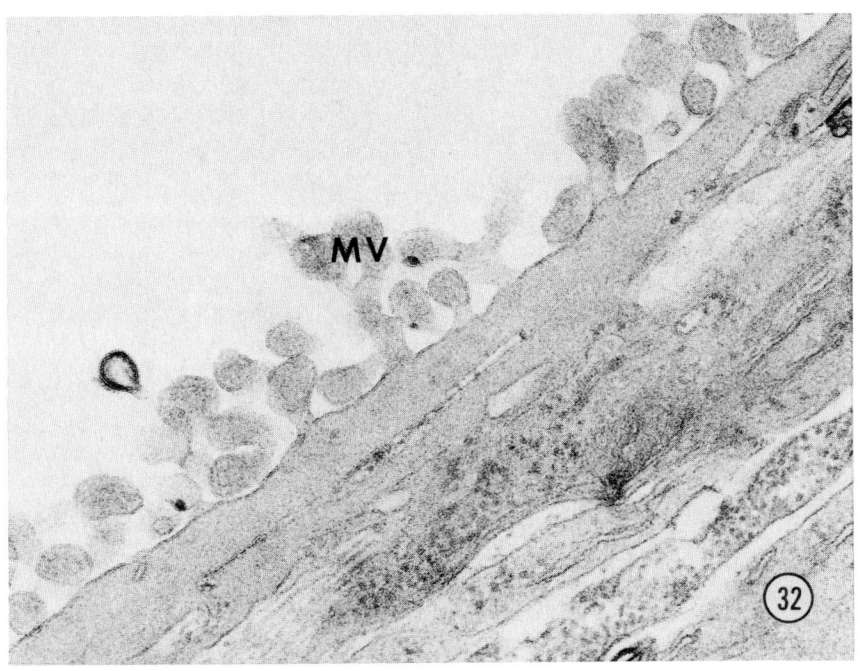

Fig. 32. Higher magnification of ductal cytoplasm of major extretory canal. Surface extended as multibranched, clavate microvilli (MV). Syncytial cytoplasm contains few organelles and is supported by withdrawn nuclei. X66,800.

arises from a basal body composed of nine triplet
microtubules and a short, transversely striated rootlet (Figs. 33 and 37). The basal 1/3 of the flame
is surrounded by a double row of digitiform cytoplasmic processes, each about 110-150 nm in diameter,
which parallel the longitudinal axis of the cilia.
The processes comprising the outer row arise from
the distal end of the capillary tubule, while those

of the inner row arise from the leading edge of the
flame cell (Fig. 34). These overlapping processes
are separated from one another by a distance of about
40 nm, but are interconnected by a thin, continuous,
amorphous diaphragm(Fig. 34). Secondary microvilliform structures (the "leptotriches" of Kummel 1964)

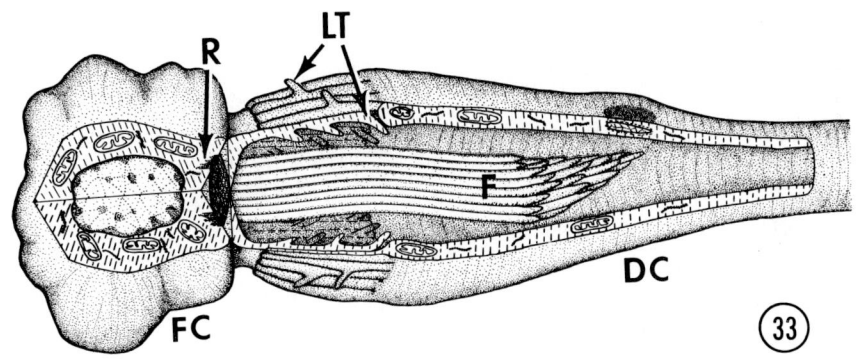

Fig. 33. Terminal organ of excretory system
flame cell (FC); flame (F) composed of approximately
50 cilia; ciliary rootlets (R); leptotriches (LT);
cytoplasm of the collecting duct (DC). (Drawing
courtesy of M.B. Hildreth).

extend laterally from the tubule processes outwardly
into the parenchyma, and from the flame cell processes
inwardly toward the ciliary tuft (Figs. 34 and 37).
The fine structure of the flame cell perinuclear
cytoplasm is unremarkable, containing a few mitochondria and profiles of granular endoplasmic reticulum,
free ribosomes, and an inconspicuous Golgi apparatus.

C. *Functional Correlates*

The contents of the canal fluid of *H. diminuta*,
as reported by Webster and Wilson (1970), include
besides water, sodium, potassium, chloride, bicarbonate, dissolved carbon dioxide, ammonia, urea, lactate,
succinate, amino acids, glucose, and soluble
protein. The amino acid and glucose concentrations

reported for the canal fluid are substantially lower than the amino acid and glucose levels of the total body fluid extracts. Webster (1972a) found evidence for some glucose resorption by the canals which apparently is phlorizin sensitive. Based on freezing point depression measurements, the total osmotic pressure of the canal fluid approximates that of the worm's external environment. Water is gained and salts are lost in proportion to the dilution of the worm's external environment (Webster 1970, 1972b).

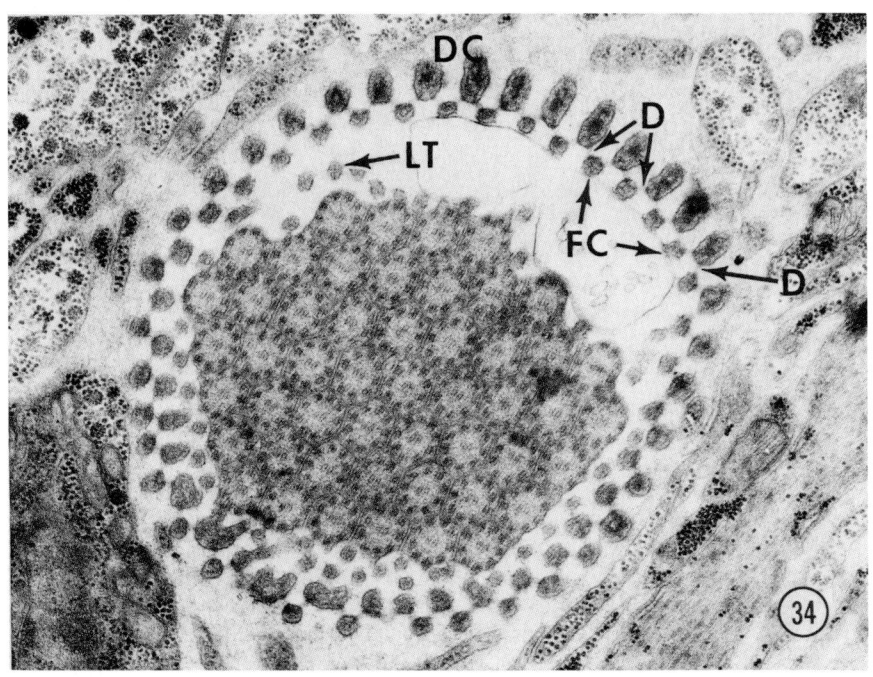

Fig. 34. Cross section of terminal organ, at level of interdigitation of flame cell (FC) and ductal cytoplasm (DC). Leptotriches (LT) from flame cell extend into lumen of terminal organ. Internal finger-like processes from flame cell (FC) and external processes from ductal cytoplasm (DC) interconnected by dense, amorphous material (D). Cilia of flame tightly packed within lumen of organ. (From Lumsden 1965a). X26,000.

Functional correlates for the fine structure of

the *H. diminuta* system of excretory ducts remain highly conjectural. Nonetheless, the thinness of the capillary tubule and canal walls would be expected to facilitate the cross-diffusion of water, ions, and small organic molecules between the surrounding connective tissue space and lumen, while the structure of the "funnel" surrounding the basal part of the "flame" is suggestive of a filter. Given their small size, the microvilli lining the ducts only modestly increase the lumenal surface area available for absorption. Their expanded tips have suggested to some observers a possible "blebbing" phenomenon, though this is not supported by any direct evidence. Morphological hallmarks of endocytotic or exocytotic activity are inconspicuous. Histochemically demonstrable phosphatase activity is associated with the collecting ducts and canals, but despite the usual conjectures about its role in transport (Parshad and Guraya 1977), the actual physiological significance of this observation remains obscure. None of the methods so far applied to tapeworms permit unequivocal diagnosis of a specific sodium-potassium ATPase activity in the excretory system. Our yet primitive knowledge of the exact microanatomical relationships of tubules, etc., precludes speculation as to any "countercurrent" mechanisms.

The ductal cytoplasm contains microfilaments generally arranged in a radial layer just below the microvilli. Microfilaments ubiquitously have been found to be composed of actin, and serve contractile functions in a wide variety of non-muscle cell types. It seems not unlikely that their function in the collecting canals and tubules is to exert a counterforce to maintain the hydrostatic fluid pressure in the lumen and, perhaps, engender microperistalsis.

Given the presence of metabolic wastes (e.g., ammonia, urea, lactate, and succinate) in the fluid of the canals (Webster and Wilson 1970; Webster 1972c), which is demonstrably discharged to the exterior (Webster 1971), an excretory function of the system would appear to be reasonably well documented. On the other hand, the "presumptive evidence" (Wardle and McLeod 1952) that it also functions to maintain a constant internal hydrostatic pressure and to regulate water balance remains highly presumptive. In isotonic saline, *H. diminuta* maintains constant weight, but gains or loses weight in more dilute or concentrated salt solutions, as a function of tissue hydration or dehydration (Chandler et al. 1950; Webster 1970). In sodium - or potassium - deficient media made iso-osmotic by the addition of mannitol,

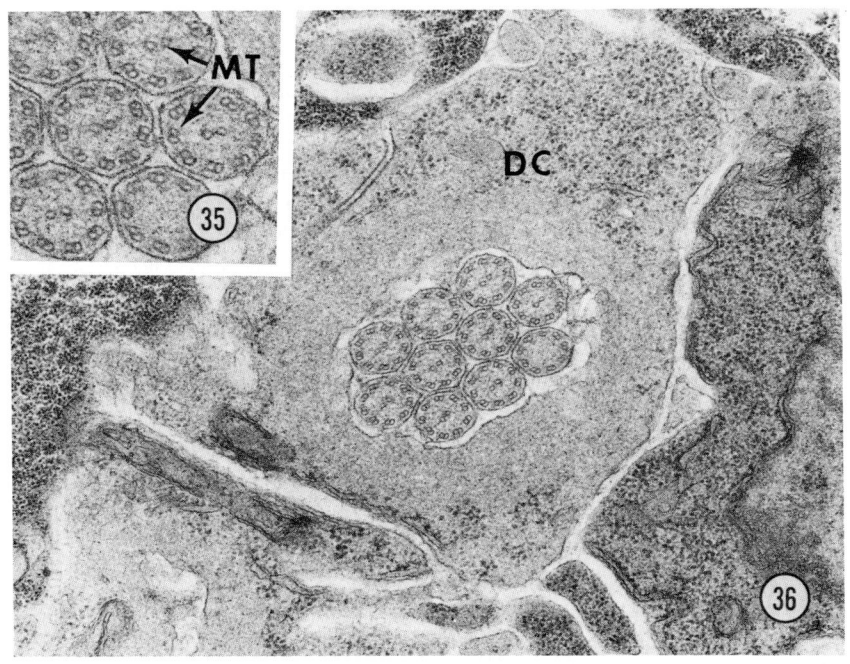

Fig. 35. Higher magnification of cilia showing typical 9 + 2 microtubular (MT) arrangement. Central microtubular pair occasionally absent from peripheral cilia. X60,000.

Fig. 36. Cross section of terminal organ. Distal portion of flame contains reduced number of cilia. Flame surrounded by ductal cytoplasm (DC). X32,000.

weight (water) changes are minimal, but there is substantial efflux of these cations from the excretory canals (Webster 1972b). By all indications, *H. diminuta* is an osmoconformer, whose excretory system exhibits little or no ability to regulate either water or salt content in response to changes in the external osmotic concentration.

The primary function of the flame cells, obviously, is to agitate fluid flow through the system. The ciliary activity of the flame cells is responsive to sudden changes in the worm's environmental chemistry (e.g., the stimulatory effect of adding urea).

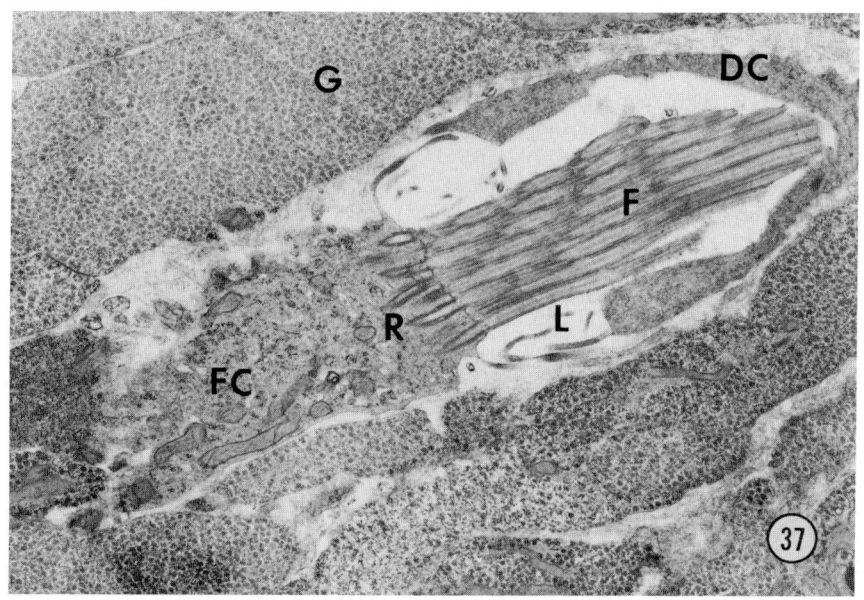

Fig. 37. Oblique sagittal section through terminal organ, missing flame cell nucleus. Flame cell (FC) cytoplasm shows numerous mitochondria, ribosomes and striated ciliary rootlets (R). Leptotriches (LT) present within the organ lumen, adjacent to flame (F). Entire organ surrounded by glycogen (G) rich myocytons. X10,700.

Morphological indices that these and other components of the excretory system may be subject to internal regulatory physiological control as well include the frequency of junctional complexes with "parenchymal" and even, though we know not to what extent, neural elements. Further, as previously noted, the structure of the "funnel" established at the overlapping of the flame cell and its collecting duct is suggestive of a primary filtration device.

VII. THE NERVOUS SYSTEM

Of the major tapeworm organ systems, the nervous system remains the least thoroughly elucidated. Most of the fixatives, embedments and staining procedures traditionally used for light microscopic study of general tapeworm histology and cytology have proven to be even more inadequate where investigations on the nervous system were attempted. A number of the techniques which have been useful for studying the microneuroanatomy of higher organisms are based on the selective staining of the capsular or glial elements, neither of which are present in tapeworms. Several others, such as the Golgi procedures, which do stain tapeworm neural elements, stain certain non-neural elements (e.g., myoblasts) as well. Specific visualization of tapeworm neural elements has been most successful employing methods which localize presumptive neurotransmitter substances or the enzymes for which they are substrates. The localization of acetycholine esterase (AChE) (Wilson and Schiller 1969) and 5-hydroxytryptamine (5-HT) (Lee *et al*. 1978) in whole mounted specimens, has revealed the distributional pattern of the major nerve tracts in *H diminuta*. While providing much useful information on the major structural features of the nervous system, these techniques provide few insights into the microneuroanatomy. Histochemical techniques sufficiently discrete to allow the identification of individual cestode neurons are currently unavailable. Thus, a comprehensive understanding of tapeworm nervous tissue can be obtained only by a methodical ultrastructural study.

Neural elements are easily recognized as such in electron micrographs, but the three-dimensional reconstruction of such complex microanatomy as represented by the tapeworm nervous system from thin sections is a more exacting and laborious task than the majority of electron microscopists to date, have been willing to undertake. With the exception of the reports by Morseth (1967), Webb and Davey (1974, 1975a, 1975b, 1976) and Webb (1976a, 1976b, 1977), accounts of the fine structure of tapeworm neural elements (other than sensilla) are fragmentary and, usually, nervous tissue is just mentioned in passing by authors addressed principally to other subjects. In any event, no systematic electron microscopic study of the adult *H. diminuta* nervous system has been published to date. The following account is based largely on the light microscopic descriptions of the adult *H. diminuta* neuroanatomy reported by Wilson and Schiller (1969) and Lee *et al.* (1978), with, where possible, fine structural correlations from the electron microscopic study of *H. microstoma* cysticercoids and adults by Webb and Davey (1974, 1975a, 1975b, 1976), Webb (1976a, 1976b, 1977) and our own, yet limited observations on the neurocytology of the adult *H. diminuta*.

A. *Neuromicroanatomy*

The cephalic nerve tissue in *Hymenolepis diminuta* is concentrated at the base of the rostellum in a pair of large lateral cerebral ganglia, connected by a flattened transverse commissure (Fig. 38). Arising from each lateral cerebral ganglion is an anteriorly directed nerve tract which enters the base of the rostellum, adjacent to the entrance of the excretory vessels, and joins a lateral rostellar ganglion. The bilateral rostellar ganglia occupy the medial basal region of the rostellum and are connected by one to three transverse rostellar commissures. Fibers extending proximally from the rostellar ganglia innervate the circular muscle constituting the inner portion of the rostellar capsule, forming the "rostellar rings" reported by Wilson and Schiller (1969). Additionally, processes extend into the musculature surrounding the anterior canal. The rostellar ganglia also receive sensory dendrites from the sensilla embedded in the rostellar tegument (Specian and Lumsden 1980).

Extending proximally from each cerebral ganglion is a major anterior nerve tract. Running between the suckers and rostellum, these tracts give rise to a number of offshoots before terminating beneath the scolex tegument in a number of fine branches. Fibers arising from these tracts innervate the outer longitudinal musculature of the rostellar capsule, the superficial musculature of the scolex proper, and appear to extend into the adjacent suckers. In addition, these tracts probably receive dendrites from the sensory endings located in the scolex tegument. Wilson and Schiller (1969) noted that a minimum of two additional nerves arise from each lateral cerebral ganglion and extend into the region between the suckers and the rostellum. One or more of these nerves undoubtedly serve to inner-

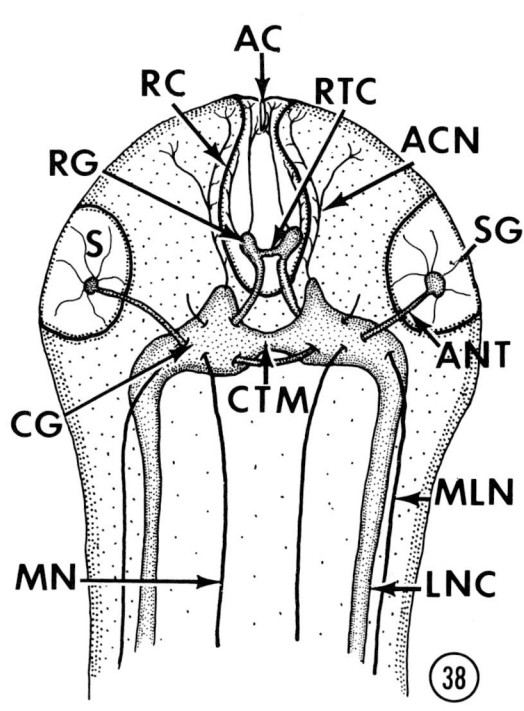

Fig. 38. Diagram of neural axis within the adult scolex. Anterior canal (AC); anterior cerebral nerve (ACN); acetabular nerve tract (ANT); cerebral ganglion (CG); cerebral transverse commissure (CTM); lateral nerve cord (LNC); minor lateral nerve (MLN); median nerve (MN); rostellar capsule (RC); rostellar ganglion (RG); rostellar transverse commissure (RTC); suckers (S); sucker ganglion (SG)

vate each sucker.

At the base of each of the suckers there is a concentration of nerve tissue from which a fine network of small processes extends throughout the musculature. In addition to the apparent neuromuscular interactions within the suckers, the distal cytoplasm of the tegument is interrupted by frequent sensory endings, especially around the rim of each sucker.

Ten longitudinal, posteriorly directed nerve tracts originate at the level of the cerebral ganglia and extend, five on each side of the body, throughout the strobila (Fig. 38). The two major lateral nerve cords are formed by a medial tapering of each cerebral ganglion. These nerve cords run parallel and external to the longitudinal excretory canals. Adjacent and parallel to each lateral nerve cord are a much smaller pair of nerve fibers, a latero-dorsal and a latero-ventral, which likewise originate from the lateral margin of each cerebral ganglion. Arising from the medio-dorsal and medio-ventral margin of each cerebral ganglion are the median nerves, which like the other longitudinal fibers, extend the length of the strobila. Wilson and Schiller (1969) reported that prior to the detachment of the first-formed terminal proglottid, the longitudinal nerve fibers terminate on either side of the excretory pore (see previous section on the excretory system). Presumably, after the onset of apolysis, these fibers end individually at the abscission face of the terminal proglottid.

Within the neck region of the worm, the ten longitudinal trunks are interconnected by transverse, bipolar neurons in the mid-dorsal and mid-ventral body plane. Adjacent to the major lateral nerve cords are what Wilson and Schiller (1969) identified as motor end plates associated with the marginal longitudinal musculature. These end plates, however, are apparently devoid of 5-HT (Lee *et al*. 1978). The germinal region of the medulla is invested with a fine network of nerve fibers.

Throughout the developing and mature region of the strobila the longitudinal nerve tracts are connected by three transverse commissures - anterior, medial and posterior - about equidistant apart in each proglottid. At the intersection of each transverse commissure and a major nerve cord, there is a small ganglion from which nerve fibers extend into the marginal musculature; this ganglion also receives dendrites from sensory endings.

Within the gravid proglottids, only the major and minor lateral nerve cords appear to remain intact, the median nerves and all of the transverse commissures become irregular and difficult to observe.

Based upon the cytochemical localization of AChE, innervation of the female reproductive tract appears to be limited to the oviduct and vitelline duct. In the male reproductive tract, all of the heavily muscularized structures (i.e., the cirrus pouch, internal seminal vesicle and genital atrium) evidence strong AChE activity, whereas only the cirral sphincter shows the presence of 5-HT (Lee *et al.* 1978).

B. *Neurocytology*

The neural elements are centralized in tapeworms to a much greater degree than in the free-living platyhelminths studied to date. Many, if not all, of the cell bodies are located within the scolex ganglia or the major strobilar nerve tracts. In the cephalic ganglia, commissures and lateral cords, the cell bodies are arranged peripherally, sometimes up to three or four layers thick, around a core of neuronal processes (axons and dendrites, or, collectively, the "neurites" of Webb and Davey 1976), constituting the so-called neuropile (Fig. 39). Autoradiographic studies by Gustafsson (1976) on the histogenesis of nervous tissue in *Diphyllobothrium dendriticum*, have shown that nerve cells are incapable of mitotic division, and thus that all new nerve cells must arise directly from the influx of germinative cells. Furthermore, those nerve cells immediately adjacent to the neuropile are the most recently differentiated.

Within the neuropile, cell junctions of three types are encountered. Synaptic junctions of the type described by Webb (1976a) from the metacestode of *H. microstoma* are observed between neurites. The

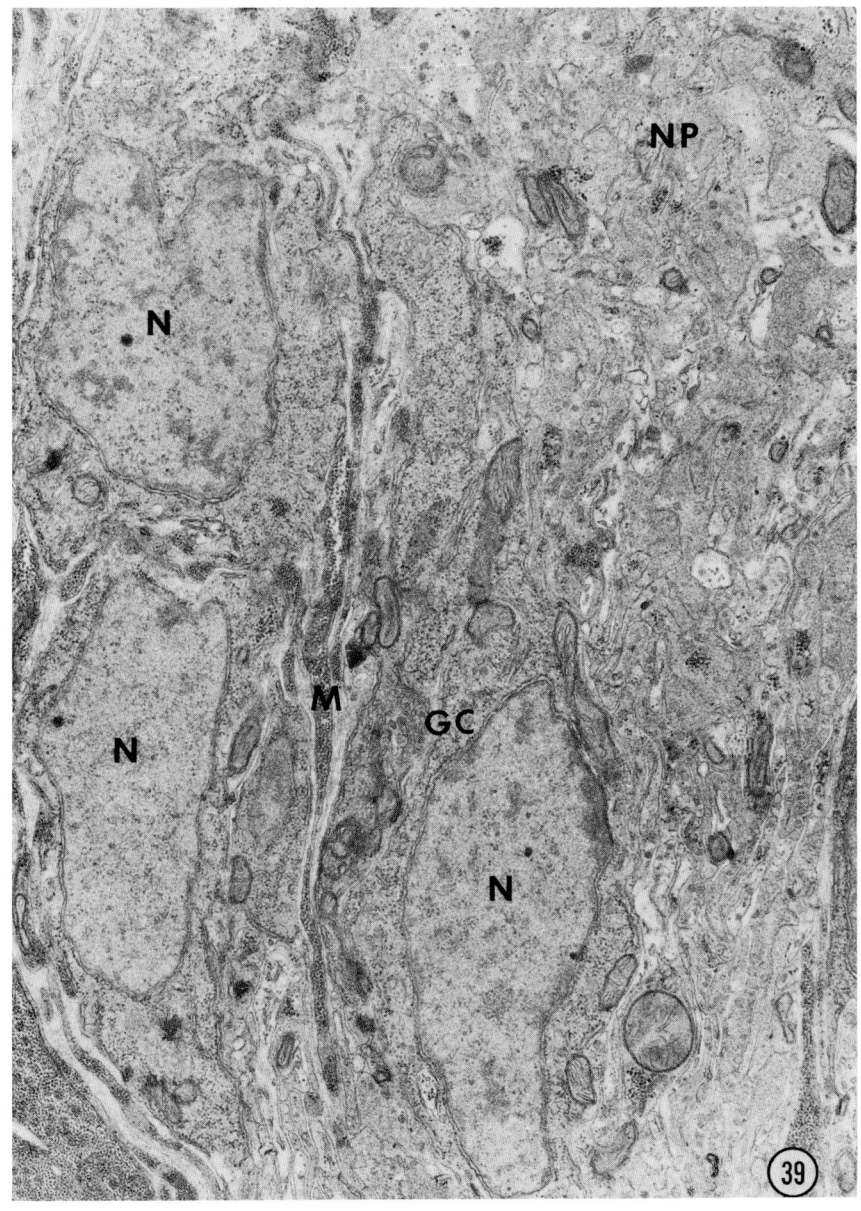

Fig. 39. Sagittal section through cerebral ganglion. Nerve perikarya located peripherally around central neuropile (NP). Nerve cells characterized by large ovoid nucleus (N) and prominent juxtanuclear Golgi complexes (GC). Muscle cell processes (M) occasionally extend into neuropile. X21,000.

junctions are characterized by a synaptic cleft of approximately 20 nm, which contains an abundance of electron dense material. Dense projections are associated with both the pre- and post-synaptic membranes. The pre-synaptic nerve endings are generally filled with numerous small (20-45 nm) electron-lucent vesicles, intermixed with dense-cored vesicles (45-100 nm). A second type of junctional complex was frequently observed within the neuropile of the lateral nerve cords. This complex, a gap junction, was described by Threadgold and Read (1970b) for cestode parenchymal and tegumental cells, but has not been heretofore reported from studies on cestode nervous tissue. Gap junctions interconnect adjacent neurites (Fig. 28) and are more commonly observed in the lateral nerve cords than is the typical synapse. The nature of these junctions and their possible function has been discussed in the previous section on muscle. Rarely a third cell junction is observed within the neuropile. As previously discussed, fine tendrillar processes often extend from the contractile portion of a muscle cell (Fig. 22), occasionally these processes extend into the neuropile of a ganglion or nerve cord (Fig. 39), where they terminate in a neuromuscular junction. In several other invertebrate groups, motor neurons receive processes from muscle cells (myocytons) such that, neuromuscular interactions take place within the nerve cords rather than within the muscular tissue (see Bullock and Horridge 1965 for review). While this is certainly not the only means of neuromuscular transmission, or even perhaps a primary mechanism, it has heretofore gone unreported for *H. diminuta*.

The nerve cell bodies (perikarya) contain a spherical or slightly ovoid nucleus with an eccentrically positioned nucleolus and scattered clumps and granules of chromatin. The perinuclear cytoplasm contains numerous free ribosomes, occasionally in polysomal arrays, juxta-nuclear Golgi complexes, profiles of granular endoplasmic reticulum, a variety of vesicles (see below), *beta*-glycogen particles, and mitochondria (Figs. 39 and 41). The endoplasmic reticulum is frequently disposed as subsurface cisterns (i.e., closely approximated to the plasma membrane), a configuration which has been noted in a variety of nerve cell bodies from other animals (see e.g., Rosenbluth 1962).

Nerve cell types have been classified for vertebrates and many invertebrates based on the size and location of the nerve perikarya, and the kinds of vesicles they contain. The nerve perikarya

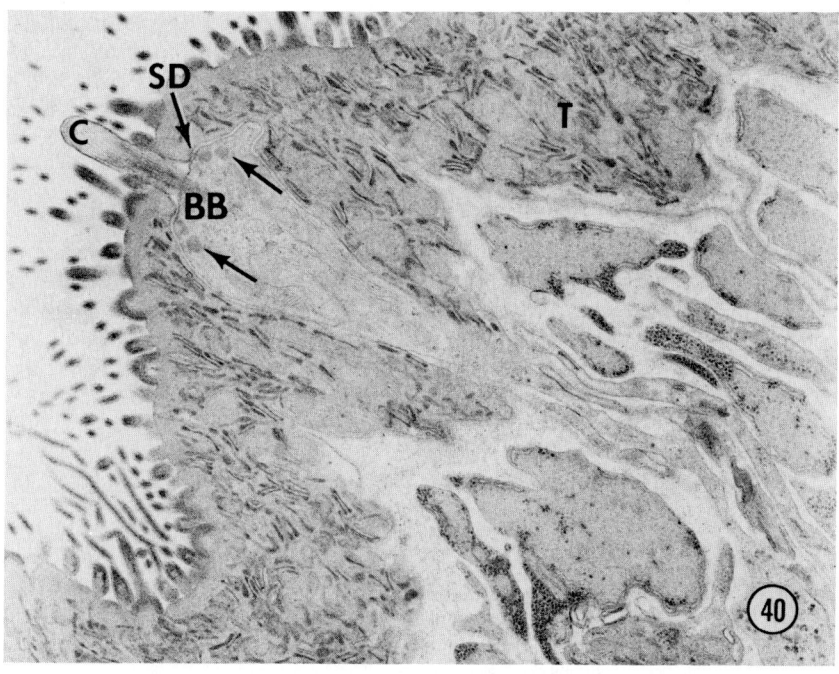

Fig. 40. Dendritic sensory ending within scolex tegument (T). Nerve terminates in apical cilium (C) which projects into surrounding environment. Basal body (BB) present. Circular septate desmosome (SD) joins tegumentary and neuronal cell membranes near base of cilium. Two prominent electron dense collars (arrows) are also present in the apical neuroplasm. Dendrite extends proximally to join cerebral ganglia. X21,700.

studied to date in hymenolepid cestodes exhibit little variation in size, though some differences in the vesicular contents of the neurons have been noted (e.g., Webb and Davey 1976). In the cephalic ganglia of *H. microstoma* metacestodes, Webb and Davey (1976) described four vesicle types: three containing electron-lucent cores and having diameters of 20-

45 nm, 45-100 nm and 90-190 nm, respectively, and a fourth type, 45-90 nm in diameter, with electron dense contents. Based on the kinds of vesicles present, Webb and Davey (1976) tentatively identified three broad categories of neurons: sensory, integrative, and motor. Webb (1976b, 1977) subsequently described some putative neurosecretory elements in *H. microstoma*. Whether by Webb's or other criteria the same kinds of neurons (motor, integrative, sensory, neurosecretory) are present in *H. diminuta* has not yet been ascertained. However, at least one of these, the sensory neuron, is readily recognizable in *H. diminuta* using Webb and Davey's (1976) criteria.

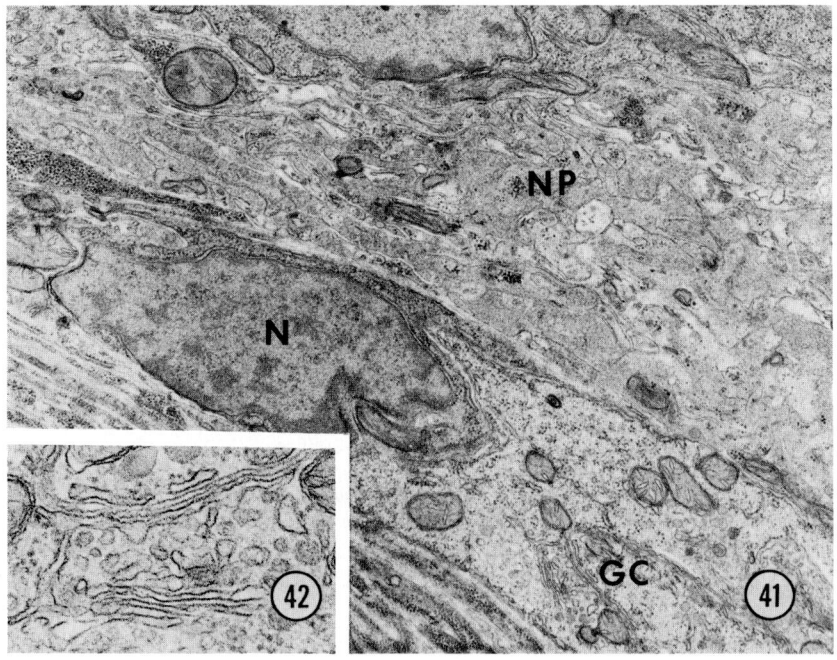

Fig. 41. Sensory nerve perikaryon from cerebral ganglion. Prominent nucleus (N) surrounded by numerous mitochondria and Golgi complexes (GC). X16,000.

Fig. 42. Higher magnification of Golgi complex from sensory nerve perikaryon. Numerous large lucent vesicles are present adjacent to Golgi cisternae. X51,000.

Sensory perikarya are frequently encountered within the rostellar and cerebral ganglia of *H. diminuta* (Fig. 41), and to a lesser degree within the lateral nerve cords. Like those so identified by Webb and Davey (1976) in *H. microstoma*, these cells in *H. diminuta* contain three vesicle types: small lucent vesicles (20-45 nm), large lucent vesicles 90-190 nm), and dense cored vesicles (45-100 nm), all apparently being formed in association with the juxtanuclear Golgi (Fig 42). By far the most characteristic feature of these neurons, however, is the uniciliate dendritic endings (sensilla) within the distal cytoplasm of the tegument. Sensory endings are remarkably uniform in structure throughout the cestodes, and have been the most frequently observed facet of cestode nervous tissue (see Webb and Davey 1974; Cooper *et al*. 1975 for review).

The terminal bulb-like expansion of the sensory dendrite contains a single cilium about 1.4 μm long, which projects beyond the tegument brush border into the external environment. The distal region of the dendritic bulb, adjacent to the base of the cilium, is attached to the distal cytoplasm of the tegument by a prominent, circumferential septate desmosome. Inside the bulb and adjacent to this point of attachment are two circular, electron dense collars. The granular cytoplasm of the sensory ending is occupied by many large electron-lucent vesicles (90-190 nm diameter) and mitchondria. *Beta*-glycogen particles are also present. The small (20-45 nm) lucent vesicles and the dense cored vesicles which occur elsewhere in the neuron are rarely observed in the terminal bulb (Fig. 40).

Although numerous authors have suggested a tactile function for this uniciliate sensory receptor, the speculation by Cooper *et al*. (1975), that they may function as chemoreceptors, appears equally justified, based on morphological criteria. Physiological studies on the sensory potential of cestodes have not yet been reported, to our knowledge.

A second type of sensory receptor, a stretch receptor, has been tentatively described as such from at least one tapeworm, the tetraphyllidean, *Acanthobothrium coronatum*, by Rees (1966). Similar receptors have not to date been observed in *H. diminuta*.

Unequivocal identification, on morphological grounds, of integrative (interneurons) and motor neurons in *H. diminuta* will require additional study, as will the significance of the various vesicle types present in the neurons generally. Based on neurocytological and biochemical studies on other organisms, the small (20-45 nm) lucent vesicles presumably contain acetylcholine, while the dense cored (45-90 nm) vesicles are usually identified with having a 5-hydroxytryptamine content. While histochemical methods applied to whole mounts (Lee *et al*. 1978) have not demonstrated 5-HT in the majority of *H. diminuta* neurons, the resolution obtainable from such preparations does not preclude, in our estimation, the possibility of minute yet physiologically significant amounts of 5-HT in a variety of *H. diminuta* neural elements. The primary catecholamines - dopamine, epinephrine, and norepinephrine - which commonly serve as neurotransmitters in vertebrates and many invertebrates - are apparently absent in cestodes (Chou *et al*. 1972; Tomosky-Sykes *et al*. 1977; Lee *et al*. 1978). A third granule type (Figs. 44 and 45), within a putative neurosecretory cell type, is similar in appearance to the "A" type or peptidergic granules described by Knowles (1965) in dogfish neural elements. Their functional significance is unknown.

The designation of neural elements as neurosecretory, from their fine structure alone, must be accepted conditionally, pending confirmation by additional cytochemical, biochemical, and physiological criteria. There is at least a modicum of fine structural evidence for the presence of neurosecretory cells in hymenolepid cestodes, as reviewed in the following paragraphs.

C. *Neurosecretion*

Despite an abundance of information on the structure and function of neurosecretory neurons in the free-living platyhelminths (see Highnam and Hill 1977, for review), similar studies on the parasitic forms are few. Based on the fine structure of their granules, elements tentatively identified as neurosecretory have been reported from cestodes and tremtodes (Dixon and Mercer 1965; Morseth 1967; Silk and

Spence 1969; Wilson 1970; Webb 1976b, 1977). Among the first reports dealing with "neurosecretory" cells in hymenolepid tapeworms were those of Davey and Breckenridge (1967) and Tofts and Meerovitch (1974). On the basis of their light microscope level staining properties, cells in the apical region of the scolex

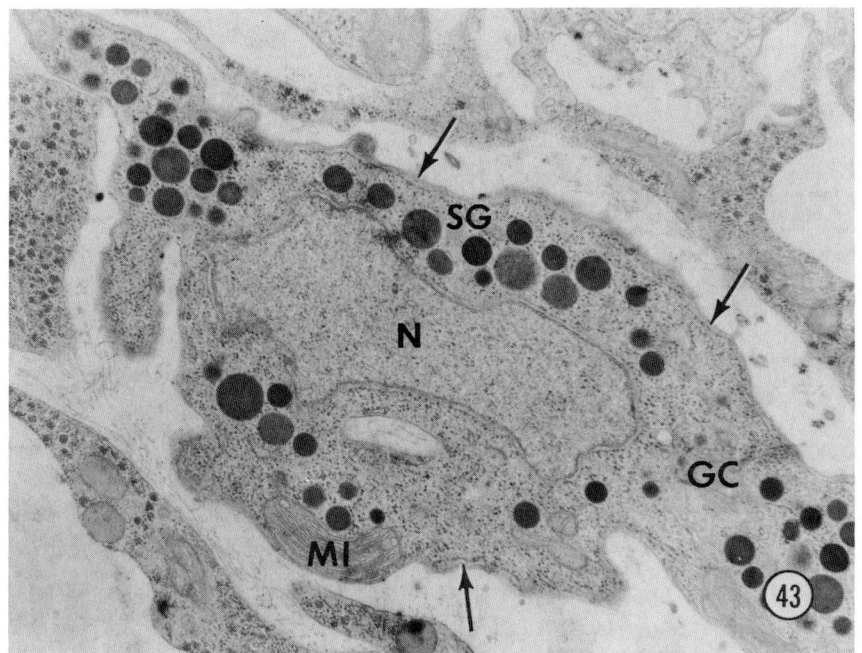

Fig. 43. Endocrine cell from anterior neck region. Multipolar cell filled with large, electron opaque, secretory granules (SG), presumably formed in association with the Golgi complex (GC). Prominent ovoid nucleus (N) surrounded by cytoplasm containing mitochondria, ribosomes and peripherally located cisternae of granular endoplasmic reticulum (arrows). (from Specian et al. 1979). X25,800.

were identified by the forementioned authors as neurosecretory; however, these particular cells have subsequently been shown instead to be specialized tegumentary perikarya (see following section on the scolex).

From their appearance in the electron microscope, Webb (1976b) described putative neurosecretory neurons within the lateral nerve cords of *H. microstoma*. The membrane bound, dense cored granules (55-90 nm diameter) appeared to be produced in association with the perinuclear Golgi complexes and transported to ostensible release sites within the lateral nerve cords. Although so-called "omega figures" characteristic of neurosecretory release in other organisms were not observed, deposits of synaptoid-like dense material, possibly aminergic, and clusters of minute electron-lucent vesicles were suggestive of release sites. In a subsequent report on *H. microstoma*, Webb (1977) described a second presumptive neurosecretory cell type. These neurons differed from those previously described (Webb 1976b) in containing significantly larger (85-125 nm) dense cored granules. Omega figures, considered by Normann (1976) diagnostic of neurosecretory release sites, were observed within the nerve terminals. One to three such release sites were found within each terminal varicosity with no corresponding adjacent "postsynaptic density" being present. These morphological features distinguish these sites from synapses. They were observed only in the neck region, in the area of proglottid proliferation. A possible role of these elements in the regulation of proglottid production and/or sexual maturation was suggested.

We have observed a neuronal type in the neck region of adult *H. diminuta* which is morphologically similar to the putative neurosecretory neurons described by Webb (1976b) in *H. microstoma* (Fig. 45). Specian *et al.* (1979) speculated that this cell type may play a role as an alternative muscle modulator (see following section on scolex); they further suggested that the vesicles in these cells (the dense cored type) contain 5-HT and were involved in motor neurotransmission. In general, cestodes appear to be able to develop a multiplicity of functions from a limited number of cell types. Accordingly, it is possible that a single cell type, in the nervous system of *H. diminuta*, is capable of transmitting information via normal synapses, as well as serving a neurosecretory function (cf. Nicoll and Barker 1971). Indeed, Webb (1977) reported the presence of synaptic junctions in the vicinity of presumptive neurosecretory release sites in *H. microstoma*.

In trematodes, 5-HT has been found to be a potent metabolic stimulator, increasing both glycolysis, and, in the absence of glucose, glycogenolysis (see Mansour 1969 for review). While similar 5-HT activity has not been reported for *H. diminuta*, a metabolic regulatory function by this or a related

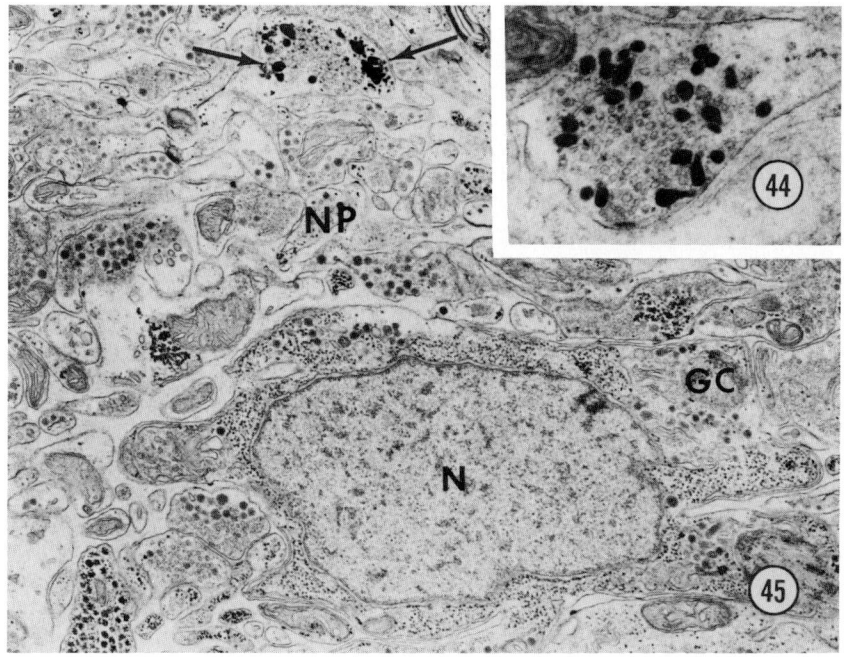

Fig. 44. Cross section of neurite from rostellar ganglion containing numerous electron dense, presumptive neurosecretory granules ("A"-type). X28,000.

Fig. 45. Cross section of lateral nerve cord from the neck region. Nerve perikaryon contains numerous dense-cored granules (DG), particularly adjacent to the Golgi complexes (GC), which are "B"-type presumptive neurosecretion granules. Adjacent neuropile (NP) contains neurite with "A"-type granules within (arrows). (from Specian et al. 1979). X20,000.

substance would not be unlikely. Such a generalized metabolic regulatory function would require the accessibility of 5-HT to the target tissue, thus necessitating the release of 5-HT from "neurosecretory" neurons into the "parenchymal" tissue.

Due to the absence of a body cavity or circulatory system in cestodes, neurosecretory material must reach its effector site(s) via diffusion through the connective tissue. From studies with other kinds of organisms (cf. Burnstock and Iwayama 1971), aminergic terminals may be separated from their target tissues by distances up to 1 µ. This feature effectively precludes the use of morphology alone to assess the functional relationships of putative neurosecretory elements to other cells. Clearly, the definitive work on this subject where cestodes are concerned will require physiological and biochemical approaches as well.

VIII. THE SCOLEX

A. *Head or Tail?*

The term "scolex" was first proposed by van Beneden, in the mid-1800's, for what most students of tapeworm anatomy since Tyson (1683) and Andry (1700) have considered to be the head of the organism. After all, for bilaterally symmetric animals, the end preceding in locomotion and containing the major neural mass is conventionally accepted as anterior, and where that end is structurally differentiated from the rest of the body, it is usually referred to as the head. Bemusing to the present authors, therefore, is that more than a few workers during the last 100 years have placed the scolex at the posterior end of the body, largely in response to the definitions of what constitutes "anterior" and "posterior" in the hexacanth larva (see Stunkard 1962, for review). The hexacanth moves with its hooked end (capsomere) in advance, while the scolex subsequently develops at the opposite end of the embryo (see Moniez 1880; Stunkard 1940, 1941; Voge and Heyneman 1957). We concur in Stunkard's (1962) view, that arguments disclaiming the scolex as the worm's head boil down to semantics, of little significance otherwise to comprehending adult tapeworm anatomy, physiology, and development. Certainly even less compelling, in our opinion, is the argument

(Wardle and McLeod 1952) to disqualify the scolex as the head because it lacks organs for handling food!

An alternative to the term scolex has been "holdfast", as in many tapeworms, including *H. diminuta*, it is the major anchorage point to the host gut. Besides that, of course, the scolex is the center of sensory and motor co-ordinative activity. These are functions which bear on many aspects of the worm's behaviour, including, no doubt, its diurnal migrations within the host's small intestine (Read and Kilejian 1969; Arai, this volume). It is also clear that in some way the scolex must exert major influence over the growth and maturation of the strobila.

B. *Overall Structure*

Adhesion is provided by two pairs of bilaterally positioned suckers, or acetabula (Fig. 1); neural co-ordination, etc., is provided by the central cephalic mass, or "brain" (Fig. 47); it has also been postulated by some workers that the apical rostellum (Figs. 1 and 47) may have functions related to behavioral and developmental phenomena.

Histologically, the scolex is comprised of tegumental, muscle, connective, nervous, and excretory tissues, with the fine structure of only the tegument differing substantially from the same tissues (see previous sections) occurring in the strobila. The scolex proper contains no germinal tissue. Consequently, there is no regrowth of surgically removed portions of the scolex (Goodchild 1958), though a degree of regenerative ability is possessed by the strobila. Indeed, where scolices detached from the strobila have been repeatedly transplanted from one host to another (Read 1967), there seems to be an inexhaustable capacity for strobilar regrowth. This phenomenon is undoubtedly due to the presence of the immediately posterior "neck", which contains the germinal anlagen. Read's (1967) observation is by no means whimsical. Under natural conditions, such as host starvation, etc., deleterious changes may take place in the strobilar tissues especially of the reproductive organs. Under such conditions, the scolex

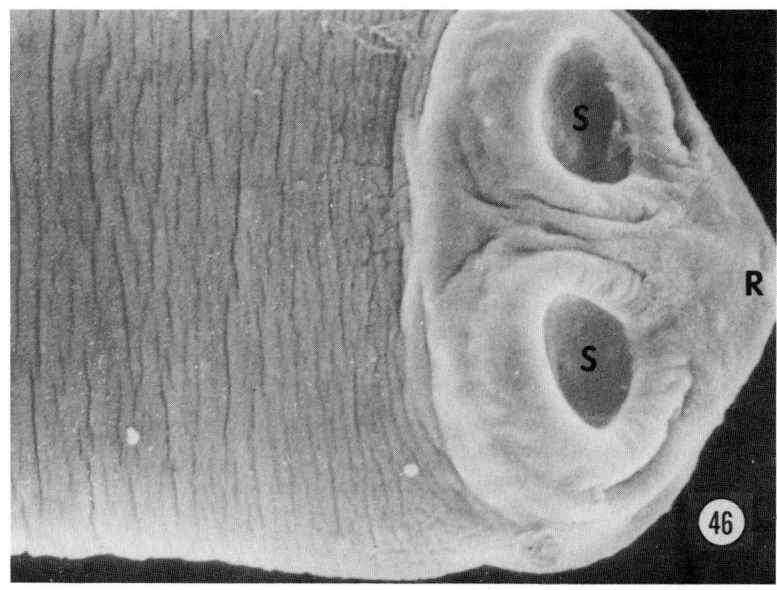

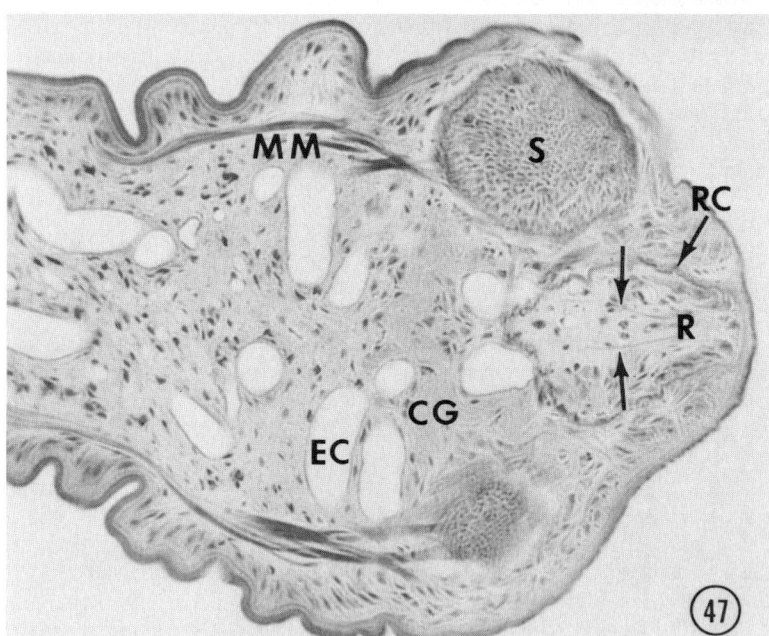

Fig. 46. Scanning electron micrograph of scolex. Apical rostellum (R) raised above bilateral suckers (S). (from Ubelaker et al. 1973). X620.

Fig. 47. Sagittal section through scolex. Pear-shaped rostellum (R) surrounded by muscular rostellar capsule (RC). Fusion of lateral excretory

simply remains attached to the gut wall, the strobila is dropped, and another one is produced when circumstances improve.

C. The Suckers

The suckers measure approximately 75 μm in diameter, and are set off from the remainder of the scolex tissues by a well-defined layer of connective tissue. The cavity of each sucker is lined by a thin tegument continuous with that of the scolex proper (Fig. 48). The intrinsic musculature consists of circular, radial, and longitudinal fibers, with the radial fibers predominating. The circular fibers are oriented around the rim of the sucker, and like a purse string, regulate the aperture of the organ. The strongly developed radial muscles extend from the tegument of the base of the sucker. The highly branched myofibrils surround the myocytons and tegumental perikarya (Fig. 48). Longitudinal fibers are irregularly distributed and relatively inconspicuous.

The extrinsic sucker musculature consists of transverse fibers inserting at the lateral margins and interconnecting adjacent suckers. Occasionally encountered diagonal fibers insert on the mediolateral margin and extend to the base of the rostellar capsule (Fig. 47). The predominate extrinsic fibers are the longitudinal medullary muscles which insert at the base of each sucker (Fig. 47). Whese undoubtedly provide for most of the sucker's mobility.

The innervation of the suckers is relatively extensive and has been described in the preceding section (Nervous System). Other cytological elements associated with the sucker musculature are the attenuated processes containing large spherical, electron opaque, PAF (paraldehyde fuchsin) positive gran-

---

canals (EC) forms bulb-like expansion at base of rostellum, with cerebral ganglia (CG) immediately beneath. Medullary muscles (MM) insert upon base of each sucker (S). Retractor muscles (arrows) for anterior canal apparent within rostellum. Plastic section stained with iron hematoxylin-triosin. (from Specian and Lumsden 1980). X650.

ules (Fig. 43). The multipolar perikarya associated with the processes are distributed through the medullary portion of the scolex and adjacent neck region (Specian *et al.* 1979). Within the perikarya, the granules are produced in association with the juxtanuclear Golgi complexes, subsequently passing into the peripheral cell processes. Ultimately these processes extend into the suckers, where they terminate below the level of the tegument. Their granules appear to be released, via exocytosis, in proximity to the acetabular myocytons and myofibrils (Fig. 48). Our present and most tentative interpretation of these cells is that they are unicellular endocrine glands, perhaps of epithelial origin. Their activity may be influenced by neurosecretory elements (see preceding seciton on nervous system), or possibly by direct communication with the adjacent muscular tissue via a gap junction (Fig. 25; see preceding section on muscle). A suggested function of the secreted material is that of a long-acting modulator of acetabular muscle activity (Specian *et al.* 1979).

D. *The Rostellum*

The rostellum is a pear-shaped organ (60 x 90 μm) located at the apex of the scolex, equidistant from the four acetabula (Figs. 47 and 49). Externally, the rostellum appears as a slight bilobed protrusion, densely covered with microtriches (Figs. 1, 46 and 50).

The capsule surrounding the rostellum is comprised of two layers of muscle, an outer layer of longitudinally oriented fibers and an inner of circularly oriented fibers. The two muscle layers are separated by a dense connective tissue layer, which is continuous with the basal lamina of the rostellar tegument. Vigorous rostellar movements are accomplished by several pairs of retractor and protractor muscles which insert upon the rostellar capsule.

Within the rostellum, the center apical portion forms an invagination of the tegument, the anterior canal (= apical organ). This structure is surrounded by two layers of muscle, an inner layer with circularly oriented fibres and an outer layer of longi-

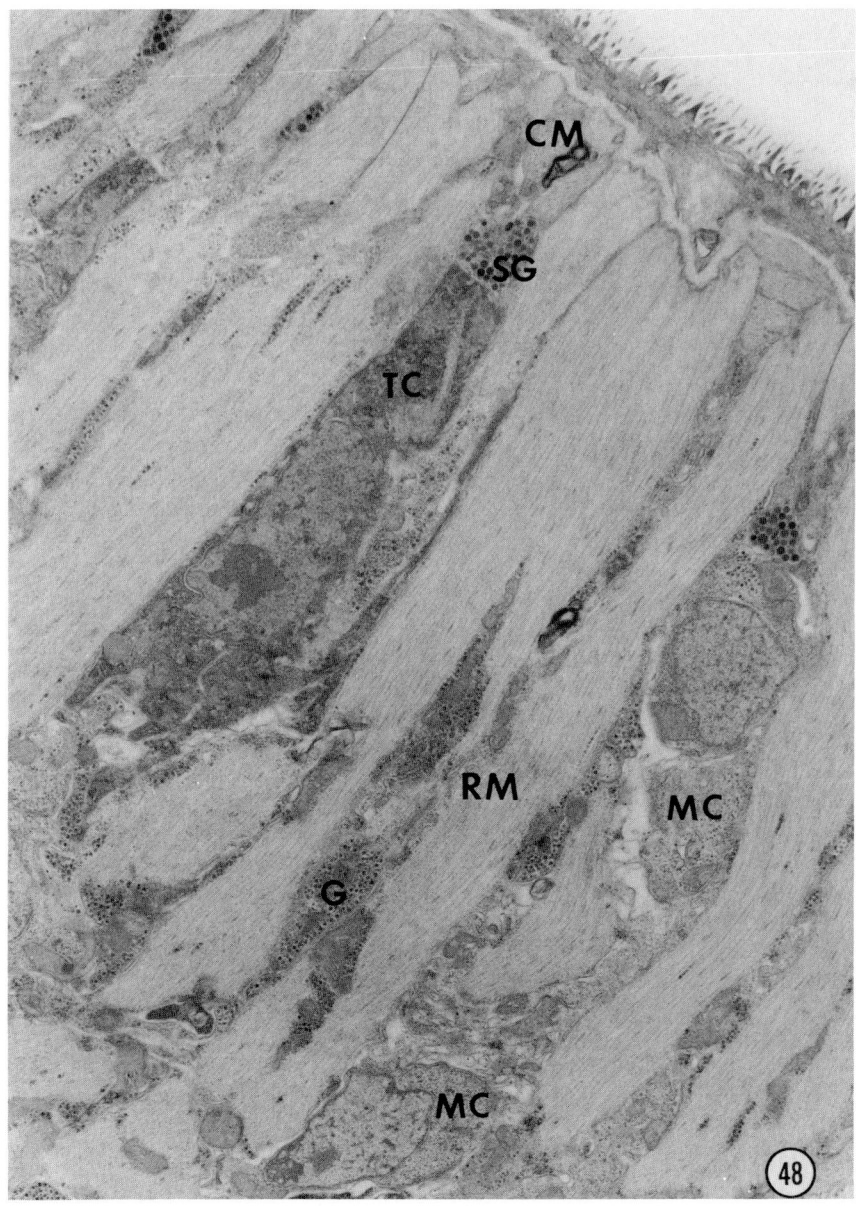

Fig. 48. Sagittal section through sucker. Tegumentary cytons (TC) and mycocytons (MC) interspersed amongst predominantly radial muscle fibers (RM). Endocrine-like cell processes filled with secretory granules (SG) frequently observed within the acetabular musculature. Circular muscles (CM) arranged beneath syncytial tegument. X20,000.

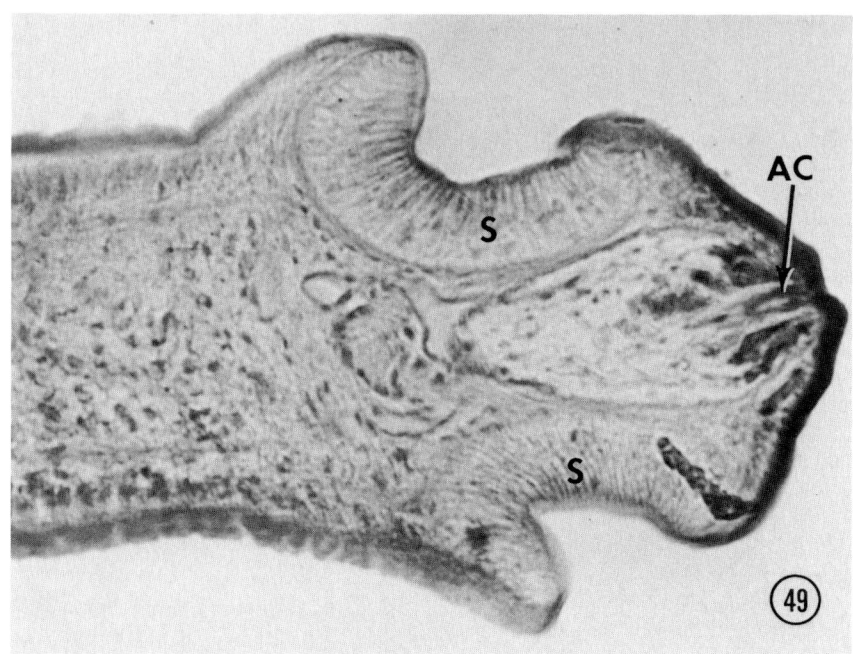

Fig. 49. Sagittal section of scolex, 14 days post-infection. Rostellar tegumentary cytons (RTC) stain positively with PAF (paraldehyde fuchsin), as does distal cytoplasm overlying the anterior canal (AC), rostellum and adjacent scolex. Paraffin section stained with PAF (Cameron and Steele 1959) and counterstained with Halmi mixture (Halmi 1950). (from Specian and Lumsden 1980). X500.

tidinal fibers (Fig. 52). In addition, two pairs of retractor muscles insert upon its base (Fig. 47).

The basal half of the rostellum is occupied by the previously described rostellar ganglia, myocytons and excretory ducts (see appropriate preceding section). Within the apical half of the rostellum lie 12-15 large and otherwise specialized tegumental perikarya, radially arranged around the anterior canal. These cells support the tegumental cytoplasm which covers the rostellum, including the anterior canal, and is continuous with the distal cytoplasm of the scolex tegument (Specian and Lumsden 1980).

Within a few days after the worm becomes established in the intestine of its mammalian host, the distal cytoplasm of the rostellum becomes filled with large (250-350 nm) ovoid, opaque granules (Figs. 51 and 53), which are elaborated by the Golgi complexes of the rostellar tegumentary cytons (Fig. 52). Coincident with the production of the large ovoid vesicles, the rostellar tegument stains differentially with PAF (Fig. 49). After approximately 18 days

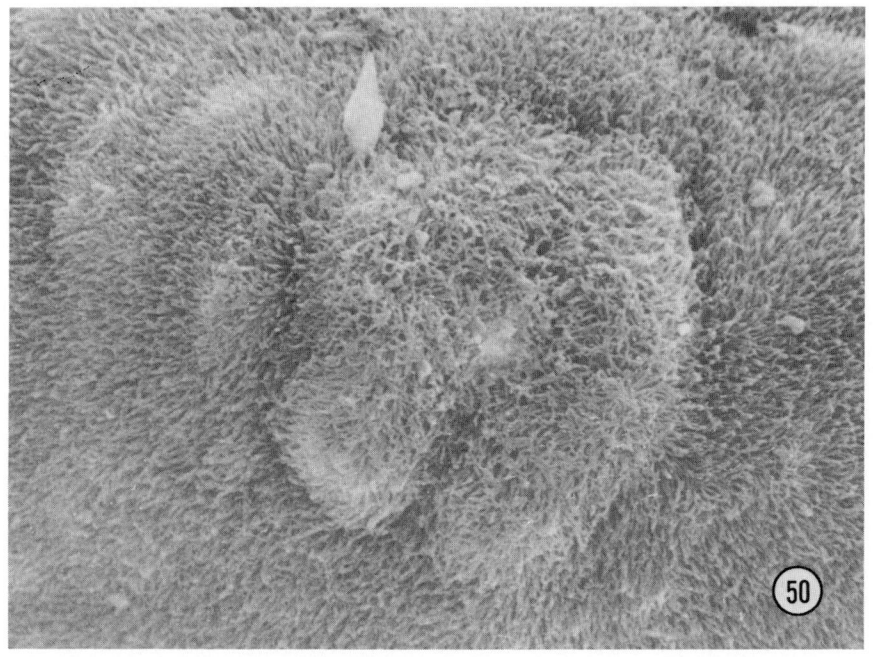

Fig. 50. Scanning electron micrograph of rostellum. Slightly protruding organ densely covered with microtriches. (from Ubelaker et al. 1973). X4,100.

post-infection, at the onset of apolysis, PAF-staining within the rostellar tegument begins to diminish, disappearing altogether by 35 days post-infection. The apparent association between the onset of apolysis and the PAF staining characteristics of these tegumental cells led Davey and Breckenridge

(1967) to the erroneous conclusion that they were neurosecretory elements. Interestingly, even after this region is no longer PAF positive, the ovoid vesicles persist as a characteristic feature of the rostellar tegument (Specian and Lumsden 1980). Within the distal cytoplasm of the anterior canal, these vesicles are aligned adjacent to the plasma membrane, where occasional profiles suggestive of vesicle release into the lumen are observed (Fig. 51).

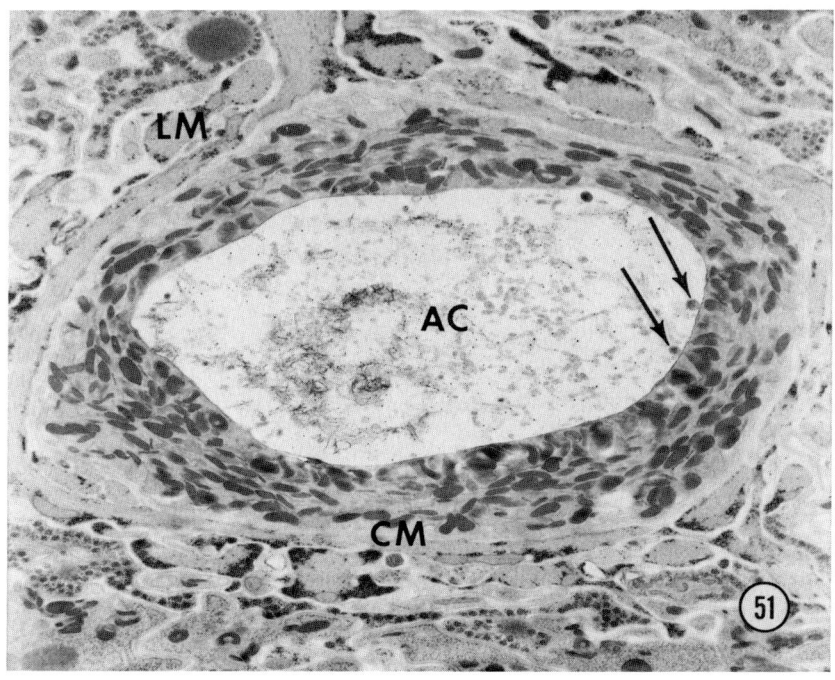

Fig. 51. Cross section of scolex 14 days post-infection. Anterior canal (AC) lined with syncytial tegument filled with ovoid granules produced in rostellar tegumentary cytons. Profiles suggestive of granule release into lumen occasionally observed (arrows). Anterior canal surrounded by inner circular (CM) and outer longitudinal (LM) muscles. (from Specian and Lumsden 1980). X16,000.

In the rostellar tegument proper, the vesicles are oriented perpendicular to the surface (Fig. 53) and extend for some distance into the scolex tegument, displacing the previously described discoidal granules (Fig. 54).

The microtriches on the rostellar tegument differ from those elsewhere on the scolex in having exceedingly elongate and filamentous tips. Those on the scolex proper are relatively short, with a thicker base than those found on the strobilar tegument (Fig. 13). Microtriches and other microvilliform projections are essentially absent within the anterior canal (Fig. 51).

D. *Neural and Excretory Components*

Basal to the rostellum is the pair of large bilateral ganglia which constitute the "brain" of

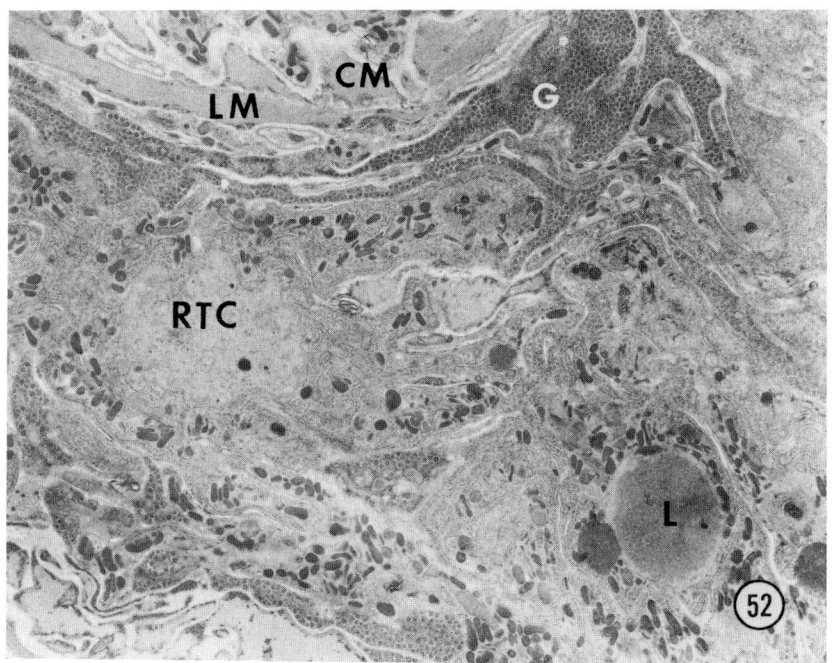

Fig. 52. Sagittal section through apical region of rostellum showing a rostellar tegumentary cyton (RTC). Perinuclear region populated by numerous ovoid granules, produced in association with the Golgi complexes. Free ribosomes and granular endoplasmic reticulum are apparent. Adjacent carbohydrate rich (G) myocytons have lipid (L) accumulations. Longitudinal (LM) and circular (CM) muscles surround ddjacent anterior canal. X11,000.

H. diminuta (Figs. 38 and 47). These ganglia, along with the adjacent rostellar ganglia co-ordinate sensory and motor activity, and may possibly be involved in the regulation of growth and maturation (for discussion, see preceding section on nervous system). Sensilla are especially abundant in the scolex tegument.

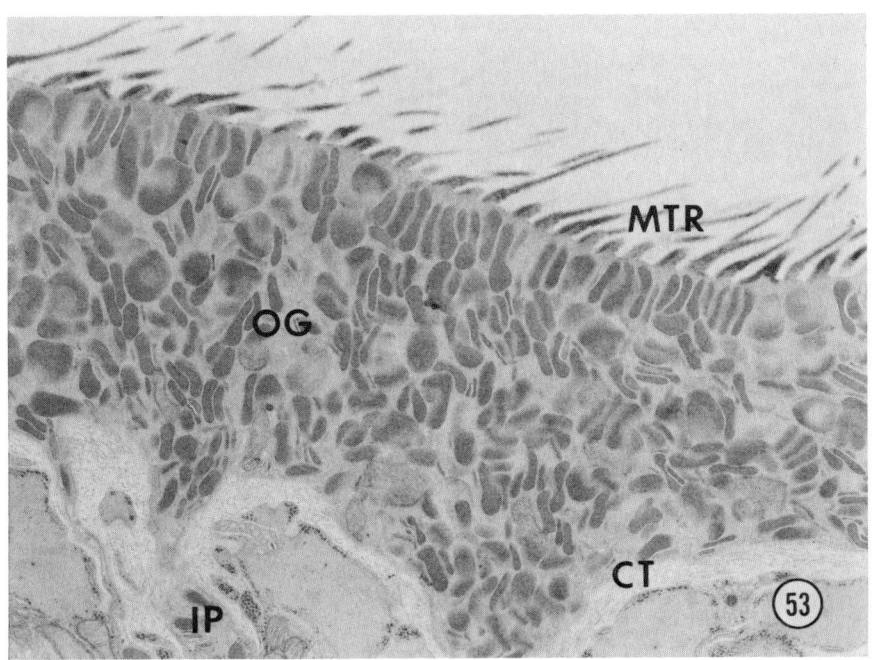

Fig. 53. Rostellar tegument filled with ovoid granules. Granules adjacent to elongate filamentous microtriches (MTR) oriented perpendicular to surface plasma membrane. Internuncial processes (IP) extend through basement lamina (CT) to join rostellar tegumentary cytons. (from Specian and Lumsden 1980). X18,700.

Although the cytological features of the excretory system within the scolex are identical to those in the strobila, the deployment of the collecting tubules and flame cells is noteworthy. Within the

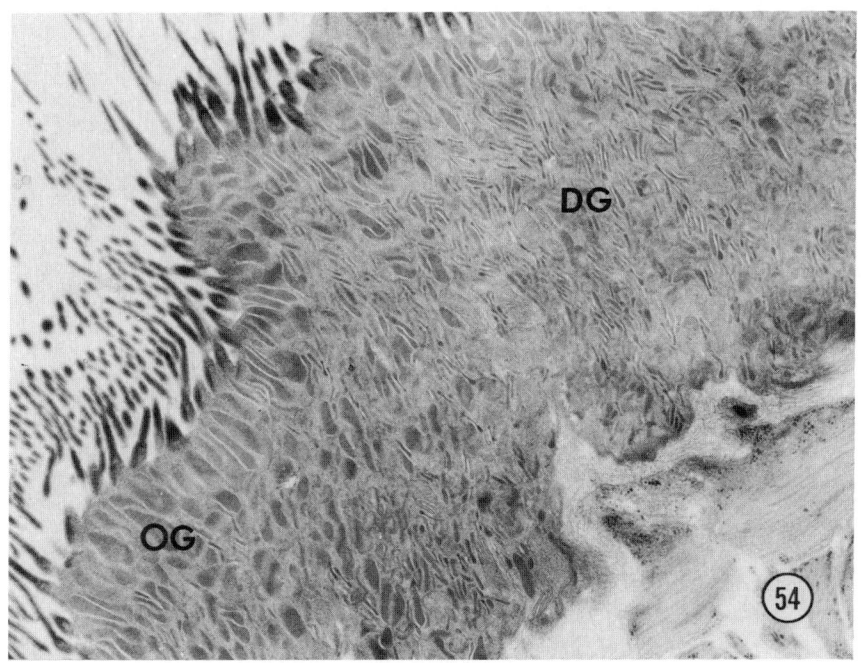

Fig. 54. Joining of scolex and rostellar teguments midway between rostellum and suckers. Rostellar ovoid granules (OG) always oriented along free surface, while scolex discoidal granules (DG) are arranged basally. (from Specian and Lumsden 1980). X17,500.

rostellum are several ducts, which, while smaller than the major vessels, are considerably larger than collecting tubules. There are apparently no flame cells or collecting tubules associated with these ducts, thus excretion presumably takes place by secretion or simple diffusion. Flame cells and collecting tubules are also absent within the suckers, occurring only basal to these organs.

IX. REPRODUCTIVE SYSTEM

As we have noted previously (see Introduction), the *raison d'être* for the adult stage in the life cycle of cestodes is reproduction. The often quoted statistics are indeed impressive: the daily egg output of *Taenia saginata* approaches 400,000; over its lifespan of 10 years or so, a single *Diphyllobothrium latum* will produce over 2 billion eggs; etc. Like the other major group of endoparasitic platyhelminths, digenetic trematodes, the life cycle of most cestodes is complex, usually requiring at least one intermediate host of a species other than the definitive host for larval development. Stunkard (1962) estimated that the odds against an individual cestode completing such a hazardous journey were approximately one million : one. Yet, despite such overwhelming odds, because of their reproductive potential, cestodes as a group have proven to be remarkably successful.

It is perhaps ironic, then, that a major focus of electron microscopists has not been the tapeworm reproductive system. The greatest amount of literature on cestode reproductive organs derives from light microscopy, and has dealt more with features for taxonomic diagnosis rather than functional morphology. Cytological descriptions at the electron microscope level are available for certain of the more obvious elements - e.g., spermatozoa, stages in spermatogenesis, vitelline cells, eggs, etc. - but for no one cestode is there a comprehensive account of the entire system. The following represents an attempt to bring together isolated reports on the reproductive system of *H. diminuta*, correlated, where feasible, with our own heretofore unpublished observations and with published accounts of reproductive fine structure in other cestodes.

A. *Organ Histogensis*

In the process of proglottid formation, cells at the base of the neck region comprising the tegument, excretory, muscular, and nervous systems are essentially differentiated. The cells which ultimately form the reproductive organs, however, remain undifferentiated here and in the anterior proglottids of the strobila. This mass of embryonic cells was termed the early primary primordium by Sulgostowska (1972, 1974).

At a distance of 3-3.5 mm behind the scolex, the early primary primordium separates, resulting in a peripheral primordium located in the outer medullary region of the proglottid, and the central primordium, which is a concentration of cells in the center of each proglottid. At this stage of strobilar development, germinative cells, germinative-somatic cells and somatic cells can be distinguished in each primordium; externally, segmentation is becoming apparent.

At a distance of 3.8-4 mm behind the scolex, another group of cells, the somatic primordium, migrates away from the central primordium toward the poral margin of the proglottid.

Since development of the reproductive organs in *H. diminuta* is protandrous, those cells responsible for the male organs differentiate closest to the neck region. The cells of the peripheral primordium agglomerate to form the testes. The cells of the somatic primordium migrate to the lateral margin of the proglottid, leaving behind a band of cells which ultimately form the sperm ducts, vagina and associated structures. At the margin of the proglottid, the cells of the somatic primordium are joined by an infolding of the tegument resulting in the formation of the genital atrium (genital pore). The genital pores are unilateral. Finally, far down the strobila (38-40 mm behind the scolex), after the male system has matured and the vagina is fully developed, the central primordium divides to form the ovarian primordium and the vitelline primordium which ultimately differentiate into the ovary and vitelline gland (Sulgostowska 1974).

B. *Male Components*

The function of the male reproductive system is to: (1) produce gametes (spermatozoa); (2) store gametes until insemination can occur; and (3) provide a mechanism for insemination. While an understanding of the basic male reproductive morphology is not difficult, a simplified overview may facilitate subsequent anatomical and microanatomical descriptions.

Gametogenesis occurs within the testes, where upon maturation spermatozoa are passed into the sperm ductules and finally into the common sperm duct. The sperm accumulate in an expanded region of the sperm duct, the external seminal vesicle. During copulation, the cirrus - the protrusible portion of the male copulatory apparatus - is inserted into the genital atrium and vagina of an appropriate proglottid of the same or another worm. Self-insemination, where by the cirrus is inserted into the vagina of the same proglottid, is not, apparently, uncommon (Nollen 1975). Movement of the spermatozoa is accomplished by their own flagellar activity and the muscular contractions of the sperm ducts.

In *H. diminuta*, spermatogenesis in an individual proglottid proceeds more or less synchronously, such that maturation of spermatozoa immediately precedes testicular involution (Kelsoe *et al*. 1977). This is possible because of the plasmodial nature of the gametogenic elements and is essential in *H. diminuta* because individual testes are functional only for about four days (Roberts 1961). Kelsoe *et al*. (1977) postulated that synchronous testicular development serves to conserve metabolic energy by providing for the maturation of the majority of testicular cells prior to testicular degeneration.

The normal testicular configuration is that of three medullary testes arranged more or less in a straight line, with two on the aporal side and one on the poral side of each proglottid (Fig. 3). Variations in this arrangement are not uncommon, however, with up to 7 or 8 testes occasionally being observed in a single proglottid, with a resulting aberrant aporal-poral distribution.

The testes arise from the germinative and germinative-somatic cells of the peripheral primordium, with the latter differentiating to form the epithelial covering of the organ. The germinative cells give rise to primary spermatogonia and thus initiate the gametogenic cell line.

As for the stages in spermiogenesis seen in higher organisms (Bloom and Fawcett 1975), following nuclear division (karyokinesis), division of the cell body (cytokinesis) is incomplete. The resulting structure is correctly termed a plasmodium (see

Introduction), not a syncytium, as it has been called by Kelsoe et al. (1977) and some other authors. This point is significant as it concerns the developmental differences between these gametogenic tissues and the syncytial tissues which occur elsewhere in cestodes.

In all studies to date, the basic pattern of cestode spermatogenesis has been found to consist of four spermatogonial mitoses and two maturation divisions, such that a single primary spermatogonium ultimately produces 64 spermatozoa (Rybicka 1962a, 1962b; Douglas 1963; Paschenko 1961; Featherston 1971; Kazacos and Mackiewicz 1972; Maamouri and Swiderski 1975; Kelsoe et al. 1977). Specifically, in *H. diminuta*, "A" spermatogonia, located around the periphery of the testis, undergo three mitotic divisions to form a plasmodial rosette of eight "B" spermatogonia. Further mitotic division results in a cluster of 16 primary spermatocytes (Fig. 55) which retain cytoplasmic continuity. At this stage, meiosis begins, with the first division yielding a large mass of 32 secondary spermatocytes and the second ultimately resulting in 64 spermatids, recognizable as a broad plasmodium with many nuclei (Fig. 58).

The diagnostic fine structural features of the spermatogonia and spermatids can be summarized as follows (after Kelsoe et al. 1977):

(1) Type A spermatogonia - large, single and with a somewhat irregularly shaped nucleus, with prominent nucleolus and abundant heterochromatin; cytoplasm dense with abundant free ribosomes and mitochondria, scant endoplasmic reticulum.

(2) Type B spermatogonia - ultimately in plasmodial rosettes; nuclei reduced in diameter, otherwise as per Type A spermatogonia; cytoplasm relatively more electron translucent, with numerous polyribosomes, mitochondria, and some juxtanuclear granular endoplasmic reticulum.

(3) Primary spermatocytes - plasmodial; nuclei larger than for Type B spermatogonia, with reduced amount of heterochromatin, and degeneration of the nucleolus; cytoplasm as for Type B spermatogonia, but even more electron translucent, and evidencing a reduction in the amount of granular endoplasmic

reticulum; peripheral centrioles (basal body precursors?) often present.

(4) Secondary spermatocytes - plasmodial; nuclei reduced in diameter, with more heterochromatin; cytoplasm containing annulate lamellae, abundant ribosomes.

(5) Spermatids - in broad plasmodial arrays, with elongate nuclei containing abundant heterochromatin; mitochondria in perpheral clusters; cell surface with marked invaginations, pockets formed thereby containing developing spermatozoa.

The reorganization of the spermatid nuclei into elongate helices marks the initiation of spermiogenesis (Fig. 56). Concommitantly, the plasma membrane of the plasmodium invaginates deeply to form arching membrane limited clefts (Rosario 1964) which ultimately delimit the forming spermatozoa from the spermatid cluster.

Mature *H. diminuta* spermatozoa are 250-300 µm long, with a broad flattened "head" region and a long cylindrical tail. Internally, there is a centrally or slightly eccentrically positioned flagellar axoneme, comprised of nine doublet microtubules surrounding and connected by spokes to a non-tubular, central cylinder or core element (Figs. 56 and 57). This rather unique pattern of axoneme substructure, possessed by other tapeworms and most other platyhelminths, is usually designated "9 + 1" to distinguish it from the more ubiquitous "9 + 2" pattern for flagella found elsewhere in the animal kingdom. However, the central element of flatworm sperm axonemes is not a microtubule (single or otherwise, as would be implied by the "9 +" designation scheme) and possesses an otherwise complex ultrastructure (see e.g., Silveira 1974). Immediately beneath the plasma membrane is a row of singlet microtubules which follows a helical course for the length of the cell (Lumsden 1965c). The nucleus is an elongate ovoid structure, helically twisted, and packed with opaque heterochromatin. Other organelles are absent from the cytoplasm of the mature *H. diminuta* spermatozoon, which otherwise contains large amounts of glycogen (Lumsden 1965a).

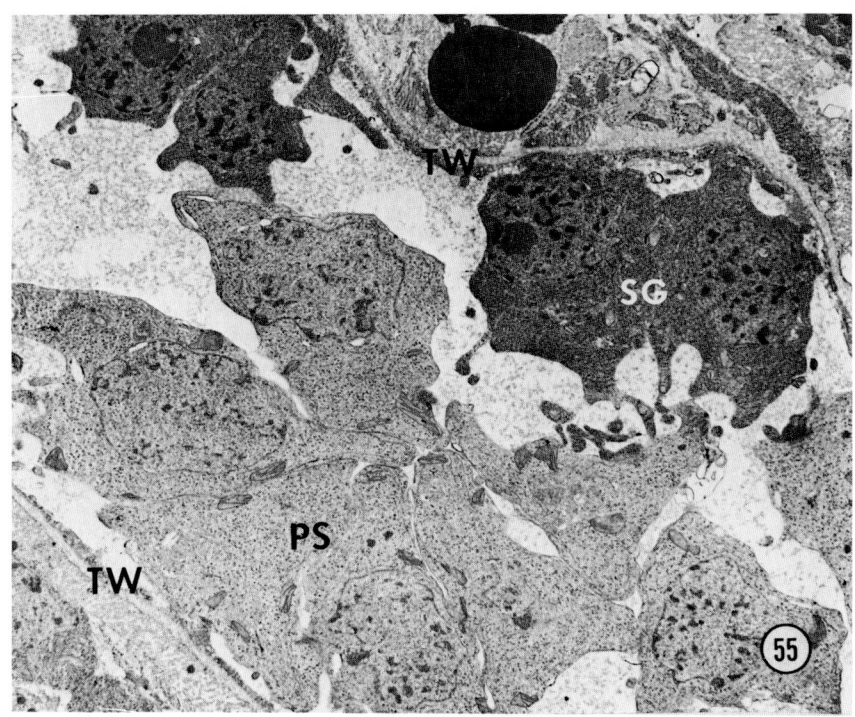

Fig. 55. Section through developing testis. Primary spermatocytes (PS) arranged in plasmodial cluster. Spermatocyte cytoplasm contains numerous mitochondria and much lighter staining than cytoplasm of adjacent spermatogium (SG). Thin epithelial elements comprise testicular wall (TW). (from Kelsoe et al. 1977). X6,050

The sperm ductules, common sperm duct and associated structures (i.e., cirrus and seminal vesicles) are all differentiated from the somatic primordium (Sulgostowska 1974). The sperm ductules (vasa efferentia) are patent with the testicular lumen and fuse midway between the poral testis (testes) and aporal testes, to form the common sperm duct (vas deferens). The sperm duct is often highly coiled and extends laterally before terminating in the male copulatory apparatus, within the genital atrium (Figs. 3 and 62). Prior to the release of

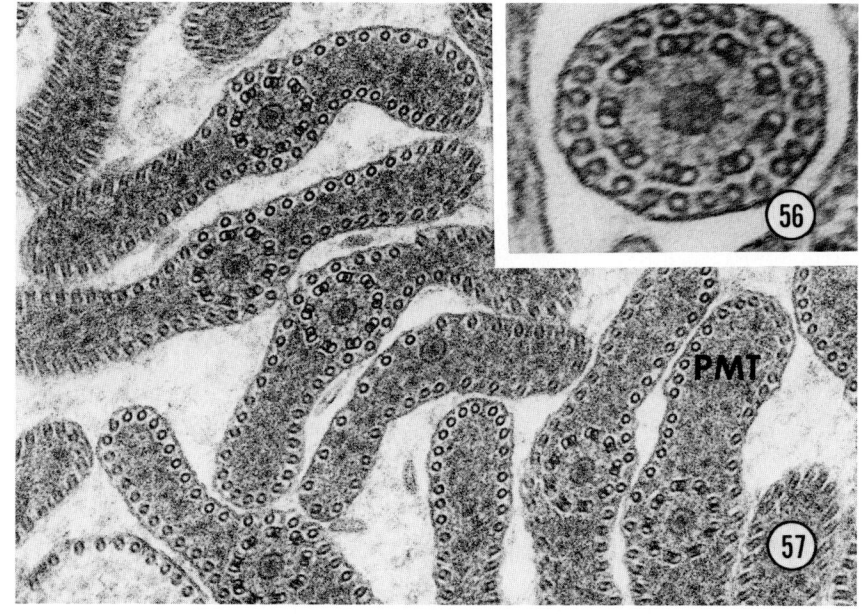

Fig. 56. Cross section of spermatozoan tail. Axonome shows 9 + 1 microtubular arrangement, with outer circle of 25 single peripheral microtubules.

Fig. 57. Cross section of several spermatozoa tails just distal to nucleus. Central axoneme has 9 + 1 microtubular arrangement. Adjacent cytoplasm devoid of organelles, except for peripheral microtubules (PMT). Number of peripheral microtubules varies between spermatozoa tails cut at same level. (micrograph courtesy of Dr. F.M. Gress). X52,100.

The Morphology, Histology, and Fine Structure of the Adult Stage   247

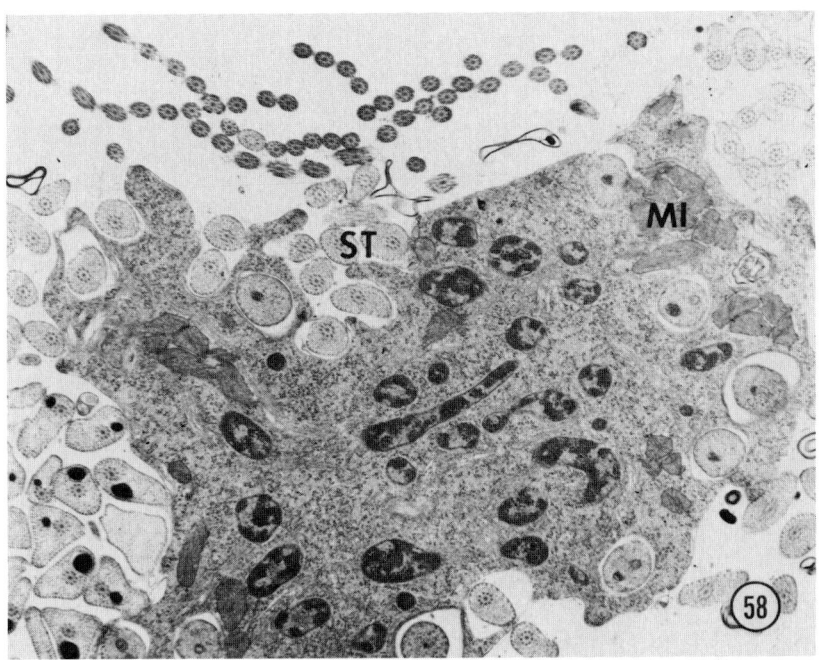

Fig. 58. Section through mature testis. Plasmodial spermatid cluster undergoing spermiogenesis. Dense staining nuclei (N) are condensing, with the cytoplasm being sequestered around individual spermatozoan. Mature spermatozoa (ST) apparent within testicular lumen. (from Kelsoe et al. 1977). X8,250.

spermatozoa from the testes, the sperm duct is slightly enlarged immediately distal to the convergence of the sperm ductules. This enlargement represents the external seminal vesicle (spermiductal vesicle of Hyman 1951), and frequently goes unnoticed at this stage of development. In mature proglottids prior to copulation, however, massive numbers of mature spermatozoa are stored here, resulting in a vesicular volume frequently in excess of that of an individual testis. When thus swollen with sperm, the seminal vesicle extends from the point of con-

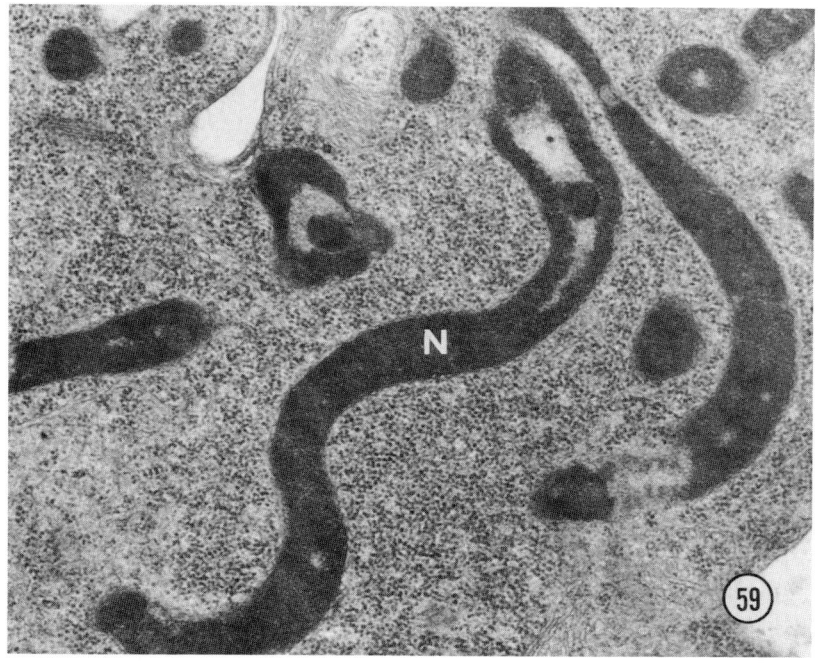

Fig. 59. Higher magnification of condensing spermatozoa nuclei (N). Nuclei elongate and assume helical configuration. (from Kelsoe et al. 1977). X28,700.

vergence of the sperm ductules, nearly to the lateral margin of the proglottid.

The lining of the sperm ducts is syncytial, with the nuclei withdrawn beneath the distal cytoplasm. The lumenal surface bears elongate, filamentous microvilli, and the adlumenal surface possesses deep and numerous infoldings (Fig. 60 and 61). The distal cytoplasm is much thicker in the common sperm duct (Fig. 60) than in either the distended seminal vesicle (Fig. 61) or in the sperm ductules. It contains a mixed population of electron dense and lucent vesicles which appear to arise from the perinuclear

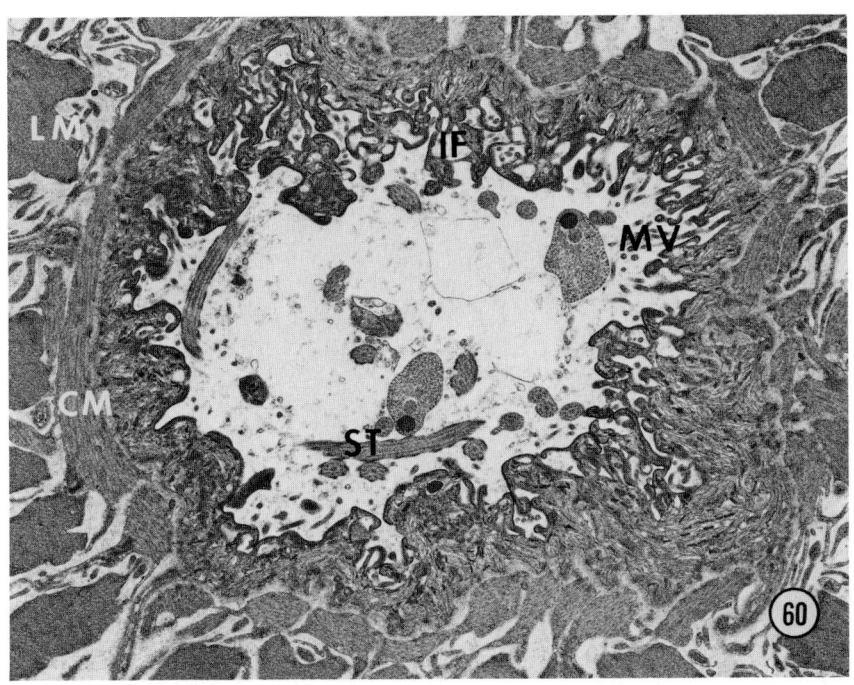

Fig. 60. Cross section of common sperm duct (vas deferens) immediately distal to fusion of sperm ductules (vasa efferentia). Lumen of duct contains mature spermatozoa (ST). Numerous infoldings (IF) and microvilli (MV) mark the free surface of syncytial duct lining. Syncytial layer populated by variety of vesicles. Duct surrounded by prominent circular (CM) and longitudinal (LM) muscle fibers. X10,300.

region of the underlying cytons. Immediately beneath the distal cytoplasm of the sperm duct is a thin layer of connective tissue followed by a well developed layer of circular muscle (this becomes somewhat reduced in sperm ductules) and an abundance of longitudinally oriented muscle fibers (Figs. 60 and 61).

The male copulatory apparatus consists of a proximal non-eversible portion - the internal seminal vesicle or ejaculatory duct - and an eversible

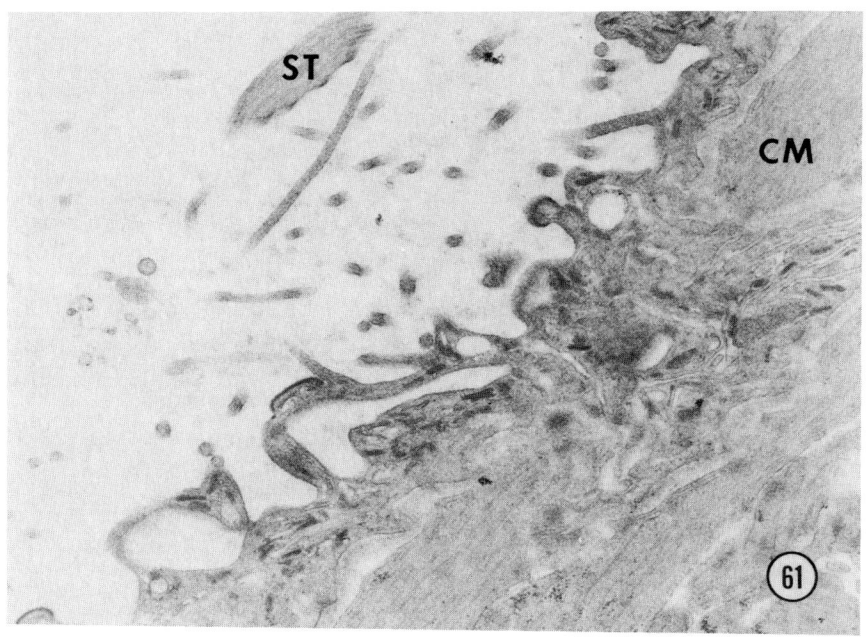

Fig. 61. Cross section of external seminal vesicle. Surface layer similar to that of common sperm duct, only thinner due to distension of vesicle by spermatozoa (ST). X17,300.

portion - the cirrus (Figs. 62 and 63). The internal seminal vesicle represents a permanently enlarged region of the common sperm duct, which terminates at the tip of the cirrus. The cirrus is a cylindrical organ (350 x 100 µm) which is covered with numerous minute spines (Fig. 63). At the base of the everted cirrus are numerous papillae which may represent sensory receptors (Fig. 63).

The entire copulatory organ lies within the muscular cirrus sac (Fig. 62). While circular muscles predominate here, protractor and retractor muscles are also present, and serve to facilitate

The Morphology, Histology, and Fine Structure of the Adult Stage 251

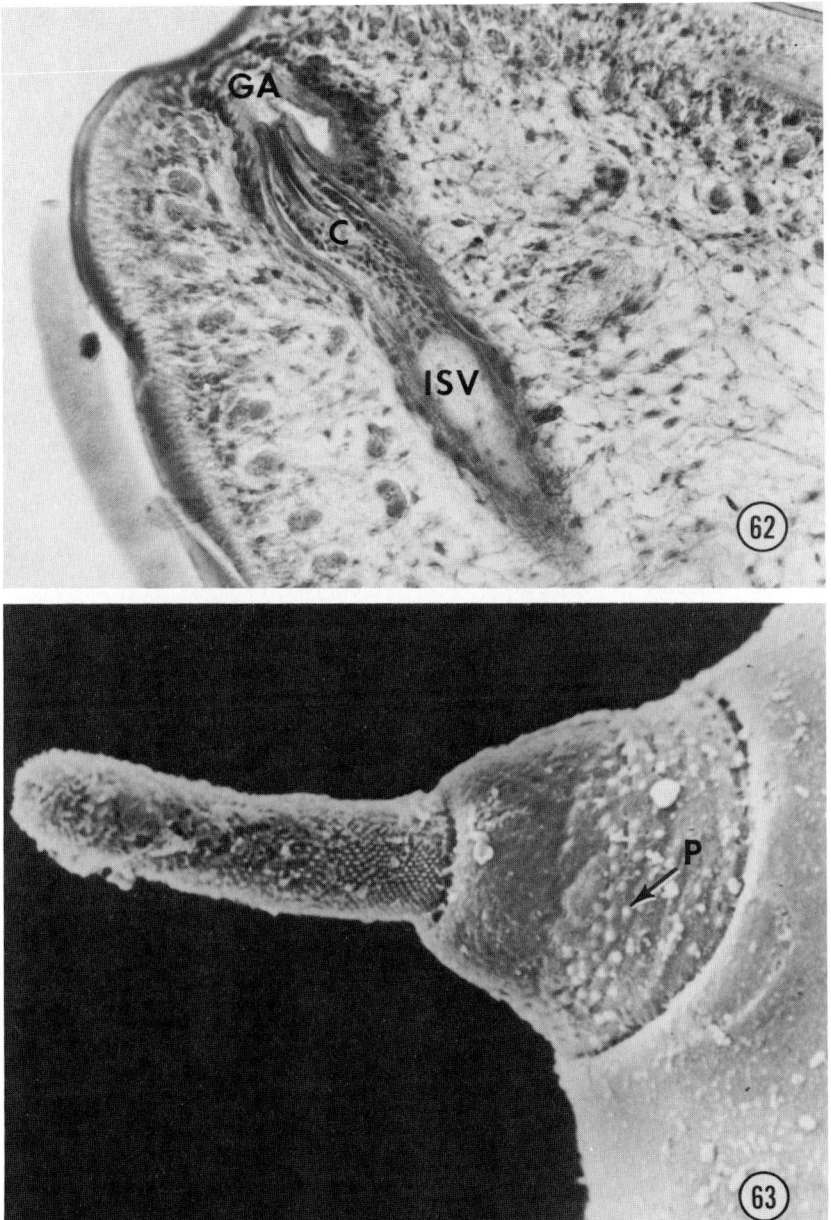

Fig. 62. Cross section through terminal genitalia of mature proglottid. Male copulatory apparatus consists of non-eversible ejaculatory duct or internal seminal vesicle (ISV) and eversible organ, the cirrus (C). Genitalia patent with exterior via gen-

ital atrium (GA). Paraffin section stained with hematoxylin and eosin. X100.

Fig. 63. Scanning electron micrograph of everted cirrus. Length of organ covered with minute spines. Basal portion possesses minute papillae (P) which may be sensory. (Micrograph courtesy of Dr. J.E. Ubelaker). X225.

movement of the cirrus. The cirrus sac stains heavily for acetylcholinesterase, suggesting a high level of neuro-muscular interaction (Wilson and Schiller 1969).

C. *Female Components*

The function of the female reproductive system is four-fold in *H. diminuta*. It serves to: (1) produce female gametes (oocytes); (2) store male gametes (spermatozoa) subsequent to insemination and prior to fertilization; (3) assist in the formation of larval capsule (eggshell) and (4) store the developing larvae until the proglottid is released. While only five organs (the ovary, vagina-seminal receptacle, oviduct, vitelline gland and Mehlis gland) accomplish all of the above functions, an understanding of even the basic anatomical features can be perplexing for the beginning student, as well as the advanced researcher. For example, the oviduct has been given no less than three distinct names for various modification along its length before becoming the uterus. Thus to facilitate subsequent anatomical and microanatomical descriptions, herein is presented an abbreviate overview of the female reproductive system.

Oocytes differentiate within the ovary, and when mature they pass into the oviduct. Fertilization takes place when spermatozoa, stored in the seminal receptacle subsequent to copulation and insemination, enter the oviduct via a muscular duct termed the seminal canal. The oviduct now contains mature oocytes and mature spermatozoa and as the site of fertilization is frequently termed the fertilization canal. Traveling down the oviduct (fertilization canal), each fertilized oocyte (zygote) fuses with a single vitelline cell which has reached the oviduct from the vitelline gland via the vitelline duct. The vitelline cell (according to certain authors, but not all) provides the zygote with two membranous coatings, the larval envelopes, and contributes to shell formation. The region of oviduct between the entrance of the vitelline duct and the next oviduct specialization, the ootype, is termed the ovovitelline canal. The ootype or "primary uterus" is surrounded by numerous unicellular glands (Mehlis or shell glands) which secrete into the ootype, but serve an otherwise unknown function. Leaving the ootype, the now fully formed eggs enter the uterus where the developing larvae mature in anticipation of proglottid release (Fig. 64).

Concurrent with the formation of the vas deferens and terminal male gentalia, the vagina is formed from cells originating in the somatic primordium. Though arising from a common germ mass, when fully differentiated the sperm ducts and vagina are independent of each other (Sulgostowska 1974).

The vagina terminates within the genital atrium, where it opens posterior to the cirrus sac. Internally, the vagina extends medially, to about the center of the proglottid, always ventral to the male ducts. Near the ovary, the vagina enlarges considerably to form the seminal receptacle, which subsequent to copulation and insemination is filled with spermatozoa (Fig. 65)

The lining of the vagina (and seminal receptacle) is syncytial, with the nuclei located basally. The cytoplasm contains numerous vesicles (Fig. 65) and the lumenal surface bears elongate, filamentous microvilli. These microvilli intertwine with the spermatozoa lying within the lumen of the organ (Fig. 65). By light microscopy, numerous authors have reported the presence of "cilia" lining the walls of the vagina and seminal receptacle of other cestodes (see Wardle and McLeod 1952), which, as reported here for *H. diminuta*, are probably, in fact, microvilli. Pinter (1934) suggested that the function of the "non-motile cilia" within the vaginal lumen was to serve as a non-return valve mechanism.

The epithelial lining of the vagina is thickest near the genital atrium, becoming much thinner around

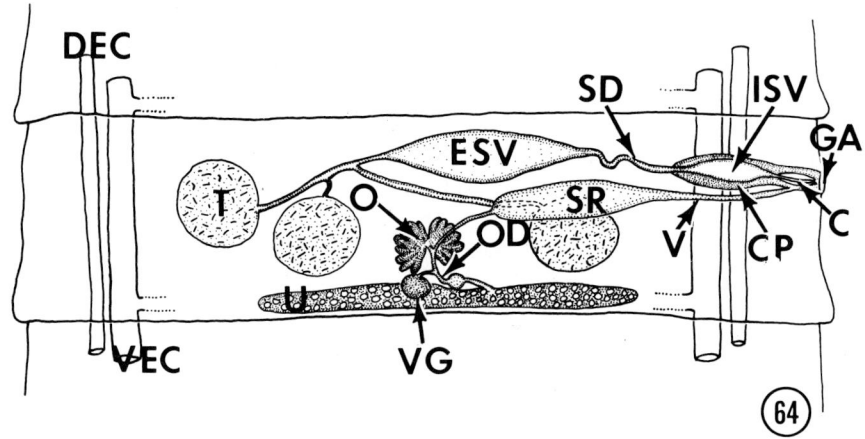

Fig. 64. Diagramatic frontal view of mature proglottid. Cirrus (C); cirrus pouch (CP); dorsal excretory canal (DEC); external seminal vesicle (ESV); internal seminal vesicle (ISV); genital atrium (GA); ovary (O); oviduct (OV); seminal receptacle (SR); spermduct (SD); uterus (U); vagina (V); ventral excretory canal (VEC); vitelline gland (VG). (After Noble and Noble 1971).

the seminal receptacle. The epithelium is surrounded by a "basement membrane" or layer of connective tissue Longitudinal muscle bundles predominate around the vagina with some oblique and transverse muscles also being present. Circular muscles are not prominent, except where they form a vaginal sphincter adjacent to the genital atrium.

Ovarian differentiation occurs subsequent to the full development of the vagina and seminal receptacle. The ovary consists of two lobes interconnected by a narrow neck region or isthmus, from which the oviduct originates. Each lobe of the ovary is composed of numerous tubular processes arranged such that the oocytes are peripherally located around the lumen of the tube. The lumen of each process is ultimately patent with the lumen of

The Morphology, Histology, and Fine Structure of the Adult Stage 255

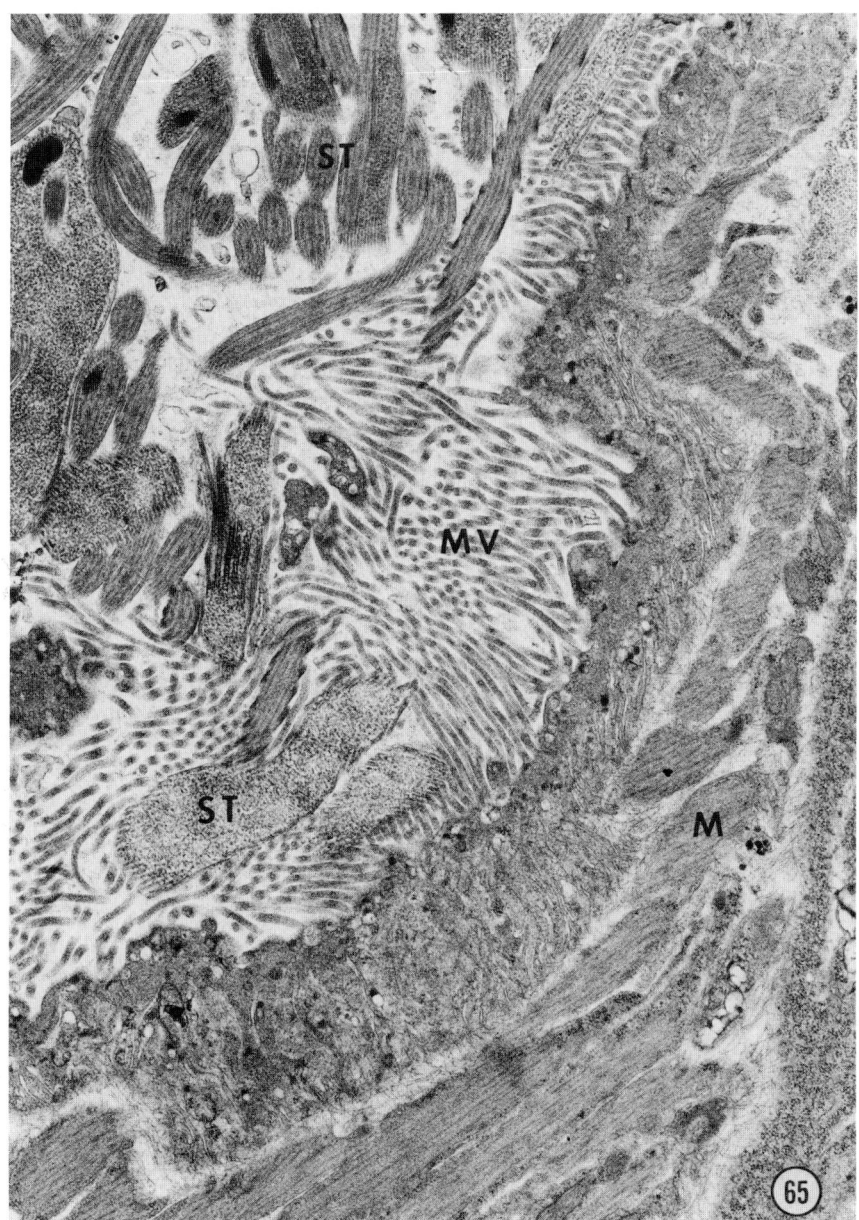

Fig. 65. Longitudinal section through seminal receptacle filled with spermatozoa (ST). Lining of organ composed of syncytial cytoplasm, nuclei withdrawn beneath muscular (M) layer. Surface cytoplasm populated by variety of vesicles. Surface extended as elongate, filamentous microvilli (MV). X19,000.

the oviduct. Similar to testicular development, the oocytes arise from the germinative cells of the ovarian primordium (derived from the central primordium), with the epithelial covering of the organ differentiating from the germinative-somatic cells of the ovarian primordium. Fine structural features for elements other than the oocyte (Fig. 68) have not been described for *H. diminuta*.

Oocytes are very large cells (12-14 μm) with a centrally located spherical nucleus (4-5 μm) and a prominent nucleolus. The cytoplasm is unremarkable, except for the presence of numerous mitochondria (Fig. 68), polyribosomes, and occasional arrays of annulate lamellae (see, e.g., Lumsden 1965a). The fine structure of developing oocytes (oogenesis) has not been described for *H. diminuta*.

The oviduct arises from a band of densely staining cells found in the central primordium, and is distinguishable prior to the formation of a discrete ovary (Sulgostowska 1974). Subsequent to ovarian differentiation, the oviduct joins the ovary at the isthmus, with apparent continuity between the epithelial covering of the ovary and the walls of the oviduct.

From the ovarian isthmus, the oviduct extends ventrally a short distance, whereupon it is joined by the muscular seminal canal arising from the terminal end of the seminal receptacle. This duct allows the passage of spermatozoa into the oviduct.

The vitelline duct joins the oviduct (or fertilization canal) a short distance beyond the entrance of the seminal canal. As previously mentioned, the vitelline duct carries the vitelline cells into the oviduct.

The vitelline gland differentiates concurrently with the ovary, arising from germinative cells in the vitelline primordium (this having previously separated from the central primordium). In the mature state, the vitelline gland is composed of numerous cells which are characterized by a holocrine secretory mechanism. The spherical vitelline cells of *H. diminuta* are large (5-6 μm) and possess a centrally located nucleus, in contrast to the peripherally located nucleus of other species (Swiderski et al. 1970a).

Maturing vitelline cells are characterized by an abundance of perinuclear granular endoplasmic reticulum and prominent Golgi complexes. Numerous mitochondria and forming secretory granules are distributed around the periphery of the cell (Fig. 66).

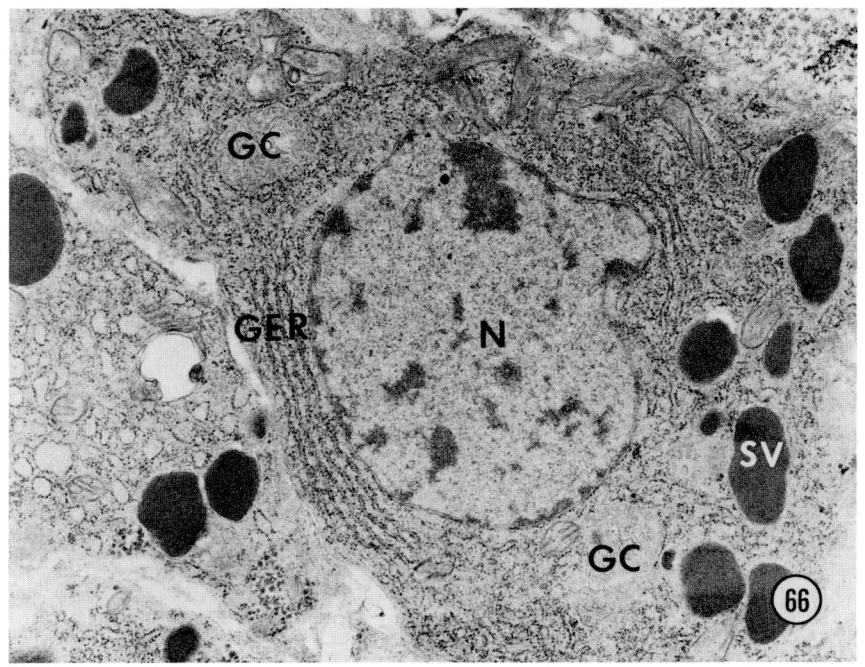

Fig. 66. Developing vitelline cell. Spherical nucleus (N) surrounded by granular endoplasmic reticulum (GER). Secretory vesicles (SV) not abundant, but forming adjacent to Golgi complexes (GC). Mitochondria (MI) peripherally located. X14,000.

Mature cells, on the other hand, exhibit a poorly defined granular endoplasmic reticulum; the cytoplasm is filled with electron dense secretory granules (Fig. 67). Vitelline cells also contain large amounts of glycogen (Lumsden 1965a).

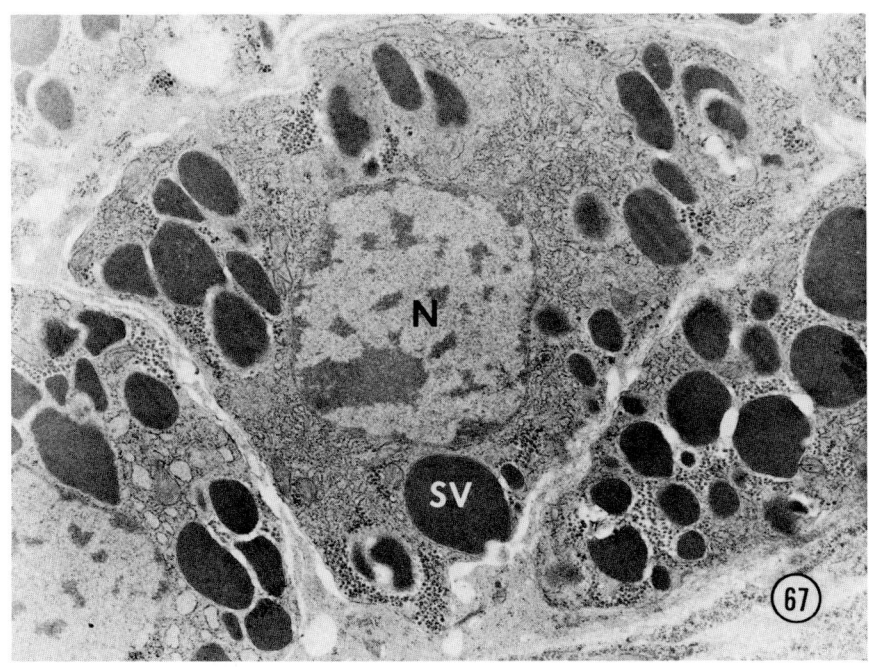

Fig. 67. Mature vitelline cell. Nucleus (N) now surrounded by numerous secretory vesicles (SV). Cytoplasm of adjacent cells also filled with vesicles. X14,000.

A mature vitelline cell passes down the vitelline duct, whereupon it degranulates in proximity to a single fertilized oocyte (Ogren, 1956; Loser 1965a, 1965b; Swiderski et al. 1970b) (Fig. 68). According to Swiderski et al. (1970b), the excess vesicular membranes associated with the degranulation process surrounds the vitelline cell and zygote (fertilized oocyte) to form the internal and external membranous envelopes of the developing larva (see also Ubelaker, this volume). On the other hand, Rybicka (1972) indicated that it is only the capsule which is formed by the vitelline secretion, the membranous envelopes arising as syncytial cytoplasmic layers formed from macromeres.

The microanatomy of the oviduct from the ovarian isthmus to the ootype is fairly uniform. The apparently syncytial epithelium is supported by basally withdrawn nuclei at infrequent intervals. The nuclei display a prominent centrally located nucleolus. The perinuclear cytoplasm is sparse and contains few formed structures other than free ribosomes. Golgi complexes are occasionally observed (Fig. 69). The lumenal surface bears small, infre-

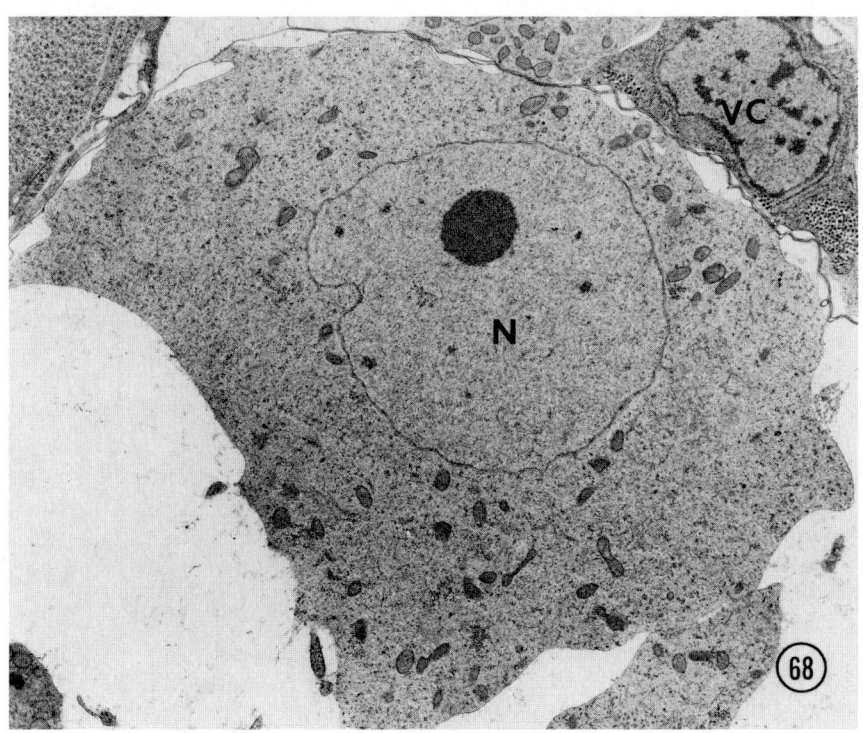

Fig. 68. Fertilized oocyte within oviduct. Cytoplasm of oocyte surrounding spherical nucleus (N) contains numerous mitochondria. Vitelline cell (VC) associated with adjacent zygote has degranulated, and embryonic envelopes have formed. X7,100.

quent microvilli, although the oviduct wall consists of only a very thin membranous layer in many areas

(Fig. 69). Underlying musculature around the oviduct is not prominent and follows no consistent pattern.

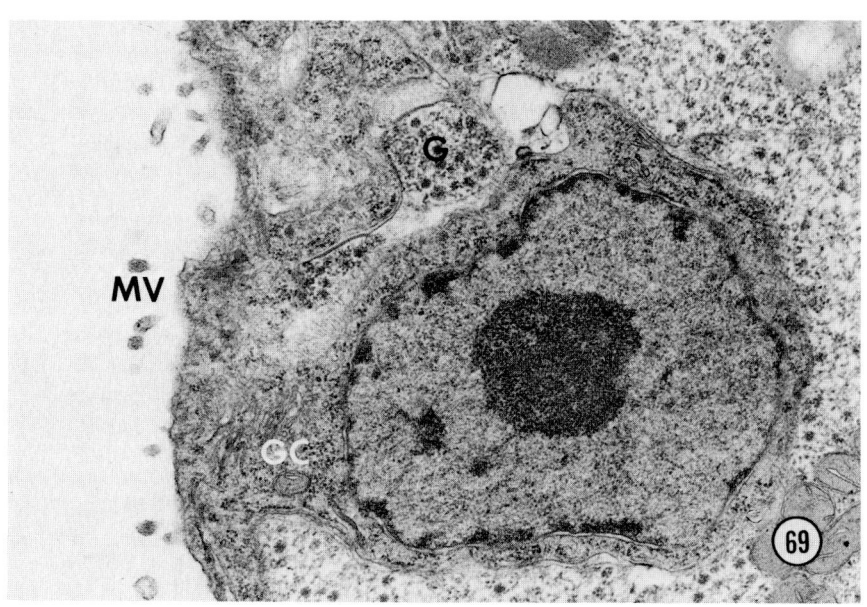

Fig. 69. *Frontal section through epithelial lining of oviduct. Thin surface cytoplasm is syncytial and extended as minute microvilli (MV). Nucleus is slightly withdrawn and surrounded by glycogen-rich (G) processes of medullary myocytons. Vesicles in surface layer appear adjacent to juxtanuclear Golgi complexes. X22,300.*

The ootype is a modified region of the oviduct into which the Mehlis glands ("shell glands") secrete. Loser (1965a, 1965b) identified two types of unicellular glands, mucous and serous, both of which consisted of club-shaped cells opening into the lumen of the ootype. The mucous secretory product was identified as a periodic acid-Schiff (PAS) positive - mucopolysaccharide in other cyclophyllidean cestodes (Johri 1957), whereas the product of the serous type gland has not been histochemically categorized. Ultrastructural studies reveal that both glandular types are unipolar cells with a single cytoplasmic process extending from the perinuclear region to the ootype.

Materials produced in the perinuclear region of the glands are transported down the cytoplasmic process to be released into the lumen of the ootype, presumably via a merocrine secretory mechanism.

The mucous glands possess a centrally placed nucleus and an abundance of juxtanuclear ribosomes and granular endoplasmic reticulum. Golgi complexes are infrequently observed. A semi-electron dense material appears to have accumulated within distended cisternae of granular endoplasmic reticulum, such that the limiting membrane is studded with ribosomes (Fig. 70).

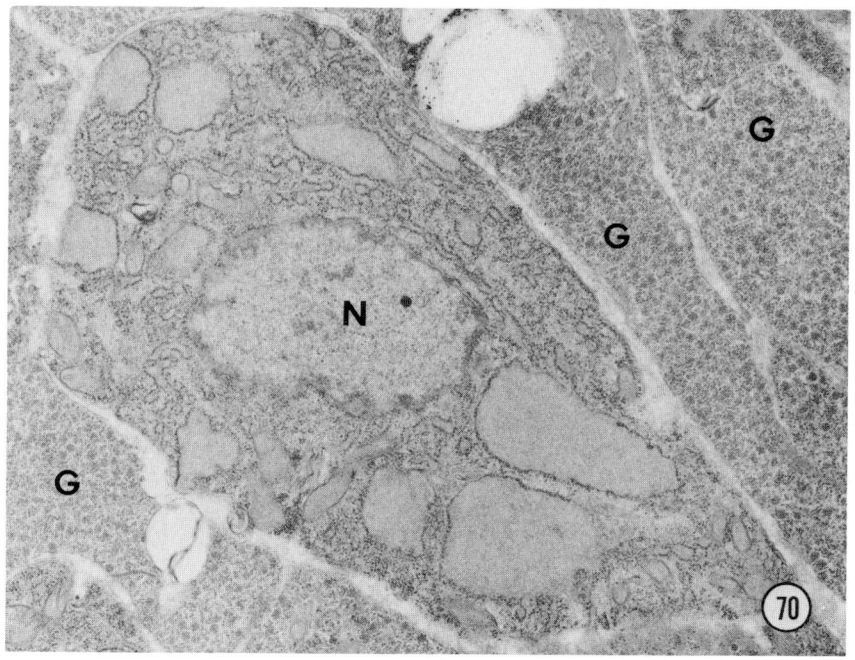

Fig. 70. Mucous type element of Mehlis gland. Pyriform cells have centrally located spherical nucleus (N). Semi-electron dense material is sequestered within distended cisternae of granular endoplasmic reticulum. Cytoplasm filled with numerous ribosomes but only infrequent Golgi complexes. Surrounding tissue composed of glycogen-rich (G) processes of medullary myocytons. X15,000.

The serous gland cells are characterized by a centrally placed nucleus and an abundance of juxtanuclear Golgi complexes. While free ribosomes are plentiful, granular endoplasmic reticulum is only rarely observed. Small (100-150 nm) membrane bound, electron dense granules are numerous adjacent to the Golgi complexes (presumably packaged there) and in the cytoplasmic extension leading to the ootype (Fig. 71).

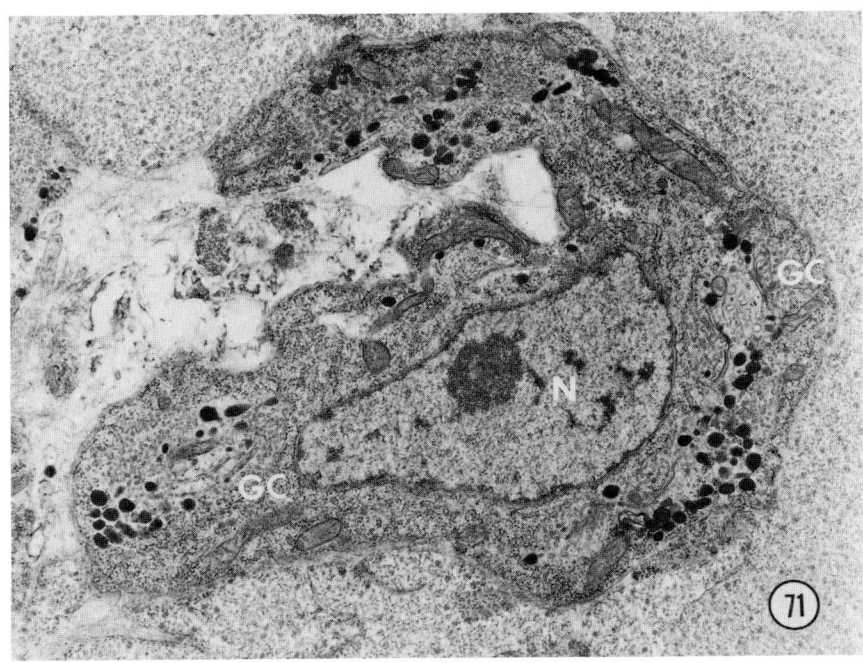

Fig. 71. Serous-type Mehlis gland. Elongate cells have centrally placed nucleus (N). Electron opaque granules appear in association with numerous Golgi complexes (GC). Dense staining cytoplasm filled with ribosomes and peripherally located mitochondria. X15,000.

The precise role of the Mehlis glands has long puzzled helminthologists. Loser (1965a, 1965b) suggested that the mucous material forms a ground lamella which surrounds the envelope produced by the

The Morphology, Histology, and Fine Structure of the Adult Stage

vitelline cell, while the serous material contributes to the formation of the outer coat. Pence (1970) reported heavy concentrations of PAS positive material in the outer coat of the egg of *H. diminuta*, lending credence to this supposition. A detailed discussion of egg formation and morphology is provided elsewhere in this volume (see Ubelaker).

Distal to the ootype the oviduct becomes the uterus. Until all other portions of the female reproductive tract have matured, the uterus consists of only a blind ending sac adjacent to the ootype. With the production of eggs however, the uterus extends rapidly to both lateral margins of the proglottid, ultimately occupying the entire posterior portion of the proglottid. The uterus then extends branches anteriorly, eventually filling the entire proglottid, occupying the space vacated by the disintegrating organs of the male and, finally, the female systems. When fully developed and ready to shed, a proglottid is packed fully with developed eggs which will be released upon the disintegration of the proglottid.

The microanatomy of the uterine wall is similar to that of the oviduct. A syncytial cytoplasm is supported by withdrawn infrequent nuclei. The luminal surface of the uterus however, possesses much larger and more frequent microvilli, many of which are flattened and formed around the eggs held within the lumen (Fig. 72).

X. SUMMARY AND CONCLUSIONS

From the foregoing account, it must be appreciated that adult tapeworms have developed a degree of anatomical specialization for enteric parasitism exceeded by no other group of metazoans. With the possible exception of the Acanthocephala, no other major group of animals is as dedicated, structurally and functionally, to life in the intestinal tract of another organism; indeed, the consequences of evolution have permitted tapeworms to live, as adults, in no other habitat *but* the vertebrate intestine or one of its major adjuncts. Nonetheless, tapeworms have been overwhelmingly successful in this regard, rivalled only by nematodes, perhaps, in the number and

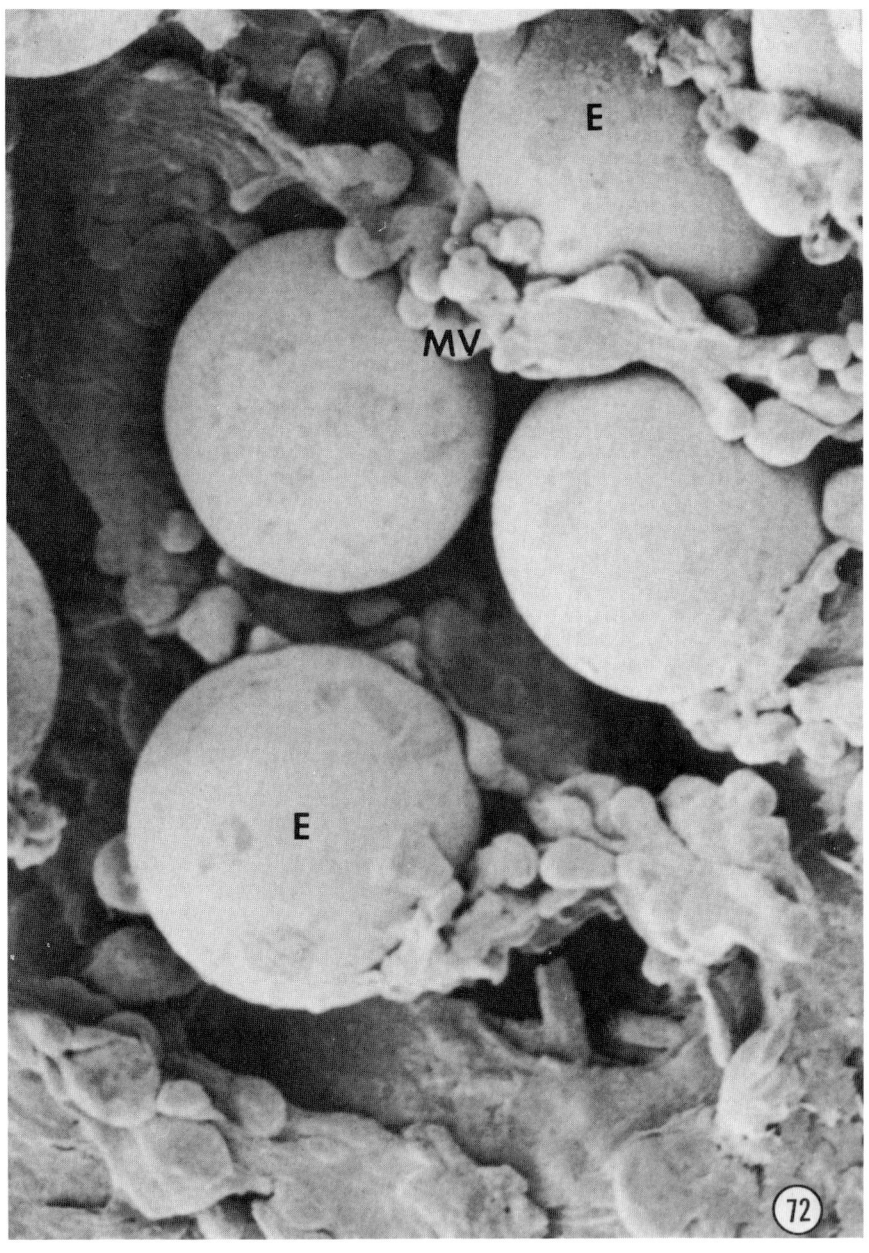

Fig. 72. Scanning electron micrograph of eggs (E) within gravid proglottid. Microvilli (MV) associated with uterine wall, flatten around each egg. X800.

diversity of vertebrate host species so parasitized.

In her design for tapeworms, Nature followed a blueprint like no other. Few other kinds of animals approach cestodes in the amount of their anatomy dedicated, in addition to sexual reproduction, to the functions of nutrient acquisition and accumulation. We would suggest that the morphological and physiological modifications of the tegument and muscle systems, for absorption and storage, respectively, constituted the major somatic contributions making possible the unique advent of proglottisation, given the magnitude of the metabolic requirements imposed by this type of growth and reproduction.

Proglottisation in most cestodes involves a high and sustained growth rate. Twenty-four hours after excystment in its definitive host, *H. diminuta* enters an exponential phase of growth with respect to increase in body length which may continue for as long as 14 days, at which time apolysis of gravid proglottids begins. The production of proglottids continues essentially unabated for the life of these and other apolytic cestodes.

Proglottisation is made possible not only by the tapeworm's capacity to acquire nutrients, but also by an abundance of syncytial structure and a limited number of somatic tissue and cell types. Surfaces, for example, are ubiquitously covered by a syncytium of common architecture - i.e., a surficial distal cytoplasm connected to underlying cell bodies - and within these syncytial epithelia (e.g., the tegument, excretory and reproductive ducts) there is very little regional specialization. Muscle fibers, irrespective of their location, are of a single type (smooth) and all have essentially the same substructure. Moreover, their myocytons serve a variety of functions which in higher organisms are delegated to discrete cell types - e.g., metabolite storage to hepatocytes or analogous cell types, connective tissue formation to fibroblasts, etc. In tapeworms, besides their primary role of supporting the contractile myofibrils, the myocytons serve as the animal's principal sites of carbohydrate metabolism and storage, and of fat deposition; also, the myocytons appear to be responsible for elaboration of connective tissue. On morphological grounds, there would appear to be a paucity of neural cell types (though it would not be surprising if future investigations revealed a greater number based on functional specializations). Only in the reproductive organs do we encounter a substantial departure from the plan of cytodifferentiative conservatism; it is here that the largest number of different cell types are found, consistent with the complexity of embryo formation.

Proglottisation is unique to the Cestoda, though certain other kinds of animals exhibit metameric repetition of somatic and reproductive organs. It is by this unorthodox route that tapeworms have achieved the reproductive potential necessary to ensure completion of their complex and statistically hazardous life histories. While faced with similarly complex and hazardous life histories, the other major group of endoparasitic platyhelminths, the Digenea, have augmented a comparatively modest reproductive potential in the adult stage by asexual propagation of larvae (polyembryony). Parasitic nematodes, equally successful at endoparasitism as tapeworms and trematodes, have, in contrast to these phylogentically lower helminths, remained rather conservative with respect to anatomical differences between them and their free living relatives. Collectively, nematode life cycles tend to be less complex that often involve a "free-living" larval stage, and, where an obligate intermediate host is involved, this is frequently an active vector (e.g., as for the mosquito-borne filarids). At the same time, the sexual reproductive capacity of parasitic nematodes compares favorably in terms of daily egg/larva output with trematodes and many cestodes.

In our estimation, no single worker in the twentieth century has surpassed the eminent Professor Horace W. Stunkard in his contributions to and perspective of tapeworm biology and morphology. Accordingly, it seems to us highly appropriate to conclude this chapter with the following quotes, from a seminar Dr. Stunkard presented at Tulane in 1962 (see also Stunkard 1962):

".... As archaic as the Palaeozoic, they (tapeworms) are as modern as tomorrow. They have attained the ideal welfare state with all its beneficience;

absolute security with an abundance of predigested food, and with a minimum of effort or exertion. .... digestive, respiratory, and circulatory organs have been discarded as superflous, (since) every essential is provided in abundance with no concern for cost or other responsibility. With no need to expend energy for food or shelter, the cestode can get down seriously to the business of reproduction ...."

".... Regarded by some as slimy, loathsome, abhorrent denizens in the bowels of other animals, they are really very intriguing and fascinating organisms".

XI. ACKNOWLEDGMENTS

We first of all dedicate this paper to our wives, Patricia and Ginger, respectively, not only for the usual reasons, but because each has also materially assisted us in its preparation. Secondly, our own research on tapeworms has been financially supported in no mean way by grants from the NIH (AI 08673, AI 23449, GM 13330) and the NSF (GB 7276, GB 17992), and by the Graduate School of Tulane University. To the latter source, we specifically acknowledge funds provided via NIH Biomedical Research Support Grant 5 SO7RR07040-11. We also thank the editors of the *Journal of Parasitology* and *Zeitschrift fur Parasitenkunde* for permission to reproduce in this chapter previously published micrographs.

Most sincerely, we acknowledge the numerous scientists whose contributions to the anatomy and fine structure of *Hymenolepis diminuta* and other tapeworms are responsible not only for the existence of this chapter, but also for its inordinate length. We hope the great majority of these men and women are appropriately cited in the references, but in a review of this scope, there inevitably will be some whose contributions appear only by inference. The knowledgable reader will readily identify these as well. Nonetheless, and with the fear of further unintentional omissions, we would list at least the following as having contributed personally to the authors' appreciation of tapeworm anatomy and fine structure:

Frank M. Fisher, Jr.; Justus F. Mueller; John A. Oaks; Charles William (Bill) Philpott; Keith R. Porter; Clark P. Read; Magdalena Reissig; Larry S. Roberts; Alvin Rothman; Krystina Rybicka; Everett Schiller; Franklin Sogandares-Bernal; Horace B. Stunkard; Lawrence Threadgold; John E. Ubelaker; Marietta Voge.

REFERENCES

1. Afzelius, B. A., Cilia and flagella that do not conform to the 9 + 2 pattern. I. Aberrant members within normal populations. *J. Ultrastructure Res.* *9*, 381-392 (1963).
2. Allee, W. C., Emerson, A. E., Park, O., Park, T. and Schmidt, K. P., "Principles of Animal Ecology." W. B. Saunders Co., Philadelphia. (1949).
3. Andry, N., "De la Generation des vers dans le Corps de l'homme." Paris (1700).
4. Angevine, J. B., The nervous system. *In:* "A Textbook of Histology" (W. Bloom and D. Fawcett, eds.), pp. 333-385. W. B. Saunders Co., Philadelphia. (1975).
5. Beguin, F., Étude au microscope électronique de la cuticle et de ses structures associées chez quelques cestodes. Essai d'histologie comparée. *Zeits. Zellforsch. Mikros. Anat.* *72*, 30-46 (1966a).
6. Beguin, F., Un intestin externe: la cuticle des cestodes et les structures qui lui sont associées. *Rev. Suisse Zool.* *73*, 521-526 (1966b).
7. Belton, C. M., Freeze-fracture study of the tegument of larval *Taenia crassiceps*. *J. Parasitol.* *63*, 306-313 (1977).
8. Bentley, A., "Studies in the Development and Regenerative Capabilities of the Tegument of Parasitic Platyhelminthes." Ph.D. Dissertation, Tulane University (1973).
9. Berger, J. and Mettrick, D., Microtrichial polymorphism among hymenolepid tapeworms as seen by scanning electron microscopy. *Trans. Am. Micros. Soc.* *90*, 393-403 (1971).
10. Blanchard, R., "Histoire Zoologique et Medicale des Teniades du genre *Hymenolepis* Weinland." Paris. (1891).

11. Blochmann, F., "Die Epithelfrage bei Cestoden und Trematoden". Hamburg. (1896).
12. Bloom, W. and Fawcett, D. W., "A Textbook of Histology." W. B. Saunders Co., Philadelphia (1975).
13. Bolla, R. I. and Roberts, L. S., Developmental physiology of cestodes. IX. Cytological characteristics of the germinative region of *Hymenolepis diminuta*. *J. Parasitol. 57*, 267-277 (1971).
14. Brand, T. von, "Chemical Physiology of Endoparasitic Animals." Academic Press, New York, (1952).
15. Bullock, T. H. and Horridge, G. A. "Structure and Function in the Nervous System of Invertebrates." Freeman and Co., San Francisco, (1965).
16. Burnstock, G. and Iwayama, T., Fine-structural identification of autonomic nerves and their relationship to smooth muscle. *Prog. Brain Res. 34*, 389-404 (1971).
17. Cain, G., Collagen from the giant acanthocephalan *Macracanthorhynchus hiradinaceus*. *Arch. Biochem. Biophys. 141*, 264-270 (1970).
18. Cameron, M. L. and Steele, J. E., Simplified aldehyde-fuchsin staining of neurosecretory cells. *Stain Tech. 34*, 265-266 (1959).
19. Carmichael, G. and Fullmer, H., The fine structure of the oxytalan fiber. *J. Cell Biol. 28*, 33-36 (1966).
20. Chandler, A., Read, C. P. and Nicholas, H. O., Observations on certain phases of nutrition and host-parasite relations of *Hymenolepis diminuta* in white rats. *J. Parasitol. 36*, 523-535 (1950).
21. Chou, T. T., Bennett, J. and Bueding, E., Occurrence and concentrations of biogenic amines in trematodes. *J. Parasitol. 51*, 1098-1102 (1972).
22. Collin, W., Electron microscopy of the postembryonic stages of the tapeworm, *Hymenolepis citelli*. *J. Parasitol. 56*, 1159-1170 (1970).
23. Colucci, A. V., Orrell, S. A., Saz, H. J. and Bueding, E., Differential glucose incorporation into glycogen by *Hymenolepis diminuta*. *J. Bio. Chem. 241*, 464-468 (1966).
24. Cooper, N. B., Allison, V. F. and Ubelaker, J. E., The fine structure of the cysticercoid of *Hymenolepis diminuta*. III. The scolex. *Zeits. Parasitenk. 46*, 229-239 (1975).

25. Cotta-Pereira, G., Rodrigo, F. and Bittencourt-Sampaio, S., Oxytalan, elaunin and elastic fibers in the human skin. *J. Investigative Dermatol.* 66, 143-148 (1976).
26. Davey, K. G. and Breckenridge, W. R., Neurosecretory cells in a cestode, *Hymenolepis diminuta*. *Science* 158. 931-932 (1967).
27. Dixon, K. E. and Mercer, E. H., The fine structure of the nervous system of the cercaria of the liver fluke, *Fasciola hepatica* L. *J. Parasitol.* 51, 967-976 (1965).
28. Douglas, L. T., The development of organ systems in nematotaeniid cestodes. I. Early histogenesis and formation of reproductive structures in *Baerietta diana* (Holfer, 1948). *J. Parasitol.* 47, 669-680 (1961).
29. Douglas, L. T., The development of organ systems in nematotaeniid cestodes. III. Gametogenesis and embryonic development in *Baerietta diana* and *Distoichometra kosloffi*. *J. Parasitol.* 49, 530-588 (1963).
30. Featherston, D. W., *Taenia hydatigena*. III. Light and electron microscope study of spermatogenesis. *Z. Parasitenk.* 37, 148-168 (1971).
31. Foster, A. O., Parasitological speculations and patterns. *J. Parasitol.* 46, 1-9 (1960).
32. Fujimoto, D., Isolations of collagens of high hydroxyproline, hydroxylysine and carbohydrate content from muscle layer of *Ascaris lumbricoides* and pig kidney. *Bioch. Biophys. Acta* 168, 537-543 (1968).
33. Fullmer, H. M., Differential staining of connective tissue fibres in areas of stress. *Science* 127, 1240 (1958).
34. Fullmer, H. M. and Lillie, R. D., The oxytalan fiber: A previously undescribed connective tissue fibre. *J. Histochem. Cytochem.* 6, 425-430 (1958).
35. Fullmer, H. M., Sheetz, J. and Warkates, A., Oxytalan connective fibres. A review. *J. Oral Pathol.* 3, 291-316 (1974).
36. Ginger, C. D. and Fairbairn, D., Lipid metabolism in helminth parasites. I. The lipids of *Hymenolepis diminuta* (Cestoda). *J. Parasitol.* 52, 1086-1096 (1966a).
37. Ginger, C. D. and Fairbairn, D., Lipid metabolism in helminth parasites. II. The major origins of lipids in *Hymenolepis diminuta* (Cestoda). *J. Parasitol.* 52, 1097-1107 (1966b).

38. Goldberg, B. and Green, H., An analysis of collagen secretion by established mouse fibroblast lines. *J. Cell Biol.* 22, 227-258 (1964).
39. Goodchild, C. G., Transfaunation and repair of damage in the rat tapeworm, *Hymenolepis diminuta*. *J. Parasitol.* 44, 345-351 (1958).
40. Gough, L. H., A monograph of the tapeworms of the subfamily Avitellinae, being a review of the genus *Stilesia* and an account of the histology of *Avitellina centripunctata* (Riv.). *Quart. J. Micros. Sci.* 56, 317-383 (1911).
41. Grassi, G. B., *Taenia flavopunctata* Weinl., *Taenia leptocephala* Creplin, *Taenia diminuta* Rud. *Atti della reale Accademia delle Scienze di Torino.* 23, 492-501 (1888).
42. Greenlee, T., Jr., Ross, R. and Hartman, J., The fine structure of elastic fibers. *J. Cell Biol.* 30, 59-71 (1966).
43. Gross, J., Comparative biochemistry of collagen. In: "Comparative Biochemistry." (Florkin, M. and Mason, H., eds.). Vol. V. pp. 307-345. Academic Press, New York. (1963).
44. Gustafsson, M. K. S., Observations on the histogensis of nervous tissue in *Diphyllobothrium dendriticum* Nitzsch, 1824 (Cestoda, Pseudophyllidea). *Z. Parasitenk.* 50, 313-321 (1976).
45. Halmi, N. S., Two types of basophils in the anterior pituitary of the rat and their cytophysiological significance. *Endocrinology* 47, 289-299 (1950).
46. Highnam, K. C. and Hill, L., "The Comparative Endocrinology of the Invertebrates." Edward Arnold Ltd., London, (1977).
47. Hyman, L. H., "The Invertebrates." Vol. II. McGraw-Hill Book Co., Inc., New York, (1951).
48. Ishikawa, H., Bischoff, R. and Holtzer, H., Formation of arrowhead complexes with heavy meromyosin in a variety of cell types. *J. Cell Biol.* 43, 312-328 (1969).
49. Johri, L. N., A morphological and histochemical study of egg formation in a cyclophyllidean cestode. *Parasitology* 47, 107-116 (1957).
50. Josse, J. and Harrington, W., Role of pyrrolidine residues in the structure and stabilization of collagen. *J. Mol. Biol.* 9, 269-287 (1964).
51. Kazocos, K. and Mackiewicz, J. S., Spermatogenesis in *Hunterella nodulosa* Mackiewicz and McCray, 1962 (Cestoidea: Caryophyllidea). *Z. Parasitenk.* 38, 21-31 (1972).

52. Kelsoe, G. H., Ubelaker, J. E. and Allison, V. F., The fine structure of spermatogenesis in *Hymenolepis diminuta* (Cestoda) with a description of the mature spermatozoon. *Zeits. Parasitenk.* 54, 175-187 (1977).
53. King, J. W. and Lumsden, R. D., Cytological aspects of lipid assimilation by cestodes. Incorporation of linoleic acid into the parenchyma and eggs of *Hymenolepis diminuta*. *J. Parasitol.* 55, 250-260 (1969).
54. Knowles, F., Neuroendocrine correlations at the level of ultrastructure. *Arch. d'Anat. Micros. Morphol. Exp.* 54, 343-357 (1965).
55. Kohn, A., Cotta-Pereira, G., Lopez-Alvarez, M. and Kattenbach, W., Oxytalan fibers in the *Schistosoma mansoni* tegument. *J. Parasitol.* IN PRESS (1979).
56. Kummel, G., Die Feinstruktur der Terminalzellen (Cyrtocyten) un den protonephridien der Priapuliden. *Zeits. Zellforsch. Mikros. Anat.* 62, 468-464 (1964).
57. Lee, M. B., Bueding, E. and Schiller, E. L., The occurrence and distribution of 5-hydroxytryptamine in *Hymenolepis diminuta* and *H. nana*. *J. Parasitol.* 64, 254-257 (1978).
58. Lentz, T. L., "Cell Fine Structure." W. B. Saunders Co., Philadelphia (1971).
59. Loser, E., Der Feinbau des Oogenotop bei Cesdoden. *Zeits. Parasitenk.* 25, 413-458 (1965a).
60. Loser, E., Die eibildung bei cestoden. *Zeits. Parasitenk.* 25, 556-580 (1965b).
61. Lumsden, R. D., Macromolecular structure of glycogen in some cyclophyllidean and trypanorhynch cestodes. *J. Parasitol.* 51, 501-515 (1965a).
62. Lumsden, R. D., "Cytological Studies on the Absorptive Surfaces of Cestodes." Ph.D. Dissertation, Rice University (1965b).
63. Lumsden, R. D., Microtubules in the peripheral cytoplasm of cestode spermatozoa. *J. Parasitol.* 51, 929-931 (1965c).
64. Lumsden, R. D., Fine structure of the medullary parenchymal cells of a trypanorhynch cestode, *Lacistorhynchus tenuis* (v. Beneden, 1858), with emphasis on specializations for glycogen metabolism. *J. Parasitol.* 52, 417-427 (1966a).
65. Lumsden, R. D., Cytological studies on the absorptive surfaces of cestodes. I. The fine

structure of the strobilar tegument. *Zeits. Parasitenk. 27*, 355-382 (1966b).
66. Lumsden, R. D., Cytological studies on the absorptive surfaces of cestodes. II. The synthesis and intracellular transport of protein in the strobilar integument of *Hymenolepis diminuta*. *Zeits. Parasitenk. 28*, 1-13 (1966c).
67. Lumsden, R. D., Surface ultrastructure and cytochemistry of parasitic helminths. *Exp. Parasitol. 37*, 267-339 (1975a).
68. Lumsden, R. D., The tapeworm tegument: A model system for studies on membrane structure and function in host-parasite relationships. *Trans. Am. Micros. Soc. 94*, 501-507 (1975b).
69. Lumsden, R. D., Acceptance of The Henry Baldwin Ward medal. *J. Parasitol. 62*, 818-820 (1976).
70. Lumsden, R. D. and Byram, J., The ultrastructure of cestode muscle. *J. Parasitol. 53*, 326-342 (1967).
71. Lumsden, R. D. and Harrington, G. W., Incorporation of linoleic acid by the cestode *Hymenolepis diminuta* (Rudolphi, 1819). *J. Parasitol. 52*, 695-700 (1966).
72. Lumsden, R. D., Oaks, J. A. and Alworth, W. L., Cytological studies on the absorptive surfaces of cestodes. IV. Localization and cytochemical properties of membrane-fixed cation binding sites. *J. Parasitol. 56*, 736-747 (1970).
73. Maamouri, F. M. and Swiderski, Z., Etude en microscopie electronique de la spermatogenese de deux cestodes *Acanthobothrium filicolle benedenii* Loennbert, 1889 et *Onchobothrium ancinatum* (Rud., 1819) Tetraphyllidea, Onchobothriidae. *Zeits. Parasitenk. 47*, 269-281 (1975).
74. Mansour, T. E., Biogenic amines as metabolic regulators in invertebrates. *In:* "Biogenic Amines as Physiological Regulators" (J. J. Blum, ed.) pp. 119-138. Prentice-Hall, Inc. New Jersey (1969).
75. McKanna, J. A., Fine structure of the protonephridial system in planaria. II. Ductules, collecting ducts and osmoregulatory cells. *Zeits. Zellforsch. Mikros. Anat. 92*, 524-535 (1968).
76. Moniez, R., Essai monographique sur les cysticerques. *Trav. l'Institut Zool.* Lillie et

Wimereux. *3*, 1-183 (1880).
77. Morseth, D. J., Observations on the fine structure of the nervous system of *Echinococcus granulosus*. *J. Parasitol.* 53, 492-500 (1967).
78. Nicoll, R. A. and Barker, J. L., The pharmacology of recurrent inhibition in the supraoptic neurosecretory system. *Brain Res.* 35, 501-511 (1971).
79. Noble, E. R. and Noble, G. A., "Parasitology: The Biology of Animal Parasites." Lea and Febiger, Philadelphia (1971).
80. Nollen, P. M., Studies on the reproductive system of *Hymenolepis diminuta* using autoradiography and transplantation. *J. Parasitol.* 61, 100-104 (1975).
81. Nordwig, A. and Hayduk, U., Invertebrate collagens: isolation, characterization and phylogenic aspects. *J. Mol. Biol.* 44, 161-172 (1969).
82. Normann, T. D., Neurosecretion by exocytosis. *Intern. Rev. Cytol.* 46, 2-77 (1976).
83. Oaks, J. A. and Lumsden, R. D., Cytological studies on the absorptive surfaces of cestodes. V. Incorporation of carbohydrate-containing macromolecules into tegument membranes. *J. Parasitol.* 57, 1256-1268 (1971).
84. Ogren, R. E., Development and morphology of the oncosphere of *Mesocestoides corti*, a tapeworm of mammals. *J. Parasitol.* 42, 414-428 (1956).
85. Pappas, P. W. and Read, C. P., Membrane transport in helminth parasites: A review. *Exp. Parasitol.* 37, 469-530 (1975).
86. Parshad, V. R. and Guraya, S. S., Comparative histochemical observations on the excretory system of helminth parasites. *Zeits. Parasitenk.* 52, 81-89 (1977).
87. Pashchenko, L. F., [Early stages of spermatogenesis in *Taenirhynchus saginata* Goeze, 1782] In Russian. *Problemy Parazitol.* 1, 112-122 (1961).
88. Pedersen, K. J., Some observations on the fine structure of planarian protonephridia and gastrodermal phagocytes. *Zeits. Zellforsch. Mikros. Anat.* 53, 609-628 (1961).
89. Pence, D. P., Electron microscope and histochemical studies on the eggs of *Hymenolepis diminuta*. *J. Parasitol.* 56, 48-97 (1970).
90. Pinter, T., Ueber entwicklungsvorgunge in der Cestodenkette. *Anz. Akad. Wissens. Wein.* 71,

256-258 (1934).
91. Porter, K. R., Cell fine structure and biosynthesis of intercellular macromolecules. *Biophys. J.* 4, 167-196 (1964).
92. Pratt, H. S., The cuticula and subcuticula of trematodes and cestodes. *Am. Nat.* 43, 705-720 (1909).
93. Prenant, M., Recherches sur le parenchyme de platyhelminthes. *Arch. Morphol. Gen. Exp.* 5, (1922).
94. Read, C. P., Intestinal physiology of the host-parasite relationship. *In:* "Some Physiological Aspects and Consequences of Parasitism. (W. Cole, ed.) pp. 27-43. Rutgers University Press, New Brunswick. (1955).
95. Read, C. P., Longevity of the tapeworm, *Hymenolepis diminuta*. *J. Parasitol.* 53, 1055-1056 (1967).
96. Read, C. P. and Kilejian, A. Z., Circadian migratory behavior of a cestode symbiote in the rat host. *J. Parasitol.* 55, 574-578 (1969).
97. Rees, G., Nerve cells in *Acanthobothrium coronatum* (Rud.) (Cestoda: Tetraphyllidea). *Parasitol.* 56, 45-54 (1966).
98. Reissig, M. and Colucci, A. V., Localization of glycogen in the cestode, *Hymenolepis diminuta*. *J. Cell Biol.* 39, 754-763 (1968).
99. Rietschel, P. E., Zur Bewegungsphysiologie der Cestoden. *Zool. Anz.* 111, 109-111 (1935).
100. Roberts, L. S., The influence of population density on patterns and physiology of growth in *Hymenolepis diminuta* (Cestoda: Cyclophyllidea) in the definitive host. *Exp. Parasitol.* 11, 332-371 (1961).
101. Robertson, J. D., The ultrastructure of cell membranes and their derivatives. *Biochem. Soc. Symposia* 16, 3-43 (1959).
102. Rosario, B., An electron microscope study of spermatogenesis in cestodes. *J. Ultrastructure Res.* 11, 412-427 (1964).
103. Rosenbluth, J., Subsurface cisternae and their relationship to the neuronal plasma membrane. *J. Cell Biol.* 13, 405-421 (1962)
104. Ross, R., The smooth muscle cell in connective tissue metabolism and atherosclerosis. *In:* "Biology of Fibroblast." (Kulonen, E. and Pikkarainen, J., eds.). pp. 627-636. Academic Press, New York. (1973).

105. Ross, R. and Klebakoff, S. J., The smooth muscle cell. I. *In vivo* synthesis of connective tissue proteins. *J. Cell Biol.* *50*, 159-171 (1971).
106. Rothman, A., The physiology of tapeworms, correlated to structures seen with the electron microscope. *J. Parasitol.* *45*, (suppl), 28 (1959).
107. Rothman, A., Electron microscopy studies of tapeworms: The surface structures of *Hymenolepis diminuta* (Rudolphi, 1819) Blanchard, 1891. *Trans. Am. Micros. Soc.* *82*, 22-30 (1963).
108. Rudolphi, C. A., "Entozoorum Synopsis cui Accedant Mantissa Duplex et Indices Locupletissimi." Berolini (1819).
109. Rybicka, K., Observations sur la spermatogenese d'un Cestode pseudophyllidean *Triaenophorus lucii* (Mull., 1776). *Bull. Soc. Neuchateloise Sci. Nat.* *85*, 177-181 (1962a).
110. Rybicka, K., La spermatogenese du Cestode *Dipylidium caninum* (L.). *Bull. Soc. Zool. France* *87*, 225-228 (1962b).
111. Rybicka, K., Ultrastructure of embryonic envelopes and their differentiation in *Hymenolepis diminuta* (Cestoda). *J. Parasitol.* *58*, 849-863 (1972).
112. Rybicka, K., Ultrastructure of macromeres in the cleavage of *Hymenolepis diminuta* (Cestoda). *Trans. Am. Micros. Soc.* *92*, 241-255 (1973).
113. Silk, M. H. and Spence, I. M., Ultrastructural studies of the blood fluke *Schistosoma mansoni* III. The nervous tissue and sensory structures. *South African J. Med. Sci.* *34*, 93-104 (1969).
114. Silveira, M., The fine structure of 9 + 1 flagella in turbellarian flatworms. *In:* "The Functional Anatomy of the Spermatozoon." (Atzelius, B., ed.), pp. 289-298. Pergamon Press, Oxford and New York (1974).
115. Singer, S. J. and Nicholson, G., The fluid mosaic model of the structure of cell membranes. *Science* *175*, 720-731 (1972).
116. Specian, R. D. and Lumsden, R. D., The microanatomy and fine structure of the rostellum of *Hymenolepis diminuta*. *Zeits. Parasitenk.* IN PRESS (1980).
117. Specian, R. D., Lumsden, R. D., Ubelaker, J. E. and Allison, V. F., A unicellular endo-

crine gland in cestodes. *J. Parasitol. 65*, 569-578 (1979).

118. Stewart, G. L., Lumsden, R. D., and Fisher, F. M., Jr., The contributions of Clark P. Read on the ecology of the vertebrate gut and its parasite. *In:* "Rice University Studies" (Byram, J. E. and Stewart, G. L., eds.), pp. 1-20 Rice University Press, Houston. (1976).

119. Stunkard, H. W., The morphology and life history of the cestode, *Bertiella studeri*. *Am. J. Trop. Med. 20*, 305-333 (1940).

120. Stunkard, H. W., Studies on the life history of the anoplocephaline cestodes of hares and rabbits. *J. Parasitol. 27*, 299-325 (1941).

121. Stunkard, H. W., The organization, ontogeny and orientation of the Cestoda. *Quart. Rev. Biol. 37*, 23-34 (1964).

122. Sulgostowska, T., The development of organ systems in cestodes. I. A study of histology of *Hymenolepis diminuta* (Rudolphi, 1819) (Hymenolepididae). *Acta Parasitol. Polon. 20*, 449-462 (1972).

123. Sulgostowska, T., The development of organ systems in cestodes. II. Histogenesis of the reproductive system in *Hymenolepis diminuta* (Rudolphi, 1819)(Hymenolepididae). *Acta Parasitol. Polon. 22*, 179-190 (1974).

124. Swiderski, Z., Huggel, H. and Schonenberger, N., Comparative fine structure of vitelline cells in cyclophyllidean cestodes. *Septieme Congres International de Microscopie Electronique*, Grenoble, pp. 825-826 (1970a).

125. Swiderski, Z., Huggel, H. and Schonenberger, N., The role of the vitelline cell in the capsule formation during embryogenesis in *Hymenolepis diminuta* (Cestoda). *Septieme Congres International de Microscopie Electronique*, Grenoble, pp. 669-679 (1970b).

126. Threadgold, L., An electron microscope study of the tegument and associated structures of *Dipylidium caninum*. *Quart. J. Micros. Sci. 103*, 135-140 (1962)

127. Threadgold, L. T. and Read, C. P., *Hymenolepis diminuta:* Ultrastructure of a unique membrane specialization in tegument. *Exp. Parasitol. 28*, 246-252 (1970a).

128. Threadgold, L. T. and Read, C. P., Cell relationships in *Hymenolepis diminuta*. *Parasitol.*

60, 181-184 (1970b).
129. Tofts, J. and Meerovitch, E., The effect of farnesyl methyl ether, a mimic of insect juvenile hormone, on *Hymenolepis diminuta in vitro*. *International J. Parasitol.* *4*, 211-218 (1974).
130. Tomosky-Sykes, T. K., Mueller, J. F. and Bueding, E., Effects of putative neurotransmitters on the motor activity of *Spirometra mansonoides*. *J. Parasitol.* *63*, 492-494 (1977).
131. Tyson, E., *Lumbricus hydrotropicus* or . . . the joynted worm . . . *Philosoph. Trans. Roy. Soc. London* *13*, 113-144 (1683).
132. Ubelaker, J. E., Allison, V. F. and Specian, R. D., Surface topography of *Hymenolepis diminuta*. *J. Parasitol.* *59*, 667-671 (1973).
133. Voge, M. and Heyneman, D., Development of *Hymenolepis nana* and *H. diminuta* (Cestoda: Hymenolepididae) in the intermediate host *Tribolium confusum*. *Univ. Calif. Publ. Zool.* *59*, 549-580 (1957).
134. Wardle, R. A. and McLeod, J. A., "The Zoology of Tapeworms." University of Minnesota Press, Minneapolis (1952).
135. Webb, R. A., Ultrastructure of the synapses of the metacestode of *Hymenolepis microstoma*. *Experientia (Basel)* *32*, 99-101 (1976a).
136. Webb, R. A., Putative neurosecretory cells of the cestode *Hymenolepis microstoma*. *J. Parasitol.* *62*, 756-760 (1976b).
137. Webb, R. A., Evidence for neurosecretory cells in the cestode *Hymenolepis microstoma*. *Can. J. Zool.* *55*, 1726-1733 (1977).
138. Webb, R. A. and Davey, K. G., Ciliated sensory receptors of the unactivated metacestode of *Hymenolepis microstoma*. *Tissue and Cell* *6*, 587-598 (1974).
139. Webb, R. A. and Davey, K. G., The gross anatomy and histology of the nervous system of the metacestode of *Hymenolepis microstoma*. *Can. J. Zool.* *53*, 661-667 (1975a).
140. Webb, R. A. and Davey, K. G., Ultrastructural changes in an uniciliated sensory receptor during activation of the metacestode of *Hymenolepis microstoma*. *Tissue and Cell* *7*, 519-524 (1975b).

141. Webb, R. A. and Davey, K. G., The fine structure of the nervous tissue of the metacestode of *Hymenolepis microstoma*. *Can. J. Zool.* 54, 1206-1222 (1976).
142. Webster, L. A., The osmotic and ionic effects of different saline conditions on *Hymenolepis diminuta*. *Comp. Biochem. Physiol.* 37, 271-275 (1970).
143. Webster, L. A., The flow of fluids in the protonephridial canals of *Hymenolepis diminuta*. *Comp. Biochem. Physiol.* 39A, 785-793 (1971).
144. Webster, L. A., Absorption of glucose, lactate and urea from the protonephridial canals of *Hymenolepis diminuta*. *Comp. Biochem. Physiol.* 41A, 861-868 (1972a).
145. Webster, L. A., Further osmotic and ionic effects of different saline conditions on *Hymenolepis diminuta*. *Comp. Biochem. Physiol.* 42A, 409-413 (1972b).
146. Webster, L. A., Succinic and lactic acids present in the protonephridial canal fluid of *Hymenolepis diminuta*. *J. Parasitol.* 58, 410-411 (1972c).
147. Webster, L. A. and Wilson, R. A., The chemical composition of protonephridial canal fluid from the cestode *Hymenolepis diminuta*. *Comp. Biochem. Physiol.* 35, 201-209 (1970).
148. Weinland, D. F., "An Essay on the Tapeworms of Man." Cambridge, Mass. (1858).
149. Westblad, E., Studien uber skandinavische Turbellaria Acoela. I. *Arkiv for Zoologi.* 3A, 1028 (1940).
150. Wetzel, B. K., Contributions to the cytology of *Dugesia tigrina* (Turbellaria) protonephridia. *Proc. Fifth Intern. Congr. Elect. Micros.* 2, Q-10 (1962).
151. Wikgren, B. J. and Knuts, G., Growth of subtegumental tissue in cestodes by cell migration. *Acta Acad. Aboenis. Series B.* 30, 1-6 (1970).
152. Wilson, R. A., Fine structure of the nervous system and specialized nerve endings in the miracidium of *Fasciola hepatica*. *Parasitology.* 60, 399-410 (1970).
153. Wilson, R. A. and Webster, L. A., Protonephridia. *Biol. Rev.* 49, 127-160 (1974).
154. Wilson, V. C. L. C. and Schiller, E. L., The neuroanatomy of *Hymenolepis diminuta* and *H.*

nana. *J. Parasitol.* *55*, 261-270 (1969).
155. Young, R. T., The histogenesis of *Cysticercus pisiformis*. *Zool. Jahrb. Abteil. Anat. Ontogen. Tiere.* *26*, 183-254 (1908).
156. Young, R. T., Some unsolved problems of cestode structure and development. *Trans. Am. Micros. Soc.* *54*, 229-239 (1935).

THE INTESTINE AS AN ENVIRONMENT FOR *HYMENOLEPIS DIMINUTA*

D. F. Mettrick

Department of Zoology
University of Toronto
Toronto, Ontario

I. INTRODUCTION

The gastrointestinal tract in general, and the small intestine in particular, is the most favoured niche for adult metazoan parasites. *Hymenolepis diminuta* is no exception and the normal site for the adult worm is the small intestine of the rat, although it can also be established in the small intestine of a few other animals such as the guinea pig, hamster and mouse. Hence an accurate description of the structure of the intestinal wall and of the physiology of the intestinal lumen is of general importance because of their influence on our current concepts of the host-parasite relationship and is of particular importance in understanding the relationship between *H. diminuta* and its host.

T. von Brand and T. L. Jahn (1941) were the first to draw attention to the importance of considering both the parasite itself and its intestinal environment. This concept was taken up by C. P. Read (1950), whose classic pamphlet is still quoted, although a number of more recent detailed descriptions of the gastrointestinal tract and the intestinal luminal environment have considerably updated our information (Rubin 1971; Allen and Snary 1972; Crompton 1973; Mettrick and Podesta 1974;

Isselbacher 1974; Argenzio and Stevens 1975; Waldram 1975; Befus and Podesta 1976). As far as space limitations will allow, the present review will deal specifically with *H. diminuta* and its environment, although the discussion will, in fact, be pertinent to a wide range of other parasites occupying the same habitat. In an earlier review (Mettrick and Podesta 1974), it was pointed out that studies dealing with the physiology of intestinal parasites had lagged behind those on intestinal physiology in both the development of theoretical concepts of helminth-host models and the practical application to helminth physiology of the advanced techniques developed in other fields. As this and other contributions to this volume will indicate, this gap is closing and we are now beginning to know and understand something of what we are talking about when discussing intestinal helminth infections.

II. INTESTINAL MUCOSA

The mammalian small intestine consists of the duodenum, jejunum and ileum. These three regions tend to merge into one another although the differences are clearly shown by histological examination. In the young adult rat ($\sim$ 150 g body weight) the small intestine averages 100 cm length, but varies between 85 and 125 cm (Mettrick and Dunkley 1969). The mucosa of the small intestine consists of three distinct regions; an inner muscularis mucosae, the lamina propria containing blood and lymph vessels and various connective tissue cellular elements, and thirdly, a single monolayer of epithelial cells lining the intestinal lumen (Trier 1971; Rubin 1971). The last monolayer of epithelia constitutes the major barrier between the body proper and the external environment as represented by the intestinal lumen. The surface area of the intestinal mucosa is increased, particularly in the proximal small intestine, by three morphological phenomena (Rubin 1971). Firstly, the intestinal mucosa and submucosa form prominent circular folds, which disappear in the mid to distal ileum. Secondly, the lamina propria and surface epithelium form numerous projections into the lumen called villi associated with many intestinal crypts formed by the surface epithelia pushing into the lamina propria as far as the muscularis mucosae. The third morphological feature increasing surface area is the microvilli on the apical surface of the epithelial surface; the microvilli are most prominent on the cells of the villi.

The epithelium of the crypts contains a number of different types of cells, but most are undifferentiated. These cells have the capacity to develop into and replace either the differentiated villous epithelial cells (Lipkin *et al*. 1963; MacDonald *et al*. 1964), the goblet cells (Troughton and Trier 1969) or the Paneth cells (Merzel and Leblond 1968; Cheng 1969). The latter are predominantly situated at the base of the crypts, whereas both the goblet and differentiating epithelial cells migrate up the villus to replace cells sloughed off into the lumen. A fourth type of cell, the argentaffine or chromaffin cells, are also predominantly found in the crypts.

There is little evidence that the epithelial cells of the crypt absorb material from the intestinal lumen. The major function of the three specialized types of cell is that of secretion. The goblet cells continually produce mucus by merocrine secretion (Trier 1968). The Paneth cells show the structural features of zymogen-secreting cells, that is, cells that synthesize protein packaged in membrane-enclosed granules for external secretion (Trier 1963, 1968; Rubin *et al*. 1966 a,b); the composition of these granules has not been determined. Similarly, the chromaffin cells synthesize peptide hormones such as secretin and cholecystokinin-pancreozymin, and pharmacologically active amines such as 5-HT (serotonin) and prostaglandins (Rubin *et al*. 1966a; Corvalheira *et al*. 1968; Trier 1968; Forssmann *et al*. 1969; Go and Summerskill 1971). The undifferentiated epithelial cells are also thought to have a secretory function apart from their role in replacing the mature epithelial cells of the villus (Trier 1964). The latter, morphologically columnar, with numerous, larger microvilli, are functionally the most important component of the epithelial layer; their primary role is one of absorption (Rubin 1971). As these cells differentiate morphologically they acquire numerous enzymes acting as either "receptors" or "carriers" for disaccharidases (Jos *et al*. 1967; Nordström *et al*. 1968), alkaline phosphatase (Dawson and Pryse-Davies 1963; Nordström *et al*. 1968), dipeptidases (Nordström *et al*. 1968), leucine amino peptidase (Nachlas *et al*. 1960) and adenosine triphosphatase (Padykula *et al*. 1961). Many of these enzymes are associated with the glycocalyx and plasma membrane of the microvilli (Nachlas *et al*. 1960; Padykula *et al*. 1961; Stirling and Kinter 1967; see Trier 1971 and Mettrick and Podesta 1974 for additional references). Trier (1971) pointed out that since the differentiated villous cells survive 1-7 days (Leblond and Messier 1958; Lipkin *et al*. 1963; MacDonald *et al*. 1964) the relatively rapid turnover of rat intestinal disaccharidases (Rubenstein *et al*. 1966; Das and Gray 1970) imply that the cells are capable of *de novo* synthesis of disaccharidases. The debate as to whether these disaccharidases are located on or within the microvillus membrane is still unresolved (Korn 1969; Kaback 1970; Isselbacher 1974). Similarly, although it is generally agreed that peptide digestion is intimately associated with the villus epithelial cells, the cellular location remains controversial (Fern *et al*. 1969; Gray and Cooper 1971; Rhodes *et al*. 1967; Peters and MacMahon 1970; Ugolev and Delaey 1973; Arvenitakis *et al*. 1976).

Comparison of the pattern of intestinal digestion of disaccharides and tripeptides indicates that in the former disaccharide digestion and absorption is associated with microvillus membrane disaccharidase, luminal accumulation of products and rapid disappearance of the disaccharide; maltose disappears faster than sucrose (Dahlqvist and Thompson 1963 a,b; Arvenitakis *et al*. 1976).

The marked difference in cellular enzymatic activity, luminal accumulation of hydrolytic products and rate of substrate disappearance of test tripeptides, indicate two different methods of digestion and absorption. In one case, microvillus membrane hydrolysis is active, while in the other hydrolysis is apparently cytoplasmic with only minimal efflux of products into the lumen (Silk *et al*. 1974; Arvenitakis *et al*. 1976).

Recent histochemical studies on rats have shown the distribution pattern of enzymes in individual villi of the proximal intestine. Aminopeptidase and leucyl-aminopeptidase activity is restricted to the base of the villus while enteropeptidase is restricted to the tip. Maltase, lactase and all phosphatase activity commences at the base of the villus (not in the crypt) increasing towards the tip of the villus (Jervis 1963; Nordström and Dahlqvist 1973; De Both et al. 1974; Gossrau 1975). These enzymes also show different levels of activity confirming that both the different regions of the intestine and individual villus can be divided into various functional zones of varying enzymatic activity (Gossrau 1975).

Migration of cells from the crypts up the villi may be so rapid that the entire intestinal mucosa is replaced in less than 48 hours, depending on the species of animal (Leblond and Messier 1958; Lipkin and Bell 1968). Shorter et al. (1964) calculated that the rate of cell renewal in the crypts was 1 cell every 3 hours while the rate of cell loss from the tip of the villus is 1 cell/hour. The disparity in these two figures is explained by Loehry et al.'s (1969) demonstration of the complex three-dimensional structure of the intestinal mucosa, showing a number of crypts associated with a single villus. The average number of crypts per villus varies between different species of animal ranging from 3 in man (Loehry and Creamer 1969) to 13 in rats (Fuji 1972). Presumably the higher the ratio the quicker the potential for a rapid turnover rate for the mucosa. As not all of the cells produced in the crypts migrate up the villi, there are qualitative differences in the composition of the cells forming the epithelium of the villus at different levels of the crypt and villus (Isselbacher 1974) lending some support to the suggestions that have been made for there being different regional loci on the villi for the absorption of amino acids and carbohydrates. There are also proximal to distal secretory and absorptive gradients in the rat small intestine (Schedl et al. 1968; Harrison and Webster 1971; Cook et al. 1973).

Weiser (1973) has shown that the crypt zone is characterized by a high degree of incorporation of labelled sugars into crypt cells, as compared with villus cells, from their respective nucleotide precursors; the only exception to this glycosyltransferase distribution was sialytransferase, which was located on the villus rather than the crypt cell surface. Other differences between crypt and villus cells were that the latter were not agglutinated by concanavalin A whereas crypt cells showed striking agglutination (Weiser 1972); there is a high correlation between concanavalin A agglutination and surface membrane galactosyltransferase activity (Podolsky et al. 1974). It appears that the surface glycoproteins of the differentiated villus cell membranes are complete whereas those of the crypt cells are incomplete and demonstrate similarities with foetal-type surface membranes (Isselbacher 1974).

Both the villi and microvilli pulsate, aiding in the dispersion of exogenous and endogenous products in the lumen (Lee 1971; Joyner and Kokas 1973). The inner core of the microvilli has both longitudinal and cross fibres, the latter being largely composed of actin (Tilney and Mooseker 1971). In addition, strong peristaltic movements in the proximal intestine ensure that the contents of the bulk aqueous phase in the lumen are homogeneous. In the distal intestine, the size of the villi decreases and peristaltic movements decline as water is re-absorbed from the bulk luminal aqueous phase leading to solidification of the undigested particulate matter.

The potential absorptive surface area of the intestinal mucosa is increased $\times$ 30-40 by the presence of the microvilli on the epithelial cells of the villi (Trier 1971). The microvilli have been implicated in intracellular digestion and glucose transport (Faust et al. 1972) although structural functions and a role in the mixing and passage of the luminal contents have also been suggested. Recently, however, Befus and Podesta (1976) have questioned the physiological significance of the increased surface area of the gut mucosa and the cestode tegument due to the presence of microvilli.

External to all biological membranes is a hydrodynamic layer of water through which solute molecules pass by diffusional forces only before they reach the plasmalemma proper. This unstirred layer of water may exert a large part of the total resistance encountered by solutes passing from the bulk luminal aqueous phase into the intracellular layer and, in the small intestine, has been shown to cause pronounced alterations in permeability coefficients; in some cases, it becomes the rate limiting step for intestinal transport (Westergaard and Dietschy 1974). Similarly, in the case of unidirectional uptake rates for nonelectrolytes across the external tegumental membrane of *Hymenolepis diminuta*, the unstirred water layer has been shown to be the major source of error in calculating uptake rates if the results are not corrected for extracellular absorbate in the unstirred layer (Podesta *et al.* 1977). This hydrodynamic layer significantly reduces the potential effective absorptive surface area of both the intestinal mucosa and the helminth tegument.

The anatomical surface area of the rat intestine varies between 1,226 and 696 cm^2 100 mg^{-1} dry wt depending upon the region of the small intestine (Wilson and Dietschy 1974; Westergaard and Dietschy 1974), while the anatomical surface area of *H. diminuta* is only 101 cm^2 100 mg^{-1} dry weight (Podesta and Mettrick 1976c). Per unit weight the anatomical surface area of the rat intestine is therefore far greater than that of the worm, but the effect of the unstirred water layer is to reduce the physiological surface area of the small intestine to only 8.2-9.5 cm^2 100 mg^{-1} dry weight and that of the worm tegument to 39 cm^2 100 mg^{-1}. Interestingly, the greater density of the intestinal villi and microvilli lead to a 1/100-1/200 reduction in effective surface area whereas the fewer tegumental microvilli of the tapeworm only reduce effective surface area to 1/3rd of the anatomical area. Per unit weight the worm effective surface area is greater than that of intestine by a factor of 3-4, which explains why cestodes are so successful in competing with the host mucosa for available luminal nutrients. In support of this conclusion, it has been pointed out that the rates of transport, per unit weight of worm tissue, for electrolytes, nonelectrolytes and water by *H. diminuta* are equivalent or greater than those of the small intestine (Podesta and Mettrick 1976 a,c). Befus and Podesta (1976) suggest that selective pressures during the evolution of the cestodes did not favour the development of a complex surface area structure which may be related to the fact that the cestode tegument is primarily designed for absorption. In contrast, the functions of the intestinal mucosal surface area involve digestion, secretion, mobility of luminal contents and absorption; these additional functions may have influenced the complex mucosal structure which is characteristic of the intestinal epithelium but not of other epithelia, such as the gall bladder, urinary bladder, kidney and Malpighian tubules, salt glands, and others which, like the helminth tegument, are primarily transporting surfaces.

III. DIGESTION IN THE SMALL INTESTINE

Acid chyme entering the duodenum from the stomach is a mixture of fat, which is semi-emulsified, protein, polypeptides and carbohydrates including a large proportion of non-hydrolyzed starch. The acidity of the chyme of rats is due to secretion of hydrochloric acid by the parietal cells of the stomach and the optimum pH for gastric pepsin activity is in the range of pH 1.2.

Many parasitologists have believed that this acidity was largely or wholly buffered by the alkaline pancreatic and intestinal juices and by bile, although even standard physiology texts have for some time indicated that this was not the case and that the normal pH of the small intestine is acidic (Bell *et al.* 1963). In animals with simple stomachs the contribution of water and electrolytes, particularly bicarbonate, from the pancreas is much greater than that from the liver (Harper 1967; Wheeler 1968). The rate of secretion of water and bicarbonate from the pancreas may be increased by the release of the gastrointestinal hormone secretin from the intestinal wall; release of this hormone is mainly in response to duodenal acidity caused by the presence of acid chyme in the intestine (Wheeler 1968; Meyer *et al.* 1970 a,b). While digestion may commence in the stomach or even the mouth, the enzymes secreted into the duodenum by the pancreas and intestinal mucosa are, together with bile, capable of initiating and completing the entire digestive process on their own.

Proteins of both exogenous and endogenous origin are attacked first by the pancreatic endopeptidases; the resulting polypeptides by the amino- and carboxy-peptidases and hydrolysis is completed by the dipeptidases of the succus entericus.

Fats are hydrolysed by the lipases of the pancreatic and intestinal juices and carbohydrates by the disaccharidases of the small intestine and exocrine pancreas. While part of the primary breakdown of nutrients in the small intestine is catalyzed by enzymes from other organs, the major portion of ingested food is catalyzed by enzymes secreted by the exocrine pancreas (Beck 1973).

The traditional view of intestinal digestion is that of a straight interaction between exogenous (and endogenous) nutritional substances and the intestinal enzymes which hydrolyse the nutrients available. The modern concept is that of adaptation of the intestinal enzymes to the diet ingested and it has now been well documented that the composition of the diet alters intestinal enzyme activity to maximize potential utilization (Rosensweig 1975).

The implications of this adaptive capability by the gut to studies on the effect of intestinal parasites on intestinal digestion are discussed elsewhere in this chapter but it adds further emphasis to the point that the environment of the gut lumen is an ever-changing milieu and that any parasite must be capable of a wide range of adaptations to its environment if it is to survive. Herein, in fact, may lie the key to specificity between host and parasite and the restricted intestinal sites occupied by some worms in contrast to the broader range exhibited by the highly mobile *Hymenolepis diminuta*. The extent to which an intestinal parasite can tolerate or adapt to its ever-changing environment determines the range of its habitat.

A. *Pancreatic Secretions*

The pancreas lies in the mesentery of the first duodenal loop, opening into the distal duodenum behind the bile duct by a number of small ducts. It is a remarkable gland in that it produces both an external and an internal secretion.

The exocrine function is well-known and the organic component of pancreatic juice represents a number of pro-enzymes (catalytically inactive) and enzymes used in the luminal hydrolysis of carbohydrates, proteins and fats. Pancreatic juice is alkaline due to the high HCO_3^- content which accounts for 50-70% of the total inorganic constituents present. In dogs, the rate of flow of pancreatic juice after feeding increases five-fold whereas in the rat the increase is only 50% (Cooke *et al*. 1967).

The principal enzymes present include trypsin, secreted as its inactive precursor trypsinogen which is converted to its active form by enterokinase secreted in the succus entericus from the duodenal mucosa. Chymotrypsinogen is the precursor of chymotrypsin, activated by trypsin in the duodenum. Both trypsin and chymotrypsin are proteolytic enzymes with pH optima about 8; thus they operate considerably below optimum activity in the highly acidic postprandial duodenum. A third endopeptidase, elastase, is also present. Carboxypeptidase A and B complete the hydrolysis of the peptides formed by tryptic action. A number of enzymes involved in hydrolytic digestion of carbohydrates and lipids are also present.

The acidic conditions of the stomach favour hydrolysis of soluble carbohydrates independently of any enzyme, which is particularly important for carbohydrates such as fructosans which are not susceptible to specific enzymes (Kronfeld and Van Soest 1976). Ptyalin or salivary amylase initiates starch hydrolysis to dextrins and maltose. While active in man, it is absent in most other species. The pancreatic amylase appears to be identical with salivary amylase and similar, if not identical, in most species. Amylase hydrolyses amylose, amylopectin, glycogen and some dextrins, but does not degrade potato-starch granules. Pancreatic amylase is adsorbed by the intestinal mucosa where it is important in membrane digestion, but not necessarily vital as the mucosa produces its own gluco-amylase. Intermediary products of starch degradation are poor substrates for amylase which is why most mammals also secrete oligosaccharidases, maltase, sucrase, lactase and other disaccharidases.

The quantity and quality of pancreatic juice are influenced by the diet. Although there is a linear relationship between the amounts of each enzyme class secreted, the total amount, and the relative proportions of the individual enzymes secreted, can vary considerably. On a high carbohydrate diet amylase is increased and the trypsins reduced; the reverse occurs on high protein diets (Harper 1967; Keller 1968; Mettrick and Podesta 1974).

The endocrine function of the pancreas involves the pancreatic islet tissue (Islets of Langerhans) accounting for only 1-2 per cent of total pancreatic volume. Each of the two main types of cells in the islets elaborates a substance that affects carbohydrate metabolism. The α-cells accounting for approximately one quarter of the islet tissue, secrete glucagon. The smaller β-cells, which account for up to 75 per cent of the tissue, secrete insulin. Glucagon is a polypeptide that promotes glycogenolysis, hypoglycaemia and increases the cellular concentration of active phosphorylase.

Pancreatic enzymes and bile have been implicated in the release of enterokinase (Nordström 1972a; Gotze *et al.* 1972) and other brush border enzymes (Nordström 1972b) from the mucosal membrane itself. Alpers and Tedesco (1975) suggested that as the disaccharidases are located on the external cell membrane, the release of brush border enzymes from their membrane might be mediated by intraluminal pancreatic proteases. Rapid disaccharidase turnover occurs along the length of the villus (James *et al.* 1971; Alpers 1972). As the disaccharidases function extracellularly, it seems reasonable for them to be located externally on the membrane and to be removed by intraluminal factors, such as the pancreatic secretion. This suggestion is supported by the increased specific activity of disaccharidases in patients with chronic pancreatitis (Arvenitakis and Olsen 1974) and the demonstration that pancreatic secretions play some role in the turnover of large brush border proteins (Alpers and Tedesco 1975). Both Nordström (1972a) and Gotze *et al.* (1972) found that cholecystokinin-pancreozymin stimulated release of enterokinase, sucrase and alkaline phosphatase from the intestinal mucosa *in vivo*, and that is was related to the presence of bile salts. While it has been thought that much of the protein turnover in all membranes was intracellular, more recent studies show that surface proteins are shed into the luminal fluid. Alpers and Tedesco (1975) in particular have demonstrated that pancreatic proteases may be involved in the release of macromolecules from the brush border surface without necessarily causing any membrane damage in the process.

Trypsin and chymotrypsin become adsorbed to intestinal debris after their secretion into the lumen. This adsorption, which does not impair their digestive capability, is pH dependent having 2 peaks at pH 5.0 and 8.5. The affinity of the luminal intestinal mucosal cells is greater for chymotrypsin than for trypsin (Goldberg *et al.* 1969). This raises the question of adsorption of these enzymes to intact mucosal cells and the close physico-chemical relationship between the enzymes involved in protein digestion and the cells absorbing the products of digestion, which would obviously be advantageous to the host and to an intestinal parasite such as *H. diminuta*.

B. *The Intestinal Juice - Succus Entericus*

The two types of glands found in the small intestine are Brunner's Glands found only in the duodenal sub-mucosa and the Crypts of Lieberkühn or intestinal glands which are present throughout the small intestine. The crypts contain a number of different types of cells which secrete a large number of enzymes and mucus; these secretions are collectively referred to as intestinal juice or *succus entericus*.

In the absence of pancreatic amylase, starch digestion is significantly reduced, which implies that the amount of amylase in the *succus entericus* is slight. Intestinal maltase, lactase and sucrase reinforce the action of the pancreatic disaccharidases. The nucleosidases and phosphatase probably originate primarily from sloughed-off mucosal cells; that is, they are essentially intracellular enzymes. Nucleases and nucleotidases are extracellularly secreted enzymes.

The proteolytic enzymes synthesized and secreted by the pancreas enter the duodenum as zymogens or proenzymes devoid of proteolytic functions (Haverback *et al*. 1960; Beck *et al*. 1962, 1965). They are activated by the duodenal enzyme, enterokinase, which is therefore the key enzyme involved in protein digestion. Normal protein digestion is not possible in the absence of enterokinase (Hadorn *et al*. 1969). Enterokinase is localized at the brush border of the duodenal mucosal cells (Nordström and Dahlqvist 1973) and released by the action of bile salts (Hadorn *et al*. 1971). The cascade reactions involved in activating the pancreatic proteases have been described by Beck (1973), but it is the action of enterokinase on trypsinogen, resulting in the active enzyme trypsin, which initiates the whole chain.

Although there are no known inhibitors of lipase and amylase activity (Beck 1973), there are a number of proteolytic enzyme inhibitors both widely described in Nature and synthesized by the pancreas itself (Huber *et al*. 1970). Despite their different composition, all proteolytic inhibitors induce pancreatic enlargement and increase secretion of trypsinogen, chymotrypsinogen and amylase by the pancreas in an attempt to compensate for the reduced luminal activity of the enzymes (Beck *et al*. 1965; Geratz and Hurt 1970; Beck 1973; Mettrick and Podesta 1974). The important physiological aspect of trypsin inhibitors is the protection of the pancreas from autodigestion; inhibition of trypsin activation of course inhibits the whole process of activation of protoeolytic enzymes in the duodenum. Obviously, in the same way that the pancreas has mechanisms to prevent autodigestion, intestinal helminths have to inhibit the action of luminal enzymes on worm tissue, and inactivation of trypsin and chymotrypsin by intact *Hymenolepis diminuta* has been described by Pappas and Read (1972 a,b) and of pancreatic lipase by Ruff and Read (1973). The inactivation of pancreatic enzymes by *H. diminuta* is apparently entirely different to their inactivation by other known inhibitors, and there is no evidence of increased proteolytic secretion by the pancreas of a parasitized host animal in response to cestode inactivation of proteolytic enzymes. The helminth inactivator is produced at a high rate at the lumen-tegument interface and then detaches from the interfacial material after combination with the proteolytic enzyme (Pappas and Read 1972 a,b). In contrast, pancreatic lipase is inhibited by an adsorption phenomenon (Ruff and Read 1973). As was pointed out by Mettrick and Podesta (1974) these studies are equivocal due to the experimental methodology employed. For example, the assay medium contained maleate which has been shown to inhibit the activity of proteolytic enzymes and of amylase and to stimulate the activity of pancreatic lipase (Webb 1966). Determination of proteolytic activity in pancreatic juice and serum presents serious technical problems which have yet to be overcome (Beck 1973). The early results of Borgstrom *et al.* (1957) and Webb (1966) on trypsin and chymotrypsin inhibition by the intestinal mucosa have not yet been substantiated; Goldberg *et al.* (1968, 1969) found no inhibitors in the mucosa of the small intestine. The colonic proteolytic enzyme mucosal inhibitor reported by Goldberg *et al.* (1969) may have been due to the presence of mucus in the fresh preparations. In the *post mortem* colon no mucus was present and no inhibition of enzyme activity was reported. Protection by *H. diminuta* against proteolytic and other enzymes may similarly depend more on the physical separation of the enzymes from tegumental proteins by the brush border membrane, as is the case in the pancreas itself (Palade *et al.* 1962), than on the action of the unique enzyme inhibitors.

C. *Bile*

Bile is secreted continuously by the parenchymal cells of the liver. In those animals which have a gall bladder - the rat does not - bile may be concentrated before being released at the appropriate time in the feeding cycle. In composition, bile is a highly complex fluid containing up to 98% water. The bile salts are formed in the liver by the conjugation of glycine or taurine with cholic acid or related components. They have a number of properties including, reacting with substances such as cholesterol to form water soluble complexes, reduction of surface tension enhancing lipase activity, and activation of lipase activity. Only small amounts of the bile conjugates are excreted in faecal material due to reabsorption in the distal small intestine and the large bowel.

Bile acids are the end products of cholesterol metabolism and, together with cholesterol itself, represent the major route for cholesterol excretion from the body. Approximately 90% of the bile acids secreted into the intestine per day are reabsorbed and returned to the liver via the enterohepatic circulation. The remainder, including cholesterol, are excreted in faecal material. Alkaline phosphatase is also present in bile but no digestive or absorptive function has been ascribed to this enzyme.

There is comparatively little information on the regulation of bile secretion in the rat. Bile formation is normally stimulated to a maximal or near-maximal extent by the recirculating bile acids (Shaw and Heath 1972) and the gastrointestinal hormones have little influence on hepatic secretion. This is in contrast to other animals, such as the dog, where feeding (Fritz and Brooks 1963; Nahrwold and Grossman 1967; Jones and Grossman 1969a) and the gastrointestinal hormones, secretin, cholecystokinin-pancreozymin and gastrin (Jones *et al.* 1971; Jones and Grossman 1969b, 1970) are important factors in the control bile flow. However, the rate of flow in rats is of the same order as that recorded for other animals (Shaw and Heath 1972). As bile enters the rat duodenum on a continuous basis due to the absence of a gall bladder, the reabsorbed bile acids in the enterohepatic circulation provide a relatively constant stimulus to bile formation which may explain the lack of dependence on a choleretic response to feeding and hormonal influence.

The functions of bile in the intestine appear to be mediated primarily by the bile salts (Hofmann 1968; Weiner and Lack 1968). Bile salts facilitate pancreatic lipase activity and aid in the digestion of dietary lipid. They facilitate the transport of dietary lipids from the lumen to the mucosal brush border and of cholesterol, lecithins and bilirubin conjugates from the liver into the duodenum. They are essential to the absorption of the fat-soluble vitamins D, E and K, and of cholesterol and β-carotene. Other functions include a role in the regulation of the intestinal microflora (Percy-Robb and Collee 1972), protection of cholesterol esterase from proteolytic attack (Vahouny et al. 1964), facilitation of triglyceride intramucosal resynthesis (Weiner and Lack 1968) and facilitation of the movement of luminal contents through the colon (Hofmann 1968). The free dihydroxy bile acids, deoxycholic and chemodeoxycholic acid may inhibit absorption of fluid and electrolytes in the rat small intestine (Forth et al. 1966) depending on their intra-luminal concentration (Harries and Sladen 1972). Certain bile salts also have an inhibitory effort on monosaccharide absorption (Gracey et al. 1971 a,b; Harries and Sladen 1972). The mechanisms involved in bile salt inhibition of monosaccharide absorption differ from those involved in inhibition of fluid and electrolyte absorption. Glycine and taurine conjugates of cholic acid increase the activities of both (Na^+, K^+) - and (Mg^{++}) - ATPase (Faust and Wu 1966) but glycocholate inhibits rat small intestine ATPase (Parkinson and Olson 1964) and deoxycholate inhibits (Na^+, K^+) - ATPase (Pope et al. 1966). The free dihydroxy and trihydroxy bile acids stimulate (Mg^{++}) - ATPase, although the glycine and taurine conjugates of the dihydroxy acids inhibit both the (Mg^{++}) - and (Na^+, K^+) - ATPase of the rat intestinal mucosa (Hepner and Hofmann 1973).

The small intestine of the rat contains approximately 80% of the body pool of bile acids with most of the remainder in the large bowel (Weiner and Lack 1968); recruitment via cholesterol catabolism balances the loss due to faecal excretion.

In the duodenum the bile salts secreted into the lumen are largely conjugated with glycine or taurine whereas in the distal small intestine and large bowel they are deconjugated and dehydroxylated into secondary bile acids by bacterial interaction (Weiner and Lack 1968; Rosenberg 1969; Schiff and Dietschy 1969). While a direct correlation has not been shown between the quality and quantity of conjugated and free bile acids and the quality and quantity of the gut microflora (Mallory et al. 1973 a,b), it is reasonable to assume that the reduced intestinal microflora associated with infections of *H. diminuta* (Mettrick 1971a) will influence the course and distribution of free and conjugated bile acids in the intestine.

Conjugated and free bile acids have differing pKa's and therefore at a given pH more of the free acids will be in a nonionic form than the conjugated bile acids (Schiff and Dietschy 1969). Non-conjugated bile acids are less soluble in the acid pH of the gut, cannot substitute functionally for the conjugated forms and cannot incorporate the products of lipolysis into micelles (Hislop et al. 1967; Hofmann 1968; Dowling and Small 1968). As a result of the complex interactions between the different bile roles, their variable form as ionic or nonionic, conjugated or nonconjugated, and the effect of various modulators such as luminal pH, the microflora, diet, etc., the form and type of the bile acids presented to the tegument of *H. diminuta* will vary enormously and have profoundly different effects on the parasite. As has been previously pointed out (Mettrick and Podesta 1974) the role, if any, of bile acids in the host-parasite relationship is obviously so complex that the major role attributed to bile acids in the biology of various host-parasite interactions (Rothman 1959; Smyth 1962; Smyth and Haslewood 1963) requires a re-evaluation taking into account the recent advances in our understanding of the role of bile in gastrointestinal function in both the normal and diseased state.

IV. PHYSICAL CHARACTERISTICS OF THE SMALL INTESTINE

A. *Hydrogen Ion Concentration (pH)*

It is over 45 years since parasitologists interested in intestinal parasites were made aware of the fact that the mammalian gut was acidic (Kofoid *et al.* 1932). Further, it has been amply demonstrated that luminal contents become even more strongly acidic after feeding and during perfusion (Wilson 1954, 1962; McHardy and Parsons 1957; Wilson and Kazyak 1957; Wormsley 1971).

Hymenolepis diminuta exhibits a number of migrational activities in the gut lumen (see Arai, this volume) and studies have been carried out relating the changes in intestinal pH and other physico-chemical characteristics of the small intestine to the migrational responses of *H. diminuta* (Mettrick 1971 a,c, d).

In the uninfected, rested (pre-prandial) rat small intestine, the duodenal-jejunal pH is slightly acidic becoming alkaline (pH 7.3) in the terminal ileum. Following feeding the pH of the proximal small intestine decreases rapidly establishing a marked gradient down the length of the small bowel (Mettrick 1971 c,d). In the parasitized gut the changes in the intestinal $[H^+]$ appear to be correlated with the migrational responses of *H. diminuta* to the experimental diet. In general, the lowest pH of any region of the intestine was matched with the highest percentage of worm biomass. Similar results have been obtained from *ad libitum* fed animals in which the duodenal pH of the parasitized gut was nearly 2 pH units more acid than in uninfected animals, with the pH gradients again being closely correlated to worm biomass distribution (Mettrick 1971c). Further studies varying the size (age) of the worms and the quantity of the carbohydrate fed indicated that the quality of ingested carbohydrate influenced the pH range and gradient in the parasitized gut, with the lowest pH being recorded for a glucose diet and the larger (older) worm infection. Intestinal pH in both uninfected and parasitized rats also changed following the feeding of dietary components such as amino acids and olive oil although in the latter the differences between the uninfected and parasitized gut were not significant. The 20% inhibitory action of olive oil on the pentagastrin and histamine-stimulated acid secretion by the stomach may be related to these observations (Schmidt et al. 1971). In all cases, there were substantial migrational responses of the worms to the diets fed (Mettrick 1971 c,d; 1972a, 1973). The magnitude of the changes in intestinal pH in the parasitized gut is also related to the quality of the diet. In uninfected glucose-fed rats the pH range was only 1.28 units; in parasitized rats 2.18 units. Dextrin and galactose were intermediate (Mettrick 1972a). Changes in worm distribution in the small intestine are probably dependent on the amount of glucose or other carbohydrate fed, as at 2 hours following the feeding of 1, 2 or 3 g glucose, 2 g dextrin or 2 g galactose, the total worm biomass in the duodenum-jejunum only varied by 3% (94-97%). Small differences in the worm biomass distribution in the duodenum and jejunum between the different diets were observed but if these differences are correlated to the intestinal glucose gradient, *H. diminuta* must be able to adjust its intestinal location in a remarkable precise manner to changing gradients in the gut lumen.

The suggestion that the lower intestinal pH of the parasitized intestine was related to the excretion by *H. diminuta* of ions and other acidic end products of carbohydrate metabolism (Mettrick 1971 c,d) has since been substantiated by *in vivo* intestinal perfusion techniques (Podesta and Mettrick 1975). Increases in acidity of the intestine occur due to either HCO_3^- transport and/or to H^+ ion secretion. The net result of HCO_3^- transport from the intestinal lumen (HCO_3^- absorption) or H^+ ion secretion into the lumen is that the luminal concentration of HCO_3^- decreases and that of H^+ ions increases, thus reducing the pH of the luminal fluid. The difference between the two mechanisms is that secretion of H^+ ions generates a high pCO_2 in the luminal fluid while HCO_3^- absorption lowers intestinal pH without increasing pCO_2.

A unique problem faced by any intestinal helminth is that in the postprandial intestine, acid chyme reacts with HCO_3^- secreted by the pancreas, liver (bile) and mucosa (Brunner's glands) producing high luminal pCO_2. This CO_2 diffuses down its concentration gradient into both the mucosa and the worm tissue, so that the poise of the HCO_3^- - CO_2 reaction tends towards the production of HCO_3^- and H^+ ions within the mucosal and worm tissues. In the case of the mucosa the CO_2 continues down its concentration gradient and enters the blood stream thus preventing acidification of the mucosal tissues. In the case of luminal dwelling worms such as *H. diminuta* there has to be a mechanism of neutralizing the acidity of their tissues in the post-prandial situation. The action of a H^+ ion secretory mechanism is one such mechanism utilized by *H. diminuta* and at least partly explains the lower pH in the infected intestine when the worms are *in situ*. The higher pCO_2 of perfusion fluids passed through the infected rat intestine is direct evidence supporting the existence of a hydrogen-ion secretory mechanism by *H. diminuta* (Podesta and Mettrick 1974a). However, as Webster and Wilson (1970) have shown that the protonephridial canals of *H. diminuta* contain a fluid with a pH of 4.5 and a pCO_2 of 120 mm Hg, obviously the hydrogen-ion secretory mechanism does not entirely solve the problem of tissue acidification in this worm. Cestodes, including *H. diminuta*, have been shown to excrete organic acids such as lactic acid, succinic acid, etc. both *in vitro* (see von Brand 1966) and *in vivo* (Mettrick 1971a). Although most of the accumulation and direction of net transport of lactate, following its formation in the mucosal cells is toward the serosal side of the epithelium (Wilson 1954; Faelli and Esposito 1971) considerable amounts of lactate are found in the intestinal lumen (Faelli and Esposito 1971; Lease and Mansford 1971). Increased luminal lactate concentration is not accompanied by lower luminal pH (Frazier and Vanatta 1973) indicating that lactate contributes little to luminal acidification and that increased $[H^+]$ in the intestinal lumen is primarily due to H^+ ion secretion (Podesta and Mettrick 1975). It is likely that *H. diminuta* uses the same mechanism as the mucosa and the apparent correlation between worm biomass distribution and the luminal lactate and pH gradients (Mettrick 1971a) can equally well be the result of H^+ ion secretion by the worms which is, of course, greatest in those regions of the gut containing the greatest amount of worm biomass.

Intestinal hydrogen-ion concentration is of major importance because of its effect upon various transport phenomena in the mucosa and mucosal cellular metabolism. Increasing [H^+] reduces transport of amino acids (Adibi et al. 1971; Fogel and Adibi 1972), sugars (Csaky 1971; Jackson et al. 1968 a,b), fluid and electrolytes (Parsons 1971; Podesta and Mettrick 1974 b,c, 1975, 1977c; Hubel 1972), IF (Intrinsic Factor) binding of vitamin B_{12} (Mackenzie and Donaldson 1972), mucosal glucose (Podesta and Mettrick 1974a) and reduces mucosal metabolism (Jackson et al. 1968 a,b).

In contrast, the effect of reduced luminal pH on H. diminuta is to increase both fluid and glucose transport (Podesta and Mettrick 1974a, 1976c) and Na^+ transport (Podesta and Mettrick 1976a); Cl^- transport by the worm is not affected by luminal pH.

B. HCO_3^-

The problems of measuring the fluxes of HCO_3^- in the small intestine are similar to those for H^+ ions. Turnberg et al.'s (1970a, 1970b) technique to measure intestinal HCO_3^- absorption and secretion in man has been applied to the rat intestine (see Podesta and Mettrick 1977a), in which considerable variation in luminal HCO_3^- did not result in significant changes in the level of luminal pCO_2; this indicates that there is a jejunal H^+ secretory mechanism in operation rather than a HCO_3^- pump.

However, both Hubel (1973) and Podesta and Mettrick (1977a) have shown that this H^+ ion secretory mechanism does not account for all of the HCO_3^- which disappeared from the lumen. HCO_3^- absorption by the mucosa which is not mediated by H^+ ion secretion may simply represent diffusion down a concentration gradient when there is high luminal [HCO_3^-]; a similar diffusion into worm tissue is also likely to occur.

The observations that luminal HCO_3^- accelerated mucosal Na^+ absorption and that Na^+ deletion reduced HCO_3^- absorption, reduced luminal acidification and reduced luminal [pCO_2] suggest a Na^+: H^+ cation exchange in the intestine (Turnberg et al. 1970b; Hubel

1973). While not all HCO_3^- absorption by the intestine is Na^+-dependent, Na^+-dependent HCO_3^- absorption becomes relatively more important as the luminal concentration of HCO_3^- decreases. The physiological importance of HCO_3^--stimulated Na^+ absorption in the acidic postprandial intestine is probably due entirely to the presence of free CO_2 in the lumen (Podesta and Mettrick 1977a).

Unlike the jejunum, the ileal lumen accumulates HCO_3^- and becomes more alkaline. Podesta and Mettrick (1977b) recently demonstrated the presence of an ileal H^+ ion secretory mechanism and suggested that HCO_3^- moves into the lumen rather than its precursor, OH^-.

HCO_3^- secretion into the lumen requires the presence of Cl^- (Binder and Rawlins 1973; Hubel 1967, 1969). Removing Na^+ and Cl^- decreases HCO_3^- absorption by 33-55% as well as decreasing the acidic change in pH. Part of the H^+ ion secretory mechanism must also be dependent on luminal Na^+ (Podesta and Mettrick 1977b). The latter authors' results using Cl^--containing and Cl^--depleted fluids showing negligible net H^+ are consistent with a Cl^- : HCO_3^- exchange mechanism operating in the rat ileum.

As luminal HCO_3^- concentrations increase, more HCO_3^- secretion is dependent upon Na^+ than could be explained by the absence of net Cl^- absorption, if there is a close coupling between Cl^- absorption and HCO_3^- secretion; this suggests that Na^+ absorption and HCO_3^- secretion are also coupled. These results are consistent with a mucosal ion transfer model in which there is primary coupled absorption of Na^+ and Cl^- which, because of the interaction between Na^+ and HCO_3^-, probably mediates $NaHCO_3^-$ secretion. Cl^- : HCO_3^- exchange may be due to this primary system. A secondary system mediates a Cl^--independent absorption of Na^+ and H^+ secretion - i.e. Na^+ : H^+ exchange (Schultz *et al.* 1974; Sheerin and Field 1975; Podesta and Mettrick 1977b).

C. *Oxidation - Reduction Potential (Eh)*

In the gastrointestinal lumen, the oxidation-reduction potential (Eh) is a measurement indicating the state of equilibrium between the oxidized and reduced metabolites present in the lumen. These metabolites are largely produced by the intestinal microflora so that Eh is influenced by factors such as the types and number of bacteria present in the lumen and the level of metabolic activities of the micro-organisms. Eh values only supply information on the relative proportions of the oxidizing and reducing agents present and it should not be considered as a quantitative measurement, particularly as the system is not in true thermodynamic balance (Hentges and Maier 1972; Podesta and Mettrick 1974 a,b).

Another factor which affects Eh both directly and indirectly is the hydrogen ion concentration of the gut. A change in $[H^+]$ is accompanied by electron uptake or release, such that an alteration (+ or -) equivalent to a change of one pH unit will directly alter the value of Eh by 57.7mV (Clark and Cohen 1923). The pH falls with increasing H^+ and the Eh increases if already positive in value or becomes less negative.

The indirect action is the effect of intestinal pH on the distribution and number of intestinal microbes; increased luminal hydrogen ion concentration enhances the antibacterial effect of the bile acids (Percy-Robb and Collee 1972; Podesta and Mettrick 1974a). There are very few studies on intestinal Eh, and it has been generally assumed that the intestinal lumen exhibits strong reducing tendencies with an Eh of -100 mV in the proximal intestine falling to -200 mV in the terminal ileum (Bergeim *et al.* 1945). This was recently confirmed by Mettrick (1975a) who showed that there was an Eh gradient in the small intestine of from -28 in the proximal duodenum to -195 mV in the distal ileum at 10.00 h in uninfected, *ad libitum* fed rats. These strong reducing tendencies may influence luminal pO_2 levels (see following section). The intestinal Eh of similar animals parasitized with *H. diminuta* ranged from +75 mV in the duodenum to -75 mV in the distal ileum. Further observations following feeding showed that in uninfected animals, the -ve Eh rapidly decreased so that the entire small intestine had a +ve Eh 2-3 h post-feed reaching + 118 mV in uninfected animals and + 189 mV in parasitized rats.

In the parasitized animals, the more strongly +ve intestinal Eh reflected the higher H^+ ion concentrations of the parasitized gut. Significant differences between the Eh of uninfected and parasitized animals and between the duodenum/jejunum and ileum were also observed in perfusion studies.

The extent of the difference in Eh between the parasitized and uninfected animals cannot be simply attributed to the difference in pH and must therefore be partly related to the reduced intestinal microflora of the parasitized animals (Burmak 1970; Mettrick 1971a) and the limiting effect that a weakly -ve or +ve Eh has upon the anaerobic microflora. While intestinal Eh may have a significance for helminth metabolism in terms of electron transport, its major importance probably lies in its relation to, and interaction with, other luminal physical characteristics.

D. *Luminal Gases*

The quality and quantity of gases in the intestinal lumen is particularly important to intestinal helminths in view of the importance of carbon dioxide in various metabolic pathways and the apparent absence of a need for oxygen.

Carbon dioxide is the most common and abundant gas present in the intestinal lumen reaching partial pressures as high as 680mm Hg (90.66 kPa.) after feeding. In the rat steady state, carbon dioxide tensions in the jejunum-ileum are 23-27 mm Hg (Powell *et al.* 1971) increasing to 44-48 mm Hg under experimental conditions (Powell *et al.* 1971; Podesta and Mettrick 1974a).

In animals parasitized with *H. diminuta*, the carbon dioxide tension is considerably increased and in perfusion studies the pCO_2 of the bulk aqueous phase in the lumen has been shown to be equivalent to 68-70 mm Hg (Podesta and Mettrick 1974a) or nearly double that of the uninfected rat intestine. This higher luminal pCO_2 is due to secretion of H^+ ions by *H. diminuta* and their subsequent transformation.

Parasitologists have generally considered the intestinal environment to be anoxic except for an ill-defined region adjacent to the mucosa which provided "access to larger amounts of oxygen---" (Read 1950). Measurements from oxygen electrodes placed in the intestinal lumen of mammals and birds indicated that the lumen was anoxic except for regions very near or touching the mucosa (Rogers 1949; Crompton *et al*. 1965). The interpretation of such data obtained by oxygen electrode-probes has been cautioned on a number of accounts by various authors (Bergofsky 1964; Lübbers 1968; Schuler and Kreuzer 1968; Hamilton *et al*. 1968; Albanese 1973; Podesta and Mettrick 1974a). Other information supporting the idea that the intestinal lumen was anoxic is that the absorption of exo- and endogenous fluid in the distal ileum and colon results in solidification of the undigested particulate matter with an anoxic core, and secondly, that biochemical studies on several intestinal helminths have shown that they are capable of anaerobic energy metabolism involving the fixation of CO_2 (for reviews see Saz 1971, 1972; Bryant 1972, 1975).

Hamilton *et al's* (1968) elegant study demonstrating the direct and practically instantaneous proportionality between arterial and luminal pO_2 levels was interpreted as indicating that the oxygen tension of the bulk aqueous phase in the intestinal lumen was equivalent to that of the mucosa, as both rapidly reached equilibria. Maggi *et al*. (1970) obtained similar results for the rat intestine and Podesta and Mettrick (1974a) determined the pO_2 of the luminal bulk liquid-phase as 40-50 mm Hg in both uninfected and parasitized animals. There was a marked tendency for the parasitized rats to have a luminal pO_2 up to 10 mm Hg higher than the corresponding uninfected control groups. In addition to the higher oxygen tension in the parasitized gut, the rates of increase and decrease of pO_2 in the perfusion fluid were greater than in the uninfected animals, suggesting that the mucosal barrier to diffusion of oxygen from artery to lumen was reduced in the parasitized gut. In support of this explanation and the possibility of an increased mucosal pO_2 in the infected animals, the mucosa of the uninfected gut has been shown to be 20% heavier in weight than that of the parasitized intestine (Podesta and

Mettrick 1974a). The reduced weight of the latter may reflect glucose metabolism associated with increased [H^+] (Thompson *et al.* 1970) and/or the reduced substrate and fluid transport in the parasitized intestine which results in less energy being expended within the epithelial cells. A third explanation involves the relationship between luminal [H^+] and Eh. In a strongly acidic parasitized intestine, the Eh is more +ve than in the uninfected gut. Thus, less oxygen would be consumed by oxidising agents as it diffuses from the blood to the intestinal lumen, resulting in the observed higher pO_2.

As arterial blood has a pO_2 of 100 mm Hg, it is impossible to rule out the possibility of there being an even higher oxygen tension in the area immediately adjacent to the brush border than in the lumen proper. While the associated unstirred water layers at the membrane-lumen interface are of great importance in determining the fluxes of ions and metabolites between mucosa and lumen (Drost-Hansen 1971; Parsons and Boyd 1972; Podesta *et al.* 1977), it is unlikely that these layers act as a barrier to the diffusion of mucosal oxygen into the bulk aqueous phase (Podesta and Mettrick 1974a).

Moreover, the pH of the unstirred water layers is 1-2 units lower than the pH of the bulk luminal phase (Smyth and Wright 1966) which would further reduce the possibility of the oxygen diffusing across the mucosa membrane and associated unstirred layers being consumed by luminal oxidising agents.

Finally, the reduced microflora in the parasitized intestine (Burmak 1970; Mettrick 1971a), associated with the changes in luminal pH and Eh would also tend to increase the availability of oxygen to intestinal helminths.

The oxygen tension of the lumen of the parasitized gut is sufficiently high to drive aerobic metabolic pathways, and at the level of the unstirred water layers adjacent to the mucosal membrane is likely to be in equilibrium with the mucosal pO_2 and may approach that of arterial blood. Earlier fears that high oxygen tensions are detrimental to intestinal helminths (Berntzen 1962;

Berntzen and Mueller 1964) have not been substantiated by Roberts and Mong (1969) who showed that *H. diminuta* grows equally well *in vitro* under zero or 20% oxygen in the gas phase of the incubation system.

V. CHEMICAL CHARACTERISTICS OF THE SMALL INTESTINE

A number of food substances have been shown to establish linear gradients in the intestinal lumen which depend on the quantity and quality ingested, the rate of stomach emptying, the rate, site, and mechanisms of absorption and on intestinal motility (Mettrick 1970). As peristalsis diminishes proceeding distally in the intestine, the transit of luminal food material through the duodenum and jejunum is more rapid than through the ileum. It is obvious that a disturbance in any of the above limiting factors will have pronounced effects on the nutrient gradients in the intestine.

A. *Protein and Amino Acid Luminal Gradients*

The gastro-intestinal tract plays a central role in protein metabolism of the whole body. Endogenous proteins are digested within the intestinal tract and largely reabsorbed. Together with exogenous protein recruitment, a large reservoir of amino acids is always present within the lumen of the intestine. The recruitment, digestion and absorption of these proteins has been extensively studied (Nasset *et al*. 1955; Gitler and Martinez-Rojas 1964; Rogers and Harper 1964; Fisher 1967; Gray and Cooper 1971; Fauconneau and Michel 1970; Alpers and Kinzie 1973). Depriving a host of exogenous dietary protein has little effect on the growth of *H. diminuta*, indicating that endogenous protein secretion into the intestinal lumen is quite sufficient to meet the protein nitrogen requirements of the worms (Chandler 1943; Mettrick and Munro 1965). The large free amino acid pool in the small intestine goes far towards explaining the negligible effects on worm growth of withdrawal of exogenous proteins. A gradient of amino acid concentrations exist in the lumen of the intestine, varying from duodenum to ileum depending on the source of the protein, time after feeding and the region of the intestine (Mettrick 1970). This differing amino acid content in the lumen may affect intracellular amino acid levels in the mucosa (Alpers and Kinzie 1973) and in *H. diminuta*. Digestion of endogenous protein is slower than exogenous so that more endogenous protein is found partially digested in the ileum (Nixon and Mawer 1970).

The source of exogenous protein significantly influences the protein-nitrogen gradients in the intestine. The changing gradients can be at least partly related to the rate of gastric digestion and release from the stomach into the duodenum; the more rapid the hydrolysis of the protein, the quicker the stomach empties (Mettrick 1970).

Under *ad libitum* feeding, the concentrations and molar ratios of the amino acids constituting the intestinal amino acid pool are significantly different in every region of the uninfected rat gut from those determined in animals infected with *H. diminuta*. Similarly, the protein nitrogen (PN) and non-protein nitrogen (NPN) gradients and concentrations were significantly different in uninfected to those in parasitized rats (Mettrick 1971a).

In contrast, ignoring regional and concentration differences, the molar proportions of the amino acids in the total free amino acid intestinal pool of the rat are similar in both parasitized and uninfected animals (Mettrick 1971a, 1975b; Read 1971).

Read *et al*. (1963) suggested that tapeworms lack control mechanisms for the regulation of free amino acid fluxes between lumen and worm tissue, and are therefore unprotected against any environmental pertubation of the pool. A number of studies indicate that *H. diminuta* has indeed little selective capacity in amino acid transport (Hopkins and Callow 1965; Arme and Read 1969; Chappell and Read 1973; Webb and Mettrick 1973; Mettrick 1975b).

With *ad libitum* feeding the total concentration of the PN amino acid pool of *H. diminuta* more than doubled between 1000 and 1600 h, indicating a diurnal periodicity in the size of both the intestinal and worm PN amino acid pools (Mettrick 1975b). Diurnal periodicity in nutrient levels in the plasma, enzyme levels in various tissues, and intestinal endocrine secretions have been well documented (see Wurtman 1969). There are also daily rhythmic changes in amino acid and glucose absorption by the rat small intestine *in vitro* and *in vivo*, (Furuya and Yugari 1971, 1974) which are directly related to the feeding cycle. Page *et al.* (1977) have shown a diurnal periodicity in uridine uptake by *H. diminuta* which also was greatest just prior to the hosts' normal active feeding period during the hours of darkness. It seems likely that diurnal migration by *H. diminuta* is related to the periodicity of uptake of metabolites which in turn is related to the diurnal periodicity and metabolism of the host.

The reduced levels of NPN and PN amino acid pools in the parasitized intestine and the increased concentration of the PN amino acid pool of *H. diminuta* provide evidence of nutritional dependency by the worm on host exogenous and endogenous protein. But for the fact that more amino acids are absorbed by the intestinal mucosa in the di-, tri, and peptide forms than as monomers (Smyth 1971; Matthews 1972; Cook 1972; Lis *et al.* 1972) the effect of the worms on the free amino acid pool would probably be even greater than that recorded.

The suggestion that intestinal helminths also transport at least some amino acids as peptides (Mettrick 1975b) is supported by the fact that the rate of increase in the concentration of amino acids in *H. diminuta* is equivalent to the worms absorbing 60% of the luminal NPN amino acid pool per hour. Secondly, proline and glycine are absorbed by the intestinal mucosa as peptides as their release as monomers following feeding is very slow (Holdsworth 1972). However, these two amino acids also exhibit rapid accumulation in the worm PN amino acid pool when there is no corresponding increase in the luminal pool (Mettrick 1975). Peptide transport by *H. diminuta* would give greater flexibility in the length or region of the intestinal tract that was habitable; *H. diminuta* is obviously not restricted in its environment, and, as has been shown in many studies, occupies and utilizes the whole of the small intestine in normal infections (Mettrick and Podesta 1974).

B. *Carbohydrate and Glucose Intestinal Gradients*

Early data on the effect of dietary carbohydrate content and quality on cestode development (Chandler 1943; Chandler *et al*. 1950; Read 1959) is unfortunately equivocal due to the methodology utilized and in particular, the fact that the diets used were not isocaloric. Further, rats have been shown to eat more (Meyer 1958; Roberts and Platzer 1967) or less (Harper 1964) in an attempt to counteract the deficiencies of experimental diets.

Hymenolepis diminuta is only able to utilize for metabolic purposes a very limited number of the carbohydrates that may be found in the intestinal lumen (Read 1955, 1956; Laurie 1957; Read and Rothman 1957 a,b). Di- and poly-saccharides are not utilizable and the dominant and most important carbohydrate source is glucose; galactose is used to a limited extent (Read and Rothman 1958) and may be incorporated directly into the sugar moiety of the cerebrosides (Webb and Mettrick 1973).

Dunkley and Mettrick (1969) using diets that were calorically and quantitatively identical confirmed that *H. diminuta* could not be supported on a galactose diet and that sucrose, dextrin and maltose were all inferior to glucose in promoting worm growth. Similarly, worm growth was greatest on a corn starch diet and least on potato starch; wheat starch was intermediate. The dextrin-maltose-glucose sequence represents the sequence of polysaccharide hydrolysis as well as increasing worm growth and it is reasonable to conclude that glucose availability in the lumen is a sensitive index to worm growth and development. The poor growth with potato starch is associated with its low level of digestibility ($\sim 50\%$) compared to 98% for cereal starches.

Quantity of dietary carbohydrate influences the growth of *H. diminuta* (Read *et al*. 1958) up to a level of 3.0g of starch per diem (Read 1959). Increasing dietary glucose content up to 7.2g per diem resulted in a linear increase of growth; with starch an asymptote was observed at 5.2g per diem (Dunkley and Mettrick 1976), indicating that available intestinal luminal glucose was not directly proportional to the quantity of corn (maize) starch fed.

If *H. diminuta* is strongly dependent on exogenous carbohydrate and glucose in particular, the differences between the carbohydrate and glucose gradients in uninfected and parasitized animals are not surprising (Mettrick 1971a, 1972b). What is perhaps surprising is that the luminal carbohydrate and glucose levels are not always reduced in the parasitized gut, attesting to the strength of the host's adaptive response to intestinal infection. Both Mettrick (1972b) and Dunkley and Mettrick (1977) attempted to correlate the migrational responses of *H. diminuta* to the changing intestinal glucose gradient through time; no direct relationship was observed although the amount of luminal glucose present in the parasitized gut averaged 50% less on a glucose diet, 19% with sucrose and 22% with corn starch; in the case of the two latter carbohydrates the gradient changes were complex, reflecting differences in the rate of hydrolysis and the region of the small intestine in which hydrolysis occurred (Blair and Tuba 1963; Dalquist and Thomson 1963b). Blood plasma glucose levels are initially hypoglycaemic in the infected animals, becoming hyperglycaemic some 2.5 h after feeding (Dunkley and Mettrick 1977). These results support the earlier studies of Podesta and Mettrick (1974c) who demonstrated that the glucose transport system in the parasitized small bowel is affected first at the level of the brush border where transport across the mucosa is decreased with increasing $[H^+]$ and secondly, at the level of the basal and lateral membranes of the mucosal tissue so that glucose transfer is inhibited and glucose accumulates in the mucosal tissue.

Several studies have indicated that the quality and quantity of exogenous carbohydrate ingested by the host regulates the growth and maturation of *H. diminuta*. The limited availability of nutrients, and of carbohydrate in particular, in the intestinal lumen has also been credited with being responsible for the so-called "crowding effect" where individual worm size decreases as population size increases (Read and Rothman 1957 a,b; Read *et al*. 1958; Roberts 1966; Read and Kilejian 1969; Dunkley and Mettrick 1969, 1976).

Castro et al.'s (1976) demonstration that *H. diminuta* does not necessarily require any enteral nutrient intake by the host for growth and development by the worm is therefore particularly intriguing. As has been shown above, amino acid requirements by *H. diminuta* for protein metabolism can be met entirely from the endogenous protein and amino acid luminal pool. But can the lumen also supply all the required glucose for energy expenditure by the worms? The answer is probably "no". The normal balance in nutrient flux across the intestinal mucosa favours serosal accumulation and transfer to the circulatory systems. Under enteral feeding, it is possible that simple diffusion gradients would allow plasma glucose to reach the intestinal mucosa and even lumen, so that some glucose would be directly available to the worms. The balance of energy requirement by the worms may be met by fatty acid and amino acid mobilization in a manner similar to that of man and other animals when faced with starvation (Olson 1975; Waterlow 1975). This explanation would depend on *H. diminuta* having the enzymatic adaptive capability to utilize alternative energy sources. As the basic turnover of proteins in the host body would continue luminal amino acids and proteins would not be limiting. Further, *H. diminuta* has been shown to readily absorb and assimilate fatty acids (Ginger and Fairbairn 1966; Lumsden and Harrington 1966). Such an adaptive capability by intestinal helminths in general would be valuable in all cases where the host was an intermittent feeder such as in the carnivores, as well as those which have a diurnal periodicity in their feeding behaviour.

A further important factor to be considered is the effect of enteral feeding on the characteristics and physiology of the gastrointestinal tract, as the small intestine itself has considerable adaptive enzyme capability.

The three common dietary disaccharides are lactose, sucrose and maltose, which on hydrolysis yield glucose, galactose and fructose. Sucrose feeding increases sucrase activity in rats (Blair et al. 1963; Deren et al. 1967). Similarly in man the specific activities of sucrase and maltase (but not lactase) can be regulated by specific dietary sugars (Rosensweig and Herman 1968, 1969, 1970).

The time interval for this adaptive enzyme activity is 2-5 days; the same time interval applied when the sugar was removed from the diet. As the time response is similar to the estimated renewal time of the human intestinal epithelium, Rosensweig and Herman (1969) postulated that the regulator effect of a dietary sugar occurs at the crypt cell level and becomes apparent as the crypt cells mature and migrate up the villus. Specific substrate is not required to produce an adaptive response as fructose produces an increase in sucrase and maltase activity identical to that observed with sucrose (Rosensweig and Herman 1968). There is a dose response of jejunal disaccharidase activity to dietary sucrose and glucose (Rosensweig and Herman 1970) using isocaloric diets.

Rosensweig and co-workers have also demonstrated that increased fructose feeding increases the enzymes involved in fructose metabolism, i.e., the glycolytic enzymes (Rosensweig *et al*. 1968, 1970; Shakespeare *et al*. 1969; Stifel *et al*. 1968 a,b; 1969). The adaptive response of the glycolytic enzymes commenced within a matter of hours and was complete in 24 hours (Rosensweig *et al*. 1969), which suggests that glycolytic enzyme adaptation occurs at the villus epithelial cell rather than the crypt cell level, as is the case with disaccharidase adaptation.

The mechanism of this adaptive response is not clear although inhibition of protein synthesis prevents adaptation (Grand and Jaksina 1973; Stifel *et al*. 1971). Folic acid produces significant increases in jejunal glycolytic enzymes but has no effect on disaccharidase activity.

Rosensweig and co-workers postulate that if dietary regulation of intestinal enzymes is a needed physiologic mechanism, malfunction of the regulation should be associated with gastrointestinal disorders. Such disorders may not be related to an enzyme deficiency but to a failure of the proper regulation of enzyme activity by normal exogenous stimuli such as diet. The possibility of an intestinal helminth contributing to that failure is an intriguing question that warrants careful consideration in any further dietary experimentation involving *H. diminuta*.

Changes in the proportions of protein, fat and carbohydrate ingested also have marked effects on the activity and level of specific enzymes. On a protein-free, high carbohydrate diet, urea cycle enzymes in the rat liver decrease 40-70% whereas under starvation conditions they are greatly increased (Schimke 1962). High carbohydrate diets decrease the concentration of enzymes controlling gluconeogenesis, the transaminases and serine dehydrogenase; the kinases involved in regulating glycolysis and acetyl-CoA-carboxylase increase (Kenney 1970).

C. Lipids

In the parasitized intestine, the total lipid content is 30% less than in uninfected rats. The lipid gradient itself, however, closely follows the pattern in uninfected animals, except for the terminal region of the ileum where the luminal lipid content in the parasitized animals increased (Mettrick 1971a).

VI. GUT MICROBIAL ECOLOGY

The microflora of the gastrointestinal tract exerts profound effects on the structure and function of the gut wall, host nutrition, ability to protect against potential pathogens, the development of the immune response and the activation of the reticuloendothelial system (Donaldson 1968; Rosenberg 1969; Broitman and Giannella 1971; Gordon and Pesti 1971; Mettrick and Podesta 1974). Bearing in mind that the evolution of the mammalian gut occurred in intimate association with the microflora (Dubos *et al.* 1963), it is not unreasonable to assume that any changes in the normal flora will result in a corresponding response by the intestinal mucosa influencing one or more of the functions enumerated above.

More than 60 bacterial species have been isolated from the gastro-intestinal tract of man and others are still being identified as experimental and diagnostic techniques improve.

In the small intestine, the flora is relatively sparse in comparison to other regions of the gut. The luminal contents of the duodenum and jejunum contain $10^1 - 10^4$ microbes/ml of gram positive organisms, i.e. aerobic and anaerobic lactobacilli, streptococci, staphylococci and yeasts (Draser et al. 1969; Gorbach et al. 1967). Small numbers of anaerobic fusiform and veilonellae may also be present.

The microflora of the terminal ileum represents a transition, both in number and type of bacteria, between the proximal small bowel and the colon. Hence, in addition to the gram positive flora characteristic of the duodenum and jejunum, facultative and true anaerobes predominate, i.e. coliforms, bacteroides and clostridia. In the colon, the flora is predominantly anaerobic and large in number (10^7/ml aerobes; 10^{10}/ml anaerobes) (Gorbach et al. 1967; Broitman and Giannella 1971; Williams et al. 1971; O'Grady and Vince 1971; Mallory et al. 1973a).

A number of factors, including diet, influence the nature of the luminal flora. In cases of intestinal resection large quantities of unabsorbed nutrients may reach the colon, with resulting changes in the composition of the colonic flora (Winawer et al. 1966). This situation is similar to the effect of *Hymenolepis diminuta* infections on luminal carbohydrate and protein digestion, which result in a significant increase of partially or non-hydrolyzed nutrient material in the distal ileum which passes into the colon in an undigested state (Mettrick 1971a).

Perhaps of greater significance to the host is the effect of the changes in the intraluminal environment, caused by the presence of *Hymenolepis diminuta*, on the intestinal bacterial population. The flora of the proximal small bowel is normally predominantly aerobic while that of the distal ileum (and colon) is anaerobic. The most important factor in the control of the size of the intestinal bacterial flora is the mechanical cleansing action due to intestinal peristalsis (Donaldson 1968). If, however, hypomotility occurs, there is bacterial overgrowth and a significant increase in the anaerobe population (Rosenberg 1969), implying that normal luminal oxygen tensions have been reduced. Motility and oxygen tensions are therefore related (Podesta and Mettrick 1974a). Aerobic intestinal microorganisms can be maintained by a pO_2 of 15 mm Hg although anaerobes are inhibited at this oxygen tension (Levitt 1970; Hentges and Maier 1972). The influence of oxygen on the bacterial fauna is mediated by its effect upon the oxidation-reduction potential (Eh) of the lumen, as anaerobes do not proliferate unless the Eh is below -200 mV (Broitman and Giannella 1971).

The low pH and high pO_2 (120 - 150 mm Hg) of the stomach maintains a gastric Eh which precludes the development of an anaerobic flora. Following feeding, highly acid oxygenated chyme is released into the proximal small intestine where rapid peristalsis and other host factors limit the development of a rich microflora. Intraluminal oxygen is therefore not sufficiently utilized by the aerobes to either reduce the Eh or to ameliorate the direct toxic effect of oxygen on the anaerobic microflora (Hentges and Maier 1972). In the terminal ileum, the flow of luminal contents is slowed by the ileocaecal valve and the population growth of aerobic and facultative anaerobes utilizes luminal oxygen, reduces the Eh and allows the anaerobes to flourish. The aerobic microorganisms are essential for this process (Levitt 1970). Water absorption from the luminal contents of the ileum results in solidification of the particulate matter and increased viscosity, leading to the development of an anoxic luminal core. This, with the action of the aerobes and facultative anaerobes in lowering the Eh, allows the obligate anaerobic bacteria to flourish (Broitman and Giannella 1971).

This sequence of interactions is upset by the presence of *Hymenolepis diminuta* in the small intestine (Podesta and Mettrick 1974a). The increased [H^+] of the parasitized gut due to H^+ secretion by the worms, enhances the antibactericidal action of the bile acids (Floch *et al.* 1970; Shimada *et al.* 1969) further reducing the flora of the proximal small bowel. Oxygen tension in the lumen therefore increases so that there are two pressures causing the Eh to approach or become positive in value; the second pressure is the [H^+] itself as an increase in [H$^+$] equivalent to one pH unit raises Eh by 57.7 mV. Water absorption by the ileal mucosa is diminished in the parasitized gut (Podesta and Mettrick 1974a, 1976a) so that the luminal contents of the distal small bowel do not increase in viscosity and oxygen is able to continue to freely diffuse into the lumen inhibiting the growth of the anaerobic bacteria. The overall result is a drastic reduction in the size of the microbial gut flora and significant changes in its composition in parasitized animals (Burmak 1970; Mettrick 1971a). What effect these changes in the microflora have on the structure and function of the gut wall, luminal nutrition, immune responses, etc. has not yet been determined.

While the intestinal microflora exerts limited effects on exogenous dietary components, they do contribute to the degradation of endogenous protein present in the lumen. A major portion of this endogenous protein is secreted digestive enzymes. Partial denaturation of these proteins occurs in the small bowel (Gitler 1964) and it has been suggested that bacterial enzymes are also important in the catabolism of proteins that reach the ileum and colon (Lundh 1958) such as occurs with *H. diminuta* infections. Amino acids liberated intraluminally during protein degradation may be carboxylated or deaminated by the intestinal microflora (Michel 1966). Similarly, the carbohydrate moieties of mucins have been shown to be degraded by the enteric flora of the rat intestine (Hoskins and Zamcheck 1968). Suggestions that the microflora contribute to or modify dietary lipids have not yet been unequivocally demonstrated (Broitman and Giannella 1971).

There is also evidence that a number of physiologically significant metabolites undergo a series of degradations in their passage through the gut. Cholesterol, bile salts, bilirubin and urea are all modified by bacterial action in the gut prior to reabsorption of the resulting metabolites. The intestinal microflora therefore plays an important role in the enterohepatic circulation of metabolites (Dietschy 1969; Drasar and Hill 1969; Lester and Troxler 1969; Phear and Ruebner 1956; Broitman and Giannella 1971). It seems likely that the reduced microflora of the parasitized gut will affect the sequence of degradation of metabolites involved in the enterohepatic circulation, resulting in changes in host physiology.

Another important aspect of the reduced microflora of the parasitized gut is the immunological mechanisms of the gastrointestinal tract and their relationship with the intestinal flora (Tomasi and Bienenstock 1968; Ginsberg 1971; Broitman and Giannella 1971; Fubara and Freter 1972; Berg and Savage 1972; Plant 1972; Quick *et al.* 1972; Tomasi and Grey 1972; Mettrick and Podesta 1974; Befus and Podesta 1976).

One aspect of the lives of parasitic animals which has no parallel among free living organisms is the capacity of the environment of a parasite to respond to that parasite in a manner detrimental to the continued survival of the parasite. Wakelin (1976) has recently reviewed the host immune responses to parasitic infections. The importance of host immune mechanisms for tissue and blood parasites has long been recognized; of much more recent recognition is the fact that intestinal parasites also have to cope with potentially lethal host immune responses (Befus and Podesta 1976). At present, we cannot answer the question whether changes in the intestinal microflora (and in mucosal structure) in helminth infections alter the potential of the immune response. It is, nonetheless, a question which will have to be answered if we are to understand further the nature of the intestinal environment for parasitic helminths. In this respect, the demonstration of mouse immunoglobulins binding to the tegumental surface of *Hymenolepis diminuta* and *H. microstoma* (Befus 1977) and of possible immunological damage to the tegument of *H. diminuta* in both mice and rats (Befus and Threadgold 1975) has confirmed that host immune mechanisms are involved in the survival of *H. diminuta* in its intestinal milieu. Befus and Podesta (1976) have suggested that pathophysiological alterations induced by parasites may depress the effectiveness of intestinal immune responses, and that the parasites' second strategy is to utilize some of the host responses as survival mechanisms. The immunoglobulins detected by Befus (1977) on the surface of *H. diminuta* may be both relatively host protective and worm protective antibodies; the interaction between them determines survival (Befus and Podesta 1976).

VII. REGULATION OF DIGESTION

The term 'homeostasis' covers the collective action of the tissues of the body in maintaining the composition of extracellular fluids constant (Cannon 1929) and a variety of feedback mechanisms have been described that are involved in the regulation of the internal environment. Olson (1975) pointed out that fluxes of metabolites and ions may change drastically as a result of environmental pressures in spite of the constancy of the concentrations in the extracellular fluid or plasma. Enzyme activity may then be activated to stabilize the intracellular milieu because not only must the constancy of the extracellular milieu be maintained, but the capacity of the tissues to perform their function must be adequate. In short, while first-order homeostasis may maintain the structure and composition of the extracellular phase, second-order homeostatic mechanisms are intracellular and may match the extent of variation that occurs in the external environment.

Exogenous food recruitment into the gastro-intestinal canal constitutes a significant perturbation of the external environment and it is well established that changes in the quality and quantity of the diet induce appropriate changes in the enzymatic activities of the tissues and organs associated with the gastrointestinal tract.

While it is possible that the dietary effects on enzyme levels could be mediated directly by the biochemical and substrate components of the diet, the evidence is that many nutritional effects on enzyme levels are mediated through hormonal regulation (Olson 1975). It is obvious that any changes in the biochemicals and substrates found in the intestinal lumen due to the presence of a parasitic organism are going to represent yet a further perturbation of the external environment and induce appropriate response by the extracellular and intracellular servomechanisms. For example, endocrine glands and the hypothalmus are very sensitive to variations in the components of blood plasma. Hypoglycaemia activates the growth hormone releasing factor (GRF) of the hypothalmus, which initiates growth hormone secretion by the anterior pituitary and glucagon secretion by the α-cells of the pancreas, but inhibits pancreatic insulin secretion. On the other hand, hypoglycaemia stimulates pancreatic insulin secretion and inhibits glucagon secretion; glucagon itself stimulates insulin release from the β-cells. Indirect effects on metabolism include the secretion of glucagon and growth hormone in response to hypoglycaemia which not only initiates reactions to return the blood sugar level to normal, but also acts to release fatty acids as an alternate fuel. In view of the fact that *H. diminuta* does affect blood plasma glucose levels (Mettrick 1972b; Dunkley and Mettrick 1977), it will be important to monitor endocrine responses to altered nutritional levels in order to fully understand the adaptive response of the host to the nutritional perturbations caused by the parasite.

Digestion is the primary event of the proximal intestine involving secretion, motility and absorption. Abnormalities in the secretory function, motility and absorption usually express themselves clinically, although it is important to realize that the reason for the abnormality may be local, that is, involved the intestine directly, or it may be due to failure of some part of the hormonal-vagal control system of digestion. The process of digestion is precisely coordinated during the passage of food through the small intestine. While the luminal conditions may not be optimum for any particular enzyme, it is assumed that the normal regional environments established through the mucosal-luminal fluxes of fluid, electrolytes, bile, etc. do provide the optimum balance allowing all of the numerous enzymes from the stomach, pancreas and mucosal epithelium to perform their allotted tasks. These secretory and propulsive activities are integrated through hormonal interaction and autonomic mechanisms which together create the appropriate luminal conditions to maximize the process of digestion.

A. *Gastrointestinal Hormones*

Recent studies on the gastrointestinal hormones suggest that they are not an isolated system, but are integrated with other secretory, endocrine and neuroendocrine systems (Dockray 1977). This view has important consequences in both the physiology of digestion and the pathology of intestinal diseases such as parasitic infections.

In the GI tract, two main groups of hormonal peptides can be distinguished on the basis of similarities in amino acid sequence. First, secretin and the pancreatic hormone glucagon (Mutt and Jorpes 1967a), and secondly, gastrin and cholecytokinin-pancreozymin (CCK-PZ) (Mutt and Jorpes 1967b). Two other polypeptides, vasoactive intestinal peptide (VIP) and gastric inhibitory polypeptide (GIP), related in structure to the first group, have also been identified (Brown and Dryburgh 1971; Said and Mutt 1972) and there may well be other peptides related to either group that are candidates for membership in the family of gut hormones (see review by Grossman and others 1974).

The biological actions shared by all members of the secretin-glucagon group include the inhibition of acid secretion and the stimulation of insulin release (Brown *et al.* 1975; Lin and Warwick 1971; Rehfeld 1972; Said 1975). The primary action of secretin is the stimulation of water and bicarbonate secretion from the exocrine pancreas, although full expression of its pancreatic effect depends on the presence of CCK-PZ (Grossman and Konturek 1974). The primary action of glucagon is stimulation of hepatic glycogenolysis and gluconeogenesis leading to hyperglycaemia (Falkner and Patent 1972).

Typical CCK-PZ actions are characterized by high potency on gall bladder and pancreas, but low potency on gastric acid secretion; those for gastrin are the reverse.

The distribution and concentration of secretin is greatest in the duodenum, decreasing with increased distance from the pyloric sphincter; there is virtually no secretin activity in the distal ileum (Friedman and Thomas 1950). There is a very close correlation between intra-duodenal pH and the degree of secretin release (Meyer *et al.* 1970 a,b) with direct correlation between the length of gut acidified and the amount of secretin released. It may confidently be predicted that secretin release is enhanced in the acidic parasitized small intestine. Vagal innervation facilitates release of secretin by acid (Henriksen and Rune 1969; Konturek *et al.* 1972).

The distribution of CCK-PZ corresponds closely to that of secretin and the hormone is believed to originate from the I-cells (Soleia *et al.* 1972). Peptone is the most potent release stimulus and one would expect to find the physiological releasers of CCK-PZ among luminal peptides, amino acids and fatty acids (Wang and Grossman 1951). Hydrochloric acid also stimulates CCK-PZ release (Barbezat and Grossman 1971). As with secretin, vagal innervation facilitates release of CCK-PZ in response to chemical agents; direct vagal action on CCK-PZ release is unlikely (Konturek *et al.* 1972; Moreland and Johnson 1971).

Gastrin I and II (Gregory and Tracy 1964) are released from the pyloric gland area of the stomach, although the duodenum may contain almost as much gastrin as the antrum (McGuigan 1968; Nilsson *et al.* 1971). The physiological release of gastrin is by vagal innervation and through chemical and mechanical stimulation of the antrum mucosa by gastric distension caused by the presence of food and protein in the stomach. There is a feedback regulatory mechanism with high stomach acidity inhibiting gastrin release; inhibition increases as pH decreases (Oberhelman *et al.* 1952; Grossman 1968). Gastrin secretion in response to cephalic stimulation involves a cholinergic release mechanism, while that associated with food includes a non-cholinergic release mechanism.

Considerable interaction among the gastrointestinal hormones obviously must occur as they are all secreted sequentially or simultaneously and all have various functions including mimicking or counteracting the effect of another hormone; pancreatic glucagon for example, mimics or counteracts most of the actions of secretin (Go and Summerskill 1971). A model for Hormonal-Neural-Gastrointestinal-Helminth interactions has been proposed, taking into account on the one hand the three major pathways for interactions presently identified between the gastrointestinal tract and the central nervous system; the gastrointestinal tract and the pancreas and between the central nervous system and the pancreas, together with the pathways by which *H. diminuta* directly or indirectly influences the digestive process (Mettrick 1973). Regulation of digestion depends on the gastrointestinal hormones acting in concert and continuously adjusting their effects on secretion, motility and absorption. The neural, hormonal and metabolic relationships with the extragastrointestinal organs further modify the coordination of digestive homeostasis; the presence of an intestinal helminth, such as *H. diminuta*, merely adds a further modulator influencing the already very complex coordination and homeostasis of digestive function. That *H. diminuta* does not cause a greater perturbation of the system than it does, reinforces the point that the gastrointestinal tract has very considerable powers of adaptation to physical, chemical and metabolic changes in the lumen.

B. *Luminal Homeostasis*

There is considerable evidence supporting homeostatic control of osmolality in the intestinal lumen (Mettrick and Podesta 1974; see above discussion). Similarly, homeostatic regulation of luminal lipids has been proposed (Karmen *et al.* 1963), although the evidence in support of such a process is weak. Cotton (1972) estimated that the lipid content of the intestinal lumen following feeding was mainly exogenous in source. Estimates of the amount of endogenous triglyceride fatty acids present in the lumen range from 15% (Blomstrand *et al.* 1964) to 43% (Karmen *et al.* 1963).

Homeostatic regulation of the luminal free amino acid pool has also proved controversial (see Mettrick and Podesta 1974). There is considerable endogenous recruitment of protein and amino acids into the lumen both via direct secretion or transport, and indirectly from exfoliated mucosal cells. Gent and Creamer (1972 a,b) suggested that endogenous protein recruitment was primarily from pancreatic secretions while endogenous amino acid recruitment was primarily by secretions from the Paneth cells. This may be the case, but such contributions do not appear to be sufficient to stabilize the diurnal changes in the luminal protein and amino acid pools (Mettrick 1970, 1971a, 1972 a,b; Nixon and Mawer 1970; Holdsworth 1972; Bielorai *et al.* 1972; Adibi and Mercer 1973; Alpers and Kinzie 1973; Grand and Jaksina 1973; Olson 1975). Intermittent feeding and fasting is characteristic of most animals and results in significant changes in the luminal environment. The counterperturbations, often mediated by the endocrine system, are equally characteristic of most animals. Diurnal changes in amino acid levels in the plasma do not relate directly to the time of feeding so that hormonal activity must play a role in their uptake and mobilization (Olson 1975). Adibi and Mercer (1973) considered that exogenous protein was primarily responsible for the increase in plasma amino acids, as well as the changes in the composition and concentration of the luminal free amino acid and peptide amino acid pools. As the mucosal concentration of amino acids is always lower than that of the lumen, a significant mucosal amino acid flux into the lumen may be discounted. Sanchez *et al.* (1972) found that the changes in the amino acid pool of the liver following a meal reflected the composition of the dietary protein, indicating that endogenous recruitment had not swamped exogenous recruitment to the luminal amino acid pool. There are, as discussed above, also significant differences in the luminal amino acid and peptide pools of uninfected and parasitized (*H. diminuta*) rats (Mettrick 1971a, 1972 a,b, 1975b). Addition of amino acid supplements to the diet or the feeding of a nutritionally unbalanced protein, affects the growth and development of *H. diminuta*, the effect of the amino acid supplement being directly related to the rate of its absorption by the intestinal mucosa (Mettrick and Munro 1965; Mettrick 1968, 1971b). This implies that the supplement was not counterbalanced by endogenous amino acids, and, as a result led to an imbalance in amino acid uptake by the worm resulting in impaired protein metabolism and growth. The positive rank correlation between the amino acids in the free amino acid pool of *H. diminuta* and that of the intestinal lumen, indicate that the worm has little selective capacity for amino acid uptake and is dependent on the composition of the luminal amino acid and peptide pools (Mettrick 1975b).

VIII. CONCLUSION

The process of digestion in the gastrointestinal canal involving hydrolysis of food products and absorption or reabsorption of exogenous and endogenous nutrients, fluids and electrolytes, is controlled at the level of the total organism through a cephalic mechanism mediated via the vagus and secondly, at the local level through intraluminal mechanisms initiated by the stimulation of mucosal receptors sensitive to chemical, osmotic and physical changes in the lumen. As the above account has indicated, individual components of the system are complex in operation; in their totality the actions and interactions occurring in the intestinal lumen are even more complex.

One of the striking things about the role and action of the gastrointestinal canal in digestion is the extent of adaptation that is possible by the organism to changes and fluctuations in the luminal environment. This is pertinent to a consideration of whether *H. diminuta* should be considered a parasite or an endocommensal.

It has been shown that at the level of the gastrointestinal tract and the extragastrointestinal organs, *Hymenolepis diminuta* markedly alters the intestinal nutritional (Mettrick 1971a, 1972 a,b, 1973) and absorptive gradients (Podesta and Mettrick 1976c), the quality and quantity of the intestinal microflora (Mettrick 1971a), the pH gradients (Mettrick 1971 c,d) and the oxidation reduction potential (Mettrick 1975b). Absorption of water, ions and glucose is markedly diminished in infected animals (Podesta and Mettrick 1974 a,b,c), resulting in alterations in blood and liver chemistry (Mettrich 1973; Dunkley and Mettrick 1977). Further, the proximal-distal absorptive gradients in the intestine are altered by *H. diminuta* (Podesta and Mettrick 1977c) as is the permeability of the parasitized intestinal mucosa (Podesta and Mettrick 1976b, 1977d). However, if one views the whole organism, there are neither clinical signs of infection and intestinal disease nor of marked weight loss with changes in feeding and excreta (Insler and Roberts 1976).

This apparent anomaly can be explained in terms of the adaptive capability of the intestine to respond to perturbations of the luminal environment. This explanation is supported by evidence of compensatory mechanisms in effect in the parasitized intestine which, for example, accelerate the glucose-stimulated component of salt and water absorption, enhance the bicarbonate-stimulated Na^+ and fluid absorption and extend the region of the gut involved in absorption of fluid, electrolytes and non-electrolytes (Podesta and Mettrick 1976a). Thus even when there is considerable maldigestion and malabsorption, alternative physiological mechanisms compensate for the defects caused by the parasite. Animal associations are a spectrum ranging from those truly free-living, through mutualism in which both partners benefit, commensalism in which the host shows no obvious ill effects to parasitism in which the host is clearly harmed by the parasite. However, to define harm or ill-effects simply in gross terms such as nutrient consumption, weight gain, etc. ignores the physiological stress that may have been placed upon the host animal by its parasite, and contributes little to our understanding of the totality of the host-parasite system in question. In the present case, *Hymenolepis diminuta* clearly causes significant changes in the physiology of digestion and may therefore be viewed as a pathophysiological agent. That the pathology is not more marked may be related to the highly-evolved and long-standing association between this worm and its host. We have come some way towards understanding the nature of this association, but as one aspect is unravelled, further complexities become exposed. It is no longer adequate to present elementary observations without attempting to relate them to physiological events occurring in the intestinal environment. Future progress in our knowledge of the biology of *H. diminuta* will go hand-in-hand with increased understanding of gastrointestinal function in health and disease.

ACKNOWLEDGMENTS

I an indebted to all my graduate students and post-doctoral associates who have contributed to the work cited in this review and to the National Research Council of Canada for their continued financial support.

REFERENCES

1. Adibi, S. A., and Mercer, D. W., Protein digestion in human intestine as reflected in luminal, mucosal and plasma amino acid concentrations after meals. *J. Clin. Invest. 52*, 1586-1594 (1973).
2. Adibi, S., Ruiz, C., Glazer, O., and Fogel, M., Effect of variation in intraluminal pH on absorption rates of amino acids, water and electrolytes in human jejunum. *Clin. Res. 19*, 654 (1971).
3. Albanese, R. A., On microelectrode distortion of oxygen tensions. *J. theor. Biol. 38*, 143-154 (1973).
4. Allen, A., and Snary, D., The structure and function of gastric mucus. *Gut 13*, 666-672 (1972).
5. Alpers, D. H., The relation of size to the relative rates of degradation of intestinal brush border proteins. *J. Clin. Invest. 51*, 2621-2630 (1972).
6. Alpers, D. H., and Kinzie, J. L., Regulation of small intestinal protein metabolism. *Gastroenterology 64*, 471-496 (1973).
7. Alpers, D. H., and Tedesco, F. J., The possible role of pancreatic proteases in the turnover of intestinal brush border proteins. *Biochim. Biophys. Acta 401*, 28-40 (1975).
8. Argenzio, R. O., and Stevens, C. E., Cyclic changes in ionic composition of digesta in the equine intestinal tract. *Am. J. Physiol. 228*, 1224-1230 (1975).
9. Arme, C., and Read, C. P., Fluxes of amino acids between the rat and a cestode symbiote. *Comp. Biochem. Physiol 24*, 1135-1147 (1969).

10. Arvenitakis, C., and Olsen, W. A., Intestinal mucosal disaccharidases in chronic pancreatitis. *Am. J. Dig. Dis. 19*, 417-421 (1974).
11. Arvenitakis, C., Ruhlen, J., Folscroft, J., and Rhodes, J. B., Digestion of tripeptides and disaccharides: Relationship with brush border hydrolysis. *Am. J. Physiol. 231*, 87-92 (1976).
12. Barbezat, G. O., and Grossman, M. I., Cholecystokinin released by duodenal acidification. *Gastroenterology 60*, 761 (1971).
13. Beck, I. T., The role of pancreatic enzymes in digestion. *Am. J. Clin. Nutr. 26*, 311-325 (1973).
14. Beck, I. T., McKenna, R. D., Zyeberszac, B., Solymar, J., and Eisenstein, S., The effect of trypsin inhibitor, trasylol, on the course of bile and trypsin induced pancreatitis in dogs. *Gastroenterology 48*, 478-483 (1965).
15. Beck, I. T., Pinter, E. J., Solymar, J., McKenna, R. D., and Ritchie, A. C., The role of pancreatic enzymes in the pathogenesis of acute pancreatitis. II. The fate of pancreatic proteolytic enzymes in the course of acute pancreatitis. *Gastroenterology 43*, 60-70 (1962).
16. Befus, A. D., *Hymenolepis diminuta* and *H. microstoma*: Mouse immunoglobulins binding to the tegumental surface. *Expl. Parasit. 41*, 242-251 (1977).
17. Befus, A. D., and Podesta, R. B., Intestine. In "Ecological Aspects of Parasitology" (C. R. Kennedy, ed.), pp. 303-325. North-Holland Publishing Company, Amsterdam, (1976).
18. Befus, A. D., and Threadgold, L. T., Possible immunological damage to the tegument of *Hymenolepis diminuta* in mice and rats. *Parasitology 71*, 525-534 (1975).
19. Bell, G. H., Davidson, J. N., and Scarborough, H., "Textbook of Physiology and Biochemistry". (5th Edit.) 1117p. Livingstone, Edinburgh, (1963).
20. Berg, R. D., and Savage, D. C., Immunological responses and microorganisms indigenous to the gastrointestinal tract. *Am. J. Clin. Nutr. 25*, 1364-1371 (1972).

21. Bergeim, O., Kleinberg, J., and Kirch, E. R., Oxidation-reduction potentials of the contents of the gastrointestinal tract. *J. Bact. 49*, 453-458 (1945).
22. Bergofsky, E. M., Determination of tissue oxygen tensions by hollow viscus tonometry: effect of breathing enriched oxygen mixtures. *J. Clin. Invest. 43*, 193-200 (1964).
23. Berntzen, A. K., *In vitro* cultivation of tapeworms. II. Growth and maintenance of *Hymenolepis diminuta* (Cestoda: Cyclophyllidea). *J. Parasit. 48*, 715-717 (1962).
24. Berntzen, A. K., and Mueller, J. F., *In vitro* cultivation of *Spirometra mansonoides* (Cestoda) from the procercoid to the early adult. *J. Parasit. 50*, 705-711 (1964).
25. Bielorai, R., Harduf, Z., and Alumot, E., The free amino acid pattern of the intestinal contents of ducks fed raw and heated soybean meal. *J. Nutr. 102*, 1377-1382 (1972).
26. Binder, H. J., and Rawlings, C. L., Electrolyte transport across isolated large intestinal mucosa. *Am. J. Physiol. 225*, 1232-1239 (1973).
27. Blair, D. G. R., and Tuba, J., Rat intestinal sucrase. I. Intestinal distribution and reaction kinetics. *Can. J. Biochem. Physiol. 41*, 905-916 (1963).
28. Blair, D. G. R., Yakimets, W., and Tuba, J., Rat intestinal sucrase. II. The effects of rat age and sex and of diet on sucrase activity. *Can. J. Biochem. Physiol. 41*, 917-929 (1963).
29. Blomstrand, R., Gurtlev, J., and Werner, B., Fatty acid esterification in man during fat absorption. *Acta chem. Scand. 18*, 1019-1021 (1964).
30. Borgström, B., Dahlquist, A., Lundh, G., and Sjovall, J., Studies of intestinal digestion and absorption in the human. *J. Clin. Invest. 36*, 1521-1536 (1957).
31. Broitman, S. A., and Giannella, R. A., Gut microbial ecology and its relationship to gastrointestinal disease. *In* "Topics in Medical Chemistry" (J. L. Rabinowitz and R. M. Myerson, eds.). Vol. 4, Absorption Phenomena, pp. 265-321. John Wiley and Sons, N.Y., (1971).
32. Brown, J. C., and Dryburgh, J. R., A gastric inhibitory polypeptide. II. The complete amino acid sequence. *Can. J. Biochem 49*, 867-872 (1971).

33. Brown, J. C., Dryburgh, J. R., Moccia, P., The current status of GIP. *In* "Gastrointestinal Hormones" (J. C. Thompson, ed.), pp. 537-547. Univ. of Texas Press, Austin, Texas, (1975).
34. Bryant, C., The utilization of carbon dioxide by *Moniezia expansa*: Aspects of metabolic regulation. *In* "Comparative Biochemistry of Parasites" (H. Van den Bossche, ed.), pp. 49-80. Academic Press, N.Y., (1972).
35. Bryant, C., Carbon dioxide utilization and the regulation of respiratory metabolic pathways in parasitic helminths. *In* "Advances in Parasitology" (B. Dawes, ed.), Vol. 13, pp. 36-70. Academic Press, London, (1975).
36. Burmak, S. A., [Interactions of *Hymenolepis nana* and microflora in the intestinal parasitocoenosis of white mice.] *Medskaya. Parazitol. 39*, 91-96 (1970).
37. Cannon, W. B., Organization for physiological homeostasis. *Physiol. Rev. 9*, 399-423 (1929).
38. Castro, G. I., Johnson, L. R., Copeland, E. M., and Dudrick, S. J., Course of infection with enteric parasites in hosts shifted from enteral to total parenteral nutrition. *J. Parasit. 62*, 353-359 (1976).
39. Chandler, A. C., Studies on the nutrition of tapeworms. *Am. J. Hyg. 37*, 123-130 (1943).
40. Chandler, A. C., Read, C. P., and Nicholas, H. O., Observation on certain phases of nutrition and host-parasite relations of *Hymenolepis diminuta* in white rats. *J. Parasit. 36*, 523-535 (1950).
41. Chappell, L. H., and Read, C. P., Studies on the free pool of amino acids of the cestode *Hymenolepis diminuta*. *Parasitology 67*, 289-305 (1973).
42. Cheng, H., Renewal of Paneth cells in the mouse intestine. *Anat. Rec. 163*, 168 (1969).
43. Clark, W. M., and Cohen, B., Studies on oxidation-reduction. II. An analysis of the theoretical relations between reduction potentials and pH. *Public Health Rep., Washington 38*, 666-670 (1923).
44. Cook, G. C., Comparison of intestinal absorption rates of glycine and glycylglycine in man and the effect of glucose in the perfusing fluid. *Clin. Sci. (Oxf.) 43*, 443-453 (1972).

45. Cook, R. M., Powell, P. M., and Moog, F., The influence of biliary stasis on the activity and distribution of maltase, sucrase, alkaline phosphatase and leucine aminopeptidase in the small intestine. *Gastroenterology 64*, 411-420 (1973).
46. Cooke, A. R., Nahrwold, D. L., and Grossman, M. I., Diversion of pancreatic response to a meal stimulus. *Am. J. Physiol. 214*, 637-639 (1967).
47. Corvalheira, A. F., Welsch, V., and Pearse, A. G. E., Cytochemical and ultrastructural observations on the argentaffine and argyrophil cells of the gastrointestinal tract in mammals, and their place in the APUD series of polypeptide-secreting cells. *Histochemie 14*, 33-42 (1968).
48. Cotton, P. B., Non-dietary lipid in the intestinal lumen. *Gut 13*, 675-681 (1972).
49. Crompton, D. W. T., The sites occupied by some parasitic helminths in the alimentary tract of vertebrates. *Biol. Rev. 48*, 27-83 (1973).
50. Crompton, D. W. J., Shrimpton, D. H., and Silver, I. A., Measurements of the oxygen tension in the lumen of the small intestine of the domestic duck. *J. Expl. Biol. 43*, 27-32 (1965).
51. Csâky, T. Z., Physiological considerations of the relationship between intestinal absorption of electrolytes and non-electrolytes. In "Intestinal Transport of Electrolytes, Amino Acids and Sugars" (W. McD. Armstrong and A. S. Nun, eds.), pp. 188-207. Thomas, Springfield, Ill., (1971).
52. Dahlquist, A., and Thomson, D. L., The digestion and absorption of sucrose by the intact rat. *J. Physiol. (Lond.) 167*, 193-209 (1963a).
53. Dahlquist, A., and Thompson, D. L., The digestion and absorption of maltose and trehalose by the intact rat. *Acta Physiol. Scand. 59*, 111-125 (1963b).
54. Das, B. C., and Gray, G. M., Intestinal sucrose: *in vivo* synthesis and degradation. *Clin. Res. 18*, 378 (1970).
55. Dawson, I., and Pryse-Davies, J., The distribution of certain enzyme systems in the normal human gastrointestinal tract. *Gastroenterology 44*, 745-760 (1963).

56. De Both, N. J., van Bongen, J. M., van Hofwegan, B., Keulemans, J., Visser, W. J., and Soljaard, J., The influence of various kinetic conditions on functional differentiation in the small intestine of the rat. A study of enzymes bound to subcellular organelles. *Dev. Biol. 38*, 119-137 (1974).
57. Deren, J. J., Broitman, S. A., and Zamcheck, N., Effect of diet upon intestinal disaccharidases and disaccharide absorption. *J. Clin. Invest. 46*, 186-195 (1967).
58. Dietschy, J. M., The role of the intestine in the control of cholesterol metabolism. *Gastroenterology 57*, 461-464 (1969).
59. Dockray, G. J., Molecular evolution of gut hormones: Application of comparative studies on the regulation of digestion. *Gastroenterology 72*, 344-358 (1977).
60. Donaldson, R. M., Role of indigenous enteric bacteria in intestinal function and disease. *In Handb. Physiol. 5* (Section 6), 2807-2837. Am. Physiol. Soc., Washington, D.C., (1968).
61. Dowling, R. H., and Small, D. M., The effect of pH on the solubility of varying mixtures of free and conjugated bile salts in solution. *Gastroenterology 54*, 1291 (1968).
62. Drasar, B. S., and Hill, M. J., Degradation of bile acids by human intestinal bacteria. *In* "Bile Salt Metabolism" (L. Schiff, J. B. Carey, and J. M. Dietschy, eds.), pp. 71-75. Thomas, Springfield, Ill., (1969).
63. Drasar, B. S., Shiner, M., and McLeod, G. M., Studies on the intestinal flora. I. The bacterial flora of the gastrointestinal tract in healthy and achlorhydric persons. *Gastroenterology 56*, 71-79 (1969).
64. Drost-Hansen, W., Role of water-structure in cell-wall interactions. *Fed. Proc. Fedn. Am. Socs. exp. Biol. 30*, 1539-1548 (1971).
65. Dubos, R., Schaedler, R. W., and Costello, R., Composition, alteration and effects of the intestinal flora. *Fedn. Proc. Fedn. Am. Socs. exp. Biol. 22*, 1322-1329 (1963).
66. Dunkley, L. C., and Mettrick, D. F., *Hymenolepis diminuta*: Effect of quality of host dietary carbohydrate on growth. *Expl. Parasit. 25*, 146-161 (1969).

67. Dunkley, L. C., and Mettrick, D. F., Effect of dietary carbohydrate intake on the growth of *Hymenolepis diminuta* (Cestoda) in the laboratory rat. *Can. J. Zool.* 54, 1073-1078 (1976).
68. Dunkley, L. C., and Mettrick, D. F., *Hymenolepis diminuta*: Migration, and the rat host's intestinal and blood plasma glucose levels following dietary carbohydrate intake. *Expl. Parasit.* 41, 213-228 (1977).
69. Faelli, A., and Esposito, G., Bicarbonate and transintestinal potential difference of the jejunum of rat intestine incubated "*in vitro*". *Proc. 1st European Biophys. Congr.* 3, 317-321 (1971).
70. Falkner, S., and Patent, G. J., Comparative and embryological aspects of the pancreatic islets. *In Handb. Physiol.* 1 (Section 7), 1-23. Am. Physiol. Soc., Washington, D.C., (1972).
71. Fanconneau, G., and Michel, M. C., Role of the gastrointestinal tract in regulation of protein metabolism. *In* "Mammalian Protein Metabolism" (H. N. Munro, ed.), Vol. 4, pp. 481-522. Academic Press, N.Y., (1970).
72. Faust, R. G., and Wu, S. L., The effect of bile salts on oxygen consumption, oxidative phosphorylation and ATPase activity of mucosal homogenates from rat jejunum and ileum. *J. Cell. Physiol.* 67, 149-158 (1966).
73. Faust, R. G., Shearin, S. J., and Misch, D. W., Sodium-dependent binding of D-glucose to filamentous fraction of tris-disrupted brush border from hamster jejunum. *Biochim. Biophys. Acta* 255, 685-690 (1972).
74. Fern, E. B., Hider, R. C., and London, D. R., The sites of hydrolysis of dipeptides containing leucine and glycine by rat jejunum *in vitro*. *Biochem. J.* 114, 855-861 (1969).
75. Fisher, R. B., Absorption of proteins. *Br. Med. Bull.* 28, 241-246 (1967).
76. Floch, M. H., Gershengoren, W., Diamond, S., and Hersh, T., Cholic acid inhibition of intestinal bacteria. *Am. J. Clin. Nutr.* 23, 8-10 (1970).
77. Fogel, M. R., and Adibi, S. A., Varied alteration in transport of free amino acids and dipeptides by the acidic intraluminal pH in human intestine. *Gastroenterology* 62, 747 (1972).

78. Forssmann, W. G., Orci, L., Pictet, R., Renold, A. E., and Rouiller, C., The endocrine cells in the epithelium of the gastrointestinal mucosa of the rat. An electron microscope study. *J. Cell. Biol. 40*, 692-715 (1969).
79. Forth, W., Rummel, W., and Glasner, H., Zur resorptions hemmenden Wirkung von Gallensaüren. Naunyn-Schmiedeberg's. *Arch. exp. Path. Pharmak. 254*, 364-380 (1966).
80. Frazier, L. W., and Vanatta, J. C., Characteristics of H^+ and NH_4^+ excretion by the urinary bladder of the toad. *Biochem. Biophys. Acta 311*, 98-108 (1973).
81. Friedman, M. H. F., and Thomas, J. E., The assay and distribution of secretin. *J. Lab. Clin. Med. 35*, 366-372 (1950).
82. Fritz, M. E., and Brooks, F. P., Control of bile flow in the cholecystectomized dog. *Am. J. Physiol. 204*, 825-828 (1963).
83. Fubara, E. S., and Freter, R., Source and protective function of coproantibodies in intestinal disease. *Am. J. Clin. Nutr. 25*, 1357-1363 (1972).
84. Fuji, R., Quantification of the number of villi and crypts in the intestine of rodent animals. *Experientia 28*, 1209-1210 (1972).
85. Furuya, S., and Yugari, Y., Daily rhythmic change in the transport of histidine by everted sacs of rat small intestine. *Biochim. Biophys. Acta 241*, 245-248 (1971).
86. Furuya, S., and Yugari, Y., Daily rhythmic changes of L-histidine and glucose absorption in rat small intestine *in vivo*. *Biochim. Biophys. Acta 343*, 558-564 (1974).
87. Gent, A. E., and Creamer, B., Paneth cell secretion. *Digestion 7*, 1-12 (1972a).
88. Gent, A. E., and Creamer, B., Amino acid homeostasis in the small intestine. I. Studies in the rat. *Digestion 7*, 13-23 (1972b).
89. Geratz, J. D., and Hurt, J. P., Regulation of pancreatic enzyme levels by trypsin inhibitors. *Am. J. Physiol. 219*, 705-711 (1970).
90. Ginger, C. D., and Fairbairn, D., Lipid metabolism in helminth parasites. II. The major origins of the lipids of *Hymenolepis diminuta* (Cestoda). *J. Parasit. 52*, 1097-1107 (1966).

91. Ginsberg, A. L., Alterations in immunologic mechanisms in diseases of the gastrointestinal tract. *Am. J. Dig. Dis. 16*, 61-80 (1971).
92. Gitler, C., Protein digestion and absorption in non-ruminants. *In* "Mammalian Protein Metabolism" (H. N. Munro and J. B. Allison, eds.), Vol. 1, pp. 35-69. Academic Press, N.Y., (1964).
93. Gitler, C., and Martinez-Rojas, D., The absorption of amino-acid mixtures from the small intestine of the rat. *In* "The Role of the Gastrointestinal Tract in Protein Metabolism" (H. N. Munro, ed.), pp. 269-281. Blackwell, Oxford, (1964).
94. Go, V. L. W., and Summerskill, W. H. J., Digestion, maldigestion and the gastrointestinal hormones. *Am. J. Clin. Nutr. 24*, 160-167 (1971).
95. Goldberg, D. M., Campbell, R., and Roy, A. D., Binding of trypsin and chymotrypsin by human intestinal mucosa. *Biochim. Biophys. Acta 167*, 613-615 (1968).
96. Goldberg, D. M., Campbell, R., and Roy, A. D., Studies on the binding of trypsin and chymotrypsin by human intestinal mucosa. *Scand. J. Gastroent. 4*, 217-226 (1969).
97. Gorbach, S. L., Plant, A. G., Nahus, L., Weinstein. L., Spanknevel, G., and Levitan, R., Studies of intestinal microflora. II. Microorganisms of the small intestine and their relations to oral and fecal flora. *Gastroenterology 53*, 856-867 (1967).
98. Gordon, H. A., and Pesti, L., The gnotobiotic animal as a tool in the study of host microbial relationships. *Bact. Rev. 35*, 390-443 (1971).
99. Gossrau, R., Enzyme histochemistry of the intestinal brush border. *Acta Histochem. Cytochem. 8*, 153-163 (1975).
100. Gotze, H., Adelson, J. H., Hadorn, H. B., Portmann, R., and Troesch, V., Hormone-elicited enzyme release by the small intestinal wall. *Gut 13*, 471-476 (1972).
101. Gracey, M., Burke, V., and Oschin, A., Reversible inhibition of intestinal active sugar transport by deconjugated bile salt *in vivo*. *Biochim. Biophys. Acta 225*, 308-314 (1971a).

102. Gracey, M., Burke, V., and Oschin, A., Influence of bile salts on intestinal sugar transport *in vivo*. *Scand. J. Gastroent.* 6, 273-276 (1971b).
103. Gracey, M., Burke, V., Oschin, A., Barker, J., and Glasgow, E. F., Bacteria, bile salts, and intestinal monosaccharide malabsorption. *Gut* 12, 683-692 (1971c).
104. Grand, R. J., and Jaksina, S., Additional studies on the regulation of carbohydrate dependent enzymes in the jejunum: changes in amino acid pools, protein synthesis, and the effect of actinomycin-D. *Gastroenterology* 64, 429-437 (1973).
105. Gray, G. M., and Cooper, H. L., Protein digestion and absorption. *Gastroenterology* 61, 535-544 (1971).
106. Gregory, R. A., and Tracy, H. J., The constitution and properties of two gastrins extracted from hog antral mucosa. *Gut* 5, 103-117 (1964).
107. Grossman, M. I., Neural and hormonal stimulation of gastric secretion of acid. *In Handb. Physiol.* 2 (Section 6), pp. 835-863. Amer. Physiol. Soc., Washington, D.C., (1968).
108. Grossman, M. I., and Konturek, S. J., Gastric acid does drive pancreatic bicarbonate secretion. *Scand. J. Gastroent.* 9, 299-302 (1974).
109. Grossman, M. I., and Others, Candidate hormones of the gut. *Gastroenterology* 67, 730-755 (1974).
110. Hadorn, B., Tarlow, M. J., Lloyd, J. K., and Wolff, O. H., Intestinal enterokinase deficiency. *Lancet* 1, 812-813 (1969).
111. Hadorn, B., Steiner, N., Sumida, C., and Peters, T. J., Intestinal enterokinase. Mechanisms of its "secretion" into the lumen of the small intestine. *Lancet* 1, 165-166 (1971).
112. Hamilton, J. D., Dawson, A. M., and Webb, J. C. W., Observations upon small gut "mucosal" pO_2 and pCO_2 in anesthetized dogs. *Gastroenterology* 55, 52-60 (1968).
113. Harper, A. A., Hormonal control of pancreatic secretion. *In Handb. Physiol.* 2 (Section 6), pp. 969-995. Am. Physiol. Soc., Washington, D.C., (1967).

114. Harper, A. E., Amino acid toxicities and imbalances. *In* "Mammalian Protein Metabolism" (H. N. Munro and J. B. Allison, eds.), Vol. II, pp. 87-134. Academic Press, N.Y., (1964).
115. Harries, J. T., and Sladen, G. E., The effects of different bile salts on the absorption of fluid, electrolytes and monosaccharides in the small intestine of the rat *in vivo*. *Gut* 13, 596-603 (1972).
116. Harrison, D. D., and Webster, H. L., Proximal to distal variations in enzymes of the rat intestine. *Biochim. Biophys. Acta* 244, 432-436 (1971).
117. Haverback, B. J., Dyce, B., Bundy, H., and Edmondson, H. A., Trypsin, trypsinogen and trypsin inhibitor in human pancreatic juice. Mechanism for pancreatitis associated with hyper-parathyroidism. *Am. J. Med.* 29, 424-433 (1960).
118. Henriksen, F. W., and Rune, S. J., Cholinergic effect on the canine pancreatic response to acidification of the duodenum. *Scand. J. Gastroent.* 4, 203-208 (1969).
119. Hentges, D. J., and Maier, B. R., Theoretical basis for anaerobic methodology. *Am. J. Clin. Nutr.* 25, 1299-1305 (1972).
120. Hepner, G. W., and Hofmann, A. F., Different effects of free and conjugated bile acids and their keto derivatives on (Na^+, K^+) - stimulated and Mg^{++} - ATPase of rat intestinal mucosa. *Biochim. Biophys. Acta* 291, 237-245 (1973).
121. Hislop, I. G., Hofmann, A. F., and Shoenfield, L. J., Determinants of the rate and site of bile acid absorption in man. *J. Clin. Invest.* 46, 1070-1071 (1967).
122. Hofman, A. F., Functions of bile in the alimentary canal. *In Handb. Physiol.* 5 (Section 6), pp. 2507-2533. Am. Physiol. Soc., Washington, D.C., (1968).
123. Holdsworth, C. D., Absorption of protein, amino acids and peptides - a review. *In* "Transport across the Intestine" (W. L. Burland and P. D. Samuel, eds.), pp. 136-152. Churchill-Livingstone, Edinburgh, (1972).
124. Hopkins, C. A., and Callow, L. L., Methionine flux between a tapeworm *(Hymenolepis diminuta)* and its environment. *Parasitology* 55, 653-666 (1965).

125. Hoskins, L. C., and Zamcheck, N., Bacterial degradation of gastrointestinal mucins. I. Comparison of mucus constituents in the stools of germfree and conventional rats. *Gastroenterology 54*, 210-217 (1968).
126. Hubel, K. A., Bicarbonate secretion in rat ileum and its dependence on intraluminal chloride. *Am. J. Physiol. 213*, 1409-1413 (1967).
127. Hubel, K. A., Effect of luminal chloride concentration on bicarbonate secretion in rat ileum. *Am. J. Physiol. 217*, 40-45 (1969).
128. Hubel, K. A., Dependence of bicarbonate absorption on intraluminal sodium in rat jejunum. *Gastroenterology 62*, 764 (1972).
129. Hubel, K. A., Effect of luminal sodium concentration on bicarbonate absorption in rat jejunum. *J. Clin. Invest. 52*, 3172-3179 (1973).
130. Huber, R., Kukla, D., Rühlmann, A., Epp, O., and Formanek, H., The basic trypsin inhibitor of bovine pancreas. I. Structure analysis and conformation of the polypeptide chain. *Naturwissenschaften 57*, 389-397 (1970).
131. Insler, G. D., and Roberts, L. S., *Hymenolepis diminuta*: Lack of pathogenicity in the healthy rat host. *Expl. Parasit. 39*, 351-357 (1976).
132. Isselbacher, K. J., The intestinal cell surface: Some properties of normal undifferentiated and malignant cells. *Ann. Int. Med. 81*, 681-686 (1974).
133. Jackson, M. M., Levin, R. J., and Thompson, E., The influence of pH on intestinal metabolism and transport *in vivo*. *J. Physiol. (Lond.) 197*, 168-178 (1968a).
134. Jackson, M. M., Levin, R. J., and Thompson, E., A comparison of the effects of pH on the absorptive and metabolic functions of the jejunum and ileum *in vitro*. *J. Physiol. (Lond.) 201*, 38p (1968b).
135. James, W. P. T., Alpers, D. H., Gerber, J. E., and Isselbacher, K. J., The turnover of disaccharidases and brush border proteins in rat intestine. *Biochim. Biophys. Acta 230*, 194-203 (1971).
136. Jervis, J. R., Enzymes in the mucosa of the small intestine of the rat, guinea-pig and the rabbit. *J. Histochem. Cytochem. 111*, 692-699 (1963).

137. Jones, R. S., and Grossman, M. I., The choleretic response to feeding in dogs. *Proc. Soc. exp. Biol. Med. 132*, 708-711 (1969a).
138. Jones, R. S., and Grossman, M. I., Choleretic effects of secretin and histamine in the dog. *Am. J. Physiol. 217*, 532-535 (1969b).
139. Jones, R. S., and Grossman, M. I., Choleretic effects of cholecystokinin, gastrin II and caerulin in the dog. *Am. J. Physiol. 219*, 1014-1018 (1970).
140. Jones, R. S., Geist, R. E., and Hall, A. D., The choleretic effects of glucagon and secretin in the dog. *Gastroenterology 60*, 64-68 (1971).
141. Jos, J., Trézal, J., Rey, J., and Lamy, M., Histochemical localization of intestinal disaccharidases: application to peroral biopsy specimen. *Nature 213*, 516-518 (1967).
142. Joyner, W. L., and Kokas, E., Effect of various gastrointestinal hormones and vasoactive substances on villous motility. *Comp. Biochem. Physiol. 46*, 171-181 (1973).
143. Kaback, H. R., Transport. *Ann. Rev. Biochem. 39*, 561-598 (1970).
144. Karmen, A., White, M., and Goodman, D. S., Fatty acid esterification and chylomicron formation during fat absorption. I. Triglycerides and cholesterol esters. *J. Lipid Res. 4*, 312-321 (1963).
145. Keller, P. J., Pancreatic proteolytic enzymes. In *Handb. Physiol. 5* (Section 6), pp. 2605-2627. Am. Physiol. Soc. Washington, D.C., (1968).
146. Kenney, F. T., Hormonal regulation of synthesis of liver enzymes. In "Mammalian Protein Metabolism" (H. N. Munro, ed.), Vol. 4, pp. 131-176. Academic Press, N.Y., (1970).
147. Kofoid, C. A., McNeil, E., and Caillean, R., Electrometric pH determination of the walls and contents of the gastro-intestinal tracts of normal albino rats. *Univ. Calif. Publs. Zool. 36*, 347-355 (1932).
148. Konturek, S. J., Radecki, T., Biernat, J., and Thor, P., Effect of vagotomy on pancreatic secretion evoked by endogenous and exogenous cholecystokinin and caerulein. *Gastroenterology 63*, 273-278 (1972).

149. Korn, E. D., Cell membranes: structure and synthesis. *Ann. Rev. Biochem. 38*, 263-288 (1969).
150. Kronfeld, D. S., and Van Soest, P. J., Carbohydrate Nutrition. *In:* "Comparative Animal Nutrition." I. Carbohydrates, lipids and accessory growth factors (M. Recheigl, Jr., ed.), pp. 23-73. S. Karger, Basel, (1976).
151. Laurie, J., The *in vitro* fermentation of carbohydrates by two species of cestodes and one species of acanthocephala. *Expl. Parasit. 6*, 245-260 (1957).
152. Lease, H. J., and Mansford, K. R. L., The effect of insulin and insulin deficiency on the transport and metabolism of glucose by rat small intestine. *J. Physiol. (Lond.) 212*, 819-838 (1971).
153. Leblond, C. P., and Messier, P., Renewal of chief cells and goblet cells in the small intestine as shown by radioautography after injection of thymidine-H^3 into mice. *Anat. Record 132*, 247-259 (1958).
154. Lee, J. S., Contraction of villi and fluid transport in dog jejunial mucosa *in vitro*. *Am. J. Physiol. 221*, 488-495 (1971).
155. Lester, R., and Troxler, R. F., Recent advances in bile pigment metabolism. *Gastroenterology 56*, 143-169 (1969).
156. Levitt, M. D., Oxygen tension in the gut. *New Engl. J. Med. 282*, 1039-1040 (1970).
157. Lin, T. M., and Warwick, M., Effect of glucagon on pentagistrin-induced gastric acid secretion and mucosal blood flow in the dog. *Gastroenterology 61*, 328-331 (1971).
158. Lipkin, M., and Bell, B., Cell proliferation. *In Handb. Physiol.* 5 (Section 6), pp. 2861-2879. Am. Physiol. Soc., Washington, D.C., (1968).
159. Lipkin, M., Sherlock, P., and Bell, B., Cell proliferation kinetics in the gastrointestinal tract of man. II. Cell renewal in stomach, ileum, colon and rectum. *Gastroenterology 45*, 721-729 (1963).
160. Lis, M. T., Crompton, R. F., and Matthews, D. M., Effect of dietary changes on intestinal absorption of L-methionine and L-methionyl-L-methionine in the rat. *Br. J. Nutr. 27*, 159-167 (1972).

161. Loehry, C. A., and Creamer, B., Three dimensional structure of the human small intestinal mucosa in health and disease. *Gut 10*, 6-12 (1969).
162. Loehry, C. A., Croft, D. N., Sing, A. K., and Creamer, B., Cell turnover in the rat small intestine mucosa: An appraisal of cell loss. *Gut 10*, 13-18 (1969).
163. Lubbers, D. W., The meaning of the tissue oxygen distribution curve and its measurement by means of Pt. electrodes. *Prog. resp. Res. 3*, 112-123 (1968).
164. Lumsden, R. D., and Harrington, G. W., Incorporation of linoleic acid by the cestode *Hymenolepis diminuta* (Rudolphi, 1819). *J. Parasit. 52*, 695-700 (1966).
165. Lundh, G., Intestinal digestion and absorption after gastrectomy. *Acta Chir. Scand.*, *Suppl. 231*, 5-80 (1958).
166. MacDonald, W. C., Trier, J. S., and Everett, N. B., Cell proliferation and migration in stomach, duodenum and rectum of man: radioisotope studies. *Gastroenterology 46*, 405-417 (1964).
167. Mackenzie, I. L., and Donaldson, R. M., Effect of divalent cations and pH on intrinsic factor mediated attachment of vitamin B_{12} to intestinal microvillous membranes. *J. Clin. Invest. 51*, 2465-2471 (1972).
168. Maggi, P., Brue, F., Broussalle, B., Bensimon, E., and Peres, G., Les tensions d'O_2 et de CO_2 au niveau de l'epithelium intestinal du rat au cours d'experiences d'absorption *in vivo*. Effects de l'hyperoxie et de l'hypercaprice. *C.R.Seanc. Soc. Biol. 164*, 2285-2287 (1970).
169. Mallory, A., Savage, D., Kern, F., and Smith, J. G., Patterns of bile acids and microflora in the human small intestine. II. Microflora. *Gastroenterology 64*, 34-42 (1973a).
170. Mallory, A., Kern, F., Smith, J., and Savage, D., Patterns of bile acids and microflora in the human small intestine. I. Bile acids. *Gastroenterology 64*, 26-33 (1973b).
171. Matthews, D. M., Rates of peptide uptake by small intestine. In "Peptide Transport in Bacteria and Mammalian Gut" (K. Elliot and M. O'Conner, eds.), pp. 71-92. Ciba Foundation Symp., Assoc. Sci. Publ., Amsterdam, (1972).

172. McGuigan, J. E., Gastric mucosal intracellular localization of gastrin by immunofluorescence. *Gastroenterology* 55, 315-327 (1968).
173. McHardy, G. J. R., and Parsons, D. S., The absorption of water and salt from the small intestine of the rat. *Q. J. exp. Physiol. 42*, 33-48 (1957).
174. Merzel, J., and Leblond, C. P., Renewal of goblet cells in the small intestine of the mouse. *Anat. Record 160*, 393-394 (1968).
175. Mettrick, D. F., Studies on the protein metabolism of cestodes. 2. Effect of free dietary amino acid supplements on the growth of *Hymenolepis diminuta*. *Parasitology 58*, 37-45 (1968).
176. Mettrick, D. F., Protein, amino acid and carbohydrate gradients in the rat intestine. *Comp. Biochem. Physiol. 37*, 517-541 (1970).
177. Mettrick, D. F., *Hymenolepis diminuta*: The microbiota, nutritional and physico-chemical gradients in the small intestine of uninfected and parasitized rats. *Can. J. Physiol. Pharmacol. 49*, 972-984 (1971a).
178. Mettrick, D. F., *Hymenolepis diminuta*: Quantity of host amino acid dietary supplement and growth. *Expl. Parasit. 29*, 13-25 (1971b).
179. Mettrick, D. F., Effect of host dietary constituents on intestinal pH and on the migrational behaviour of the rat tapeworm *Hymenolepis diminuta*. *Can. J. Zool. 49*, 1513-1525 (1971c).
180. Mettrick, D. F., *Hymenolepis diminuta*: pH changes in rat intestinal contents and worm migration. *Expl. Parasit. 29*, 386-401 (1971d).
181. Mettrick, D. F., Changes in some of the characteristics of the intestinal microcosm due to parasitic infection. *West Ind. Med. J. 21*, 95-104 (1972a).
182. Mettrick, D. F., Changes in the distribution and chemical composition of *Hymenolepis diminuta*, and in the intestinal nutritional gradients of uninfected and parasitized rats following a glucose meal. *J. Helminth. 46*, 407-429 (1972b).
183. Mettrick, D. F., Competition for ingested nutrients between the tapeworm *Hymenolepis diminuta* and the rat host. *Can. J. Pub. Health 64*, 70-82 (1973).

184. Mettrick, D. F., *Hymenolepis diminuta*: Effect of oxidation-reduction potential in the mammalian gastrointestinal canal. *Expl. Parasit. 37*, 223-232 (1975a).
185. Mettrick, D. F., Correlations between the amino acid pools of *Hymenolepis diminuta* and the rat intestine. *Can. J. Zool. 53*, 320-331 (1975b).
186. Mettrick, D. F., and Dunkley, L. C., Variation in the size and position of *Hymenolepis diminuta* (Cestoda: Cyclophyllidea) within the rat intestine. *Can. J. Zool. 47*, 1091-1101 (1969).
187. Mettrick, D. F., and Munro, H. N., Studies on the protein metabolism of cestodes. I. Effect of host dietary constituents on the growth of *Hymenolepis diminuta*. *Parasitology 55*, 453-466 (1965).
188. Mettrick, D. F., and Podesta, R. B., Ecological and Physiological Aspects of Helminth-Host interactions in the Mammalian Gastrointestinal Canal. *Advances in Parasitology* (B. Dawes, ed.), Vol. 12, pp. 183-278. Academic Press, London (1974).
189. Meyer, J. H., Interactions of dietary fibre and protein on food intake and body composition of growing rats. *Am. J. Physiol. 193*, 488-494 (1958).
190. Meyer, J. H., Way, L. W., and Grossman, M. I., Pancreatic bicarbonate response to various acids in the duodenum. *Am. J. Physiol. 219*, 964-970 (1970a).
191. Meyer, J. H., Way, L. W., and Grossman, M. I., Pancreatic response to acidification of various lengths of proximal intestine in the dog. *Am. J. Physiol. 219*, 971-977 (1970b).
192. Michel, M. C., Metabolisme de la flore intestinale du porc. Degradation des formes L et D des acides amines. *Ann. Biol. Animale Biochem. Biophys. 6*, 33-42 (1966).
193. Moreland, H. J., and Johnson, L. R., Effect of vagotomy on pancreatic secretion stimulated by endogenous and exogenous secretin. *Gastroenterology 60*, 425-431 (1971).
194. Mutt, V., and Jorpes, J. E., Contemporary developments in the biochemistry of the gastrointestinal hormones. *Recent Prog. Horm. Res. 23*, 483-495 (1967a).

195. Mutt, V., and Jorpes, J. E., Isolation of aspartyl-phenylalanine amide from cholecystokinin-pancreozymin. *Biochem. Biophys. Res. Commun.* 26, 392-397 (1967b).
196. Nachlas, M. M., Monis, B., Rosenblatt, D., and Seligman, A. M., Improvement in the histochemical localization of leucine aminopeptidase with a new substrate, L-leucyl-4-methoxy-Z-naphthylamide. *J. Biophys. Biochem. Cytol.* 7, 261-264 (1960).
197. Nahrwold, D. L., and Grossman, M. I., Secretion of bile in response to food with an without bile in the intestine. *Gastroenterology* 53, 11-17 (1967).
198. Nasset, E. S., Schwartz, P. S., and Weiss, H. V., The digestion of proteins in $vivo$. *J. Nutr.* 56, 83-94 (1955).
199. Nilsson, G., Yalow, R. S., and Berson, S. A., Distribution of gastrin in the gastrointestinal tract of human, dog, cat and hog. *In* "Nobel Symposium XVI, Frontiers in Gastrointestinal Hormone Research" (S. Andersson, ed.), pp. 95-101. Almquist and Wiksell, Uppsala, Sweden, (1971).
200. Nixon, S. E., and Nawer, G. E., The digestion and absorption of proteins in man. I. The site of absorption. *Br. J. Nutr.* 24, 227-240 (1970).
201. Nordström, C., Enzymic release of enteropeptidase from isolated rat duodenal brush borders. *Biochim. Biophys. Acta* 268, 711-768 (1972a).
202. Nordström, C., Release of enteropeptidase and other brush-border enzymes from the small intestinal wall in the rat. *Biochim. Biophys. Acta* 289, 367-377 (1972b).
203. Nordström, C., and Dahlqvist, A., Quantitative distribution of some enzymes along villi and crypts of the small intestine. *Scand. J. Gastroent.* 8, 407-416 (1973).
204. Nordström, C., Dahlqvist, A., and Josefsson, L., Quantitative determination of enzymes in different parts of the villi and crypts of rat small intestine. Comparison of alkaline phosphatase, disaccharidases and dipeptidases. *J. Histochem. Cytochem.* 15, 713-721 (1968).
205. Oberhelman, H. A., Woodward, E. R., Zubiran, J. M., and Dragstedt, L. R., Physiology of the gastric antrum. *Am. J. Physiol.* 169, 738-748, (1952).

206. O'Grady, F., and Vince, A., Clinical and nutritional significance of intestinal bacterial overgrowth. *J. Clin. Path.* 24, suppl. 5, 130-137 (1971).
207. Olson, R. E., Introductory remarks: nutrient, hormone, enzyme interactions. *Am. J. Clin. Nutr.* 28, 626-637 (1975).
208. Padykula, H. A., Strauss, E. W., Ladman, A. J., and Gardner, F. H., A morphologic and histochemical analysis of the human jejunal epithelium in non-tropic sprue. *Gastroenterology* 40, 735-763 (1961).
209. Page, C. R., MacInnis, A. J., and Griffith, L. M., Diurnal periodicity of uridine uptake by *Hymenolepis diminuta*. *J. Parasit.* 63, 91-95 (1977).
210. Palade, G. E., Siekevitz, P., and Caro, L. G., Structure, chemistry and function of the pancreatic exocrine cell. In "Ciba Foundation Symposium on Exocrine Pancreas" (A. V. S. DeReuck and M. P. Cameron, eds.), pp. 23-49 Churchill, London, (1962).
211. Pappas, P. W., and Read, C. P., Trypsin inactivation by intact *Hymenolepis diminuta*. *J. Parasit.* 58, 864-871 (1972a).
212. Pappas, P. W., and Read, C. P., Inactivation of α- and β-chymotrypsin by intact *Hymenolepis diminuta* (Cestoda). *Biol. Bull.* 143, 605-616 (1972b).
213. Parkinson, T. M., and Olson, J. A., Inhibitory effects of bile acids on adenosine triphosphatase, oxygen consumption and the transport and diffusion of water soluble substances in the small intestine of the rat. *Life Sci.* 3, 107-112 (1964).
214. Parsons, D. S., Salt transport. *J. Clin. Path.* 24, suppl. 5, 90-98 (1971).
215. Parsons, D. S., and Boyd, C. A. R., Transport across the intestinal mucosal cell: Hierarchies of function. *Int. Rev. Cytol.* 32, 209-255 (1972).
216. Percy-Robb, I. W., and Collee, J. G., Bile acids: A pH dependent antibacterial system in the gut? *Br. Med. J.* 3, 813-815 (1972).
217. Peters, T. J., and MacMahon, M. T., The absorption of glycine oligopeptides by the rat. *Clin. Sci.* 39, 811-821 (1970).

218. Phear, E. A., and Ruebner, B., *In vitro* production of ammonia and amines by intestinal bacteria in relation to nitrogen toxicity as factors in hepatic coma. *Brit. J. Exp. Pathol. 37*, 253-262 (1956).
219. Plant, A. G., A review of secretory immune mechanisms. *Am. J. Clin. Nutr. 25*, 1344-1350 (1972).
220. Podesta, R. B., and Mettrick, D. F., Pathophysiology of cestode infections: Effect of *Hymenolepis diminuta* on oxygen tensions, pH and gastrointestinal function. *Int. J. Parasit. 4*, 277-292 (1974a).
221. Podesta, R. B., and Mettrick, D. F., The effect of bicarbonate and acidification on water and electrolyte absorption by the intestine of normal and infected (*Hymenolepis diminuta*: Cestoda) rats. *Am. J. Digest. Dis. 19*, 725-735 (1974b).
222. Podesta, R. B., and Mettrick, D. F., Components of glucose transport in the host-parasite system, *Hymenolepis diminuta* (Cestoda) and the rat intestine. *Can. J. Physiol. Pharmacol. 52*, 183-197 (1974c).
223. Podesta, R. B., and Mettrick, D. F., *Hymenolepis diminuta*: Acidification and bicarbonate absorption in the rat intestine. *Expl. Parasit. 37*, 1-14 (1975).
224. Podesta, R. B., and Mettrick, D. F., Pathophysiology and compensatory mechanisms in a compatible host-parasite system. *Can. J. Zool. 54*, 794-803 (1976a).
225. Podesta, R. B., and Mettrick, D. F., Permeability alterations in the diseased small intestine. *In* "Biochemistry of Parasites and Host-Parasite Relationships" (H. Van den Bossche, ed.), pp. 373-377. North Holland, Amsterdam, (1976b).
226. Podesta, R. B., and Mettrick, D. F., The interrelationships between *in situ* fluxes of water, electrolytes and glucose by *Hymenolepis diminuta*. *Int. J. Parasit. 6*, 163-172 (1976c).
227. Podesta, R. B., and Mettrick, D. F., HCO_3 transport in rat jejunum: relationship to NaCl and H_2O transport *in vivo*. *Am. J. Physiol. 232* (1): E 62-68 (1977a).

228. Podesta, R. B., and Mettrick, D. F., HCO_3^- and H^+ in rat ileum *in vivo*. Am. J. Physiol. *232* (6): E 574-579 (1977b).
229. Podesta, R. B., and Mettrick, D. F., Proximal-distal absorptive gradients in the *in vivo* intestine of normal and infected (*Hymenolepis diminuta*: Cestoda) rats. Can. J. Physiol. Pharmacol. *55*, 791-803 (1977c).
230. Podesta, R. B., and Mettrick, D. F., Permeability changes in the parasitized (*Hymenolepis diminuta*: Cestoda) rat intestine. Comp. Biochem. Physiol. *57*, 265-273 (1977d).
231. Podesta, R. B., Stallard, H. E., Evans, W. S., Lussier, P. E., Jackson, D. J., and Mettrick, D. F., *Hymenolepis diminuta*: Determination of unidirectional uptake rates for nonelectrolytes across the surface "epithelium" membrane. Expl. Parasit. *42*, 300-317 (1977).
232. Podolsky, D. K., Weiser, M. M., and Lamont, J. T., Galactosyltransferase and concanavalin A agglutination of cells. Proc. Nat. Acad. Sci. U.S.A. *71*, 904-908 (1974).
233. Pope, J. L., Parkinson, T. M., and Olson, J. A., Action of bile salts on the metabolism and transport of water-soluble nutrients by perfused rat jejunum *in vitro*. Biochim. Biophys. Acta *130*, 218-232 (1966).
234. Powell, D. W., Goldberg, L. I., Plotkin, G. R., Catlin, D. H., Maenza, R. M., and Formal, S. B., Experimental diarrhea. III. Bicarbonate transport in rat *Salmonella* enterocolitis. Gastroenterology *60*, 1076-1086 (1971).
235. Quick, J. D., Goldberg, H. S., and Sonnenwirth, A. C., Human antibody to *Bacteroidaceae*. Ann. J. Clin. Nutr. *25*, 1351-1356 (1972).
236. Read, C. P., The vertebrate small intestine as an environment for parasitic helminths. Rice Inst. Pamph. *37*, No. 2, 94p. (1950).
237. Read, C. P., Intestinal physiology and the host-parasite relationship. *In* "Some Physiological Aspects and Consequences of Parasitism" (W. H. Cole, ed.), pp. 27-43. Rutgers Univ. Bur. Biol. Research, Ann. Conf. Protein Metabolism, (1955).
238. Read, C. P., Carbohydrate metabolism of *Hymenolepis diminuta*. Expl. Parasit. *5*, 344-352 (1956).

239. Read, C. P., The role of carbohydrates in the biology of cestodes. VIII. Some conclusions and hypotheses. *Expl. Parasit. 8*, 365-382 (1959).
240. Read, C. P., The microcosm of intestinal parasites. *In* "Ecology and Physiology of Parasites" (A. M. Fallis, ed.), pp. 188-197. Univ. Toronto Press, Toronto, (1971).
241. Read, C. P., and Kilejian, A. Z., Circadian migratory behaviour of a cestode symbiote in the rat host. *J. Parasit. 55*, 574-578 (1969).
242. Read, C. P., and Rothman, A. H., The role of carbohydrates in the biology of cestodes. I. The effect of dietary carbohydrate quality on the size of *Hymenolepis diminuta*. *Expl. Parasit. 6*, 1-7 (1957a).
243. Read, C. P., and Rothman, A. H., The role of carbohydrates in the biology of cestodes. IV. Some effects of host dietary carbohydrate on growth, and reproduction of *Hymenolepis diminuta*. *Expl. Parasit. 6*, 294-305 (1957b).
244. Read, C. P., and Rothman, A. H., The role of carbohydrates in the biology of cestodes. VI. The carbohydrates metabolized *in vitro* by some cyclophyllidean species. *Expl. Parasit. 7*, 217-223 (1958).
245. Read, C. P., Rothman, A. H., and Simmons, J. E., Studies on membrane transport, with special reference to parasite-host integration. *Ann. N.Y. Acad. Sci. 113*, 154-205 (1963).
246. Read, C. P., Schiller, E. L., and Phifer, K., The role of carbohydrates in the biology of cestodes. V. Comparative studies on the effect of host dietary carbohydrates on *Hymenolepis* spp. *Expl. Parasit. 7*, 198-216 (1958).
247. Rehfeld, J. F., Gastrointestinal hormones and insulin secretion. *Scand. J. Gastroent. 7*, 289-292 (1972).
248. Rhodes, J. B., Eichholz, A., and Crane, R. K., Studies on the organization of the brush border in intestinal epithelial cells. IV. Aminopeptidase activity in microvillus membranes of hamster intestinal brush borders. *Biochim. Biophys. Acta 135*, 959-965 (1967).

249. Roberts, L. S., Developmental physiology of cestodes. I. Host dietary carbohydrate and the "crowding effect" in *Hymenolepis diminuta*. *Expl. Parasit.* 18, 305-310 (1966).
250. Roberts, L. S., and Mong, F. N., Developmental physiology of cestodes. IV. *In vitro* development of *Hymenolepis diminuta* in the presence and absence of oxygen. *Expl. Parasit.* 26, 166-174 (1969).
251. Roberts, L. S., and Platzer, E. G., Effects of changes in host dietary carbohydrate and roughage on previously established *Hymenolepis diminuta*. *J. Parasit.* 53, 85-93 (1967).
252. Rogers, Q. R., and Harper, A. E., Transfer rates along the gastrointestinal tract. In "The Role of the Gastrointestinal Tract in Protein Metabolism" (H. N. Munro, ed.), pp. 3-24. Blackwell, Oxford, (1964).
253. Rogers, W. P., On the relative importance of aerobic metabolism in small nematode parasites of the alimentary canal. I. Oxygen tensions in the normal environment of the parasites. *Aust. J. Scient. Res.* 2B, 157-165 (1949).
254. Rosenberg, I. H., Influence of intestinal bacteria on bile acid metabolism and fat absorption. *Am. J. Clin. Nutr.* 22, 284-291 (1969).
255. Rosensweig, N. S., Diet and intestinal enzyme adaptation: implications for gastrointestinal disorders. *Am. J. Clin. Nutr.* 28, 648-655 (1975).
256. Rosensweig, N. S., and Herman, J., Control of jejunal sucrase and maltase activity by dietary sucrose or fructose in man. A model for the study of enzyme regulation in man. *J. Clin. Invest.* 47, 2253-2262 (1968).
257. Rosensweig, N. S., and Herman, J., Time response of jejunal sucrase and maltase activity to a high sucrose diet in normal man. *Gastroenterology* 56, 500-505 (1969).
258. Rosensweig, N. S., and Herman, J., Dose response of jejunal sucrase and maltase activities to isocaloric high and low carbohydrate diets in man. *Am. J. Clin. Nutr.* 23, 1373-1377 (1970).

259. Rosensweig, N. S., Herman, R. H., and Stifel, F. B., Dietary regulation of glycolytic enzymes. VI. Effect of dietary sugars and oral folic acid on human jejunal pyruvate kinase, phosphofructokinase and fructosediphosphatase activities. *Biochim. Biophys. Acta* 208, 373-380 (1970).
260. Rosensweig, N. S., Stifel, F. B., Herman, R. H., and Zakim, D., The dietary regulation of the glycolytic enzymes. II. Adaptive changes in human jejunum. *Biochim. Biophys. Acta* 170, 228-234 (1968).
261. Rosensweig, N. S., Stifel, F. B., Zakim, D., and Herman, R. H., Clofibrate-induced changes in the activity of human intestinal enzymes. *Gastroenterology* 56, 496-499 (1969).
262. Rothman, A. H., Studies on the excystment of tapeworms. *Expl. Parasit.* 80, 336-364 (1959).
263. Rubenstein, M., Weser, E., and Sleisenger, M. H., Effect of puromycin on rat intestinal disaccharidases. *Clin. Res.* 14, 305 (1966).
264. Rubin, W., The epithelial "membrane" of the small intestine. *Am. J. Clin. Nutr.* 24, 45-64 (1971).
265. Rubin, W., Ross, L. L., Jeffries, G. H., and Sleisenger, M., Intestinal heterotopia. A fine structural study. *Lab. Invest.* 15, 1024-1049 (1966a).
266. Rubin, W., Ross, L. L., Sleisenger, M., and Wesser, E., An electron microscope study of adult celiac disease. *Lab. Invest.* 15, 1520-17 (1966b).
267. Ruff, M. D., and Read, C. P., Inhibition of pancreatic lipase by *Hymenolepis diminuta*. *J. Parasit.* 59, 105-111 (1973).
268. Said, S. I., Vasoactive intestinal peptide (VIP): current status. In "Gastrointestinal Hormones" (J. C. Thompson, ed.), pp. 591-597. Univ. of Texas Press, Austin, Texas, (1975).
269. Said, S. I., and Mutt, V., Isolation from porcine intestinal wall of a vasoactive octacosapeptide related to secretin and glucagon. *Eur. J. Biochem.* 28, 199-204 (1972).
270. Sanchez, A., Swendseid, M. E., Clark, A. J., and Umezawa, C., Amino acid pools and hepatic enzyme activities in rats fed a meal of high or low methionine content. *Am. J. Clin. Nutr.* 25, 550-554 (1972).

271. Saz, H. J., Facultative anaerobiasis in the invertebrates: pathways and control systems. *Am. Zool. 11*, 125-135 (1971).
272. Saz, H. J., Comparative biochemistry of carbohydrates in nematodes and cestodes. In "Comparative Biochemistry of Parasites" (H. Van den Bossche, ed.), pp. 33-48. Academic Press, N.Y., (1972).
273. Schedl, H. P., Wilson, H. D., and Miller, D. L., Proximal to distal secretory and absorptive gradients of the rat small intestine. *Proc. Soc. Exp. Biol. Med. 129*, 511-515 (1968).
274. Schiff, E. R., and Dietschy, J. M., Current concepts of bile acid absorption. *Am. J. Clin. Nutr. 22*, 273-278 (1969).
275. Schimke, R. T., Differential effects of fasting and protein-free diets on levels of urea cycle enzymes in rat liver. *J. Biol. Chem. 237*, 1921-1924 (1962).
276. Schmidt, H. A., Johannson, F., and Goebell, H., [The influence of acid, fat, secretin and cholecystokinin on the pentagastrin stimulated and the histamine stimulated acid secretion in the rat - German text.]. *Z. ges. exp. Med. 156*, 23-33 (1971).
277. Schuler, R., and Kreuzer, F., Properties and performance of membrane covered rapid polarographic oxygen catheter electrodes for continuous oxygen recording *in vivo*. *Progr. resp. Res. 3*, 64-78 (1968).
278. Schultz, S. G., Frizzell, R. A., and Nellans, H. N., Ion transport by mammalian small intestine. *Ann. Rev. Physiol. 36*, 51-91 (1974).
279. Shakespeare, C., Srivastava, Z. M., and Hubscher, G., Glucose metabolism in the mucosa of the small intestine. The effect of glucose on hexokinase activity. *Biochem. J. 111*, 63-67 (1969).
280. Shaw, H. M., and Heath, T., The significance of hormones, bile salts and feeding in the regulation of bile and other digestive secretion in the rat. *Aust. J. Biol. Sci. 25*, 147-154 (1972).
281. Sheerin, H. E., and Field, M., Ileal HCO_3 secretion: relationship to Na and Cl transport and effect of theophylline. *Am. J. Physiol. 228*, 1065-1074 (1975).

282. Shimada, K., Bricknell, K. S., and Finegold, S. M., Deconjugation of bile acids by intestinal bacteria: Review of the literature and additional studies. *J. Infect. Dis. 119*, 273-281 (1969).
283. Shorter, R. G., Moertel, C. G., Titus, J. L., and Reitmeier, R. J., Cell kinetics in the jejunum and rectum of man. *Am. J. Dig. Dis. 9*, 760-763 (1964).
284. Silk, D. B. A., Perrett, D., Webb, J. P. W., and Clark, M. L., Absorption of two tripeptides by the human small intestine: a study using a perfusion technique. *Clin. Sci. 46*, 393-402 (1974).
285. Smyth, D. G., Energetics of intestinal transfer. *In:* "Intestinal Transport of Electrolytes, Amino Acids and Sugars." (W. McD. Armstrong and A. S. Nunn, eds.), pp. 52-75. Thomas, Springfield, Ill., (1971).
286. Smyth, D. H., and Wright, E. M., Streaming potentials in the rat small intestine. *J. Physiol. (Lond.) 182*, 591-602 (1966).
287. Smyth, J. D., Lysis of *Echinococcus granulosus* by surface-active agents in bile and the role of this phenomenon in determining host specificity in helminths. *Proc. R. Soc. Lond. B 156*, 553-572 (1962).
288. Smyth, J. D., and Haslewood, G. A. D., The biochemistry of bile as a factor in determining host specificity in intestinal parasites, with particular reference to *Echinococcus granulosus*. *Ann. N.Y. Acad. Sci. 113*, 234-260 (1963).
289. Soleia, E., Capella, C., Vezzadini, P., and Barbara, L., Immunohistochemical and ultrastructural detection of the secretin cell in the pig intestinal mucosa. *Experientia 28*, 549-550 (1972).
290. Stifel, F. B., Herman, R. H., and Rosensweig, N. S., Dietary regulation of galactose-metabolizing enzymes: Adaptive changes in rat jejunum. *Science 162*, 692-693 (1968a).
291. Stifel, F. B., Rosensweig, N. S., Zakim, D., and Herman, R. G., Dietary regulation of glycolytic enzymes. I. Adaptive changes in rat jejunium. *Biochim. Biophys. Acta 170*, 221-227 (1968b)

292. Stifel, F. B., Herman, R. H., and Rosensweig, N. S., Dietary regulation of glycolytic enzymes. IV. Differential hormonal effects in male and female rat jejunum. *Biochim. Biophys. Acta 184*, 495-501 (1969).
293. Stifel, F. B., Herman, R. H., and Rosensweig, N. S., Dietary regulation of glycolytic enzymes. XI. Effect of inhibitors of protein synthesis on the adaptation of certain jejunal glycolytic and folate-metabolizing enzymes to diet and sex steroids. *Biochim. Biophys. Acta 237*, 484-489 (1971).
294. Stirling, C. E., and Kintner, W. B., High resolution radiautography of galactose − ^{3}H accumulation in rings of hamster intestine. *J. Cell. Biol. 35*, 585-593 (1967).
295. Thompson, E., Levin, R. J., and Jackson, M. J., The stimulating effect of low pH on the amino acid transferring systems of the small intestine. *Biochim. Biophys. Acta 196*, 120-122 (1970).
296. Tilney, L. G., and Mooseker, M., Actin in the brush border of epithelial cells of the chicken intestine. *Proc. Nat. Acad. Sci. U.S.A. 68*, 2611-2615 (1971).
297. Tomasi, T. B., and Bienenstick, J., Secretory immunoglobulins. *Adv. Immunol. 9*, 2-96 (1968).
298. Tomasi, T. B., and Grey, H. M., Structure and function of immunoglobulin A. *Progr. Allergy 16*, 81-213 (1972).
299. Trier, J. S., Studies on the small intestinal crypt epithelium. I. The fine structure of crypt epithelium of the proximal small intestine of fasting humans. *J. Cell. Biol. 18*, 599-620 (1963).
300. Trier, J. S., Studies on small intestinal crypt epithelium. II. Evidence for and mechanisms of secretory activity by undifferentiated crypt cells of the human small intestine. *Gastroenterology 47*, 480-495 (1964).
301. Trier, J. S., Morphology of the epithelium of the small intestine. *In Handb. Physiol. 3* (Section 6), pp. 1125-1175. Am. Physiol. Soc. Washington, D.C., (1968).

302. Trier, J. S., Functional morphology of the mucosa of the small intestine. *In:* "Intestinal Transport of Electrolytes, Amino Acids and Sugars." (W. McD. Armstrong and A. S. Nun, eds.), pp. 12-23. Thomas, Springfield, Ill., (1971).
303. Troughton, W. D., and Trier, J. S., Paneth and goblet cell renewal in mouse duodenal crypts. *J. Cell. Biol. 41*, 251-268 (1969).
304. Turnberg, L. A., Fordtran, J. S., Carter, N. W., and Rector, F. C., Mechanisms of bicarbonate absorption and its relationship to sodium transport in the human jejunum. *J. Clin. Invest. 49*, 548-556 (1970a).
305. Turnberg, L. A., Bieberdorf, F. A., Morawski, S. G., and Fordtran, J. S., Interrelationships of chloride, bicarbonate, sodium and hydrogen transport in the human ileum. *J. Clin. Invest. 49*, 557-567 (1970b).
306. Ugolev, A.M., and Delaey, P., Membrane digestion. A concept of enzymatic hydrolysis on cell membranes. *Biochim. Biophys. Acta 300*, 105-128 (1973).
307. Vahouny, G.V., Weersing, S., and Treadwell, C. R., Taurocholate protection of cholesterol esterase against proteolytic inactivation. *Biochim. Biophys. Res. Commun. 15*, 224 (1964).
308. von Brand, T., "Biochemistry of Parasites." Academic Press, N.Y., (1966).
309. von Brand, T., and Jahn, T. L., Chemical composition and metabolism of nematode parasites of vertebrates, and the chemistry of their environment. *In:* "An Introduction to Nematology." (B. G. Chitwood and M. B. Chitwood, eds.), pp. 356-371. Monumental Printing Co., Baltimore, Md., (1941).
310. Waldram, R., Mechanisms of lipid loss from the small intestinal mucosa. *Gut 16*, 118-124 (1975).
311. Wang, C. C., and Grossman, M. I., Physiological determination of release of secretin and pancreozymin from intestine of dogs with transplanted pancreas. *Am. J. Physiol. 164*, 527-545 (1951).
312. Wakelin, D., Host responses. *In:* "Ecological Aspects of Parasitology." (C.R. Kennedy, ed.), pp. 115-141. North Holland Publishing Co., Amsterdam, (1976).

313. Waterlow, J. C., Adaptation to low-protein intakes. *In* "Protein-Calorie Malnutrition" (R. E. Olson, ed.), pp. 23-35. Academic Press, N.Y., (1975).
314. Webb, J. L., "Enzyme and Metabolic Inhibitors", Vol. III, Academic Press, N.Y., (1966).
315. Webb, R. A., and Mettrick, D. F., The role of serine in lipid metabolism of the rat tapeworm *Hymenolepis diminuta*. *Int. J. Parasit. 3*, 47-58 (1973).
316. Webster, L. A., and Wilson, R. A., The chemical composition of protonephridial canal fluid from the cestode *Hymenolepis diminuta*. *Comp. Biochem. Physiol. 35*, 201-209 (1970).
317. Weiner, I. M., and Lack, L., Bile salt absorption; enterohepatic circulation. *In Handb. Physiol. 3* (Section 6), pp. 1439-1455. Am. Physiol. Soc., Washington, D.C., (1968).
318. Weiser, M. M., Concanavalin A agglutination of intestinal cells from the human fetus. *Science 177*, 525-526 (1972).
319. Weiser, M. M., Intestinal epithelial cell surface membrane glycoprotein synthesis. II. Glycosyltransferases and endogenous acceptors of the undifferentiated cell surface membrane. *J. Biol. Chem. 248*, 2542-2548 (1973).
320. Westergaard, H., and Dietschy, J. M., Delineation of the dimensions and permeability characteristics of the two major diffusion barriers to passive mucosal uptake in the rabbit intestine. *J. Clin. Invest. 54*, 718-732 (1974).
321. Wheeler, H. O., Water and electrolytes in bile. *In Handb. Physiol. 5* (Section 6), pp. 2409-2432. Am. Physiol. Soc., Washington, D.C., (1968).
322. Williams, R. E. O., Hill, M. J., and Draser, B. S., The influence of intestinal bacteria on the absorption and metabolism of foreign compounds. *J. Clin. Path. 24*, suppl. 5, 125-129 (1971).
323. Wilson, F. A., and Dietschy, J. M., The intestinal unstirred layer. Its surface area and effect on active transport kinetics. *Biochim. Biophys. Acta 363*, 112-126 (1974).
324. Wilson, T. H., Concentration gradients of lactate, hydrogen and some other ions across the intestine *in vitro*. *Biochem. J. 56*, 521-527 (1954).

325. Wilson, T. H., "Intestinal Absorption". W. B. Saunders, London, (1962).
326. Wilson, T. H., and Kazyak, L., Acid-base changes across the wall of hamster and rat intestine. *Biochim. Biophys. Acta 24*, 124-132 (1957).
327. Winawer, S. J., Broitman, S. A., Wolochow, D. A., Osborne, M. H., and Zomcheck, N., Successful management of massive small bowel resection based on assessment of absorptive defects and nutritional needs. *New Engl. J. Med. 274*, 72-78 (1966).
328. Wormsley, K. G., Reactions to acid in the intestine in health and disease. *Gut 12*, 67-84 (1971).
329. Wurtman, R. J., Diurnal rhythms in mammalian protein metabolism. *In* "Mammalian Protein Metabolism" (H. N. Munro, ed.) Vol. 4, pp. 445 Academic Press, N.Y., (1969).

DEVELOPMENT OF *HYMENOLEPIS DIMINUTA* IN ITS DEFINITIVE HOST

Larry S. Roberts[1]

Department of Zoology
University of Massachusetts
Amherst, Massachusetts

I. THE SYSTEM

Cestodes are a unique group among the Metazoa in their possession of a segmented strobila as adults. In *H. diminuta* and in many other species, the development and growth of the strobila is extremely rapid after infection of the definitive host. These characteristics of its development, combined with its ease of maintenance and manipulation in the laboratory, make *H. diminuta* a very useful model for developmental studies. When the worm excysts in the small intestine of the rat, it consists of little more than a relatively tiny scolex and germinative region. Thereupon it undergoes a growth that can be described as explosive; the growth rate must rival or surpass that of any other metazoan tissue, including embryonic and neoplastic. Within 15 days after infection of the rat, a normal *H. diminuta* will have produced up to 2200 proglottids and will have increased its length by up to 3400 times and its weight by up to 1.8 million times (Roberts 1961). That development and the factors which affect it are the subject of this review.

[1]*Present address: Department of Biological Sciences, Texas Tech University, Lubbock, Texas*

Other aspects of the worm's development, such as oncospheral and cysticercoid through excystment, and development of the adult worm in mice, are covered elsewhere in this volume.

II. GERMINATIVE AREA

In most cyclophyllidean cestodes, new proglottids are produced in an area of cell proliferation just behind the scolex referred to variously as the "neck", "growth zone", "Keimzone", or "germinative area". Based on observation of mitotic activity in *H. diminuta*, Bolla and Roberts (1971a) delimited the area as beginning about 0.2 mm from the apex of the scolex and extending posteriorly to the region where genital primordia could be observed (about 5.6 mm). No dividing cells were seen in the scolex itself, and, other than in the gonads and embryos, mitotic activity was scant or absent posterior to the germinative area. Thus, the area is quite small in comparison to the rest of the strobila, particularly in later stages of development.

A. *Stem Cells*

The stem cells were described by Bolla and Roberts (1971a) as having characteristics similar to unspecialized cells in other systems (e.g., Herlant-Meewis 1964; Hay 1958). The cells have a large nucleus, a nucleolus, and an intensely basophilic cytoplasm (Fig. 1,2). Ultrastructurally, the relatively large, granular nucleolus and densely clumped chromatin can be observed in the nucleus (Fig. 3). The cytoplasm contains an abundance of densely packed free ribosomes and some ovoid mitochondria. Neither Golgi regions nor smooth or rough endoplasmic reticula are found. Similar cells have also been described in plerocercoids of *Diphyllobothrium dendriticum*, plerocercoids of *Triaenophorus nodulosus*, cysts of *Echinococcus multilocularis*, and adults of *E. granulosus* (Bonsdorff et al. 1971; Wikgren and Gustafsson 1971; Gustafsson 1973, 1976 a,b, 1977; Sakamoto and Sugimura 1970). Further, cells of that type have been described in embryos and cysticercoids of *Hymenolepis* (Ogren 1962, 1967,

Development of *Hymenolepis diminuta* in Its Definitive Host

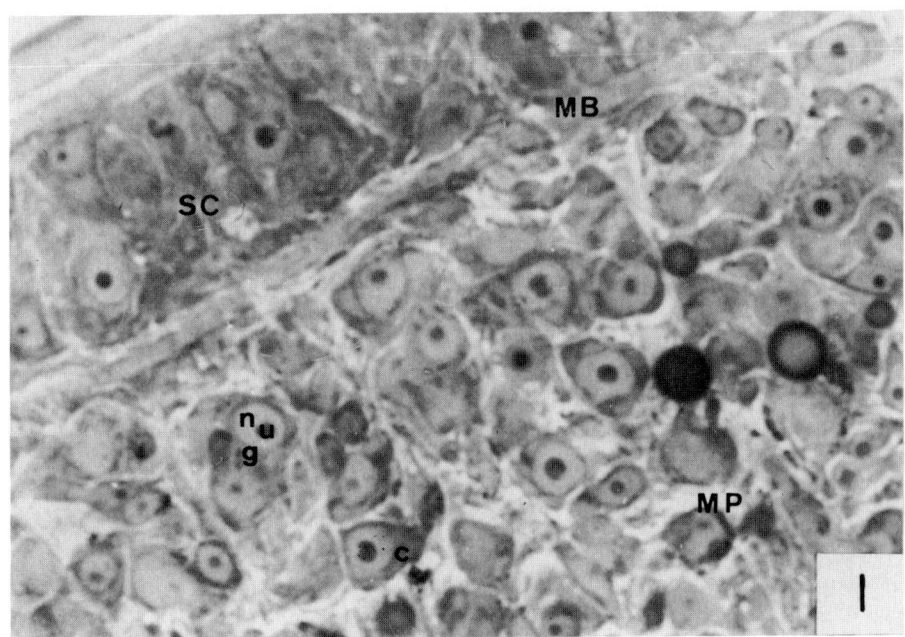

Fig. 1. Light micrograph of a section through the anterior part of a 4-day-old H. diminuta. A major part of the cell population is comprised of stem or germinative cells (g), characterized by a large nucleus (n) with a large, centrally located nucleolus (u), and a basophilic cytoplasm (c). MB = parenchymal muscle, MP = medullary parenchyma, SC = subtegumental region. X2,125. (from Bolla 1970; Bolla and Roberts 1971a).

1968 a,b; Rybicka 1966 a,b, 1967 a,b; Collin 1970). A variety of terms have been used to refer to these cells, though "germinative" has been the most common. However, as Wikgren and Gustafsson (1971) pointed out, "The term stem cells ... perhaps most exactly describes the actual role of these cells in cell population kinetics", and is, therefore, here accepted as most appropriate.

It has been shown that the stem cells in *Diphyllobothrium dendriticum* give rise to all other cell types in the strobila: nerve cells, binding cells, tegumental cells, muscle cells, and cells in the

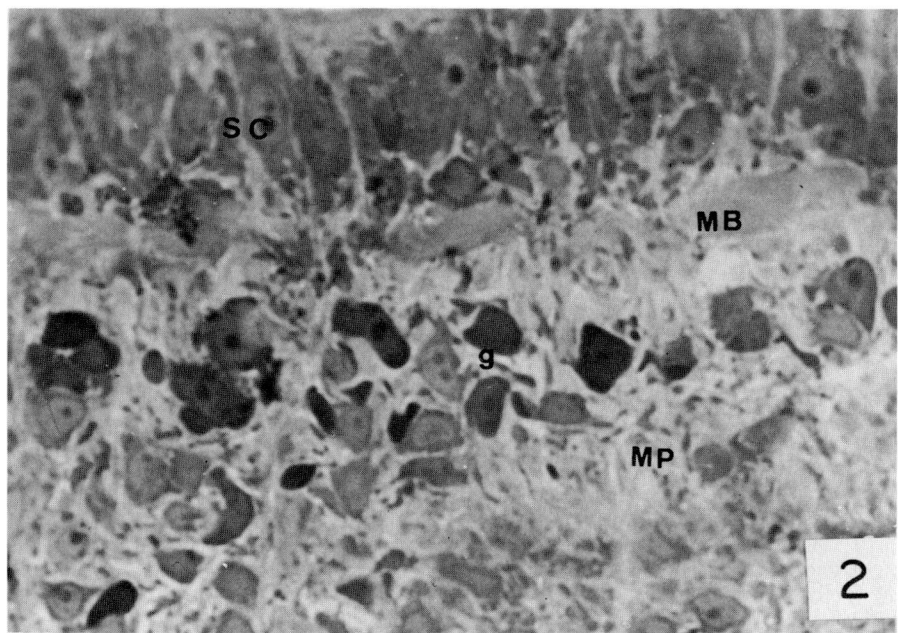

Fig. 2. Light micrograph of a section through the anterior part of a 10-day-old H. diminuta. The stem cells are now concentrated in a region just internal to the parenchymal muscle layer. Labelling as in Fig. 1. X2,125. (from Bolla 1970).

genital anlagen (and ultimately, one must assume, to the gametes) (Wikgren and Knuts 1970; Wikgren *et al.* 1971; Gustafsson 1976 a,b, 1977). Though differentiation of the stem cells has not been studied in *H. diminuta*, it is highly probable that these cells give rise to all other cell types in that species as well. In a light microscope study, Sulgostowska (1972) described three types of undifferentiated cells, one of which Gustafsson (1977) considered the same as the stem cell described by Bolla and Roberts (1971a). The significance of the other two types is problematic; Sulgostowska (1972) did not mention observation of division stages. Gustafsson (1977) suggested that these two types might have developed as a "side line" from the primary stem cells.

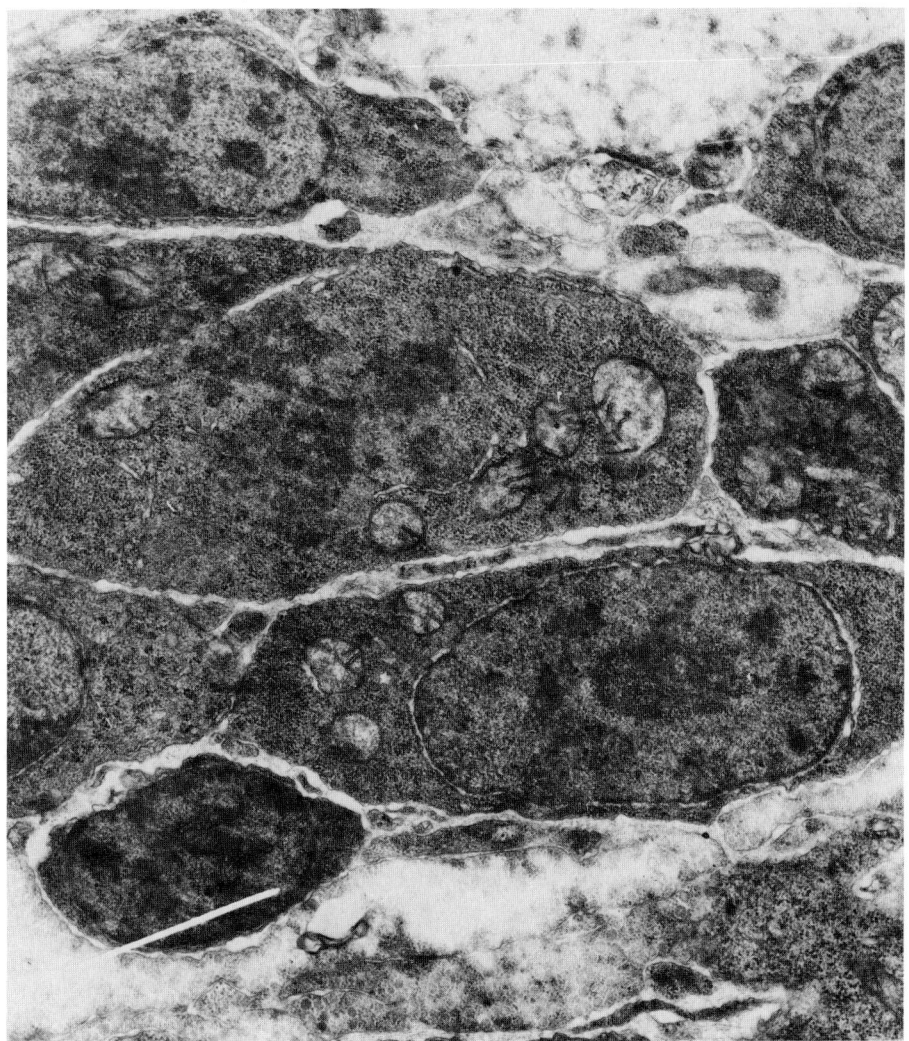

Fig. 3. Electron micrograph showing two stem cells in a 4-day-old H. diminuta. The upper cell in the micrograph is in prometaphase of mitosis, showing a breakdown of the nuclear membrane and organization of the chromatin into early chromosomal arrangements. The lower cell demonstrates the large nucleus with clumped chromatin and centrally located nucleolus. The cytoplasm contains densely packed free ribosomes and a paucity of membranous organelles. X23,900 (from Bolla and Roberts 1971a).

B. Cell Cycle and Mitotic Activity

The stem cells described by Bolla and Roberts (1971a) were the only cell type they observed in mitosis. Using the method of Wikgren (1964), the duration of mitosis from late prophase to early telophase can be calculated as 3.4 min (the figure of 1.2 min given in Bolla and Roberts [1971a] is in error). The graphic method of Sisken (1964) was used to estimate times for phases of the cell cycle after pulse labelling in ^{3}H-thymidine: G_1 as 3.0 hr; S as 2.3 hr; and G_2 as 3.2 hr; with the entire cell cycle requiring 8.5 hr in 4-day-old worms. For comparison, Wikgren and Gustafsson (1967) reported the following estimates of the cell cycle in stem cells of *Diphyllobothrium dendriticum*: G_1, 6 hr; S, 10 hr; G_2, 3 hr or a total of 19 hr in plerocercoids removed from fish and incubated at 39 C.

Correlated with the period of most rapid specific growth, which the worm undergoes between 2 days postinfection and 8 days postinfection (see Section III.A), Bolla and Roberts (1971a) observed the highest mitotic activity in the stem cells in 2-day-old worms, decreasing with time until 10 days postinfection. Thereafter, mitotic activity did not diminish significantly. The same result was obtained whether the activity was scored as percent arrested metaphases after colchicine treatment or as number of mitoses observed per square millimeter in sections from untreated worms (Bolla 1970).

III. GROWTH IN LENGTH AND WEIGHT

A. Growth Curve

The first systematic examination of growth of *H. diminuta* in the definitive host was that of Chandler (1939). Basing his conclusion on observation of arithmetic increase in length, Chandler stated that *H. diminuta* grew "... very slowly during the first 5 to 7 days in rats, but rapidly thereafter". Data obtained by subsequent workers (Goodchild and Harrison 1961; Roberts 1961) agreed with those of Chandler, but Roberts (1961) noted that plotting the logarithm of size as a function of time, rather than the absolute value, emphasized the multiplicative aspects of growth. From this perspective, the worms are in a phase of exponential growth in length between 1 and 7 days postinfection (Goodchild and Harrison 1961; Roberts 1961), after which they enter a phase of retardation, reaching maximal size by about 14 days (Fig. 4) (Roberts 1961). It is to be emphasized, nevertheless, that a very substantial absolute increase in size occurs during the phase of retardation. Curves of specific growth in weight follow essentially the same pattern although data for the first three days in the rat were not included because of manipulative problems (Fig. 5).

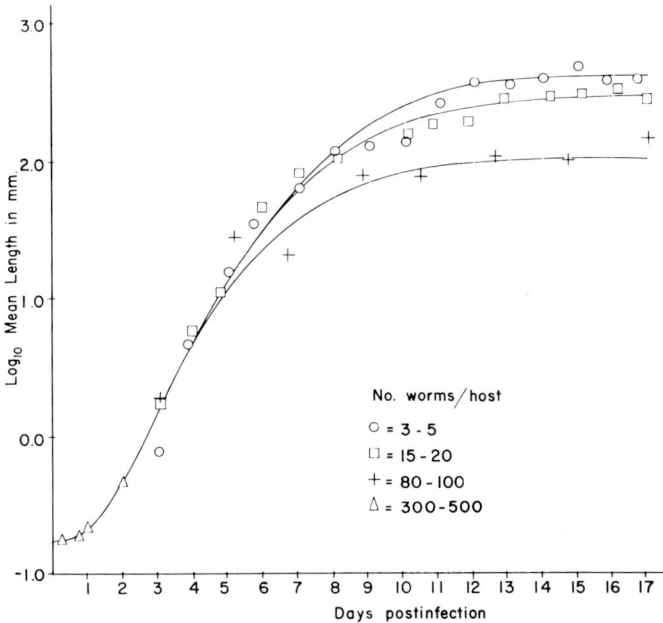

Fig. 4. Curve of specific growth in length of H. diminuta, showing effect of population density. The curves were fitted to the Pearl-Verhulst logistic equation. (from Roberts 1961).

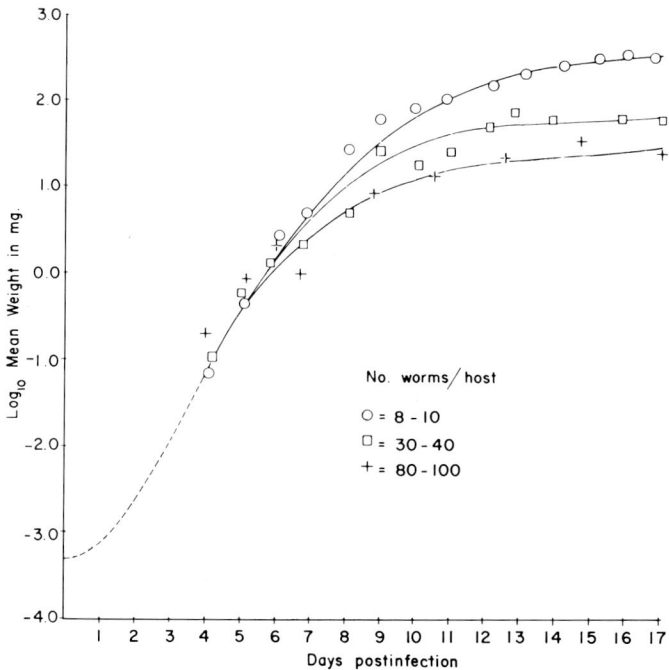

Fig. 5. Curves of specific growth in fresh weight, also fitted to the logistic equation. Early characteristics of the growth curves are suggested by the dotted line (from Roberts 1961).

B. The Crowding Effect

Growth in length and weight of *H. diminuta* in its definitive host both reflect the effect of the population density within the host, commonly called the "crowding effect". Chandler (1939) characterized the crowding effect by noting that the size attained by the worms at maturity was in inverse proportion to the number of worms harbored. This generalization has been confirmed, with certain reservations, by subsequent workers (Read 1951; Read and Phifer 1959; Weinmann 1958; Roberts 1961, 1966). Thus, a plot of size as a function of population density forms a rectangular hyperbola (Read 1959). The curve adequately describes the average weight and length attained from about 5 worms per host up to at least 100 worm populations; size attained is independent of worms present if there are fewer than

4 per host, since maximum size per worm is reached in populations of that size (Roberts 1961). Furthermore, worm growth is independent of population density during the exponential phase, but the effect of crowding becomes detectable between 8 and 10 days postinfection (Figs. 4,5).

C. *Preformed Informational RNA During Early Development*

Bolla and Roberts (1970, 1971c) used actinomycin-D to study the role of preformed informational RNA in development of *H. diminuta*. They found that about 75% of the protein synthesis in 4-day-old worms and in the germinative area of 6-day-old worms was independent of the synthesis of new mRNA. This figure decreased to about 25% at 8 days and 5% at 12 days postinfection. Thus, much of the informational RNA for protein synthesis during early development in the rat is produced prior to 4 days postinfection, perhaps even in the cysticercoid. Bolla and Roberts (1971c) suggested that one reason that the crowding effect is not manifested prior to 8 days might be related to the early synthesis of mRNA. Such a relationship would imply that the mechanism of the crowding effect operates during transcription or at some point prior to that, e.g., in DNA replication.

IV. PROGLOTTISATION AND MATURATION OF PROGLOTTIDS

Proglottid production and maturation were studied by Roberts (1961). The first proglottids, distinguished by the presence of genital primorida, were observed at 4 days postinfection, and segmentation was observed in 5-day-old worms. Mature proglottids, defined as those in which the ovary had become lobate, were seen by day 6, and the first gravid proglottids, defined as those containing shelled embryos, were observed by day 12 postinfection. Apolysis began in some worms by day 15, and in most by day 16 or 17. Eggs were present in the feces of the host by day 16 or 17, regardless of numbers of worms in the infection, though some worms lagged behind in development in hosts carrying higher population densities.

Numbers of proglottids increased relatively most rapidly between 4 and 6 days postinfection up to about 400 to 600 proglottids, then rose more slowly up to a total of about 2000 by day 17 in populaton sizes of one to ten worms per host (Fig. 6) (Roberts 1961). Effects of crowding were observed: cestodes from 20 worm populations had a total of about 1600 to 1700 proglottids at 17 days, those from 40 worm populations, 1100 to 1400 proglottids, and those from 100 worm populations 1100 to 1200. Numbers of immature proglottids were independent of population density, reaching about 600 to 700 by 8 days post-infection and remaining constant thereafter. Numbers of mature and gravid proglottids were, however, decreased in worms from high population densities. Proglottid counts for worms from 10 worm populations of *H. diminuta* between 5 and 16 days postinfection were reported by Mettrick and Cannon (1970), and their data were in close agreement with those of Roberts (1961).

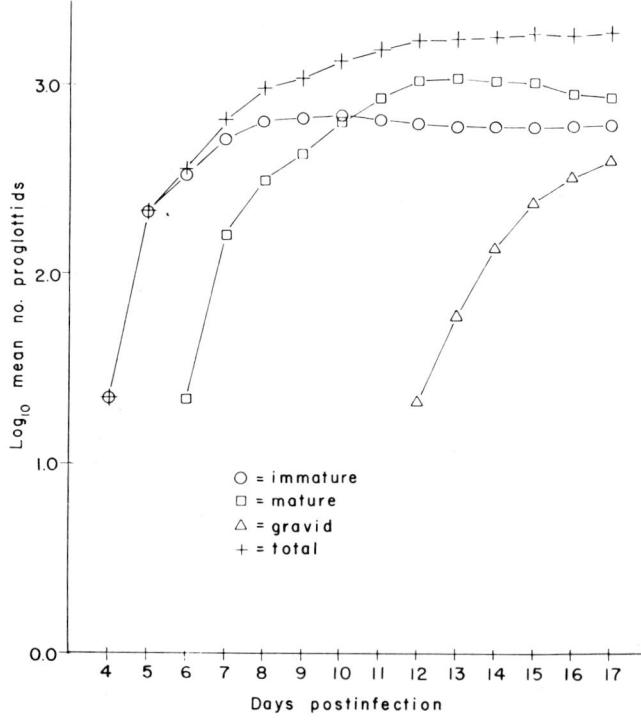

Fig. 6. Increase in number of proglottids during growth, 3-5 worms per host (from Roberts 1961).

There have been a number of suggestions that strobilation and growth of cestodes might be under neuroendocrine control (Smyth 1969; Smyth 1964; Smyth *et al.* 1967; Davey and Breckenridge 1967; Wilson and Schiller 1969), and neurosecretory cells were reported in a short paper by Davey and Breckenridge (1967). They observed a cluster of bipolar fuchsinophilic cells in the rostellum. In the cysticercoid, the cells did not display fuchsinophilia, but fuchsinophilic material began to accumulate by 3 days postinfection, rapidly becoming maximal as the cells increased in size. The material began to move out into the axons at 16-18 days postinfection and disappeared completely by 40 days postinfection. Davey and Breckenridge suggested that the putative neurosecretory material might be involved with initiation of proglottisation (at 3 days) or apolysis (at 16-18 days). Hitcho and Roberts (unpublished) observed cells in the rostellum which became paraldehyde-fuchsin positive at 3 days postinfection but the fuchsinophilia did not decrease in older worms, at least up to 82 days postinfection, nor were the fuchsinophilic granules observed to move posteriorly in the axons. The existence of any neuroendocrine control in the development of *H. diminuta* has yet to be confirmed.

V. SUPERINFECTION AND LONG TERM MAINTENANCE IN THE RAT

A. *Premunition and Superinfection*

Premunition, or a resistance to superinfection conferred by the presence of the infectious agent in the host, was believed to prevail in cestode infections by earlier authors (reviewed by Roberts and Mong 1968). However, experimental evidence for the existence of the phenomenon in tapeworm infections is meager. In the case of *H. diminuta*, Chandler (1939) reported that the presence of 36 worms in a host precluded establishment of additional tapeworms and that below that number (36) of primary worms, the percentage of secondaries established was in inverse proportion to the number of primaries present. At 10 days after secondary infection, the size of the secondary worms was in inverse proportion to the number of primaries. Chandler concluded that since establishment and growth of secondary worms was normal in rats from which the primaries had been chemically or mechanically removed, the premunition was due to crowding and not to the immune response of the host.

Roberts and Mong (1968) confirmed Chandler's (1939) observation that the size of secondaries was in inverse proportion to the number of primaries present at 10 days after the secondary infection, but they found only a slightly reduced secondary establishment correlated with numbers of primary worms present up to 40 primaries. The rate of growth and maturation of secondary worms was retarded by the presence of primaries, but by 30 days after the secondary infection, the secondaries were reaching maximum size, and the primaries were being reduced in size so as to make the two populations indistinguishable. Roberts and Mong (1968) concluded that there was no evidence for premunition in *H. diminuta* in the sense of resistance to superinfection, and that the effects on the growth of the secondary worms were a manifestation of the crowding effect.

B. Fate of Worms in Long Term Infections

Roberts and Mong (1968) infected rats with 50 cysticercoids each and recovered the cestodes at periods from 30 to 150 days postinfection. Effects of host age on worm establishment and recovery were controlled by infecting other groups of rats of the same age with 50 worms and recovering the worms at 30 days to coincide with the autopsies of the rats in each of the long term maintenance groups. Some rats maintained their high density infections for as long as 150 days, but in some the worm populations were spontaneously reduced to 10 worms or less as early as 90 days postinfection. Immune response of the host was not suggested as a possible explanation for the spontaneous loss of worms. Worms recovered were of a size to be expected from infections of that density, i.e., they were not small, destrobilated worms as reported by Hopkins *et al.* (1972) from long term infections of mice. However, it is possible that such worms escaped notice.

Subsequent to Roberts and Mong (1968), several authors have reported spontaneous loss of *H. diminuta* from multiple worm infections. Harris and Turton (1973) reported a loss of worms from 25 worm infections over a period of 14 weeks. Since no such loss was observed in 5 worm infections, though the antibody titer in the rats was similar to those bearing 25 worm infections, Harris and Turton did not attribute the worm loss to host immunological response. Andreassen *et al.* (1974) observed loss of cestodes from 100 worm infections and an increasing incidence of destrobilated worms up to 75% at 6 weeks postinfection. Since they were able to prevent the worm loss by treatment of the hosts with cortisone, and because a challenge infection after the primary infection had been expelled by an anthelminthic resulted in earlier destrobilation and worm loss, these authors concluded that the mechanism of the loss was the host immune response. Hesselberg and Andreassen (1975) recovered only 2 - 10% "normal" (i.e., not destrobilated) worms from 50 and 100 cysticercoid infections at 8 weeks. Chappell and Pike (1976) reported that average fresh weight decreased in worms from 5, 15, and 30 worm infections from day 19 to day 50 postinfection. Spontaneous loss of worms occurred in 30 worm infections, reducing the average number of worms per host to from 5 to 15 over an 85 day period. Only slight losses occurred in the 15 worm populations, and no losses were observed when hosts were infected with a single worm. Mean recovery was higher and weight loss was less in juvenile rats compared to adult hosts. These authors were not prepared to attribute the results to host immune response.

Further consideration of host immunity and its relation to the biology of *H. diminuta* is found elsewhere in this volume.

VI. CHANGES IN CHEMICAL COMPOSITION THROUGH DEVELOPMENT

The changes in the concentrations of several major chemical constituents have been followed during the developmental period by Roberts (1961) and by Mettrick and Cannon (1970): total carbohydrate (or glycogen), nitrogen, total lipid, phospholipid, RNA, and DNA.

Roberts (1961) reported that the protein concentration of *H. diminuta* fell from 60-70% of dry weight at 4 days postinfection to about 30% of dry weight at 17 days (protein estimated by N X 6.25), and that there was no effect of crowding on the overall decrease nor on the final protein concentration. In contrast, total carbohydrate rose from between 10 and 20% of dry weight to about 40% in low population densities (Fig. 7), and the increase in

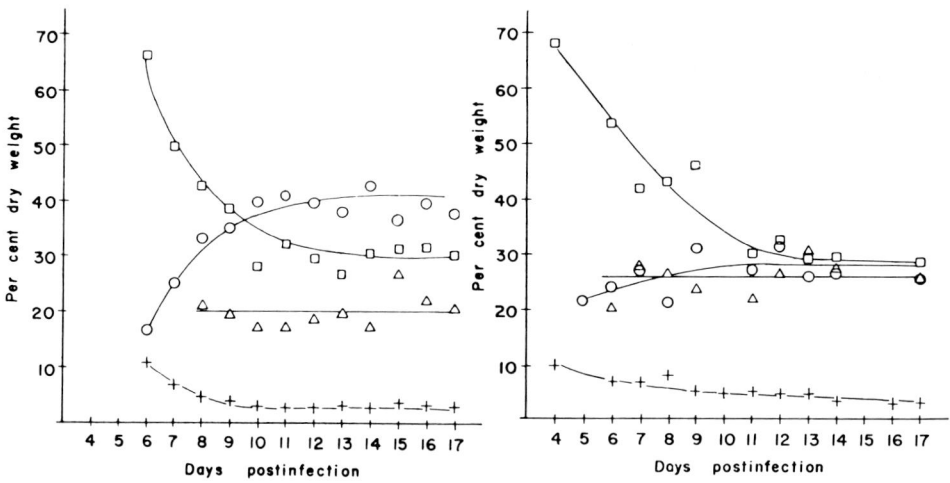

Fig. 7. Comparison of changes in gross chemical composition of H. diminuta during development as affected by population density. Fig. 7a, 3-5 worms per host; Fig. 7b, 15-20 worms per host. □= 'protein', O= carbohydrate; △= lipid, += phospholipid (from Roberts 1961).

carbohydrate was lower with higher numbers of worms per host. Cestodes from 100 worm populations contained only 24% carbohydrate at 17 days postinfection. Total lipid concentration changed relatively little during development, but the level of lipid generally increased with increasing population density and decreasing carbohydrate concentration. Phospholipid fell from a concentration of about 10% at 4 days to about 3% at 17 days, independent of population density.

Mettrick and Cannon (1970) measured non-protein and protein nitrogen, *lyo-* and *desmo-*glycogen, and total lipid in immature, mature and gravid portions of worms from 10 worm infections through development and concentrations of RNA and DNA in whole worms from a similar population density. The changes between *lyo-* and *desmo-*glycogen which they reported must be disregarded since the distinction between those two types of glycogen is an artifact of the extraction procedure (Roe *et al.* 1961). Calculating from their data, however, the concentrations of total carbohydrate and total lipid are in good agreement with those given by Roberts (1961), but their values for nitrogen are much lower, particularly in the younger worms. The reasons for the discrepancy are not apparent.

In cestodes from a 10 worm infection, RNA concentration fell from about 3.5% of dry weight at 5 days to 1.2% at 16 days, while the DNA concentration fell from 0.9% to 0.03% in the same period, with a consequent increase in the ratio of RNA to DNA from about 4:1 to 40:1 (Mettrick and Cannon 1970). These figures doubtless reflect the overall increase in differentiation of the strobila during that period.

VII. EFFECTS OF HOST DIET

A. *Carbohydrates*

That carbohydrates play a crucial role in the biology of cestodes has been recognized for some years (see Read 1959). The fact that the worms can absorb and ferment an extremely limited variety of carbohydrates, plus the fact that they have a large metabolic requirement for carbohydrate, makes the quality and quantity of these substances in the host diet critical to growth and development of the worms.

The earliest observations indicated that restriction in host diet decreased proglottid production in cestodes or caused destrobilation (autotomy) (Levine 1938; Reid 1942), and it became clear that such effects were due to inadequate dietary carbohydrate, not protein or fat (Chandler 1943; Mettrick and Munro 1965). Chandler (1943) observed that the absence or restriction of dietary carbohydrate resulted in reduced establishment of *H. diminuta* and stunting in size, and Chandler *et al.* (1950) reported similar effects whether the worms were previously established or the rats infected subsequent to being fed low carbohydrate diets. Further, they found that neither sucrose nor glucose were adequate substitutes for starch in the host diet, although worms were larger in rats fed glucose than in those fed diets with sucrose as the only carbohydrate. They believed that the difference between starch and glucose diets could be explained by the rapidity of glucose absorption when it was present in the diet in that form versus the longer availability of the substance as starch was digested. These results were confirmed and extended by Read and Rothman (1957 a,b), Read *et al.* (1958), Roberts (1966), and Roberts and Platzer (1967). In addition to sucrose, diets containing only dextrins-maltose or fructose were deleterious to worm growth, and egg production was much lower in worms from rats fed diets suboptimal in carbohydrate quality (Read and Rothman 1957 a,b). Similar effects were found in *H. citelli* and *H. nana*, but growth was inhibited in *H. nana* only if the experimental diets were fed during the time the worms were in active growth, not during the senescent period (Read *et al.* 1958). There was a positive correlation between size and egg production of *H. diminuta* and increase in the amount of starch fed per host each day in the range 0.1 to 3.0 g, and the effects of carbohydrate deprivation in the worms could be reversed by changing the rat to an adequate diet (Read *et al.* 1958). Roberts (1966) observed that low starch and sucrose diets inhibited proglottisation, as well as stunting the worms, and that these diets resulted in lower carbohydrate concentration and higher lipid than in worms from rats fed high starch diets. Roberts and Platzer (1967) confirmed that change to suboptimal carbohydrate diets reduced the size of previously established adult *H. diminuta*. They also observed that deletion of roughage from the diets and increase of starch content (from 30% to 50%) resulted in larger worms. No synthetic diet in the foregoing work, however, produced cestodes as large as those from rats fed normal laboratory ration (Purina Laboratory Chow). It should be emphasized that all the dietary formulations (used by Read, Roberts, and their co-workers) were suboptimal for the worms only; they appeared completely adequate for the rat hosts, at least for the period of the experiment. Furthermore, the hosts were fed *ad lib.* and/or with controls not fed isocalorically.

In contrast, Dunkley and Mettrick (1969) reported that worms from rats fed a glucose diet grew more rapidly than did those from rats fed a maltose diet, while maltose was more effective in supporting growth than starch. They used an isocaloric feeding regime, but one which was suboptimal for the rats (protein free, causing 18% loss in weight in 8 days) and a starch (potato) which rats do not digest completely. The results of Komuniecki and Roberts (1975), using nutritionally adequate diets and isocaloric controls, confirmed that diets containing glucose as the sole carbohydrate retarded growth as compared to diets containing adequate amounts of corn starch. One dietary formulation reported by Komuniecki and Roberts (1975) (containing 56% starch and 6% cellulose roughage) produced worm development that was entirely equal to that of the Chow ration. It was shown also that worms from rats fed diets with glucose as the sole carbohydrate produced fewer proglottids and had a higher lipid and lower carbohydrate concentration in their bodies.

Since Mead and Roberts (1972) had reported that the Purina Laboratory Chow contained some sucrose and lactose (about 6% of the total diet), Komuniecki and Roberts (1975) tested high starch diets with those components added. No beneficial effect on worm development was observed.

Roberts (1966) had reported that feeding diets *ad lib.* containing sucrose as the sole carbohydrate did not affect the growth of worms by 5 days post-infection. However, Komuniecki and Roberts (1975), feeding experimental animals isocalorically with controls, showed that a glucose diet inhibited growth of the worms as early as five days postinfection, or well within the logarithmic growth phase.

Read (1959), with considerable insight, emphasized the critical role of carbohydrates in the biology of cestodes, pointing out that these parasites and perhaps many others "have a <u>requirement for</u> <u>carbohydrate</u>" (emphasis his), and that this was in contrast to most free-living organisms. Clearly, this requirement must be met not only when the worms are increasing in size, but also when growth suffices only for maintenance, i.e., replaces proglottids lost in apolysis (Read *et al.* 1958; Roberts and Platzer 1967). The magnitude of stored carbohydrate (up to around 50% of dry weight) is impressive, and the worms rapidly deplete their glycogen during host starvation. However, the worm dry weight is still 10% carbohydrate after a 48 hr host starvation (Fairbairn *et al.* 1961). The full ramifications and implications of this large amount of stored carbohydrate in the development and maintenance of the worm are yet to be fully explored, but they are doubtless related to the primarily glycolytic energy pathways of the worm (see Fioravanti and Saz, this volume). As pointed out by Schmidt and Roberts (1977), the large amount of stored glycogen would serve as an effective cushion between host feeding periods.

B. *Vitamins*

Clear conclusions are difficult to draw from the earlier investigations of vitamin requirements of cestodes, partly because of the failure of these workers to appreciate the role of the host's cecal microflora in vitamin supply.

1. Early Work and Interaction with Host Sex Hormones. Hager (1941) found that some component of brewer's yeast in the diet of the host was necessary for normal egg production. Her observation that this component was heat stable led her to the conclusion that its identity was not vitamin B, but "vitamin G". Chandler (1943) found that *H. diminuta* was smaller when the host diet did not contain components rich in "vitamin G complex" (rice bran concentrate or autoclaved brewer's yeast), but this was true only in female rats. He reported that the size of the worms was apparently independent of vitamins A, D, E, and B_1. Addis and Chandler (1944) reported that the effects of vitamin deficient diets on the worms were greater if the hosts were fed such diets for a period before infection. They confirmed the observation that something in the "G complex" was necessary for normal development, and they found evidence that lack of vitamins A, D, and E resulted in lower worm infection in rats. If the "G complex" was also absent, the average number of worms per rat was further reduced. They suggested that the secretion of bile may have been affected by lack of the fat-soluble vitamins, and, consequently, the worms may not have excysted normally. Addis and Chandler (1946) were not able to substitute any or all of the then known components of the G complex for yeast in the diet and produce normal worm growth. The components included riboflavin, nicotinic acid, pyridoxine, pantothenic acid, biotin, p-aminobenzoic acid, inositol, choline, and folic acid. The lack of other vitamin sources in the diet was not compensated by a commercial yeast concentrate and only partially by a liver extract. Addis (1946) reported more fully on the interaction of sex hormones and host diet on growth of *H. diminuta*. He confirmed that worms grew normally in male rats whether on a complete diet or one deficient in G complex, while they were stunted in females on a deficient diet. He found that worms were smaller in castrated males, and this effect could be nullified by giving testosterone to the hosts whether or not on a deficient diet. Progesterone also produced normal worm growth in castrated males, but theelin (estrone) did not. A vitamin deficient diet resulted in smaller worms whether normal or spayed females were used. Supplementation of normal or spayed females with progesterone, theelin, stilbesterol or testosterone did not produce maximum tapeworm growth if a deficient diet was used. Conditions of pregnancy, however, allowed the worms to attain normal size, even on a deficient diet.

Beck (1951, 1952) studied egg production of *H. diminuta* under several conditions of diet and hormonal treatment of hosts. He found that egg production of worms in female hosts declined on a vitamin deficient diet, in agreement with Chandler and Addis. He also observed that if male hosts were fed deficient diets for about 3 months, worm egg production finally declined to about the same level as in females on the same diet. In contrast to the result in female hosts, however, worm size was about the same even though egg production was decreased. The decline in egg production of worms in castrated males on a complete diet was comparable, after about 3 months, to the decline observed in normal males on a deficient diet. Testosterone and progesterone raised egg production to normal in castrated males and testosterone but not progesterone had this effect in females on a deficient diet. Chorionic gonadatropin raised egg production of worms in males and females on deficient diets, but not in gonadectomized hosts. For 22 days, he injected 0.5 µg of vitamin B_{12} daily into 2 female hosts which had been on a deficient diet for 34 days. No increase in worm egg production was observed. The significance of the effects of host sex hormones and their interaction with vitamin requirements remains conjectural. The work has not been pursued with more recent nutritional methodology, using carefully controlled conditions.

Chandler *et al*. (1950) studied the effect of thiamine on worm size. The growth of the worm was not affected by elimination of thiamine from the host diet. They found that the thiamine concentration in the small intestinal mucosa was decreased on thiamine-free diets. Fecal thiamine was about the same as that in the mucosa on the thiamine-free diet but mucosal thiamine increased after parenteral injection of this vitamin, while fecal concentration did not. Thiamine in *H. diminuta* was fairly constant whether the vitamin was in the diet or not or whether parenteral injections were administered. Upon the parenteral injection of ^{35}S-labelled thiamine, specific activity of the worms was identical to that of the mucosa. On that basis, they concluded that thiamine was absorbed by the worms from the host gut mucosa.

2. *Coprophagy Prevention and the B_6 Requirement*. Subsequent to the reports cited above, it was discovered that rats may consume up to 50% or more of their feces, even when maintained on raised wire cages (Barnes et al. 1957). Furthermore, effects of unequal food intake by hosts on complete and vitamin deficient diets were not controlled in the earlier work. Platzer and Roberts (1969) examined the effects of feeding diets deficient in B vitamins on the development of *H. diminuta*, while preventing coprophagy with tail cups and feeding experimentals isocalorically with controls. Under these conditions, establishment and growth of the worms were severely inhibited when hosts were fed diets deficient in all B vitamins (biotin, cyanocobalimin, folic acid, inositol, niacin, p-aminobenzoic acid, pantothenate, pyridoxine, riboflavin, and thiamine) (Fig. 8). If coprophagy was not prevented, worms from vitamin deficient hosts were not different from controls. By a process of elimination, it was found that the lack of pyridoxine (vitamin B_6) was responsible for most of the effect. Also, production of proglottids was severely inhibited in worms from rats in which coprophagy was prevented and which were fed B_6-deficient diets. As earlier workers had implicated sex hormones in the effects produced by vitamin deficient diets, Platzer and Roberts (1969) attempted to assess the hormonal level of rats fed diets deficient in pyridoxine. The weights of the seminal vesicles and associated coagulating glands, which accurately reflect the sex hormonal status of the rat (Turner 1966), did not differ in groups fed pyridoxine-deficient diets and controls. Other experiments yielded strong evidence that the worms could obtain sufficient pyridoxine for growth via the exocrino-enteric circulation: if the rats were fed B_6-deficient diets (coprophagy prevented) and were injected with 50 or 200 µg pyridoxine daily, worm development was the same as controls fed B_6 in their diets, and daily injections of 10 µg into hosts on B_6-deficient diets produced moderate stunting of the worms.

In common with other animal tissues, the major forms of vitamin B_6 in *H. diminuta* are pyridoxal (85%) and pyridoxamine (15%) with only small amounts of pyridoxine (Platzer and Roberts 1970b). The content of vitamin B_6 measured in the tissues of

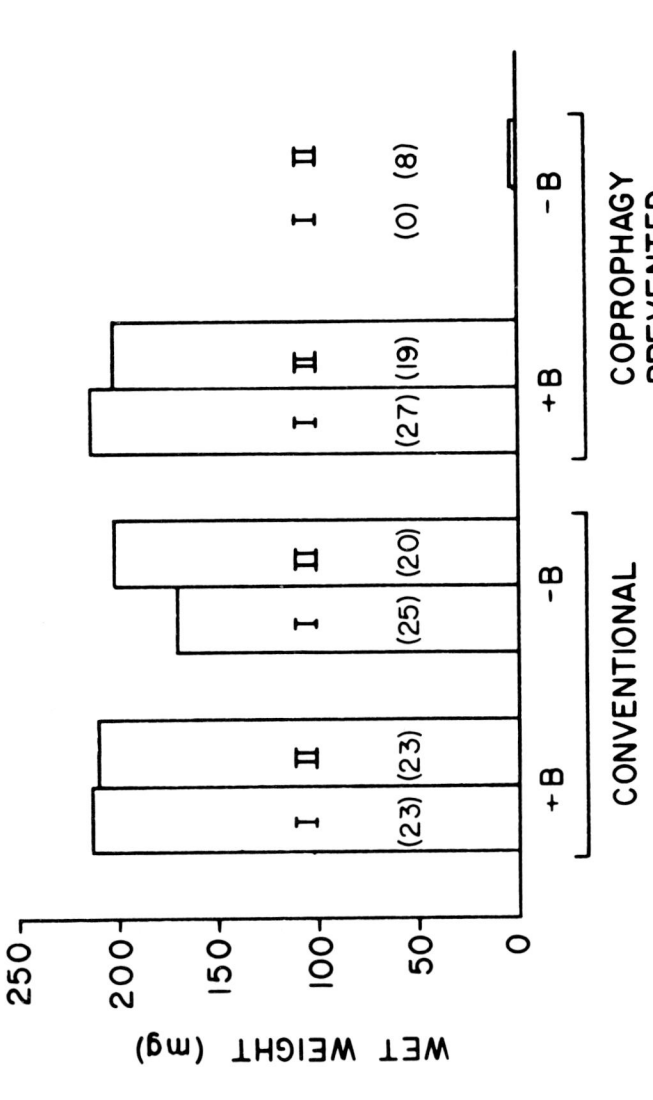

Fig. 8. Effects of coprophagy prevention and deletion of all B vitamins from host diet on mean weight attained by H. diminuta. Rats were fed test diets from 5 days prior to infection to 15 days postinfection when the worms were recovered. I, II denote results from separate experiments. Numbers in parentheses indicate total number of worms recovered from each group of 6 rats given 5 cysticercoids per host (data from Platzer and Roberts 1969).

H. diminuta was 1.6 - 2.0 ng/mg wet weight in worms from rats fed pellet diet or complete test diets; this level was reduced to 0.2 - 0.3 ng/mg in worms fed B_6-deficient diets or injected with limiting amounts of B_6 (coprophagy prevented) (Platzer and Roberts 1970b). By comparison, this level was comparable to that previously reported in *Moniezia benedeni* by Chance and Dirnhuber (1949), but only 0.2 of that in rat liver (Caldwell and McHenry 1953; Thiele and Brin 1966).

Of the many enzymes which are known to require pyridoxal phosphate as a cofactor in other systems, glycogen phosphorylase and glutamic pyruvic transaminase were chosen for assay by Platzer and Roberts (1970b) in *H. diminuta*. The worms were from hosts given diets lacking vitamin B_6 and from those given limiting amounts (10 μg per day) by injection. The specific activity of phosphorylase was 31% lower than controls in cestodes from both pyridoxine deficient and limited rats and that of glutamic pyruvic transaminase was 66% lower than controls in worms from B_6-limited hosts.

Roberts and Mong (1973) tested the effects of an antimetabolite of pyridoxine, deoxypyridoxine on the development of *H. diminuta in vitro* using a modification of the culture method of Schiller (1965). Increase in weight in vitro was substantially inhibited by the presence of 200 μM deoxypyridoxine in the medium and completely inhibited at the 400 μM level (Fig. 9). The presence of pyridoxine equal in concentration to the deoxypyridoxine reversed the inhibition. Concentrations of 200 μM deoxypyridoxine and above interfered with proglottisation and reproduction.

3. The Riboflavin Effect. In marked contrast to the foregoing, when hosts are fed a diet lacking riboflavin, *H. diminuta* grow much larger than those from hosts fed isocaloric complete diets (Platzer and Roberts 1970a). The effect was observed whether or not coprophagy was prevented. To assess the hormonal status of the rats fed riboflavin deficient diets, the seminal vesicles with attached coagulating glands and the adrenal glands were weighed, but they were not different from controls. Of the several possible explanations for the riboflavin-deficiency effect, the most likely seems to be that more glucose was available to the worms; glucose absorption is impaired in rats on riboflavin-deficient diets (Althausen *et al.* 1946).

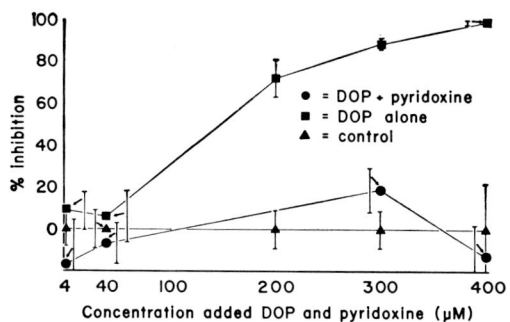

Fig. 9. Inhibition of increase in weight of H. diminuta cultured in vitro by 4-deoxypyridoxine HCl (DOP).

Per cent inhibition = 100

$$- \frac{(Final\ wt\ of\ experimental\ -\ initial\ wt) \times 100}{(Final\ wt\ of\ control\ -\ initial\ wt)}$$

Vertical lines represent ± 1 standard error, expressed as per cent of control mean. Initial weights of worms in experimental groups for each level of DOP tested did not differ from initial weights of worms in corresponding control groups.
▲ = *control, no added vitamin or antimetabolite;* ■ = *deoxypyridoxine added to Hanks' solution overlay;* ● = *deoxypyridoxine plus equimolar pyridoxine added to overlay. (from Roberts and Mong 1973).*

4. *Other Possible Requirements.* Platzer and Roberts (1970a) pointed out that the riboflavin-deficiency effect does not mean necessarily that *H. diminuta* has no requirement for an exogenous source of riboflavin or that such requirement could not be demonstrated under other conditions. Neither does the lack of any effect upon deletion of other vitamins from the host diet, even with coprophagy prevented, lead to a similar conclusion. Even in the case of vitamin B_6 in which the evidence for a requirement is very strong, rather extreme measures

must be taken to demonstrate an effect. The threshold at which the host shows symptoms of vitamin deficiency is lower than that for the worm, i.e., the rats show pyridoxine deficiency on a B_6-free diet, even without coprophagy prevention. It may be that levels of some of the other vitamins at which effects on worm development could be detected would not be compatible with continued life of the host. It is at least suggestive that the most severe effects observed by Platzer and Roberts (1969) were when the hosts were fed diets deficient in <u>all</u> B vitamins, rather than B_6 alone. *H. diminuta* absorbs thiamine, pyridoxine, riboflavin and nicotinamide (Pappas 1972; Pappas and Read 1972 a,b), but not vitamin B_{12} (Tkachuck *et al.* 1976). Pyridoxine and nicotinamide are absorbed by diffusion only, but thiamine and riboflavin are taken up, at least in part, by relatively specific mediated transport mechanisms.

C. *Other Dietary Substances*

1. *Proteins and Lipids.* Chandler (1943) reported that *H. diminuta* grew larger when rats were fed a protein-free diet than those worms from rats fed a complete diet, but his protein-free diet contained additional starch to replace the deleted casein. Mettrick and Munro (1965) confirmed that result, and they concluded that the omission of the protein from the diet was not responsible for the effect, because if the starch was replaced by lipid instead of carbohydrate, the worms from rats fed protein-free diets were not larger than controls. They believed that worm growth was not affected by protein quality since replacement of the casein with zein in the test diet did not apparently affect development.

Considering the amount of amino acids and lipids entering the gut via the exocrino-enteric circulation (see Read 1971), it is unremarkable that dietary alterations in lipid and protein should have little effect. The lack of effect on the worms of low protein in the host diet was confirmed by Morcock and Roberts (unpublished), who used 14 g daily meals of diets low in protein (5% casein) or high in protein (30% casein). The casein deleted from the low protein diet was replaced by corn starch. However, worms from rats fed the low protein diet were not larger than controls, as was found by Mettrick and Munro (1965), probably because of the very different feeding regime. Moreover, Morcock and Roberts (unpublished) found that when the meal size was decreased to 10 g/day, the size attained by worms from hosts on low protein diets was substantially less than controls (Table I). These findings were in conjunction with experiments on the effects of concurrent infections with a pathogenic nematode (*Nippostrongylus brasiliensis*) and will be discussed further below.

2. Amino Acids. Mettrick and Munro (1965) obtained varying results from experiments with tryptophan and lysine added to test diets, growth being stimulated or inhibited depending on whether the amino acids were fed together with or separately from other components of the test diet, added to carbohydrate-rich or fat-rich, protein-free diets, etc. Hopkins and Young (1967) used much larger groups of rats and failed, in replicated experiments to obtain any effect on growth by adding lysine and/or tryptophan to a protein-free diet. Mettrick (1971) suggested this was "possibly due to the variability ... in the size of worms", but calculations of standard error in Hopkins and Young's experiments give much lower values than those shown in Mettrick and Munro's (1965) and Mettrick's (1968, 1971) experiments. There is considerable doubt therefore, whether in the quantities used and as administered, l-lysine or l-tryptophan affects growth. This does not preclude other amino acids from having an effect, though Mettrick (1971) found that l-cysteine had no significant effect even at 81 mg. With other amino acid additives, Mettrick (1971) reported a consistent, small depression of growth varying up to 24% when 0.235 mmoles of the amino acid were given each day. It may be noted, however, that tryptophan in this amount had the lowest and statistically not significant, effect. This may explain why Hopkins and Young (1967) found no effect on growth by adding tryptophan. Therefore, different amino acids may affect growth of *H. diminuta* to different extents. Surprisingly, the quantity added seems to be less important: 35 mg methionine daily retarded growth by 17%, 112 mg by 26%; 25 mg of serine by 15%, 50 mg by 12%. In fact, only with tryptophan was there a large increase from 7%

TABLE I. Effect of Low Protein Diet and of Concurrent Infection with Nippostrongylus brasiliensis on Establishment and Size of Hymenolepis diminuta[a]

Protein and carbohydrate in diet	Experiment number	Nematodes recovered (Mean ± SE)	Cestodes recovered (Mean ± SE)	Mean fresh weights of cestodes (mg ± SE)
30% casein, 55% corn starch	I	—	10.0 ± 0.6	207.5 ± 17.1
	II	—	10.0 ± 0.2	158.0 ± 17.6
	I	3,383 ± 149	4.3 ± 1.1	112.4 ± 8.0
	II	3,611 ± 200	7.2 ± 1.2	99.3 ± 13.3
5% casein, 80% corn starch	I	—	10.3 ± 0.2	111.8 ± 6.0
	II	—	10.8 ± 0.8	88.8 ± 7.8
	I	3,300 ± 100	5.0 ± 1.7	52.5 ± 7.2
	II	2,255 ± 424	2.7 ± 2.2	44.8 ± 6.9

[a] Rats given 11 cysticercoids of H. diminuta, then 4000 third stage juveniles of N. brasiliensis after 5 days, worms recovered 15 days later. (Here and where applicable in other tables and figures, day of infection is day 0).

(insignificant) to 24% when the amount of tryptophan was doubled from 48 to 96 mg. This is noteworthy as a further doubling of the tryptophan to 192 mg/day led to no further retardation of worm growth. If the 96 mg tryptophan value was by chance a high result, the last discrepancy between Hopkins and Young's (1967) and Mettrick's (1968, 1971) results disappears.

The feeding regime differed slightly in these experiments, but in all experiments, two meals were given daily, morning and evening. The bulk of the carbohydrate was glucose; the other carbohydrate was potato starch, and the daily meals were less than 9 g total per rat. The amino acids were given with the morning meal along with glucose, and the rats were fed the test diet for 7 days when the worms were 168-336 hr post infection (Mettrick) and for 8 days, from a worm age of 120 to 312 hr post infection (Hopkins and Young), after which the worms were removed and weighed.

Two hypotheses why an amino acid imbalance in the diet might retard growth have been suggested. The first arose from the work of Read *et al.* (1963), in which the important concept that a tapeworm parasitizes the homeostatic mechanism of its host was first propounded, and massive evidence was presented that the amino acid pool in *H. diminuta* is in a complex equilibrium with the amino acids in the medium around the worm. Hopkins and Callow (1965) verified that free amino acids in a worm are in dynamic equilibrium with the amino acids in the lumen of the intestine and suggested "It may, therefore, become possible to inhibit the growth of a tapeworm by altering the amino acid balance in the intestine". Although, as discussed above, the evidence, at least up to the late 1960's, that an amino acid imbalance could be achieved by dietary means in the rat's small intestine sufficient to retard growth of *H. diminuta* was weak, Hopkins (1969) wrote "The hypothesis that it should be possible to inhibit growth of the tapeworm by altering the balance of amino acids in the intestine is nevertheless, still valid, and the failure to inhibit growth in practice could have been due to the dietary amino acids affecting the level of amino acids normally present in the intestine for too short a period to cause a detectable inhibition in the growth of the tapeworm". In support of this he showed that methionine in a protein-free diet does affect the amino acid pool of a tapeworm, but only for about 3 hr after the diet is eaten and only in that part of the tapeworm lying in the anterior half of the small intestine. He suggested, therefore, that to have an appreciable effect on growth, it might be necessary to give meals with an amino acid imbalance every 3 hr. It is possible, however, that other amino acids might have a more prolonged effect than did methionine, and Mettrick (1971) correlated the degree of inhibition he observed in worm growth with the speed at which the amino acids tested were absorbed by the host. The more slowly the host absorbed an amino acid, the longer it would be in contact with the worm, thus affecting the amino acid pool of the worm. The hypothesis is still attractive but needs experimental evidence to show that protein metabolism really is deranged before the notion can be considered anything more than a hypothesis.

A second explanation for the retarding effect on growth resulting from feeding an amino acid imbalanced diet was suggested by Mettrick (1971): "That the dietary amino acid supplements either directly or indirectly inhibit carbohydrate uptake and metabolism by the tapeworm". On the basis that transport of some hexoses and amino acids may be mutually inhibitory in the rat intestine, Mettrick favored the second hypothesis. Much work on the absorption of amino acids by cestodes has now been done, and it appears that such transport is not by ion-coupled mechanisms, in contrast to mammalian systems and to glucose transport by *H. diminuta* (Pappas and Read 1975). It must be concluded that this second hypothesis, like the first, is at present unproven.

VIII. EFFECTS OF BILE SALTS

Bile salts are an important physiological trigger for the development of the adult from the cysticercoid, stimulating excystment, and that role will be considered elsewhere in this volume. Other than their role in excystment, the importance of bile salts in development of cestodes has received scant attention.

Goodchild (1958, 1960, 1961 a,b) made rats bileless by cannulation of the bile duct to the outside or by rerouting bile to the cecum. He found that *H. diminuta* was seriously affected, either failing to establish in the host gut or being severely stunted. Egg production and carbohydrate concentration of worms from bileless hosts were greatly depressed. Goodchild's (1958) conclusion was that "bile contains a factor, or factors, apparently necessary for normal growth and maturation of adult *H. diminuta* in the rat host". In reference to that conclusion, Smyth and Haslewood (1963) pointed out that the effects observed could have been indirect results of disturbances in digestive function of the hosts. Smyth (1969) remarked that a bile requirement for growth of *H. diminuta* is refuted by the fact that worms can be cultured *in vitro* in the absence of bile (Berntzen 1961; Schiller 1965; Roberts and Mong 1969; Roberts 1973). However, in our hands, at least, the growth of *H. diminuta* is not "normal" *in vitro* (Roberts and Mong 1969; Roberts 1973), and Berntzen's (1961) results have yet to be duplicated. Hence, the notion that normal development of *H. diminuta* may require the presence of bile salts cannot yet be discarded.

Rather than a stimulatory effect as would be implied by the results of Goodchild, Rothman (1958) reported that the anaerobic fermentation of glucose by *H. diminuta* was inhibited by sodium cholate, taurocholate and glycocholate. Phifer (1960) found an inhibition of glucose uptake by sodium taurocholate of 65 to 70% when the worms were preincubated 15 min in the bile salt. On the other hand, using purified bile salts, Surgan and Roberts (1976b) found only 15 to 25% inhibition of glucose uptake by sodium taurocholate and no inhibition by sodium glycocholate in *H. diminuta*. Tkachuck and MacInnis (1971) observed no effect of sodium taurocholate on the glucose metabolism of *H. diminuta*. The bile salts themselves do not enter the tapeworm but adsorb to its tegument, each apparently to a specific site (Surgan and Roberts 1976a). It is more likely that the importance of bile salts in the development of cestodes will be found in their facilitation of the absorption of fatty acids by the worms (Bailey and Fairbairn 1968; Surgan and Roberts 1976b), and that conclusion must await further elucidation of the importance of lipids in the cestode's metabolism.

IX. CONCURRENT INFECTION OF THE HOST WITH OTHER HELMINTHS

The growth of *H. diminuta* in rats simultaneously infected with other helminth species has been studied. The results suggest that the presence of either an acanthocephalan, *Moniliformis dubius*, or a nematode, *Nippostrongylus brasiliensis*, can modify the habitat and affect the growth of the cestode.

A. *Moniliformis dubius*

Holmes (1961) infected rats with 5 cysticercoids of *H. diminuta* and 10 cystacanths of *Moniliformis dubius*, recovered the worms at 8 weeks postinfection and compared the size attained and position in the intestine with worms from rats given varying numbers of either species singly. *H. diminuta* from single species infections showed the crowding effect with increasing infection size, as did *M. dubius*, except that the reduction in size attained was not so marked in the acanthocephalan as in the cestode. The tapeworms were attached (position of scolex) generally in the anterior half of the intestine, spreading to the posterior half in more crowded infections (20 worms/host). The acanthocephalans were attached in the anterior third of the gut, even in the higher population densities (ca. 30 worms/host). In concurrent infections, the size attained by both species was much lower than would have been expected had the worms of the other species not been present, strongly suggesting that individuals of both species were exerting a crowding effect on the other. The number of worms recovered, however, was independent of the presence of the other species. The individuals of both species seemed to segregate into separate regions of the intestine: the acanthocephalans were attached almost entirely in the anterior quarter, with the tapeworms moving back and being attached from about 28 to 65% down the intestinal length. The growth rate of *H. diminuta* was lowered when rats were infected simultaneously with *M. dubius* and was retarded more markedly when the hosts were infected with the tapeworms after the *M. dubius* were already mature (Holmes 1962a). If the rats carried patent *H. diminuta* infections when they were given cystacanths of the acanthocephalan, the tapeworms decreased in size as the *M. dubius* grew and took up their position anterior to the cestodes. All of these results are consistent with a conclusion that *M. dubius* exerts a crowding effect on *H. diminuta* just as if there were additional tapeworms present, presumably, but not necessarily, by the same mechanism. Curiously, no such crowding effect (on either species) was observed in concurrent infections in hamsters (Holmes 1962b).

B. *Nippostrongylus brasiliensis*

Morcock and Roberts (unpublished) studied concurrent infections of *H. diminuta* and *Nippostrongylus brasiliensis* with regard to effects on the host and on tapeworm development. Rats were infected with 10 cysticercoids each of *H. diminuta*, and after five days they were given 4000 third stage juveniles of *N. brasiliensis* subcutaneously. These were compared with groups of hosts given single species infections of each worm, and all groups were divided so that half were fed 10 g/day portions of a high protein diet (30% casein, 55% corn starch) or of a low protein diet (5% casein, 80% corn starch) (Table I). The worms were recovered 10 days later. As noted above, the protein deficient diet reduced the size attained by *H. diminuta*, though number of tapeworms established was not affected by protein deficiency. The size attained by the tapeworms in the presence of the nematodes was markedly reduced, and the reduction was compounded when the rats were fed protein deficient diets (Table I). Numbers of cestodes recovered from the rats given concurrent infections, were lower than those from single species infections and since the nematode infection occurred five days later than the cestode infection, the lower recoveries presumably reflect loss of tapeworms from the rats. In another experiment, rats fed 10 g/day portions of the high and low protein diets were infected with 4000 juveniles of *N. brasiliensis* then given 11 cysticercoids of *H. diminuta*, and the worms were recovered 15 days thereafter. The effects on the size attained by the tapeworms were similar to those in the previous experiments, but the numbers of cestodes recovered were even lower (Table II). In this experiment, the location of the tapeworms in the host intestine was noted. The length of the intestine occupied by cestode tissue was less in rats with *N. brasiliensis*, irrespective of diet, with the anterior limit more posterior (Table III). In light of the reduced establishment and/or loss of *H. diminuta* from rats infected with the nematode, it would appear that the effects are not the result of crowding in this case, but rather of inhospitable conditions induced by the pathogenic effects of the nematode, stimulation by the nematode of the immune responses of the host, or both.

X. DEVELOPMENTAL ASPECTS OF CARBOHYDRATE METABOLISM IN *H. DIMINUTA*

To paraphrase Smyth (1969), the role of carbohydrates in the biology of cestodes can be considered at three interrelated levels: 1) dietary carbohydrate of the host and digestion and absorption of this carbohydrate, 2) absorption of carbohydrate by the worm, i.e., transport of carbohydrate molecules from the intraluminal locus into the worm tissue, and 3) metabolism of the carbohydrate by the worm. Effects of dietary carbohydrate on development have been reviewed above, and certain developmental aspects of the second two levels will be considered below.

A. Carbohydrate Absorption

It has been known for some time that *Hymenolepis diminuta* can absorb and metabolize only two saccharides: glucose and galactose (Laurie 1957; Read and Rothman 1958). Though it seems clear that the optimal source of glucose supply to the worm is as a digestive product of dietary starch, there is as yet no evidence that the cestodes can absorb any of the other products of starch digestion, such as maltose, maltotriose, or α-dextrin, *in vivo* or *in vitro*. Reducing conditions, as might prevail in the

TABLE II. Effect of Low Protein Diet and of Concurrent Infection with Nippostrongylus brasiliensis on Establishment and Size Attained by Hymenolepis diminuta

Protein and carbohydrate in diet	Nematodes recovered (Mean ± SE)	Cestodes recovered (Mean ± SE)	Mean fresh weights of cestodes (mg ± SE)
30% casein, 55% corn starch	608 ± 171 —	7.3 ± 0.4 1.8 ± 0.5	222.0 ± 13.3 60.3 ± 17.0
5% casein, 80% corn starch	645 ± 90 —	9.3 ± 0.3 2.0 ± 0.6	92.0 ± 7.8 35.1 ± 9.9

[a]Rats given 4000 third stage juveniles of N. brasiliensis, then 11 cysticercoids of H. diminuta after 5 days, worms recovered 15 days later.

TABLE III. Effect of Low Protein Diet and of Concurrent Infection with Nippostrongylus brasiliensis on Location of Hymenolepis diminuta in Host Intestine[a]

Protein and carbohydrate in diet	Nematodes present	Position of H. diminuta in small intestine (% of intestinal length ± SE)		
		Anterior limit[b] (% of distance from pyloric valve)	Posterior limit[b] (% of distance from pyloric valve)	Length of intestine occupied by cestode tissue
30% casein, 55% corn starch	−	9.3 ± 1.5	75.2 ± 3.0	65.8 ± 2.4
	+	27.2 ± 2.8	62.5 ± 6.8	35.3 ± 6.8
5% casein, 80% corn starch	−	14.4 ± 5.6	72.4 ± 3.3	58.0 ± 4.1
	+	40.7 ± 6.6	62.5 ± 8.4	21.7 ± 6.4

[a] Results from same experiment as Table II.

[b] Anterior and posterior limits were the anteriormost and posteriormost locations, respectively, where cestode tissue was present in the intestine.

host's intestine, do not allow maltose absorption by *H. diminuta in vitro* (Roberts, unpublished).

The characteristics of glucose absorption by *H. diminuta* as a function of development have been studied by Starling and Roberts (unpublished) and by Henderson (1977; discussed below). Some of the data of Starling and Roberts were published by Starling (1975). Their experiments compared the kinetics of hexose transport in 6, 10 and 20-day-old worms. The cestodes were collected, washed and preincubated for 30 min in balanced saline (Krebs-Ringers-Tris) at 37 C. They were then incubated 2 min in media containing ^{14}C-glucose or ^{14}C-galactose at appropriate concentrations, blotted, and extracted for 24 hr in 70% ethanol. Initial transport velocities were calculated on the basis of ethanol extractable radioactivity and expressed as micromoles of sugar absorbed per gram ethanol extracted dry weight per 2 min. Glucose uptake is a saturable function of substrate concentration and obeys Michaelis-Menten kinetics (Fig. 10). Since transport is a surface dependent phenomenon, it was not surprising that the much smaller 6-day-old worms with their greater surface to volume ratio, showed a higher transport rate on the basis of worm weight (Fig. 10). However, the hexose concentration for half-maximal absorption velocity (K_t) is a function of the kinetics of binding and translocation by individual transport sites and is, therefore, independent of the number of transport sites on the surface of worms of different sizes. The apparent K_t's for the different worm ages were calculated from Lineweaver-Burk plots and showed an increase with increasing worm age (Table IV).

In addition to the differences in K_t for glucose and galactose uptake by worms at different stages of development, there appear to be age-dependent changes in the cation binding sites of the sodium-dependent monosaccharide transport system. Hexose absorption in *H. diminuta* is absolutely dependent on the presence of sodium ions (Dike and Read 1971; Read *et al*. 1974; Pappas *et al*. 1974; Starling 1975). When Na^+ was completely replaced by K^+, no glucose transport occurred, regardless of worm age (Fig. 11). For 20-day-old worms, the Na^+ requirement was essentially saturated above 60 mM, but the need for much higher

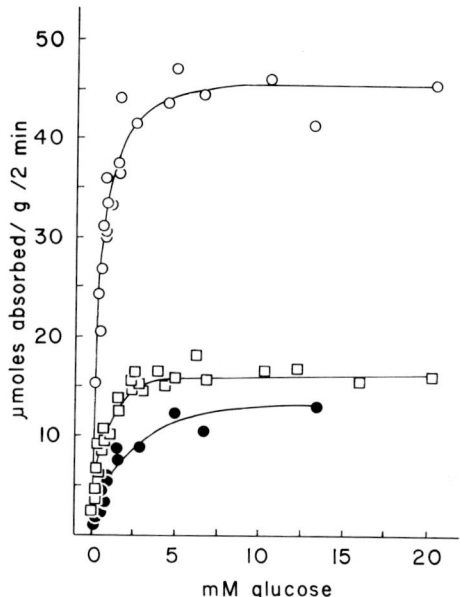

Fig. 10. Effect of worm age on glucose uptake as a function of substrate concentration. ○ = 6-day-old worms; □ = 10-day-old worms; ● = 20-day-old worms.

Na^+ levels in 6 day worms was apparently an artifact resulting from the use of K^+ as the substituting cation. When choline was used as the replacing cation, the dependence of glucose uptake on $[Na^+]$ in 6 day worms was more similar to that observed for 20 day worms, i.e., reached near saturation above 60 mM Na^+. The lower velocity observed when K^+ was the substituting cation indicated that the K^+ was an inhibitor of glucose uptake in 6 day worms. Glucose absorption in 6 day worms was measured as a function of $[K^+]$ at constant $[Na^+]$ (20 mM) for two different glucose concentrations. The Dixon plot of 1/v for glucose absorption showed common intersection of the lines on the abscissa, indicating that K^+ is a non-competitive inhibitor of glucose uptake (Fig. 12). In similar experiments at two different Na^+ concentrations, lines on the Dixon plot intersected at an ordinate value of 0.08, which is approximately equal to the reciprocal of the velocity one would expect

TABLE IV. *Transport Parameters for Glucose and Galactose Uptake by Hymenolepis diminuta of Different Ages*

Worm Age (Days Post-Infection)	Apparent K_t ± SE (mM)		V_{max} ± SE (µmoles/gram / 2 minutes)	
	Glucose	Galactose	Glucose	Galactose
6	0.43 ± 0.03	1.89 ± 0.06	49.8 ± 3.2	62.3 ± 3.3
10	0.74 ± 0.08	2.70 ± 0.44	20.1 ± 0.5	25.2 ± 2.2
20	1.84 ± 0.08	4.27 ± 0.25	16.4 ± 1.1	23.4 ± 0.9

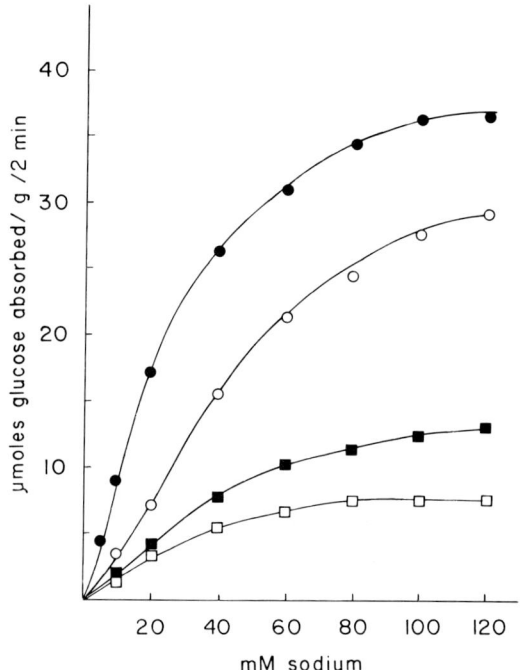

Fig. 11. Effect of worm age on rate of glucose uptake as a function of $[Na^+]$. ● = 6 day worms with choline as the replacing cation; ○ = 6 day worms with K^+ as the replacing cation; ■ and □ = 10 and 20 day worms, respectively, with K^+ as the replacing cation.

at saturating $[Na^+]$. Thus, it appeared that K^+ was a competitive inhibitor with respect to Na^+, and that K^+ competes with Na^+ for binding to the transport system. Therefore, it is confirmed that Na^+ is a velocity activator for hexose transport in *H. diminuta*, i.e., lowering the $[Na^+]$ or increasing the $[K^+]$ reduces the maximal rate of glucose transport, but has no effect on the apparent K_t (Read et al. 1974).

For any system in which the inhibitor interacts with all the transport sites and is completely effective, a double reciprocal plot of the fractional inhibition (1/i) versus the inhibitor concentration must have an ordinate intercept of 1.0, equivalent

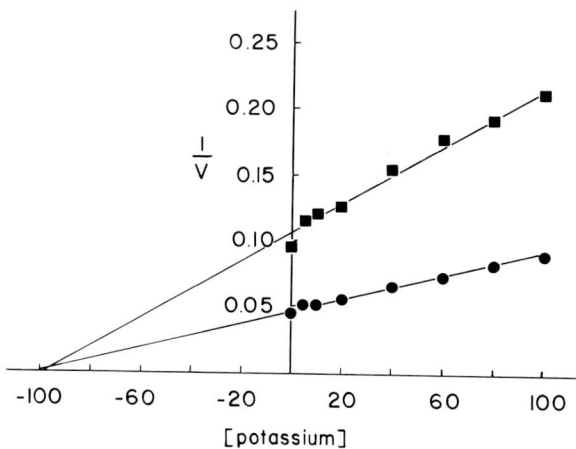

Fig. 12. Dixon plot for glucose absorption in 6 day worms as a function of [K$^+$] (in mM) at constant [Na$^+$] (20 mM) at two different glucose concentrations. ■ = 0.2 mM glucose; ● = 1.0 mM glucose.

to 100% inhibition at infinite inhibitor concentration. An intercept greater than 1 indicates that either (1) the inhibitor is only partially effective, or (2) some of the apparent activity is mediated by one or more systems which are not sensitive to the inhibitor. Such a plot for K$^+$ inhibition of glucose uptake in 6-day-old worms has an ordinate intercept of 1.2 (Fig. 13). Partial inhibition would require that some transport of glucose occur when Na$^+$ is totally replaced by K$^+$, but that is not the case (Fig. 11). Thus, additional evidence is provided that there are two systems mediating glucose transport in 6-day-old *H. diminuta*, one of which is insensitive to K$^+$. Similar experiments on 10- and 20-day-old worms showed that inhibition by K$^+$ was much lower in 10 day and not discernible in 20 day worms. These observations are consistent with the hypothesis that the increase in K_t with worm maturation reflects changes in the proportion of kinetically distinct transport sites.

We have been unable to distinguish the two transport sites by using glucose analogs as transport inhibitors. Of the analogs tested, none inhibited

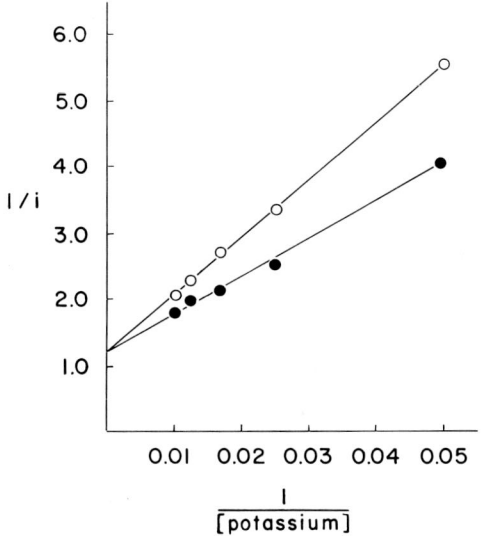

Fig. 13. *Double reciprocal plot of the fractional inhibition versus inhibitor concentration (mM) for 6-day-old worms at two glucose concentrations.* ○ = *1.0 mM glucose;* ● = *0.2 mM glucose.*

glucose uptake in 6 day worms without also inhibiting transport in more mature worms to the same degree.

Experiments were performed to determine whether occurrence of either of the two sites was correlated with degree of maturity of the proglottids. If the low K_t site was characteristic of immature proglottids and germinative region, while the high K_t site was predominant in mature and gravid segments, the high K_t site would be the one detectable at 20 days because the germinative and immature regions would constitute such a small fraction of the strobila. The smaller, 10 day worms might reflect roughly half of each site. Therefore, 10-day-old worms were cut in half, and the kinetics for glucose transport in the posterior portions were determined. The saturation kinetics for the posterior halves did not differ from those of whole worms; hence, it appears that the differentiation from the low K_t site to the high K_t site occurs continuously along the strobila as the cestode matures, i.e., it is a function of whole worm's development rather than individual proglottid development.

Henderson (1977) performed some related experiments. He reported that, for worms of unspecified age, as worm dry weight increased from 5 to 60 mg, K_t increased from approximately 1 to 2 mM, while V_{max} fell from 42 to 15 μmoles/g dry weight/2 min (compare with Table IV). He compared glucose absorption of 10-day-old worms to that of anterior ends of 24-day-old worms cut to a similar size and found higher rates with the younger worms. The rate of glucose absorption by the anterior ends of the 24-day-old worms was not different from intact 24-day-old worms. Thus, apart from the difference in values of K_t reported by Henderson, which may have been due to worm age, his results are in essential agreement with those of Starling and Roberts (unpublished). His conclusion was also similar, i.e., that there may be a low K_t and a high K_t system for glucose absorption, the ratios of which change during worm growth. Interestingly, Henderson found a higher rate of glucose uptake in worms from uncrowded infections than that in crowded worms of the same age, even though the uncrowded worms were much larger in size.

The physiological significance of the two transport sites is of considerable interest. The young worm will be able to absorb glucose more effectively at low ambient concentrations, and presumably it will compete more effectively with host mucosa for its glucose supply. For example, after a 2 hr incubation in 2 mM glucose, 6-day-old worms accumulated a concentration of 56 mM free glucose in their tissue fluid, while 10- and 20-day-old worms accumulated only 28.5 and 20 mM, respectively (Starling and Roberts, unpublished).

B. *Glycogen Synthesis*

One aspect of carbohydrate metabolism of the worm that has received some attention related to development is glycogen metabolism. It was pointed out that the concentration of stored carbohydrate in *H. diminuta* increases dramatically during the developmental period of the worm, at least in low population densities (Roberts 1961).

Like the glycogen of a number of other species and tissues examined, "native" glycogen of *H. diminuta* is highly polydisperse, but the molecular heterogeneity is destroyed by traditional extraction methods (Orrell and Bueding 1958, 1964). If the glycogen is extracted by a mild method using cold buffer, the product appears to reflect the *in vivo* state more closely (Bueding and Orrell 1964). Unlike the glycogen of other species examined, a greater proportion of the cestode glycogen is of very high molecular weight. A spectrum of molecular weight species is present, the low molecular weight species (LMWS, average 25 - 60 million) accounting for about 60% of the glycogen, the high molecular weight species (HMWS, average 900 million) for about 30% and intermediate molecular weight species (IMWS) being present in much lower concentrations. Roberts *et al.* (1972) studied the incorporation of glucose into native glycogen of *H. diminuta* as a function of development. They incubated 9-, 12-, 15-, and 84-day-old worms in ^{14}C-glucose, extracted the glycogen, separated it into fractions according to molecular weight by rate-zonal centrifugation (Barber *et al.* 1967), and determined specific radioactivity of the outer branches and phosphorylase limit-dextrins of each fraction. In all cases, the outer branches showed a higher activity than the limit-dextrin and in the 9, 12 and 15 day worms, the IMWS had much the highest specific activity (Fig. 14). There was a much more uniform incorporation of glucose into all molecular weight species of glycogen in the 84-day-old worms, except that the activity in the limit-dextrin of the HMWS was somewhat higher. A trend toward higher incorporation into the dextrins of the HMWS was also shown with increasing age from 9 to 15 days. The fact that the IMWS had the highest specific activity in worms 9 to 15 days old, in spite of being present in lowest concentration, shows that the glycogen undergoes repackaging or reassembly in those worms after initial synthesis; otherwise, the IMWS would soon be highest in concentration, rather than lowest.

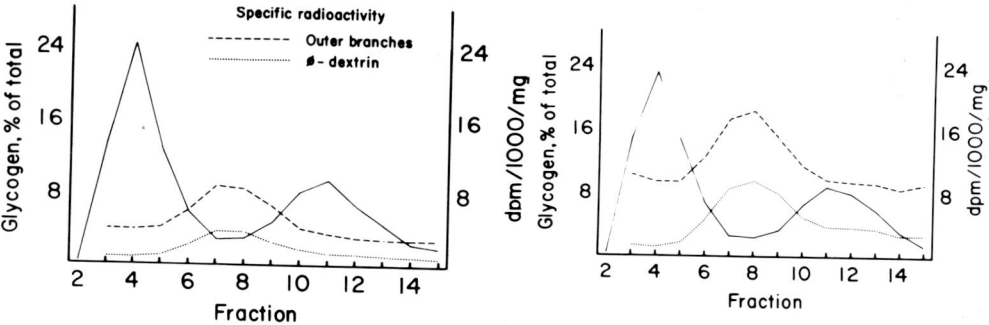

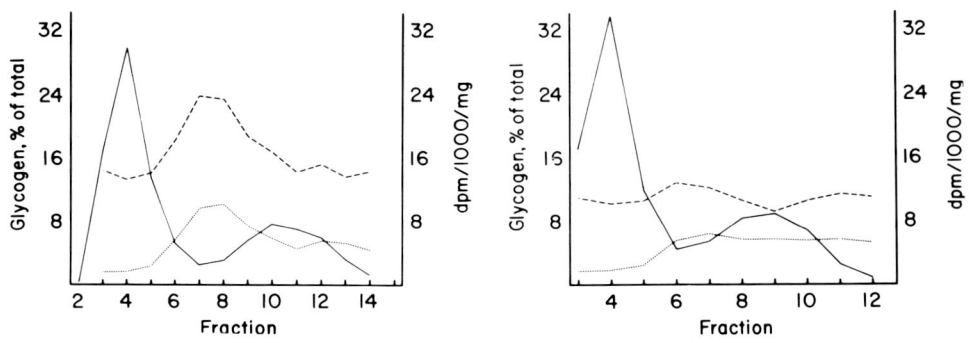

Fig. 14. Effect of worm age on incorporation of ^{14}C-glucose into glycogen as a function of molecular weight of the glycogen. (a) 9-day-old worms. (b) 12-day-old worms. (c) 15-day-old worms. (d) 84-day-old worms. Solid line is the percent of the total glycogen in the respective molecular weight fractions; the dotted line is specific activity in the phosphorylase limit-dextrin of the fractions; and the dashed line is the specific activity in the outer branches of the positions. (from Roberts et al. 1972). Approximate molecular weights represented by the fractions are given in the text.

Roberts et al. (1972) observed that worms in all age groups consumed glucose at about the same rate and retained about the same proportion of radioactive carbon that they absorbed. However, much less of the glucose consumed by the 9-day-old worms was incorporated into glycogen. They concluded that a larger proportion of the glucose in the 9-day-old worms must have been incorporated into other types of molecules. Supporting results were reported by Dendinger and Roberts (1977a), who studied the activity of glycogen synthase (E.C. 2.4.1.11) as a function of development. The activities of both the I (glucose- 6-phosphate independent) and D (glucose-6-phosphate dependent) forms of the enzyme were determined at 6, 10 and 15 days postinfection. The activities of both forms increased during the growth period of the worm, and the increase apparently reflected a synthesis of new enzyme, rather than a conversion of the D form to the physiologically active I form. Thus, the lower concentration of stored carbohydrates in younger worms (Roberts 1961) and their lower incorporation of glucose into glycogen (Roberts et al. 1972) is correlated with and probably explained by lower activity of glycogen synthase. Curiously, that explanation for the lower glycogen concentration in crowded worms does not pertain. The activity of glycogen synthase I in worms from 100 worm infections was consistently equal to or greater than that of worms from 10 worm infections at each of the three ages tested. A possible explanation for this finding may be that since high concentrations of glycogen inhibit the synthase D to I conversion (Dendinger and Roberts 1977b), the lower glycogen in crowded worms would result in a higher proportion of synthase in the I form.

XI. MECHANISM OF OPERATION OF THE CROWDING EFFECT

The crowding effect, a limitation of individual tapeworm size with increasing population density, was mentioned above. In addition to *H. diminuta*, the crowding effect has been reported in *Raillietina cesticillus*, *Hymenolepis nana* and *H. microstoma* (Reid 1942; Woodland 1924; Shorb 1933; Hunninen 1935; Litchford 1963). The important developmental implication of the crowding effect is that worms in the host's intestine are, by whatever means, influencing growth, cell division, DNA synthesis and numerous other physiological parameters of other worms. As pointed out by Chappell and Pike (1976), "No wholly satisfactory explanation for the 'crowding effect' has yet been provided despite the attention it has attracted".

A. Competition Hypotheses: Host Dietary Carbohydrate

Historically, the most appealing and simplest explanation for the crowding effect has been that the individual worms in an infection would compete for nutritive or other substances and that this competition would impose a limitation on the availability of one or more of such substances to the individual worm, thus limiting its growth. In light of the importance of host dietary carbohydrate to the normal development of *H. diminuta*, competition for carbohydrate would be a likely suspect. Read (1959) constructed a hypothetical curve of worm weight as a function of population density based on the following assumptions: (1) that host dietary carbohydrate was shared equally by all worms, (2) that host digestive physiology was not affected by varying numbers of worms, and (3) that the weight of the worm was a function of the carbohydrate it obtained. These assumptions assured that the curve would be a rectangular hyperbola, similar to that constructed from data derived from experiments in which the numbers of worms per host were varied. Further, with the discovery that *H. diminuta* could not directly utilize starch or maltose (Read 1956), it became apparent that the amount of carbohydrate available to the worms at a given time would be less than had been estimated previously by Reid (1942) and that the carbohydrate supply would indeed be limiting. These considerations led Read (1959) to conclude that the "crowding effect in cestode infections may be interpreted in terms of competition for utilizable carbohydrate by the individual worms in the populations".

While Read's explanation was reasonable, it was not adequate since evidence available at that time did not exclude the possibility that the worms could be competing for some other equally vital substance or even that competition for any substance was the causative mechanism. The following types of evidence could be adduced to support a competition hypothesis for the crowding effect, whether for carbohydrate or otherwise: (1) all physiological and developmental characteristics of crowded worms could be compared with the effects produced by suboptimal host dietary carbohydrate or other substances, (2) any substances other than carbohydrate for which the worms might be competing could be sought, and (3) it must be determined that any such vital substance would in fact be limiting *in vivo* when the crowding effect was manifested. Thus, if the effects of experimentally limiting a given substance were similar in detail to the effects observed in crowded worms and supplies of the substance *in vivo* would be limiting under conditions of crowding, the likelihood would be increased that competition for that substance was the mechanism of the crowding effect.

Very few of the many possible substances other than carbohydrate have been examined, nor has it seemed potentially fruitful to pursue such a survey. Earlier, Read (1951) suggested that competition for oxygen might be the mechanism of the crowding effect. However, since oxygen from 0% to 19% has no effect on *in vitro* development of *H. diminuta* (Roberts and Mong 1969), it seems most unlikely that competition for that substance could explain the crowding effect. Likewise, though the worms require an external source of vitamin B_6, the requirement is so low that host coprophagy prevention is necessary for its demonstration (Platzer and Roberts 1969).

The body of evidence accumulated so far tends to support the view (1) that competition for host dietary carbohydrate plays some role in the crowding effect and is a plausible explanation for at least some aspects of the phenomenon, but (2) that explanation for the developmental control in the crowding effect in terms of a single factor is probably an oversimplification. Effects produced in the worms by feeding their hosts diets with sucrose as the carbohydrate instead of starch, or with low starch content, parallel the crowding effect to a remarkable degree, i.e., lower size attained and fewer proglottids produced, low carbohydrate concentration in the worms and high lipid concentration (Roberts 1966). It is difficult to reconcile the lowered proglottid production with the carbohydrate competition hypothesis; one would reason that since there is sufficient carbohydrate available to nourish the great majority of the strobilar mass, even in crowded infections, there should be enough to allow the very small (in comparison) germinative area to produce the same number of proglottids, regardless of population size. The lower rate of cell proliferation in the germinative area (Bolla and Roberts) 1971b) shows that proglottid production is indeed a reflection of cell division in the germinative area. It has been found, however, that suboptimal carbohydrate can, in fact, decrease proglottisation and that such conditions can inhibit growth even earlier than crowding (Roberts 1966; Komuniecki and Roberts 1975). Thus, evidence in the first category listed above is strong, though that in the third category must be much more qualified. In a study of starch digestion in the rat, Mead and Roberts (1972) showed that starch in solid meals is essentially completely digested and substantial amounts of glucose are available to the worms; however, based on known rates of glucose utilization of *H. diminuta in vitro*, the glucose supply should be limiting only as the worms approach their maximal size. Nevertheless, the crowding effect can be detected at 6-8 days post-infection, when the worms weigh a maximum of about 30 mg (Roberts 1961), and the size they attain by 15 days is several times that value, even in crowded infections.

The possibility that carbohydrate supply could be limiting in very young worms is made even less likely by the observation, cited above, that the apparent K_t for glucose is only about one fourth that in mature worms. Thus, younger worms are better equipped to cope with low glucose concentration than older ones, since they can take up glucose against a steeper concentration gradient. Conversely, the increase in apparent K_t with maturation would mean that limitation in carbohydrate might become a more effective control of growth as the worms grew larger.

The observation that carbohydrate concentration in the germinative and immature regions of crowded worms is not lower than those in the same regions of uncrowded ones (Bolla and Roberts 1971b) lends further support to the contention that the carbohydrate competition hypothesis cannot, by itself, explain the manifestations of the crowding effect.

B. *Secretion of Growth Inhibitor Substances*

Roberts (1961) suggested the possibility of a feedback mechanism in the crowding effect and that an inhibitory substance, perhaps an excretory product, might be released by the worms. The amount of such substance(s) could be proportional to the mass or number of worms present, or both, and its effects could result in the inverse proportionality of size and numbers present observed in the crowding effect. To test this hypothesis, we have investigated the effects of various treatments on the *in vitro* incorporation of ^{3}H-thymidine into the DNA of anterior ends of *H. diminuta* (Insler and Roberts, unpublished).

Worm conditioned saline (WCS) was prepared by incubating 10-day-old worms from 50 worm infections for 12 hr in balanced saline with 25 mM glucose and antibiotics under a gas phase of $N_2:CO_2$, 95:5. After 12 hr the worms were recovered, and the WCS and control saline were equalized with respect to pH (usually about 6.0-6.3) and glucose concentration (12 mM). *H. diminuta* from 10-day-old, 10 worm infections were then incubated 3 hr in these two media, then 30 min in the media supplemented by 5 µCi/ml ^{3}H-thymidine, 30 min in 0.1 mM unlabelled thymidine and 4 hr more in the unsupplemented media. Thus, the worms were incubated through a length of time almost equal to that required for one entire cell cycle (Bolla and Roberts 1971a). DNA was isolated from the anterior 5 cm of the worms by a modification of Burton's (1956) colorimetric method (Giles and Myers 1965).

Incubation of the worms in WCS caused a reduction in specific activity of DNA compared to controls varying from over 50% to up to 80% in different experiments. The reduction in DNA synthesis caused by the WCS was not due to depression of thymidine uptake since absorption of thymidine in worms in WCS was equal to that of controls.

As the major end products of energy metabolism in *H. diminuta* are succinic, acetic and lactic acids, the effect on incorporation of thymidine into DNA of these substances was examined. Succinate in the WCS and in the intestinal contents of rats infected with *H. diminuta* was measured by the method of Kmetec (1966), and lactate in the WCS was determined by the method of Hohorst (1965). Watts and Fairbairn (1974) reported that 14-day-old *H. diminuta* secrete succinate, acetate and lactate in the proportions 5.0:2.5:1, respectively. We found 10-12 mM concentrations of succinate and 2-3 mM lactate in the WCS, and succinate in the intestinal contents of rats infected with *H. diminuta* (50 worm infection, 10 days old) was 9.8 mM. Acetate was not determined. Incubation of the worms in media containing 12 mM succinate, 12 mM acetate, or a combination of the acids decreased the incorporation of ^{3}H-thymidine into DNA, but only about 1/2 as much as a parallel incubation in WCS (Table V). A separate experiment showed that incubation in 12 mM lactate did not affect DNA synthesis.

In some experiments, WCS prepared from worms from 50 worm infections was compared to that prepared from worms from 10 worm infections. Equal ratios of worm mass to medium volume in the preparation of the WCS were used. DNA synthesis of cestodes incubated in WCS from crowded worms was only about 1/2 that in WCS prepared from less crowded worms, and the "10 worm" WCS itself inhibited DNA synthesis by about 2/3 (Table VI). Since the succinate concentration in the two WCS preparations was almost the same, the greater inhibition in the "50 worm" WCS may have been due to some other, as yet unidentified factor(s).

Addition of ammonia and urea to control media in concentrations equal to those found in the WCS (determined by the method of Bernt and Bergmeyer [1965]) produced no inhibition of DNA synthesis.

TABLE V. Effects of Worm-Conditioned Saline and Excretory Acids on Incorporation of ^{3}H-thymidine into DNA[a]

Medium	Specific Activity DNA dpm/μg DNA ± S.E.	% of Control
KRT-B[b]	9745 ± 122	100
WCS	4265 ± 612	43
KRT-B + 12 mM Succinate	6856 ± 172	70
KRT-B + 12 mM Acetate	7633 ± 504	78
KRT-B + 12 mM Succinate 5 mM Acetate 2 mM Lactate	6163 ± 430	63

[a] DNA recovered from anterior 5 cm of worms after incubation in the respective media, see text.

[b] Krebs Ringer Tris buffer (Read et al. 1963) modified by substitution of 25 mM sodium bicarbonate for an equimolar quantity of sodium chloride (=KRT-B).

It was of some concern whether the conditions of the experiments *in vitro* were a valid reflection of conditions prevalent during crowding *in vivo*. The fact that the concentration of succinate in the WCS was approximately the same as that in the intestinal contents with a large mass of worms present indicated that that substance was at a physiological level and by extension, probably other excreted products as well. It appears that the 12 hr incubation *in vitro* to prepare the WCS is necessary so that excreted substances will accumulate to levels approximating those to which the worm are subjected in the much more confined conditions of the infected rat intestine.

Several other kinds of determinations lend support to the physiological validity of the observations. Preliminary electron microscopy suggests

TABLE VI. Comparative Inhibitory Effects of WCS Prepared with Worms from Uncrowded and Crowded Infections of Hymenolepis diminuta[a]

Medium	Specific Activity DNA dpm/μg DNA ± S.E.	% of Control	mM Succinate	mM Lactate
KRT-B[b]	3745 ± 382	100	—	—
"10 Worm" WCS	1249 ± 163	33	10.6	2.9
"50 Worm" WCS	683 ± 88	18	12.1	1.8

[a] WCS prepared by incubation of worms from 10 worm and 50 worm infections, equal tissue: medium volume ratio; results from typical experiment.

[b] See Table V.

that the cellular integrity of worms used to prepare the WCS is still good after the 12 hr incubation: the microtriches are intact and the distal cytoplasm and perikarya of the tegument resemble those of unincubated worms. However, these observations must be extended with a larger sample size to determine their general applicability.

ATP levels in worms incubated in WCS and control media were measured by the method of Ebadi et al. (1971). There was no difference between the groups in the ATP pool, and both were equal to the value reported by Scheibel et al. (1968) in unincubated worms.

Bolla and Roberts (1971b) reported that H. diminuta from crowded infections had lower rates of protein and RNA synthesis, as well as DNA synthesis, when compared with worms from uncrowded infections. We incubated anterior portions of worms in WCS with a mixture of tritiated amino acids and in WCS with ^{3}H-uridine. Uptake of amino acids was slightly inhibited by WCS but protein synthesis was substantially lower than controls (Table VII). Uptake of uridine was inhibited by WCS but incorporation of the label into new RNA by worms in WCS was only 38% of controls (Table VIII). Since the effects parallel those observed in crowded worms, the circumstantial evidence is that inhibitors present in the WCS may be operating physiologically in a manner similar to those *in vivo*.

TABLE VII. *Radioactivity of Homogenates and Protein from H. diminuta after Incubation in ^{3}H-amino acid mixture*

Medium	Protein Fraction[a] dpm/mg protein	Homogenate dpm/mg dry weight
KRT- B[b]	15,913 ± 1,841	23,712 ± 941
WCS	9,579 ± 667	20,155 ± 785
WCS as % of control	60%	85%

[a] Precipitated with 0.4 N $HClO_4$.
[b] See Table V.

TABLE VIII. Radioactivity of Homogenates and RNA from H. diminuta after Incubation in ^{3}H-uridine

Medium	RNA Fraction dpm in RNA/mg dry wt	Homogenate dpm/mg dry wt.
KRT-B[a]	25,244 ± 2,420	418,432 ± 23,650
WCS	9,627 ± 997	396,179 ± 13,871
WCS as % of Control	38%	NSD

[a]See Table V.

Investigation of the identity of the inhibitory substances is continuing. Treatment of the WCS at 80 C for 30 min did not destroy the activity and, in some experiments, appeared to enhance it. Treatment of the WCS with insoluble proteases (trypsin on polyacrylamide, *Streptomyces* protease on carboxymethyl cellulose) for 30 min with 5 µg/200 ml (sufficient to hydrolyze 200 ml of 1.5 mM protein), with the proteases then removed by centrifugation, did not affect activity. Dialysis of the WCS in tubing to retain substances of above 3,000 molecular weight resulted in loss of activity. Treatment of the WCS with desoxyribonuclease or ribonuclease did not affect inhibitory activity.

The foregoing evidence suggests that succinate and probably acetate are active inhibitory substances, but since these acids alone cannot account for all the inhibition, we have tentatively concluded that there are other relatively small non-protein molecules involved as well. Such substances might be secreted by crowded worms or secreted in greater quantities by crowded worms and further inhibit DNA synthesis of other individuals. Succinate and the other substances could be present in sufficient concentration at 8 days postinfection to depress growth because there is much more worm tissue present at 8 days in a crowded infection than in an uncrowded one, even though the individuals become several times larger in both types of infection at maturity. The mode of action of these substances awaits investigation.

ACKNOWLEDGMENTS

Research from the author's laboratory has been supported in part by the United States Public Health Service, National Institutes of Health, Grants AI-06153, 5 TO1 AI-226, and AI-155278. I am grateful to Drs. Jane A. Starling, Robert E. Morcock and Gayle Dranch Insler for permitting me to use heretofore unpublished results of collaborative work. The technical assistance of Ms. Cynthia Ellis and Ms. Helen Boland is gratefully acknowledged. I very much appreciate the careful reading of the manuscript by Dr. C. A. Hopkins, University of Glasgow and the many helpful suggestions he made.

REFERENCES

1. Addis, C. J., Jr., Experiments on the relation between sex hormones and the growth of tapeworms (*Hymenolepis diminuta*) in rats. *J. Parasit.* 32, 574-580 (1946).
2. Addis, C. J., Jr., and Chandler, A. C., Studies on the vitamin requirement of tapeworms. *J. Parasit.* 30, 229-236 (1944).
3. Addis, C. J., Jr., and Chandler, A. C., Further studies on the vitamin requirement of tapeworms. *J. Parasit.* 32, 581-584 (1946).
4. Althausen, T. L., Eiler J. J., and Stockholm, M., The effect of B vitamins on intestinal absorption and food utilization. I. Studies in rats on diets deficient in certain B vitamins and during recovery from such diets. *Gastroenterology* 7, 469-476 (1946).
5. Andreassen, J., Hindsbo, O., and Hesselberg, C. A., Immunity to *Hymenolepis diminuta* in rats: destrobilation and expulsion in primary infections, its suppression by cortisone treatment and increased resistance to secondary infections. *Proc. Third Internatl. Cong. Parasit.* 2, 1056-1057 (1974).
6. Bailey, H. H., and Fairbairn, D., Lipid metabolism in helminth parasites. V. Absorption of fatty acids and monoglycerides from micellar solution by *Hymenolepis diminuta* (Cestoda). *Comp. Biochem. Physiol.* 26, 819-836 (1968).

7. Barber, A. A., Orrell, S. A., Jr., and Bueding, E., Association of enzymes with rat liver glycogen isolated by rate-zonal centrifugation. *J. Biol. Chem. 242*, 4040-4044 (1967).
8. Barnes, R. H., Fiala, G., McGehee, B., and Brown, A., Prevention of coprophagy in the rat. *J. Nutr. 63*, 489-498 (1957).
9. Beck, J. W., Effect of diet on singly established *Hymenolepis diminuta* in rats. *Exp. Parasit. 1*, 46-59 (1951).
10. Beck, J. W., Effect of gonadectomy and gonadal hormones on singly established *Hymenolepis diminuta* in rats. *Exp. Parasit. 1*, 109-117 (1952).
11. Bernt, E., and Bergmeyer, H. U., Urea. *In* "Methods of Enzymatic Analysis" (H. U. Bergemeyer, ed.), pp. 401-406. Verlag Chemie, Weinheim, (1965).
12. Berntzen, A. K., The *in vitro* cultivation of tapeworms. I. Growth of *Hymenolepis diminuta* (Cestoda: Cyclophyllidea). *J. Parasit. 47*, 351-355 (1961).
13. Bolla, R. I., Genic control of development in *Hymenolepis diminuta* (Cestoda: Cyclophyllidea) and its relation to the crowding effect. Ph.D. Thesis, University of Massachusetts, Amherst, (1970).
14. Bolla, R. I., and Roberts, L. S., Developmental physiology of cestodes. VIII. Inhibition of ribonucleic acid synthesis by actinomycin-D in developing *Hymenolepis diminuta*. *J. Parasit. 56*, 1151-1158 (1970).
15. Bolla, R. I., and Roberts, L. S., Developmental physiology of cestodes. IX. Cytological characteristics of the germinative region of *Hymenolepis diminuta*. *J. Parasit. 57*, 267-277 (1971a).
16. Bolla, R. I., and Roberts, L. S., Developmental physiology of cestodes. X. The effect of crowding on carbohydrate levels and on RNA, DNA and protein synthesis in *Hymenolepis diminuta*. *Comp. Biochem. Physiol. 40A*, 777-787 (1971b).
17. Bolla, R. I., and Roberts, L. S., Developmental physiology of cestodes. XII. Role of preformed RNA in development of *Hymenolepis diminuta*. *Comp. Biochem. Physiol. 40B*, 885-892 (1971c).

18. Bonsdorff, C. H. von, Forssten, T., Gustafsson, M. K. S., and Wikgren, B. J., Cellular composition of plerocercoids of *Diphyllobothrium dendriticum* (Cestoda). *Acta Zool. Fennica 132*, 1-25 (1971).
19. Bueding, E., and Orrell, S. A., Jr., A mild procedure for the isolation of polydisperse glycogen from animal tissues. *J. Biol. Chem. 239*, 4018-4020 (1964).
20. Burton, K., A study of the conditions and mechanism of the diphenylamine reaction for the colorimetric estimation of deoxyribonucleic acid. *Biochem. J. 62*, 316-323 (1956).
21. Caldwell, E. F., and McHenry, E. W., Studies on vitamin B_6 and transamination in rat liver. *Arch. Biochem. 45*, 97-104 (1953).
22. Chance, M. R. A., and Dirnhuber, P., The water-soluble vitamins of parasitic worms. *Parasitology 39*, 300-301 (1949).
23. Chandler, A. C., The effects of number and age of worms on development of primary and secondary infections with *Hymenolepis diminuta* in rats, and an investigation into the true nature of "premunition" in tapeworm infections. *Amer. J. Hyg. 29(D)*, 105-114 (1939).
24. Chandler, A. C., Studies on the nutrition of tapeworms. *Amer. J. Hyg. 37*, 121-130 (1943).
25. Chandler, A. C., Read, C. P., and Nicholas, H. O., Observations on certain phases of nutrition and host parasite relations of *Hymenolepis diminuta* in white rats. *J. Parasit. 36*, 523-535 (1950).
26. Chappell, L. H., and Pike, A. W., Loss of *Hymenolepis diminuta* from the rat. *Inter. J. Parasit. 6*, 333-339 (1976).
27. Collin, W. K., Electron microscopy of postembryonic stages of the tapeworm, *Hymenolepis citelli*. *J. Parasit. 56*, 1159-1170 (1970).
28. Davey, K. G., and Breckenridge, W. R., Neurosecretory cells in a cestode, *Hymenolepis diminuta*. *Science 158*, 931-932 (1967).
29. Dendinger, J. E., and Roberts, L. S., Glycogen synthase in the rat tapeworm, *Hymenolepis diminuta*. I. Enzyme activity during development and with crowding. *Comp. Biochem. Physiol. 58B*, 215-219 (1977a).

30. Dendinger, J. E., and Roberts, L. S., Glycogen synthase in the rat tapeworm, *Hymenolepis diminuta*. II. Control of enzyme activity by glucose and glycogen. *Comp. Biochem. Physiol.* 58B, 231-236 (1977b).
31. Dike, S. C., and Read, C. P., Relation of tegumentary phosphohydrolase and sugar transport in *Hymenolepis diminuta*. *J. Parasit.* 57, 1251-1255 (1971).
32. Dunkley, C. L., and Mettrick, D. F., *Hymenolepis diminuta*: Effect of quality of host dietary carbohydrate on growth. *Exp. Parasit.* 25, 146-161 (1969).
33. Ebadi, M. S., Weiss, B., and Costa, E., Microassay of adenosine-3', 5'-monophosphate (cyclic AMP) in brain and other tissues by the luciferin-luciferase system. *J. Neurochem.* 18, 183-192 (1971).
34. Fairbairn, D., Wertheim, G., Harpur, R. P., and Schiller, E. L., Biochemistry of normal and irradiated strains of *Hymenolepis diminuta*. *Exp. Parasit.* 11, 248-263 (1961).
35. Giles, K. W., and Myers, A., An improved diphenylamine method for the estimation of deoxyribonucleic acid. *Nature* 206, 93 (1965).
36. Goodchild, C. G., Growth and maturation of the cestode *Hymenolepis diminuta* in bileless hosts. *J. Parasit.* 44, 352-362 (1958).
37. Goodchild, C. G., Effects of starvation and lack of bile upon growth, egg production and egg viability in established rat tapeworms, *Hymenolepis diminuta*. *J. Parasit.* 46, 615-623 (1960).
38. Goodchild, C. G., Carbohydrate contents of the tapeworm *Hymenolepis diminuta* from normal, bileless, and starved rats. *J. Parasit.* 47, 401-405 (1961a).
39. Goodchild, C. G., Protein contents of the tapeworm *Hymenolepis diminuta* from normal, bileless and starved rats. *J. Parasit.*, 830-832 (1961b).
40. Goodchild, C. G., and Harrison, D. L., The growth of the rat tapeworm, *Hymenolepis diminuta*, during the first five days in the final host. *J. Parasit.* 47, 819-829 (1961).
41. Gustafsson, M. K. S., The histology of the neck region of plerocercoids of *Triaenophorus nodulosus* (Cestoda, Pseudophyllidea). *Acta Zool. Fennica* 138, 1-16 (1973).

42. Gustafsson, M. K. S., Observations on the histogenesis of nervous tissue in *Diphyllobothrium dendriticum* Nitzsch, 1824 (Cestoda, Pseudophyllidea). *Zeitsch. Parasitenk. 50*, 313-321 (1976a).
43. Gustafsson, M. K. S., Studies on cytodifferentiation in the neck region of *Diphyllobothrium dendriticum* Nitzsch, 1824 (Cestoda, Pseudophyllidea). *Zeitsch. Parasitenk. 50*, 323-329 (1976b).
44. Gustafsson, M. K. S., "Aspects of the cytology and histogenesis in cestodes with special reference to the genus *Diphyllobothrium*". Dissertation, Abo Akademi, Abo, Finland, (1977).
45. Hager, A., Effects of dietary modifications of host rats on the tapeworm *Hymenolepis diminuta*. *Iowa St. Coll. J. Sci. 15*, 127-153 (1941).
46. Harris, W. G., and Turton, J. A., Antibody response to tapeworm (*Hymenolepis diminuta*) in the rat. *Nature, London 246*, 521-522 (1973).
47. Hay, E. C., The fine structure of blastema cells and differentiating cartilage cells in regenerating limbs of *Amblystoma* larvae. *J. Biophys. Biochem. Cytol. 4*, 538-592 (1958).
48. Henderson, D., The effect of worm age, weight and number in the infection on the absorption of glucose by *Hymenolepis diminuta*. *Parasitology 75*, 277-284 (1977).
49. Herlant-Meewis, H., Regeneration in annelids. *Adv. Morphogen. 4*, 155-215 (1964).
50. Hesselberg, C. A., and Andreassen, J., Some influences of population density on *Hymenolepis diminuta* in rats. *Parasitology 71*, 517-523 (1975).
51. Hohorst, H., L(+)-lactate determination with lactate dehydrogenase and DPN. *In* "Methods of Enzymatic Analysis" (H. U. Bergmeyer, ed.), pp. 266-270. Verlag Chemie, Weinheim, (1965).
52. Holmes, J. C., Effects of concurrent infections on *Hymenolepis diminuta* (Cestoda) and *Moniliformis dubius* (Acanthocephala). I. General effects and comparison with crowding. *J. Parasit. 47*, 209-216 (1961).
53. Holmes, J. C., Effects of concurrent infections on *Hymenolepis diminuta* (Cestoda) and *Moniliformis dubius* (Acanthocephala). II. Effects on growth. *J. Parasit. 48*, 87-96 (1962a).

54. Holmes, J. C., Effects of concurrent infections on *Hymenolepis diminuta* (Cestoda) and *Moniliformis dubius* (Acanthocephala). III. Effects in hamsters. *J. Parasit.* 48, 97-100 (1962b).
55. Hopkins, C. A., The influence of dietary methionine on the amino acid pool of *Hymenolepis diminuta* in the rat's intestine. *Parasitology* 59, 407-427 (1969).
56. Hopkins, C. A., and Callow, L. L., Methionine flux between a tapeworm (*Hymenolepis diminuta*) and its environment. *Parasitology* 55, 653-666 (1965).
57. Hopkins, C. A., Subramanian, G., and Stallard, H., The development of *Hymenolepis diminuta* in primary and secondary infections in mice. *Parasitology* 64, 401-412 (1972).
58. Hopkins, C. A., and Young, R. A. L., The effect of dietary amino acids on the growth of *Hymenolepis diminuta*. *Parasitology* 57, 705-717 (1967).
59. Hunninen, A. V., Studies on the life history and host-parasite relations of *Hymenolepis fraterna* (*H. nana*, var. *fraterna* Stiles) in white mice. *Amer. J. Hyg.* 22, 414-443 (1935).
60. Kmetec, E., Spectrophotometric method for the enzymic microdetermination of succinic acid. *Anal. Biochem.* 16, 474-480 (1966).
61. Komuniecki, R., and Roberts, L. S., Developmental physiology of cestodes. XIV. Roughage and carbohydrate content of host diet for optimal growth and development of *Hymenolepis diminuta*. *J. Parasitol.* 61, 427-433 (1975).
62. Laurie, J. S., The *in vitro* fermentation of carbohydrates by two species of cestodes and one species of Acanthocephala. *Exp. Parasit.* 6, 245-260 (1957).
63. Levine, P. P., Observations on the biology of the poultry cestode *Davainea proglottina* in the intestine of the host. *J. Parasit.* 24, 423-431 (1938).
64. Litchford, R. G., Observations on *Hymenolepis microstoma* in three laboratory hosts: *Mesocricetus auratus*, *Mus musculus*, and *Rattus norvegicus*. *J. Parasit.* 49, 403-410 (1963).
65. Mead, R. W., and Roberts, L. S., Intestinal digestion and absorption of starch in the intact rat: Effects of cestode (*Hymenolepis diminuta*) infection. *Comp. Biochem. Physiol.* 41A, 749-760 (1972).

66. Mettrick, D. F., Studies on the protein metabolism of cestodes. 2. Effect of free dietary amino acid supplements on the growth of *Hymenolepis diminuta*. *Parasitology 58*, 37-45 (1968).
67. Mettrick, D. F., *Hymenolepis diminuta*: Quantity of host amino acid dietary supplement and growth. *Exp. Parasit. 29*, 13-25 (1971).
68. Mettrick, D. F., and Cannon, C. E., Changes in the chemical composition of *Hymenolepis diminuta* (Cestoda: Cyclophyllidea) during prepatent development within the rat intestine. *Parasitology 61*, 229-243 (1970).
69. Mettrick, D. F., and Munro, H. N., Studies on the protein metabolism of cestodes. 1. The effect of host dietary constituents on the growth of *Hymenolepis diminuta*. *Parasitology 55*, 453-466 (1965).
70. Ogren, R. E., Continuity of morphology from oncosphere to early cysticercoid in the development of *Hymenolepis diminuta* (Cestoda: Cyclophyllidea). *Exp. Parasit. 12*, 1-6 (1962).
71. Ogren, R. E., The cellular pattern in invasive oncospheres of *Hymenolepis diminuta* as revealed by an enzyme-acetic acid-orcein method. *Trans. Amer. Microsc. Soc. 86*, 250-260 (1967).
72. Ogren, R. E., Characteristics for two classes of embryonic cells in oncospheres of *Hymenolepis diminuta*. *Trans. Amer. Microsc. Soc. 87*, 82-97 (1968a).
73. Ogren, R. E., The basic cellular pattern for undifferentiated oncospheres of *Hymenolepis diminuta*. *Trans. Amer. Microsc. Soc. 87*, 448-463 (1968b).
74. Orrell, S. A., Jr., and Bueding, E., Sedimentation characteristics of glycogen. *J. Amer. Chem. Soc. 80*, 3800 (1958).
75. Orrell, S. A., and Bueding E., A comparison of products obtained by various procedures used for the extraction of glycogen. *J. Biol. Chem. 239*, 4021-4026 (1964).
76. Pappas, P. W., *Hymenolepis diminuta*: Absorption of nicotinamide. *Exp. Parasit. 32*, 403-406 (1972).
77. Pappas, P. W., and Read, C. P., Thiamine uptake by *Hymenolepis diminuta*. *J. Parasit. 58*, 235-239 (1972a).

78. Pappas, P. W., and Read, C. P., The absorption of pyridoxine and riboflavin by *Hymenolepis diminuta*. *J. Parasit*. *58*, 417-421 (1972b).
79. Pappas, P. W., and Read, C. P., Membrane transport in helminth parasites: a review. *Exp. Parasit*. *37*, 469-530 (1975).
80. Pappas, P. W., Uglem, G. L., and Read, C. P., Anion and cation requirements for glucose and methionine accumulation by *Hymenolepis diminuta*. *Biol. Bull*. *146*, 56-66 (1974).
81. Phifer, K., Permeation and membrane transport in animal parasites: further observations on the uptake of glucose by *Hymenolepis diminuta*. *J. Parasit*. *46*, 137-144 (1960).
82. Platzer, E. G., and Roberts, L. S., Developmental physiology of cestodes. V. Effects of vitamin deficient diets and host coprophagy prevention on development of *Hymenolepis diminuta*. *J. Parasit*. *55*, 1143-1152 (1969).
83. Platzer, E. G., and Roberts, L. S., Developmental physiology of cestodes. VI. Effect of host riboflavin deficiency on *Hymenolepis diminuta*. *Exp. Parasit*. *28*, 393-398 (1970a).
84. Platzer, E. G., and Roberts, L. S., Developmental physiology of cestodes. - Part VII. Vitamin B_6 and *Hymenolepis diminuta*: vitamin levels in the cestode and effects of deficiency on phosphorylase and transaminase activities. *Comp. Biochem. Physiol*. *35*, 535-552 (1970b).
85. Read, C. P., The "crowding effect" in tapeworm infections. *J. Parasit*. *37*, 174-178 (1951).
86. Read, C. P., Carbohydrate metabolism of *Hymenolepis diminuta*. *Exp. Parasit*. *5*, 325-344 (1956).
87. Read, C. P., The role of carbohydrates in the biology of cestodes. VIII. Some conclusions and hypotheses. *Exp. Parasit*. *8*, 365-382 (1959).
88. Read, C. P., The microcosm of intestinal helminths. *In* "Ecology and Physiology of Parasites (A. M. Fallis, ed.), pp. 188-200. University of Toronto Press, Toronto, (1971).
89. Read, C. P., and Phifer, K, The role of carbohydrates in the biology of cestodes. VII. Interactions between individual tapeworms of the same and different species. *Exp. Parasit*. *8*, 46-50 (1959).

90. Read, C. P., and Rothman, A. H., The role of carbohydrates in the biology of cestodes. I. The effect of dietary carbohydrate quality on the size of *Hymenolepis diminuta*. *Exp. Parasit.* 6, 1-7 (1957a).
91. Read, C. P., and Rothman, A. H., The role of carbohydrates in the biology of cestodes. IV. Some effects of host dietary carbohydrate on growth and reproduction of *Hymenolepis*. *Exp. Parasit.* 6, 294-305 (1957b).
92. Read, C. P., and Rothman, A. H., The role of carbohydrates in the biology of cestodes. VI. The carbohydrates metabolized *in vitro* by some cyclophyllidean species. *Exp. Parasit.* 7, 217-223 (1958).
93. Read, C. P., Rothman, A. H., and Simmons, J. E., Jr., Studies on membrane transport, with special reference to parasite-host integration. *Ann. N. Y. Acad. Sci.* 113(1), 154-205 (1963).
94. Read, C. P., Schiller, E. L., and Phifer, K., The role of carbohydrates in the biology of cestodes. V. Comparative studies on the effects of host dietary carbohydrate on *Hymenolepis* spp. *Exp. Parasit.* 7, 198-216 (1958).
95. Read, C. P., Stewart, G. L., and Pappas, P. W., Glucose and sodium fluxes across the brush border of *Hymenolepis diminuta* (Cestoda). *Biol. Bull.* 147, 146-152 (1974).
96. Reid, W. M., Certain nutritional requirements of the fowl cestode *Raillietina cesticillus* (Molin) as demonstrated by short periods of starvation of the host. *J. Parasit.* 28, 319-340 (1942).
97. Roberts, L. S., The influence of population density on patterns and physiology of growth in *Hymenolepis diminuta* (Cestoda: Cyclophyllidea) in the definitive host. *Exp. Parasit.* 11, 332-371 (1961).
98. Roberts, L. S., Developmental physiology of cestodes. I. Host dietary carbohydrate and the "crowding effect" in *Hymenolepis diminuta*. *Exp. Parasit.* 18, 305-310 (1966).
99. Roberts, L. S., Modifications in media and surface sterilization methods for *in vitro* cultivation of *Hymenolepis diminuta*. *J. Parasit.* 59, 474-479 (1973).

100. Roberts, L. S., and Mong, F. N., Developmental physiology of cestodes. III. Development of *Hymenolepis diminuta* in superinfections. *J. Parasit.* 54, 55-62 (1968).
101. Roberts, L. S., and Mong, F. N., Developmental physiology of cestodes. IV. *In vitro* development of *Hymenolepis diminuta* in presence and absence of oxygen. *Exp. Parasit.* 26, 166-174 (1969).
102. Roberts, L. S., and Mong, F. N., Developmental physiology of cestodes. XIII. Vitamin B_6 requirement of *Hymenolepis diminuta* during *in vitro* cultivation. *J. Parasit.* 59, 101-104 (1973).
103. Roberts, L. S., and Platzer, E. G., Developmental physiology of cestodes. II. Effects of changes in host dietary carbohydrate and roughage on previously established *Hymenolepis diminuta*. *J. Parasit.* 53, 85-93 (1967).
104. Roe, J. H., Bailey, J. M., Gray, R. R., and Robinson, J. N., Complete removal of glycogen from tissues by extraction with cold trichloroacetic acid solution. *J. Biol. Chem.* 236, 1244-1246 (1961).
105. Rothman, A. H., Role of bile salts in the biology of tapeworms. I. Effect on the metabolism of *Hymenolepis diminuta* and *Oochoristica symmetrica*. *Exp. Parasit.* 7, 328-337 (1958).
106. Rybicka, K., Embryogenesis in cestodes. In "Advances in Parasitology" (B. Dawes, ed.), Vol. 4, pp. 107-178. Academic Press, N.Y., (1966a).
107. Rybicka, K., Embryogenesis in *Hymenolepis diminuta*. I. Morphogenesis. *Exp. Parasit.* 19, 366-379 (1966b).
108. Rybicka, K., Embryogenesis in *Hymenolepis diminuta*. II. Glycogen distribution in the embryos. *Exp. Parasit.* 20, 98-105 (1967a).
109. Rybicka, K., Embryogenesis in *Hymenolepis diminuta*. III. Distribution of ribonucleic acid. *Exp. Parasit.* 20, 177-185 (1967b).
110. Sakamoto, T., and Sugimura, M., Studies on echinococcosis. XXIII. Electron microscopical observations on histogenesis of larval *Echinococcus multilocularis*. *Jap. J. Vet. Res.* 18, 131-144 (1970).

111. Scheibel, L. W., Saz, H. J., and Bueding, E., The anaerobic incorporation of ^{32}P into adenosine triphosphate by *Hymenolepis diminuta*. *J. Biol. Chem.* 243, 2220-2235 (1968).
112. Schiller, E. L., A simplified method for the *in vitro* cultivation of the rat tapeworm, *Hymenolepis diminuta*. *J. Parasit.* 51, 516-518 (1965).
113. Schmidt, G. D., and Roberts, L. S., *Foundations of Parasitology*. C. V. Mosby Co., St. Louis, (1977).
114. Shorb, D. A., Host-parasite relations of *Hymenolepis fraterna* in the rat and the mouse. *Amer. J. Hyg.* 18, 74-113 (1933).
115. Sisken, J. E., Methods for measuring the length of the mitotic cycle and the timing of DNA synthesis for mammalian cells in culture. In "Methods in Cell Physiology" (D. M. Prescott, ed.), Vol. 1, pp. 387-401. Academic Press, (1964).
116. Smyth, J. D., Observations on the scolex of *Echinococcus granulosus*, with special reference to the occurrence and cytochemistry of secretory cells in the rostellum. *Parasitology* 54, 515-526 (1964).
117. Smyth, J. D., *The Physiology of Cestodes*. W. H. Freeman, San Francisco, (1969).
118. Smyth, J. D., and Haslewood, G. A. D., The biochemistry of bile as a factor in determining host specificity in intestinal parasites, with particular reference to *Echinococcus granulosus*. *Ann. N. Y. Acad. Sci.* 113(1), 234-260 (1963).
119. Smyth, J. D., Morgan, J., and Howkins, A. B., Further analysis of the factors controlling strobilization, differentiation and maturation of *Echinococcus granulosus in vitro*. *Exp. Parasit.* 21, 31-41 (1967).
120. Starling, J. A., Tegumental carbohydrate transport in intestinal helminths: Correlation between mechanisms of membrane transport and the biochemical environment of absorptive surfaces. *Trans. Amer. Microsc. Soc.* 94, 508-523 (1975).
121. Sulgostowska, T., The development of organ systems in cestodes: I. A study of histology of *Hymenolepis diminuta* (Rudolphi 1819) (Hymenolepididae). *Acta Parasit. Pol.* 20, 449-462 (1972).

122. Surgan, M. H., and Roberts, L. S., Adsorption of bile salts by the cestodes, *Hymenolepis diminuta* and *H. microstoma*. *J. Parasit. 62*, 78-86 (1976a).
123. Surgan, M. H., and Roberts, L. S., Effect of bile salts on the absorption of glucose and oleic acid by the cestodes, *Hymenolepis diminuta* and *H. microstoma*. *J. Parasit. 62*, 87-93 (1976b).
124. Thiele, V. F., and Brin, M., Chromatographic separation and microbiological assay of vitamin B_6 in tissues from normal and vitamin B_6-depleted rats. *J. Nutr. 90*, 347-353 (1966).
125. Tkachuck, R. D., and MacInnis, A. J., The effect of bile salts on the carbohydrate metabolism of two species of hymenolepidid cestodes. *Comp. Biochem. Physiol. 40B*, 993-1003 (1971).
126. Tkachuck, R. D., Weinstein, P. P., and Mueller, J. F., Comparison of the uptake of vitamin B_{12} by *Spirometra mansonoides* and *Hymenolepis diminuta* and the functional groups of B_{12} analogs affecting uptake. *J. Parasit. 62*, 94-101 (1976).
127. Turner, C. D., *General Endocrinology*. 4th ed. Saunders Co., Philadelphia, (1966).
128. Watts, S. D. M., and Fairbairn, D., Anaerobic excretion of fermentation acids by *Hymenolepis diminuta* during development in the definitive host. *J. Parasit. 60*, 621-625 (1974).
129. Weinman, C. J., Egg-production by *Hymenolepis nana* var. *fraterna* and egg infectivity after passage from mice with light, moderate, and heavy worm burdens. *J. Parasit. 44(4, Sec. 2)*, 16 (1958).
130. Wikgren, B.-J. P., Studies on the mitotic activity in plerocercoids of *Diphyllobothrium latum* L. (Cestoda). *Commentat. Biol. Soc. Sci. Fenn. 27*, 1-33 (1964).
131. Wikgren, B.-J. P., and Gustafsson, M. K. S., Duration of the cell cycle of germinative cells in plerocercoids of *Diphyllobothrium dendriticum*. *Zeitschr. Parasitenk. 23*, 275-281 (1967).
132. Wikgren, B.-J. P., and Gustafsson, M. K. S., Cell proliferation and histogenesis in diphyllobothriid tapeworms (Cestoda). *Acta Acad. Aboensis, Ser. B. 31*, 1-10 (1971).

133. Wikgren, B.-J. P., Gustafsson, M. K. S., and Knuts, G. M., Primary anlage formation in diphyllobothriid tapeworms. *Zeitschr. Parasitenk. 36*, 131-139 (1971).
134. Wikgren, B.-J. P., and Knuts, G. M., Growth of the subtegumental tissue in cestodes by cell migration. *Acta Acad. Aboensis, Ser. B. 30*, 1-6 (1970).
135. Wilson, V. C. L. C., and Schiller, E. L., The neuroanatomy of *Hymenolepis diminuta* and *H. nana*. *J. Parasit. 55*, 261-270 (1969).
136. Woodland, W. N. F., On the life cycle of *Hymenolepis fraterna* (*H. nana* var. *fraterna* Stiles) in the white mouse. *Parasitology 16*, 69-83 (1924).

THE CULTIVATION OF
HYMENOLEPIS IN VITRO

William S. Evans

Department of Biology
University of Winnipeg
Winnipeg, Manitoba

I. INTRODUCTION

The need for adequate *in vitro* methods as tools for the investigation of cestode physiology was stressed by Wardle in 1934. He outlined the problems involved in developing such techniques and subsequently described a method for maintaining, apparently axenically, adult *Hymenolepis nana* var. *fraterna* alive and active in a nutrient medium for 20 days, several days longer than the life expectancy of the adult *in vivo* (Green and Wardle 1941). Since then, many attempts have been made to maintain and grow tapeworms *in vitro* and the now considerable literature on the subject has been reviewed by Silverman (1965), Weinstein (1966), Clegg and Smyth (1968), Taylor and Baker (1968), Silverman and Hansen (1971) and most recently by Voge (1978).

Prominent among the species used in this research are members of the genus *Hymenolepis*, including of course, the species that is the subject of this book. However, though research with *H. diminuta* has produced some very important achievements *in vitro*, the literature concerning its cultivation is not extensive. For this reason, information about culturing other members of this genus will also be presented in this chapter.

Initially, researchers working with these species concentrated on culturing the strobilate stage of the life cycle and the first case of a hymenolepidid cestode being grown *in vitro* was published by Schiller et al. (1959). These workers successfully induced adult *H. diminuta* fragments, composed only of scolex and neck, to increase 30-fold in size and begin gonad differentiation in a mixture of horse serum and tapeworm extract at 38 C. The next year, Berntzen (1960, 1961) announced the successful growth of *H. diminuta* from *in vitro* excysted larvae to adults containing preoncospheres and averaging 20.8 cm in length. Berntzen (1962) modified this technique, applied it to *H. nana*, and became the first to succeed in culturing a cyclophyllidean tapeworm from a larva to a patent adult with viable eggs.

Berntzen's culture method has subsequently been discussed by him (Berntzen 1966), examined and criticised by Hopkins (1967), and redescribed by Taylor and Baker (1968). It has proven useful for cultivating the pseudophyllidean *Spirometra mansonoides* (Berntzen and Mueller 1964, 1972) and the nematode *Trichinella spiralis* (Berntzen 1965). Unfortunately, subsequent attempts by others to use this method for culturing cycclophyllidean species (Smyth 1962; Webster and Cameron 1963; Taylor 1963a, 1963b; Voge 1963; Hopkins 1967; Sinha and Hopkins 1967) were unexplainably unsuccessful. Berntzen himself (Thorson et al. 1968) failed to obtain consistent results with *H. diminuta* that were as good as those he reported in 1961. As a consequence of this, alternative techniques have been developed for culturing the strobilate phase of *H. diminuta* and other hymenolepidids and these are the methods that will be dealt with in this chapter.

The first successful technique for culturing oncospheres to cysticercoids *in vitro* was reported by Graham and Berntzen (1970). They hatched the eggs of *H. diminuta* according to Berntzen and Voge (1965), separated the hatched oncospheres from egg debris in a sugar gradient, and grew them monoxenically in monolayer cultures of mouse fibroblasts. Cysticercoids recovered from culture were excysted *in vitro* by the Rothman (1959) method and cultured to gravid adults according to Berntzen (1966). This was the first report of the entire life cycle of a tapeworm being completed *in vitro*.

Axenic cultivation of precysticercoid stages was attempted by Taylor (1961) but growth and differentiation of this phase of the hymenolepidid life cycle was not achieved axenically until 1972 when Voge, working with *H. citelli*, managed to get oncospheres, hatched *in vitro* (Berntzen and Voge 1965), to develop to the hollow ball stage. Subsequently, modifications of this technique have been used in the successful axenic cultivation of *H. citelli*, *H. diminuta*, *H. nana* and *H. microstoma* from oncospheres to infective cysticercoids. The procedures for culturing these species are dealt with in section II.

II. CULTIVATION FROM ONCOSPHERE TO CYSTICERCOID

The first successful axenic culture method for growing oncospheres, hatched *in vitro*, to infective cysticercoids was described for *H. citelli* (Voge and Green 1975). Since then, Voge and her colleagues have successfully applied this technique, with some modifications in each case, to *H. diminuta* (Voge 1975), *H. nana* (Seidel and Voge 1975) and *H. microstoma* (Seidel 1975).

in general, the culturing procedure is the same for each of these parasites. First, fresh tapeworm eggs are collected, sterilized and induced to hatch *in vitro*. The activated oncospheres are then transferred to a medium in culture vessels where, under suitable circumstances, become infective cysticercoids. However, the conditions necessary for maximum hatching and development *in vitro* are different for each species. A comparison of the particular requirements of these species during each phase of the culturing process is the subject of this section. Unless otherwise stated, the data presented for each species in the following subsections have been drawn from the four articles cited above.

A. *Collection and Sterilization of Eggs*

Fresh gravid proglottids of *H. diminuta*, *H. nana* or *H. citelli* are collected from hosts and given three washes (10 to 15 min each time) in sterile 0.85% NaCl that contains 300 µg and units of units of streptomycin and penicillin, respectively, per mL. Washed segments are transferred to sterile depression slides and teased apart in Earle's saline at pH 7.0-7.2 (adjusted with $NaHCO_3$). The method is the same with *H. microstoma* except that Earle's saline with 60 μg and units of the respective antibiotics per mL was used throughout the procedure.

B. Hatching Procedure

Hatching tapeworm eggs *in vitro* is a two-step process developed from the method of Berntzen and Voge (1965).

Eggs, free of proglottid debris and suspended in Earle's saline, are added to sterile screw cap tubes containing glass beads (3 mm in diameter). The shells are broken and removed from the eggs by shaking the suspension manually for about 4 min. The fluid containing the eggs and empty shells is then transferred to a Petri dish containing the hatching fluid which activates the oncospheres and enables them to escape their embryonic membranes. The hatching medium differs for each species. For *H. citelli*, a solution of 25,000 units of tryptar per mL of Earle's saline is used. *H. diminuta* is placed in Earle's saline with 1% trypsin (or 25,000 units tryptar per mL) and 1% bacterial amylase. Both species are hatched under air at room temperature (26-28°C) and the contents of the Petri dish are checked every 5 min for free oncospheres. When most have hatched, the unhatched eggs and empty shells and other debris are concentrated in the centre of the dish by gentle swirling, removed by pipette and discarded. The hatched organisms are washed once in culture medium (without serum, see below) and transferred in groups of 100 to 200 parasites each to 130 x 10 mm screw cap culture tubes containing 6 mL of culture medium.

H. nana eggs, shells broken, are placed in a centrifuge tube with approximately 15 mL of Earle's saline containing 300 units of tryptar per mL adjusted to pH 3.0 with 0.1 N HCl. Following the addition of the eggs, the pH is raised slightly every 5 min with 0.1 $NaHCO_3$ reaching 7.0 within 20 min. During this period, 5% CO_2/95% N_2 is continuously bubbled through the solution. *H. microstoma* eggs are also hatched in a centrifuge tube. The hatching medium contains 5% $NaHCO_3$, 0.85 NaCl and 50,000 units of tryptar per mL. The solution is bubbled with 5% CO_2/94% N_2 for 10 min before and for 20 min after being inoculated with eggs. When hatching has occurred, the suspensions of *H. nana* and *H. microstoma* are centrifuged, the oncospheres are washed with culture medium, and transferred to culture tubes as described for *H. citelli* and *H. diminuta*.

C. Culture Media

Regardless of species, the culture tubes contain the following solution, a modification of a medium designed for growing coackroach cells (Landureau 1966, 1968):

MEDIUM COMPOSITION

Amino acids	Grams
L-arginine HCl	2.0
L-aspartic acid	0.200
L-glutamic acid	1.0
α-alanine	0.12
β-alanine	0.0445
L-cysteine	0.101
L-glutamine	0.559
glycine	0.200
L-histidine HCl	0.404
L-leucine	0.249
L-lysine	0.0124
L-methionine	0.492
L-proline	0.748
L-serine	0.083
L-threonine	0.020
L-tyrosine	0.362
L-valine	0.152

Salts	
$MgSO_4 \cdot 7 H_2O$	0.670
KCl	0.894
$CaCl_2$	0.484
NaCl	7.42
$NaHCO_3$	0.424
$NaH_2PO_4 \cdot H_2O$	0.010

Sugars	Grams
Glucose	2.5
Trehalose	6.9

Organic acids	
α-ketoglutaric acid	0.365
Citric acid	0.0153
Fumaric acid	0.0058
L-malic acid	0.058
Succinic acid	0.0059

1 g yeast extract

3.5 g lactalbumin hydrosate

The above ingredients are dissolved in 900 mL of double distilled water, sterilized by millipore filtration (pore size: 0.22 µ) and made up to 1 litre with non-inactivated foetal calf serum. The pH is adjusted to 7.0 with 5% $NaHCO_3$ and the addition of 300 µg and units of streptomycin and penicillin, respectively, per mL constitutes the medium for *H. nana* and *H. microstoma*. *H. citelli* and *H. diminuta* will not fully develop unless the medium contains L-cyteine at levels of 1.9×10^{-3} M per mL for the former and 8.93×10^{-4} to 1.62×10^{-3} M per mL for the latter species. This reducing agent is added to the cultures after they have been inoculated and the role it plays in stimulating growth of these species is not understood. It has been suggested that its effect is a triggering action (Voge *et al.* 1976). Apparently, uptake of L-cysteine by the parasites rapidly depleted the supply in the medium but developemnt, once started, continues in its absence.

Incidentally, L-cysteine produces abnormal growth in cultures of *H. nana* and *H. microstoma*.

D. *Gas Phase*

H. citelli, *H. microstoma* and *H. diminuta* develop fully to infective cysticercoids when cultured under air. *H. nana*, on the other hand, is inhibited by air but reaches full development to infectivity under 5% CO_2/95% N_2. This gas phase is established by bubbling the gas mixture through the medium for one minute, closing the culture tube immediately and sealing it with paraffin. When 5% CO_2/95% N_2 are used instead of air, the developmental rate of *H. diminuta* is doubled (Voge *et al.* 1976).

E. *Maintenance of Cultures*

Cultures are kept stationary in a slightly inclined position. *H. citelli* is maintained at 26°C and the other species are kept at 28°C. Structural abnormalities occur and growth is inhibited when *H. diminuta* is cultured at 25°C. The medium is changed and the gas phase is renewed three times a week after the first 5 days for *H. nana* and after the first week with the other species.

F. *Development in vitro*

The developmental pattern during the transition from oncosphere to cysticercoid *in vitro* is similar to that reported from these species *in vivo* (Voge and Heyneman 1957; Rothman 1957; Voge 1964). All species pass through four easily recognized developmental stages. First, the oncosphere increases in size and becomes a spherical structure with an internal cavity, the hollow ball stage. This elongates to become the ovoid or pear-shaped bipartite stage. Elongation continues and three regions of the body become apparent as the larvae differentiate into scolex, cyst and cercomer forming the tripartite stage. Finally, the scolex is withdrawn into the midportion or cyst which eventually completely encloses it. Cysticercoids do not become infective *in vitro* until several days after the withdrawal stage has been reached. The rate of development varies according to the species and is generally slower *in vitro* than *in vivo* (Table I).

The observation of larvae growing *in vitro* has revealed that both underdeveloped and fully differentiated cysticercoids are motile. Beginning with the tripartite stage, their bodies display waves of contractions that result in shape changes and folding of the body wall. Also, as the withdrawal stage is approached by *H. citelli*, the scolex is pulled in and out of the cyst several times before it becomes enclosed. These larval movements can be initiated by slightly disturbing the culture medium which, in the case of *H. nana*, stimulates very active twisting and turning of the scolex inside the cyst as well as contractions of the cyst wall. Motility has never been reported for cysticercoids grown *in vivo*.

III. CULTIVATION OF THE STROBILATE STAGE

Cultivation of the strobilate phase of the hymenolepidid cestodes begins either with worms recovered from their definitive hosts or with larvae recovered from cysticercoids that have been excysted *in vitro*.

A. *Cysticercoid Excystment in Vitro*

Rothman (1959) published the results of an extensive series of experiments in which he studied the effects of temperature, proteolytic enzymes and bile salts on several tapeworms including *H. nana*, *H. diminuta* and *H. citelli*. He reported that at 37°C these hymenolepidids will readily excyst in Krebs Ringer's phosphate solution that contains trypsin (0.05%) and bile salt (0.3 to 0.6% taurocholate, glycocholate or cholate) at pH 6.7 and that the excystment rate was increased when cysticercoids were treated with 1.0% pepsin in Ringer's (pH 1.5 adjusted with 1.0 N HCL) before being exposed to the trypsin-bile salt solution. Most techniques that have been developed for excysting larvae for cultivation are based on these findings. The precise details vary from one author to the next and will be dealt with later but in general, the procedure is

TABLE I

RATE OF DEVELOPMENT OF FOUR HYMENOLEPIDID CESTODES FROM ONCOSPHERES TO CYSTICERCOIDS *IN VITRO*

Species	Development Stage (age of worms in days)					Reference
	hollow ball	bipartite (ovoid)	tripartite	withdrawal	infective	
H. citelli	6	7-8	12-16	16-30	45	Voge & Green 1975
H. diminuta	3 (2)	7 (3)	9 (4-6)	14-18 (6-9)	24-25 (10)	Voge 1975
H. nana	4 (2)	6 (3)	11 (5)	14 (6-8)	22 (10)	Seidel and Voge 1975
H. microstoma	3 (2)	5 (3)	9 (5)	13-16 (6-8)	21 (10)	Seidel 1975

Throughout the culture period, *H. citelli* was kept at 26°C; the other species were maintained at 28°C. Numbers in brackets give the days of occurrence of the various stages in *Tribolium confusum* as determined in the author's laboratory.

the same for all cases. Cysticercoids are dissected free of their insect hosts and washed in sterile saline (Hanks', Ringer's or 0.85% NaCl). Thereafter, all procedures are conducted between 37 and 39°C in solutions that may or may not contain antibiotics. The washed cysticercoids are transferred to the acid-pepsin solution. After 10 to 15 min they are washed several times with sterile saline to remove the pepsin and transferred to the sterile trypsin-bile salt solution (taurocholate or tauroglycocholate) where they excyst. The larvae are then washed in sterile fluid (saline or culture medium) and transferred to culture vessels. Variations of this procedure have been used to excyst *H. nana* (Berntzen 1962; Sinha and Hopkins 1967) and *H. microstoma* (DeRycke and Berntzen 1967; Evans 1970; Seidel 1971) for cultivation.

Schiller (1965) induced *H. diminuta* to excyst in ox bile and Berntzen (1961) apparently excysted this species in sterile Tyrode's solution at pH 7.8 to 9.0 at 37°C.

B. *Cultivation Procedures*

1. *Hymenolepis diminuta.* The first technique for culturing *H. diminuta* from cysticercoids to adults that produced infective oncospheres was described by Schiller (1965). Cysticercoids were excysted incubating them in undiluted ox bile for 30 min at 37°C. Excysted larvae were washed 3 times in sterile normal saline containing 100 units and μg of penicillin and streptomycin, respectively, per mL and transferred to 50 mL Erlenmeyer flasks with culture medium. The diphasic medium consisted of a blood agar layer overlaid with Hanks' balanced salt solution. The agar was prepared by dissolving 16 g of Difco nutrient agar and 3.5 g NaCl in 700 mL of distilled water. The solution was autoclaved, mixed thoroughly with 300 mL of sterile, defibrinated, inactivated, rabbit blood and dispensed in 10 mL volumes into culture flasks. After gelation, 10 mL of Hanks', containing 100 μg and units of streptomycin and penicillin, respectively , per mL and adjusted to pH 7.5 with $NaHCO_3$, were added to each flask. The medium was pre-incubated at 32°C for 24 h. The fluid phase was saturated with 97% N_2/3% CO_2 and readjusted to pH 7.5 with NaOH. Ten to 15 larvae

were placed in each flask. The flasks were closed with cotton plugs and shaken continously in a Dubnoff shaking incubator at 37°C under 97% N_2/3% CO_2. The young worms were transferred to fresh medium on day 6, 8, 10 and every day thereafter. On days 10 and 20, 1 mg of powdered glucose per mL of fluid overlay was added to the medium. On day 10, each worm was transferred to a separate flask and on day 20, the volume of Hanks' was increased to 20 mL per flask. Worms began shedding proglottids with viable, infective eggs on day 24. Though *in vitro* grown worms were smaller than those grown for a similar time *in vivo*, no other morphological differences could be discerned. However, Schiller found 6-day-old worms obtained from rats (details not given) grew as large *in vitro* as might be expected during an equivalent time *in vivo*.

This method was modified after consultation with Schiller by Roberts and Mong (1969) and successfully used by them to study the growth and development of worms under mixtures of 0, 1, 5, or 20% oxygen with nitrogen. The medium was prepared according to Schiller except that the Hanks' solution was gassed with the appropriate gas mixture for 10 min at room temperature with a fritted gas dispersion tube and sealed until it was added to the blood agar in the culture flasks. The Hanks' was dispensed with a Cornwall automatic pipette, the flasks were sealed and preincubated for 24 h at 34 instead of 32°C.

Six-day-old worms recovered from rats were rinsed in Krebs' or Ringer's phosphate (pH 7.1) and examined under a dissecting microscope. Those not obviously damaged were rinsed 4 times in sterile Hanks', transferred to Hanks' with 5000 units of penicillin, 500 mg streptomycin and 5000 units mycostatin (Squibb mystatin) per 10 mL, incubated for 1 h at 37°C, gently blotted on clean filter paper, weighed individually and placed into culture (one worm per flask). The flasks were closed with cotton plugs and placed in a Dubnoff incubator under the appropriate gas phase. For the first five days the worms were cultured in 25 mL Erlenmeyer flasks with 5 mL blood agar and 5 mL Hanks' overlay. Then they were transferred to 50 mL flasks with 10 mL of each medium phase for the subsequent 7 days of the experiment.

Worms were transferred to flasks with fresh medium every 24 h. As in Schiller's (1965) experiments, they grew and produced viable, infective eggs by the twelfth day of culture. The worms were unaffected by the O_2 concentration tested as equivalent growth and development occurred under all gas phases.

The Roberts and Mong technique has subsequently been used successfully as an experimental tool on several occasions. Roberts and Mong (1973) used it to study the significance of vitamin B_6 in the metabolism of *H. diminuta*. Their findings suggest that the parasite has a direct nutritional requirement for an external source of this metabolite.

Tofts and Meerovitch (1974) used it to show that farnesol methyl ether (FME) markedly inhibited the development of *H. diminuta in vitro*. This was confirmed by Fioravanti and MacInnis (1976) who, using this technique, showed that farnesol and several of its derivatives have no growth promoting effect and at high concentrations inhibit the development of *H. diminuta in vitro*. These findings contradict the report of Thorson *et al*. (1968) that farnesol stimulates the growth of this tapeworm.

Roberts (1973) reported that defibrinated sheep blood was an adequate replacement for rabbit blood in Schiller's (1965) medium. Turton (1972) successfully replaced the latter diphasic medium with a serum agar overlaid with medium containing yeast extract, liver extract and horse serum. Turton's medium has the advantage of being transparent, thereby enabling workers to examine worms macroscopically and microscopically without removing them from the culture flask.

One of the difficulties associated with culturing worms recovered from rats is that, in spite of the many rinses they receive in sterile solutions with antibiotics, contaminant organisms from the gut are often carried into culture vessels on the surface of the worms. To overcome this problem, Roberts (1973) studied the effects of various surface active agents on bacterial and other contaminants of the worm's surface. He reported that worms from rats can be sterilized by a 2 to 3 s rinse in 0.1% Phisophex (Winthrop Lab.) without impairing their ability to grow and differentiate *in vitro*. Turton (1974)

approached the problem by investigating the effect
of various concentrations of broad spectrum antibacterial and antifungal antibiotics included in the
culture medium. He reported that the growth of 3-day-
old worms removed from rats was unimpaired by concentrations of mystatin (Squibb Mycostatin) and
amphotericin B (Squibb Fungizon) that were well above
levels required to control fungal contaminants.
The worms were markedly inhibited by cyclohexamide
(Koch-Light, Actidione) but unaffected by concentrations of streptomycin and penicillin ranging from
30 µg and 30 units, respectively, to 5,000 µg and
5,000 units, respectively, per mL of culture medium.
H. diminuta is considerably more resistant than
H. microstoma is to the last two compounds (Evans
1978).

2. *Hymenolepis nana*. Sinha and Hopkins (1967),
unable to repeat Berntzen's (1962) results with *H.
nana*, published a less complex method for cultivating
this parasite to patency in roller tubes, in a medium
composed of 45% Hanks' balanced salt solution, 30%
horse serum (Burroughs Wellcome No. 2, oxalated and
inactivated), 50% yeast extract (Oxoid), and 10% liver
extract (rat or lamb). Though some growth occurred
in a medium without liver extract, only when the latter was present did worms become gravid.

Liver extract was prepared using a modification
of Stoll's (1959) technique. Fresh lamb liver was
transported in crushed ice, chopped into 20 g pieces
and stored at -15°C. After thawing for 48 h at 4°C
one part by weight of liver was homogenized with 4
parts by volume of de-ionized water at 4°C. The
brei was adjusted to pH 4.0 with N HCl, squeezed
through muslin and centrifuged at 5,420 g for 1 h at
4°C. The supernatant was sterilized by millipore
filtration and stored in 5 or 10 mL aliquots at -15°C
until needed. The culture medium was dispensed in
5 mL quantities in 125 × 25 mm roller tubes and
gassed for 40 s with 95% N_2/5% CO_2. The tubes were
sealed immediately, placed in a roller drum incubator
and rotated (0.15 rpm) for 2 h before being inoculated with parasites.

Cysticercoids recovered from infected *Tribolium
confusum* were washed twice in sterile Hanks'. From
this point all procedures were conducted at 37°C in
solutions that contained 100 µg of streptomycin and

100 units of penicillin per mL. Washed parasites were pretreated in 1% pepsin in Hanks' (pH 1.7 with 0.2 N HCl) for 12-15 min and excysted in trypsin-bile salt (0.3% sodium tauroglycocholate) in Hanks' (pH adjusted to 7.0 with 0.2 N NaOH and to 7.2 with 1.4% $NaHCO_3$). After 8 to 10 min, the excysted larvae are washed three times in sterile Hanks' and transferred to roller tubes with culture medium (16-20 worms per tube). Upon receiving the worms, the tubes were gassed again with 95% N_2/5% CO_2, sealed and returned to the incubator. The medium was changed on days 3, 6, 9, 11 and 13. By the fourteenth day of culture, the worms ranged from 7 to 30 mm long. Sixty to 70% of them were mature and 20 to 30% had produced infective oncospheres. Similar results were obtained by Evans (1973) with a more defined medium in which the Hanks' and yeast extract of the Sinha-Hopkins medium were replaced by Eagle's medium (Table III).

3. *Hymenolepis microstoma*. DeRycke and Berntzen (1967) were first to succeed in growing *H. microstoma in vitro*. The worms were cultured under air in a medium consisting of HM67, a defined solution prepared from stock solutions of Medium 115 (Berntzen and Mueller 1964), Earle's glucose, serum (unspecified) and hamster bile (1%). Under these conditions, the parasites strobilated, developed gonads and grew to an average length of 4.75 mm in 12 days.

Evans (1970), using a modification of the Sinha and Hopkins (1967) method for *H. nana*, reported the first successful technique for cultivating *H. microstoma* to egg-producing adults. The culture medium was prepared by mixing 60 mL of modified Eagle's medium (Table II) with 10 mL of sheep or hamster liver extract [prepared according to the method described by Sinha and Hopkins (1967)] and 30 mL of horse serum (Burroughs Wellcome No. 2, oxalated and inactivated). One to 10 mL of whole ox bile was added, the medium was adjusted to pH 7.6 with 0.2 N NaOH and dispensed in 5 mL volumes into roller tubes. The tubes were gassed for 30 s with 95% N_2/5% CO_2, immediately sealed with Esco RHW rubber bungs, placed in a roller drum incubator and rotated 9 rph at 37.5°C for 2.5 h.

TABLE II
MODIFIED[a] EAGLE'S MEDIUM

Ingredient	Quantity (grams/litre)
L arginine mono HCl	0.042
L cystine (dissolved in 5ml of N-NaOH)	0.024
L histidine mono HCl	0.0192
L isoleucine	0.0524
L leucine	0.0524
L lysine mono HCl	0.0731
L phenylalanine	0.033
L threonine	0.0476
L tryptophan	0.008
L tryosine	0.0362
L valine	0.0468
L methionine	0.015
L glutamine	0.292
choline chloride	0.002
folic acid (dissolved in 5ml of N-NaOH)	0.002
nicotinamide	0.002
DL Ca pantothenate	0.002
pyridoxal HCl	0.002
thiamine HCl (aneurine)	0.002
riboflavin	0.0002
inositol	0.0035
<u>Salts</u>	
NaCl	6.4
KCl	0.4
$CaCl_2$	0.2
$MgSO_4 \cdot 7 H_2O$	0.2
$NaH_2PO_4 \cdot 2 H_2O$	0.14
$Fe(NO_3)_3 \cdot 9 H_2O$	0.0001
$NaHCO_3$	2.75
dextrose	4.5
streptomycin sulphate (Glaxo)	0.1
n-butyl-p-hydroxybenzoate	0.0002
penicillin (Glaxo, Crystapen)	100,000 units/litre
phenol red	0.0015%

The above ingredients are dissolved in distilled water, sterilized by Millipore and stored at 4°C.

[a] Prepared by the University of Glasgow, Department of Virology.

Cysticercoids, obtained from *Tribolium confusum*, were excysted at 38.5°C in sterile solutions without antibiotics. Solutions of digestive enzymes were prepared with modified Hanks' saline (Table III). Cysticercoids, washed 3 times in sterile modified Hanks', were pretreated with acid pepsin (pH 1.6) for 11 min, washed 3 times with modified Hanks' and placed in 2.5 mL of trypsin-bile salt (0.3% sodium tauroglycocholate) pH 7.2 (adjusted to 7.0 with 0.2 N NaOH and to 7.2 with 1.4% $NaHCO_3$), for 3.0 to 3.5 min. Then the solution was diluted to half strength with modified Hanks' and 1 min later to quarter strength; after another minute the excysted larvae were washed 3 times with sterile Hanks' and transferred to roller tubes with culture medium (20 to 30 per tube). The tubes were gassed again for 30 s, sealed and returned to the roller drum. The medium was changed on day 6 (about 144 h). On day 7, the larger worms in each culture (at least half were between 8 and 14 mm long) were transferred to roller tubes with fresh medium (1 to 3 worms per tube). The tubes were gassed, sealed and placed in the roller drum. The medium was changed on day 9, 11 and daily thereafter. In the medium with or without bile, the worms developed rapidly. By day 7, 80 to 100% had strobilated and 38 to 100% showed developing gonads. Worms cultured beyond day 7 averaged 7.9 cm in length and had complete male and female reproductive systems and active sperm by day 9. However, even when cultured to day 16 and growth continued, worms failed to become gravid unless the medium contained ox bile. Attempts to replace ox bile with sheep bile were unsuccessful as the latter was toxic to *H. microstoma* (Evans 1973).

Gravid worms were also recovered from cultures with bile supplemented medium in which gas phases containing 5 and 10% oxygen were used. No difference in size was observed between these worms and those grown simultaneously in cultures gassed with 95% N_2/5% CO_2. However, the growth and development of worms cultivated also at the same time, in cultures gassed with mixtures containing 15, 20 and 30% oxygen, was markedly retarded.

There was batch-to-batch variation in the degree to which a sample of horse serum (Burroughs Wellcome No. 2) would support the growth of *H. microstoma* and

TABLE III

MODIFIED HANKS' BALANCED SALT SOLUTION (SINHA 1967)

Solution	Ingredients	Quantity
I	NaCl	8.40 g
	KCl	0.40 g
	$Na_2H_2PO_4$	0.10 g
	$Na_2HPO_4 \cdot 2H_2O$	0.10 g
	de-ionized H_2O	900 mL
	[a]0.2% phenol red	10 mL
II	$CaCl_2$ (dried)	0.14 g
	$MgCl_2 \cdot 6H_2O$	0.10 g
	de-ionized H_2O	100 mL

Following autoclave sterilization, 1 part of solution II is combined with 9 parts of solution I to complete the balanced salt solution.

[a]The phenol red solution is prepared by dissolving 2.0 g in 100 mL of 0.2 N-NaOH and increasing this to one litre with de-ionized water.

H. nana. This variable effect was due to inherent differences in the serum batches and not to deterioration of the serum during storage at 4°C (Evans 1973). By testing new batches of serum before using them experimentally, consistent results were obtained from one experiment to the next.

Khan and DeRycke (1975) found that Eagle's basal medium (BME, Flow Laboratories, Scotland) was an adequate replacement for modified Eagle's (Table II) in Evans' (1970) medium. They confirmed the toxicity of sheep bile but reported that worms became gravid in the absence of ox bile when cultured to day 18. They verified the serum problem reported by Evans (1970, 1973) and attempted, unsuccessfully, to replace horse serum No. 2 (Burroughs Wellcome) with a variety of different blood product preparations. These workers have also reported that worm development can be improved by the addition of Oxoid yeast extract (0.1 to 2.0%) to the culture medium (Khan and DeRycke 1976b).

An alternative technique for culturing *H. microstoma* was published by Seidel (1971). Cysticercoids, excysted according to Rothman's (1959) technique (details not given), were cultivated in screw cap tubes on a 20 mL nutrient agar (Difco) slant overlaid with 20 mL of fluid under air. He tried a variety of solid and fluid phase combinations and his best results were obtained when the agar base contained 5% human blood and the overlay was 70% triple Eagle's medium (TEM GIBCO) and 30% horse serum (inactivated). Worms reached an average length of 52 mm and developed preoncospheres but did not become gravid. With the exception that the worms were smaller, similar results were obtained when nutrient agar without blood was used as long as the fluid overlay contained 0.1 mg of hemin per 100 mL. However, when the hemin was absent and the agar did not contain blood, strobilation would not occur. By simultaneously including hemin in the overlay and blood in the agar, the author induced larvae, grown and excysted *in vitro*, to become gravid, thereby completing the entire life cycle of *H. microstoma in vitro* (Seidel 1975). Khan and DeRycke (1976a) obtained results which confirm the beneficial effect of hemin on the development of *H. microstoma*.

IV. CONCLUSION

Research on culturing hymenolepidid tapeworms *in vitro* has not been profitless. It has revealed the existence of metabolic differences between the species studied, particularly in the larval forms (see Section II, C and D). It has produced valuable investigative tools for studying the influence of various factors on worm growth and differentiation. The use of these tools has been demonstrated with *H. diminuta* (see Section III, B 1) and *H. microstoma* (DeRycke and Evans, 1972). The latter authors studied the development of young adults in media of various freezing point depressions (FDP). Their results suggest that *H. microstoma* is homoiosmotic in media with FDP values ranging from 0.50 to 0.73°C. Also, *in vitro* cultivation has been applied to the study of host-parasite interaction. Lackie (1976) injected *H. diminuta* cysticercoids grown *in vitro* (according to Voge 1975) into various insects and studied the haemocytic defense reactions of the latter. Her results imply that the surface of the parasite bears an inherent similarity to the surface of the host tissues. Because of this, they escape recognition as "non-self" and are not attacked by the host's haemocytes.

One would expect *in vitro* cultivation methods to be particularly useful in studying cestode nutrition. However, all the known culture media require the addition of natural products (serum, blood, liver extract) of unknown chemical composition before they will support growth. Consequently, apart from the beneficial effect of hemin on *H. microstoma* (Seidel 1971, 1975 and Khan and DeRycke 1976a) and the implication that an external source of vitamin B_6 is required by *H. diminuta* (Roberts and Mong 1973), no precise information on the nutrition of the hymenolepidids has been gained by growing them *in vitro*. This situation will probably persist until fully defined media capable of supporting growth have been discovered.

REFERENCES

1. Berntzen, A. K., An effective method for the *in vitro* culture of *Hymenolepis diminuta*. J. Parasitol. 46 (5. Sect. 2, Suppl.), 47 (1960).
2. Berntzen, A. K., The *in vitro* cultivation of tapeworms. I. Growth of *Hymenolepis diminuta* (Cestoda: Cyclophyllidea). J. Parasitol. 47, 351-355 (1961).
3. Berntzen, A. K., *In vitro* cultivation of tapeworms. II. Growth and maintenance of *Hymenolepis nana* (Cestoda: Cyclophyllidea). J. Parasitol. 48, 785-797 (1962).
4. Berntzen, A. K., Comparative growth and development of *Trichinella spiralis in vitro* and *in vivo*. Exp. Parasitol. 16, 74-106 (1965).
5. Berntzen, A. K., A controlled culture environment for axenic growth of parasites. Ann. N.Y. Acad. Sci. 139, 176-189 (1966).
6. Berntzen, A. K., and Mueller, J. F., *In vitro* cultivation of *Spirometra mansonoides* (Cestoda) from the procercoid to the early adult. J. Parasitol. 50, 705-711 (1964).
7. Berntzen, A. K., and Mueller, J. F., *In vitro* cultivation of *Spirometra* spp. (Cestoda) from the plerocercoid to the gravid adult. J.

Parasitol. 58, 750-752 (1972).

8. Berntzen, A. K., and Voge, M., *In vitro* hatching of oncospheres of four hymenolepidid cestodes. *J. Parasitol. 51*, 235-242 (1965).

9. Clegg, J. A., and Smyth, J. D., Growth, development and culture methods: parasitic platyhelminths. In "Chemical Zoology" (B. T. Scheer, ed.), Vol. II, pp. 395-466. Academic Press, New York, (1968).

10. DeRycke, P. H., and Berntzen, A. K. Maintenance and growth of *Hymenolepis microstoma* (Cestoda: Cyclophyllidea) *in vitro*. *J. Parasitol. 53*, 352-354 (1967).

11. DeRycke, P. H., and Evans, W. S., Osmoregulation of *Hymenolepis microstoma* II. Influence of the osmotic pressure on the *in vitro* development of the young adult. *Z. Parasitenk. 38*, 147-151 (1972).

12. Evans, W. S., The *in vitro* cultivation of *Hymenolepis microstoma* from cysticercoid to egg-producing adult. *Can. J. Zool. 48*, 1135-1137 (1970).

13. Evans, W. S., The *in vitro* cultivation of *Hymenolepis nana* and *H. Microstoma*. Ph.D. thesis, University of Glasgow, Glasgow, Scotland (1973).

14. Evans, W. S., The effect of streptomycin and penicillin on the growth and differentiation *in vitro Hymenolepis microstoma*. *Can. J. Zool. 56*, 1210-1211 (1978).

15. Fioravanti, C. F., and MacInnis, A. J., The *in vitro* effects of farnesol and derivatives on *Hymenolepis diminuta*. *J. Parasitol. 62*, 749-755 (1976).

16. Graham, J. J., and Berntzen, A. K., The monoxenic cultivation of *Hymenolepis diminuta* cysticercoids with rat fibroblasts. *J. Parasitol. 56*, 1184-1188 (1970).

17. Green, N. K., and Wardle, R. A., The cultivation of tapeworms in artificial media. *Can. J. Res. 19*, 240-244 (1941).

18. Hopkins, C. A., The *in vitro* cultivation of cestodes with particular reference to *Hymenolepis nana*. In "Problems of *In vitro* Culture" (A.E.R. Taylor, ed.), pp. 24-47. Blackwell Scientific Publications, Oxford, (1967).

19. Khan, Z. I., and DeRycke, P. H., The *in vitro* cultivation of *Hymenolepis microstoma* with

particular reference to the role of serum for strobilization and gametogenesis. *Biol. Jb. Dodonaea 43*, 151-172 (1975).
20. Khan, Z. I., and DeRycke, P. H., Studies on *Hymenolepis microstoma in vitro*. I. Effect of heme compounds on growth and reproduction. *Z. Parasitenk. 49*, 253-261 (1976a).
21. Khan, Z. I., and DeRycke, P. H., Studies on *Hymenolepis microstoma in vitro* II. Effect of yeast extract on development and maturation. *Z. Parasitenk. 50*, 73-79 (1976b).
22. Lackie, A. M., Evasion of the haemocytic defence reaction of certain insects by larvae of *Hymenolepis diminuta* (Cestoda). *Parasitology 73*, 97-107 (1976).
23. Landureau, J. C., Cultures *in vitro* de cellules embryonnaires de blattes (insects dictyopteres). *Exp. Cell Res. 41*, 545-556 (1966).
24. Landureau, J. C., Cultures *in vitro* de cellules embryonnaires de blattes (insects dictyopteres). II. Obtention de lignes cellulaires a multiplication continue. *Exp. Cell Res. 50*, 323-337 (1968).
25. Roberts, L. S., Modifications in media and surface sterilization methods for *in vitro* cultivation of *Hymenolepis diminuta*. *J. Parasitol. 59*, 474-479 (1973).
26. Roberts, L. S., and Mong, F. N., Developmental physiology of cestodes. IV. *In vitro* development of *Hymenolepis diminuta* in presence and absence of oxygen. *Exp. Parasitol. 26*, 166-174 (1969).
27. Roberts, L. S., and Mong, F. N., Developmental physiology of cestodes. XIII. Vitamin B_6 requirement of *Hymenolepis diminuta* during *in vitro* cultivation. *J. Parasitol. 59*, 101-104 (1973).
28. Rothman, A. H., The larval development of *Hymenolepis diminuta* and *H. citelli*. *J. Parasitol. 43*, 643-648 (1957).
29. Rothman, A. H., Studies on the excystment of tapeworms. *Exp. Parasitol. 8*, 336-364 (1959).
30. Schiller, E. L., A simplified method for the *in vitro* cultivation of the rat tapeworm, *Hymenolepis diminuta*. *J. Parasitol. 51*, 516-518 (1965).
31. Schiller, E. L., Read, C. P., and Rothman, A. H., Preliminary experiments on the growth of a cyclophyllidean cestode *in vitro*. *J.*

Parasitol. 45, (4, sect. 2, suppl.), 45 (1959).
32. Seidel, J. S., Hemin as a requirement in the development *in vitro* of *Hymenolepis microstoma* (Cestoda: Cyclophyllidea). *J. Parasitol. 57*, 566-570 (1971).
33. Seidel, J. S., The life cycle *in vitro* of *Hymenolepis microstoma* (Cestoda). *J. Parasitol. 61*, 677-681 (1975).
34. Seidel, J. S., and Voge, M., Axenic development of cysticercoids of *Hymenolepis nana*. *J. Parasitol. 61*, 861-864 (1975).
35. Silverman, P. H., In vitro cultivation procedures for parasitic helminths. In "Advances in Parasitology" (B. Dawes, ed.) Vol. 3 pp. 159-222. Academic Press, London, (1965).
36. Silverman, P. H., and Hansen, E. L., *In vitro* cultivation for parasitic helminths: recent advances. In "Advances in Parasitology" (B. Dawes, ed.) Vol. 9, pp. 227-259. Academic Press, London, (1971).
37. Sinha, D. P., The *in vitro* cultivation of cestodes. Ph.D. Thesis, University of Glasgow, Glasgow, Scotland (1967).
38. Sinha, D. P., and Hopkins, C. A., *In vitro* cultivation of the tapeworm *Hymenolepis nana* from larva to adult. *Nature 215*, 1275-1276 (1967).
39. Smyth, J. D., Studies on tapeworm physiology. X. Axenic cultivation of the hydatid organism *Echinococcus granulosus*; establishment of a basic technique. *Parasitology 52*, 441-457 (1962).
40. Stoll, N. R., Axenic cultivation of *Entamoeba invadens* in cell-free medium. *Fifteenth International Congress of Zoology*, Sect. VIII, 639-641 (1959).
41. Taylor, A. E. R., Axenic culture of the rodent tapeworms *Hymenolepis diminuta* and *H. nana*. *Exp. Parasitol. 11*, 176-187 (1961).
42. Taylor, A. E. R., Maintenance of larval tapeworms (*Taenia crassiceps*) in a chemically defined medium. *Parasitology 53*, 5P (abstract) (1963a).
43. Taylor, A. E. R., Maintenance of larval *Taenia crassiceps* (Cestoda: Cyclophyllidea) in a chemically defined medium. *Exp. Parasitol. 14*, 304-310 (1963b).
44. Taylor, A. E. R., and Baker, J. R., "The Cultivation of Parasites *in vitro*". pp. 195-248.

Blackwell Scientific Publications, Oxford, (1968).
45. Thornson, R. E., Digenis, G. A., Berntzen, A., Konyalian, A., Biological activities of various lipid fractions from *Echinococcus granulosus* scolices on *in vitro* cultures of *Hymenolepis diminuta*. *J. Parasitol.* 54, 970-973 (1968).
46. Tofts, J., and Meerovitch, E., The effect of farnesyl methyl ether, a mimic of insect juvenile hormone, on *Hymenolepis diminuta in vitro*. *Int. J. Parasitol.* 4, 211-218 (1974).
47. Turton, J. A., The *in vitro* cultivation of *Hymenolepis diminuta*: the culture of 6-day-old worms removed from the rat. *Z. Parasitenk.* 40, 333-346 (1972).
48. Turton, J. A., *In vitro* cultivation of *Hymenolepis diminuta*: effect of antibiotics on the growth of three-day-old worms removed from the rat. *Exp. Parasitol.* 36, 62-69 (1974).
49. Voge, M., Maintenance *in vitro* of *Taenia crassiceps* cysticerci. *J. Parasitol.* 49 (5 sect. 2, suppl.), 59 (1963).
50. Voge, M., Development of *Hymenolepis microstoma* (Cestoda: Cyclophyllidea) in the intermediate host *Tribolium confusum*. *J. Parasitol.* 50, 77-80 (1964).
51. Voge, M., Axenic development of post-embryonic stages of *Hymenolepis citelli* (Cestoda). Am. Soc. Parasitol., 47th Annual Meeting, Abst. No. 203 (1972).
52. Voge, M., Axenic development of cysticercoids of *Hymenolepis diminuta* (Cestoda). *J. Parasitol.* 61, 563-564 (1975).
53. Voge, M., Cestoda. In "The Cultivation of Parasites *in vitro*" (A. E. R. Taylor and J. R. Baker, eds.) Second ed., pp. 193-225. Blackwell Scientific Publications, Oxford, (1978).
54. Voge, M., and Green, J., Axenic growth of oncospheres of *Hymenolepis citelli* (Cestoda) to fully developed cysticercoids. *J. Parasitol.* 61, 291-297 (1975).
55. Voge, M., and Heyneman, D., Development of *Hymenolepis nana* and *Hymenolepis diminuta* (Cestoda: Hymenolepididae) in the intermediate host *Tribolium confusum*. *Univ. Calif. Publ. Zool.* 59, 549-580 (1957).
56. Voge, M., Jaffe, J., Buckner, D. A., and Meymarian, E., Synergistic growth promoting action of L-cysteine and nitrogen upon

Hymenolepis diminuta cysticercoids *in vitro*. *J. Parasitol.* 62, 951-954 (1976).
57. Wardle, R. A., The viability of tapeworms in artificial media. *Physiol. Zool.* 7, 36-61 (1934).
58. Webster, G. A., and Cameron, T. W. M. Some preliminary observations on the development of *Echinococcus in vitro*. *Can. J. Zool.* 41, 185-195 (1963).
59. Weinstein, P. P., The *in vitro* cultivation of helminths with reference to morphogenesis. *In* "Biology of Parasites" (E. J. L. Soulsby, ed.) pp. 143-154, Academic Press, London (1966).

NUCLEIC ACIDS FROM HYMENOLEPIDIDS

Austin J. MacInnis

Department of Biology
The University of California
Los Angeles, California

Clint Carter

Department of Biology
Vanderbilt University
Nashville, Tennessee

I. INTRODUCTION

The past twenty years have produced a great revolution in biology, revealing the intricacies of the genetic code and the Central Dogma of informational flow from DNA to the synthesis of protein. Further highlights of this program, common presumably to all functional units of life, are being discovered practically on a daily basis, especially in the areas of regulation and the molecular and supramolecular architecture of cellular components wherein the machinery for replication, transcription, translation and rectification (=repair synthesis of DNA) reside. Most of this information has been derived from investigations on simple procaryotes and their symbionts, the phages or viruses. Such information concerning the complex eucaryotes has been more difficult to gain. Accordingly, acquisition of similar information on eucaryotic parasites has lagged even farther behind the frontiers. This lack of progress on parasites can also be attributed to the absence of model systems which are amenable to attack by the powerful tools of molecular biology. We have no established cell lines from helminths for *in vitro* culture. In fact, *in vitro* culture systems of intact helminths are complex, expensive, and do not yield the quantities of tissues required for investigations on DNA, RNA or protein synthesis. Yet knowledge of these central pathways in parasitic helminths (or protozoa) can be expected to yield as much potential for developing an understanding of parasitism and chemotherapy as has been achieved with procaryotes. Procaryotic systems for DNA, RNA, and protein synthesis have evolved aspects and details of the machinery for these pathways which differ from eucaryotes. Perhaps eucaryotic parasites also have evolved differences from the eucaryotic host's machinery, and when discovered, such differences may yield to chemotherapeutic attack just as successfully as those in the procaryotic bacteria.

Furthermore, the complex integration and co-evolution of eucaryotic parasite and host provide mysteries which most likely will be unravelled (perhaps we should say "uncoiled") only when the genetic interactions between host and parasite are revealed (see Parker and MacInnis 1977). Clearly, we must forge into the unknowns of the Central Dogma concerning parasites.

Surprisingly, the tapeworm *Hymenolepis diminuta* provides a very useful model for beginning studies of DNA, RNA and protein synthesis in parasitic flatworms, primarily because it can be obtained in sufficient quantities for isolating the components in question. For example, Parker and MacInnis (1977) have demonstrated that a single rat provides tapeworm tissue equivalent to the yield of a one-liter culture of *Escherichia coli*, the mainstay of molecular biology.

The following review of research on nucleic acids of hymenolepidids, conducted primarily by AJM and associates during the past ten years, establishes the groundwork for future studies of tapeworms and other helminths and illustrates some of the intriguing basic questions concerning parasites that can be approached at this level. This chapter will be limited to a review of the macromolecular DNA and

RNA of *Hymenolepis diminuta*. It documents results of isolation and characterization of these macromolecules with limited comments on their synthesis. Details of procedures are not given. Those interested in techniques should consult the references cited. Occasionally we may suggest newer techniques not yet applied to cestodes, which should be considered in future investigations. Where possible, we have compared results obtained with *H. diminuta* to other helminth groups.

II. ISOLATION OF TOTAL NUCLEIC ACIDS FROM *H. DIMINUTA*

There are many simple experiments on tapeworms such as *H. diminuta* which require determination of total content of DNA or RNA without requiring further knowledge of particular details of the origin of the molecules. Such determinations can ignore whether or not DNA is from nuclei or mitochondria, or whether RNA is ribosomal or messenger, etc. For example, growth of the worm entails increased nucleic acid production, but caution must be prescribed in establishing baseline data since many variables impinge on the state of the worm. Age of worm, presence or absence of eggs, number of worms per host, sex and age of host, species of host and numerous other parameters undoubtedly affect nucleic acid content. However, if one carefully regulates these parameters, reasonably accurate and repeatable results can be obtained by standardization. Well established procedures for assay of DNA and RNA were summarized in MacInnis and Voge (1970). Nucleic acid content can be calculated on the basis of wet weight of worms, but is less reliable than dry weight, especially with very young or small worms, since blotting time introduces a hazardous variable in obtaining wet weights. Ratios of nucleic acid content to protein content may be useful at times. An excellent baseline of protein and glycogen content/wet weight of 8-day-old *H. diminuta* ranging in weight from 6 to 26 mg is provided in Fioravanti and MacInnis (1976). Mettrick and Cannon (1970) have assessed DNA and RNA content for worms of several ages. They report that a 5-day-old worm contains

3.5. μg RNA and 9.2 μg DNA/mg dry tissue under the conditions of their infections.

When seeking large quantities of DNA for various purposes from hymenolepidids or other worms available in quantity (e.g. 100 gms wet weight) we have used a combination of several published procedures, as described in Kilejian and MacInnis (1976). Using this procedure, starting with 20 rats, each infected with 30 *H. diminuta*, 2-3 weeks old, one can recover 200-250 grams wet weight of worms from which 70-80 mg of DNA can be obtained.

III. ISOLATION AND CHARACTERIZATION OF NUCLEAR DNA

A. *Isolation*

In certain instances it may be desirable to ascertain nuclear DNA content of worms separately from mtDNA or vice versa. Two options are available to accomplish this. Worms can be homogenized and cell fractions obtained by zonal centrifugation as described by Carter, Wells, and MacInnis (1972). Mitochondria are exceedingly sparse in adult *H. diminuta* and best obtained by zonal centrifugation from which the nuclear or other fractions might also be saved (Carter *et al.* 1972). Alternatively, total DNA can be isolated as described by Kilejian and MacInnis (1976) and the mtDNA separated from nuclear DNA by centrifugation in cesium chloride gradients. Recently we have obtained excellent recoveries of DNA from small batches of tissues of *Schistosoma mansoni* (Tanaka *et al.* 1980) by collecting the DNA on a hydroxyapatite column as reported by Meinke *et al.* (1974). This procedure should be considered for use in future studies on *H. diminuta* DNA, especially if some shearing of the DNA is acceptable to the experiment.

B. *Buoyant Density*

When total DNA from adult *H. diminuta* is isolated and then centrifuged to equilibrium in neutral CsCl using an analytical centrifuge, the resulting banding pattern is asymmetrical, being skewed towards higher buoyant density. This suggests the presence of buoyant density "satellite DNAs." These satellites can be purified by repeated preparatory centrifugations and collection of appropriate fractions (Carter 1972). The main nuclear band of *H. diminuta* DNA, in the absence of satellites, has a buoyant density of 1.696 gm/cc. The buoyant density of individual satellites is 1.706, 1.708 and 1.717, referred to hereafter as S_1, S_2, and S_3, respectively. These satellites are present in very small recoverable amounts. Typically, 200 gm wet weight of worms yields 70-80 mg of total DNA from which 70-80 µg of satellite DNA can be recovered. When S_2 is centrifuged to equilibrium in alkaline CsCl one main band and two minor components are revealed. Under similar conditions, S_3 bands as one broad peak. S_1 has not yet been examined by this technique. GC content calculated from buoyant density data are shown in Table I. All three satellites were sensitive to treatment with deoxyribonuclease and insensitive to ribonuclease or α-amylase, confirming that this material was indeed DNA.

C. *Thermal Profiles and GC Content*

Thermal denaturation (T_m) results are shown in Table I, as well as GC content calculated from T_m for the main band and each satellite. Renaturation of satellites (sonicated to an $S_{20,w}$ of 5S) at 70.5° C was rapid, more than 75% renatures during the first 30 min. Second order rate plots of these data were linear, with rate constants of 3.6 and 5.7 for S_2 and S_3 respectively, suggesting highly repetitive DNA. S_1 appears to renature faster than main band DNA, but has not been recovered in sufficient quantity for accurate measurement. Electron micrographs of these satellites contained only linear molecules, hence none was considered to contain mtDNA which was shown to be on the light side of main band DNA (Carter *et al.* 1972).

TABLE I. Characterization of H. diminuta DNA

Source	Buoyant density in CsCl (gm/cc) (N)*	% G+C from buoyant density	T_m in SSC (deg. C)	% G+C from T_m
main band	1.696 ± 0.0002 (10)	36.7	83.6 ± 0.4 (5)	34.9
S_1	1.705 ± 0.0002 (3)	45.9	87.0 ± 0.5 (3)	43.1
S_2	1.708 ± 0.0003 (3)	48.9	89.1 ± 0.7 (3)	47.9
S_3	1.717 ± 0.0002 (3)	58.1	92.0 ± 0.5 (3)	55.3

*(N) = number of observations

D. Kinetic Complexity and Genome Size

Searcy and MacInnis (1970) have measured the kinetic complexity of a number of parasitic organisms, including *H. diminuta* and related free living species. These experiments were designed to estimate genome size and to determine if parasites have evolved by loss of genetic information. Using the rate of renaturation of DNA to estimate genome size they calculated the genome of *H. diminuta* to be 9.2×10^{10} daltons. Interestingly, this is larger than their estimate for the genome size of a free living planarian *Dugesia tigrina* at 4.6×10^{10} daltons. About 16% of the *H. diminuta* DNA was estimated as repetitive in these experiments (Searcy and MacInnis 1970).

E. Satellite DNA in Related Species of Hymenolepidids

Kilejian and MacInnis (1976) have analysed DNA from *H. citelli* and *H. microstoma*. Main band DNA from both of these two species has a buoyant density of 1.698 gm/cc. The light fraction of *H. microstoma* DNA contained a satellite at 1.692 gm/cc (perhaps similar to the mitochondrial satellite from *H. diminuta* described later). The presence or absence of this light satellite in *H. citelli* has not yet been determined. In the heavy fractions from *H. citelli* and *microstoma*, in addition to the three satellites similar in density to those reported from *H. diminuta*, there is a satellite at 1.722 gm/cc. The latter has not yet been observed in *H. diminuta*.

Satellite DNA from *Ascaris* has been studied in some detail by Kilejian and MacInnis (1976). Simmons et al. (1972) reported the presence of satellite DNA in monogeneids of the genus *Gyrocotyle*. The latter paper also illustrates the use of DNA hybridization to study similarities and differences amongst species within a genus using a technique developed by Searcy (1968) to prepare radioactive DNA by tritiating it *in vitro*. This technique is useful if live worms (or other organisms) are not available for incubation in radioactive substrates. The more recent technique of "nick" labelling could also be used. The many species of hymenolepidids are amenable to comparative studies such as those just described.

IV. ISOLATION AND CHARACTERIZATION OF MITOCHONDRIAL DNA

Carter *et al.* (1972) isolated mtDNA from adult *H. diminuta*. Since none of the previously described satellites (S_1, S_2, or S_3) contained circular DNA, it was suspected that mtDNA was either present in very small quantities as a light satellite, or had the same buoyant density as main band DNA. To circumvent this problem, mitochondria were first isolated by zonal centrifugation, then mtDNA purified from this fraction. Reorienting gradient zonal centrifugation enables isolation of large quantities of mitochondria from tissues in which they are sparse, provided that ample quantities of tissue are at hand. The mtDNA from mitochondria obtained by this procedure and subsequently purified by centrifugation in CsCl has a buoyant density of 1.690 gm/cc. Estimates made from buoyant density measurements and thermal transition values indicated a GC content of 32% for mtDNA. The T_m of mtDNA was 82.2°C. Electron micrographs of mtDNA released from osmotically shocked mitochondria revealed circular molecules with an average contour length of 4.76 µm. It is of interest that this cestode's mitochondria contain typical, circular DNA molecules even though the adult worm is anaerobic, with no functional Krebs cycle.

V. POSSIBLE FUNCTIONS OF THE HEAVY SATELLITES

A possible role for one of the satellite DNAs in *H. diminuta* could be coding for rRNA. Amplification of genes coding for rRNA is known to occur in many organisms. When purified rRNA from *H. diminuta* (made radioactive by methylation) was hybridized to satellites and other control DNA (Table II) most hybridization occurred with S_2. The S_1 satellite DNA used in these experiments was not completely pure, showing the presence of some S_2. This probably accounts for some hybridization to this fraction.

Amplification of rDNA may occur during development of *H. diminuta* as it does in many other organisms. We have analysed by analytical ultracentrifugation the DNA from six-day-old worms (no oocytes), mature four-week-old worms, the anterior portion of mature worms (no oocytes), the posterior two-thirds of mature (oocytes), and young developing eggs. Our results suggest increased amounts of the heavy satellites in older tissue containing eggs or oocytes, as well as in developing eggs.

TABLE II. Hybridization of rRNA with Various DNA Fractions from H. diminuta. Specific Activity of rRNA was 2,800 cpm/µg.

DNA source	µg DNA filter	counts/min µg DNA
salmon DNA	17 (4)*	1
H-DNA	7 (4)	14
S_1 DNA	6 (3)	46
S_2 DNA	6 (2)	80
S_3 DNA	5 (2)	3
total DNA	9 (8)	7

*(N) = number of filters

VI. RIBOSOMES, tRNA AND PROTEIN SYNTHESIS

Parker and MacInnis (1977) have described procedures for isolation, purification, and reconstruction of an *in vitro* cell-free system for protein synthesis from *H. diminuta*. These authors described an active S-30 system, purification of functional ribosomes and tRNA, but little progress has been made on the synthetases for acylation of tRNA. *H. diminuta* ribosomes were also shown to accept tRNAs from heterologous species such as rat, yeast or *E. coli*. Synthetic messenger was shown to function in the system, and the *in vitro* system could be inhibited by Puromycin. Those interested in this system should consult the paper cited for details.

VII. SYNTHESIS OF RNA AND DNA

No messenger RNA has yet been purified from *H. diminuta*. Bolla and Roberts (1971) reported that initial development of *H. diminuta* uses preformed mRNA for the first 6 days, following which new mRNA synthesis begins. No studies have yet been performed on polymerases. DNA and RNA can be labelled by incubation of worms in radioactive thymidine or uridine, respectively, as the worms actively accumulate these molecules. Farland and MacInnis (1978) have demonstrated the presence of thymidine kinase activity in *H. diminuta*. This key enzyme is a possible regulatory site for synthesis of DNA and warrants investigation in conjunction with experiments such as those reported by Insler and Roberts (1980 a,b) in which the worms apparently produce a substance which inhibits DNA synthesis.

VIII. NUCLEASES

To our knowledge, no studies have been performed on endogenous nucleases. However, Pappas *et al.* (1973) have demonstrated ribonuclease activity apparently associated with the external surface of the worm.

IX. CONCLUSIONS

Thus far the main thrust of investigations on nucleic acids of hymenolepidids has been concerned with the beginnings of physical characterizations of the macromolecules. These studies have revealed similarities with DNA and RNA of other eukaryotic organisms, but much remains to be accomplished. Very little is yet known about cestode ribosomes and associated proteins, structural and/or enzymatic. Surely there are initiation and termination factors to be identified. Nothing is known about the physical characterizations of tRNA, nor can we yet approach sequencing these molecules. Key enzymes such as DNA and RNA polymerase remain mysteries to be explored, as do other enzymes and factors concerned with protein synthesis. Does repair synthesis of DNA occur in these worms? Hymenolepidids are excellent models for the study of development, each worm being a complete system, yet we know essentially nothing about its mRNA.

All of the enzymes or molecules discussed represent potential sites for chemotherapeutic attack. We should not be obsessed by directing all of our research efforts towards neuromuscular or energy metabolism as the only potential systems for anthelmintic action. Techniques are now available so that portions of the hymenolepidid genome could be sequenced, such as mtDNA, or a satellite. We should not be satisfied until we fully understand metabolic regulation and we know the DNA sequence of the entire organism. Even then, new frontiers will exist, limited only by our insight, curiosity, and imagination.

ACKNOWLEDGMENTS

Reports cited from the laboratory of AJM were supported by grants from the NIH, NSF, and the UCLA Biomedical Support Grant. Current studies by AJM and associates are supported by grant NIH AI 13,228. Dr. Carter's current studies are supported by NIH AI 12996.

REFERENCES

1. Bolla, R. I., and Roberts, L. S., Developmental physiology of cestodes - XII. Role of preformed informational RNA in development of *Hymenolepis diminuta*. Comp. Biochem. Physiol. 40B, 885-892 (1971).
2. Carter, C. E., Purification and characterization of *Hymenolepis diminuta* DNA. Doctoral dissertation. The University of California, Los Angeles, (1972).

3. Carter, C. E., Wells, J. R., and MacInnis, A. J., DNA from anaerobic adult *Ascaris lumbricoides* and *Hymenolepis diminuta* mitochondria isolated by zonal centrifugation. *Biochim. Biophys. Acta 262*, 135-144 (1972).
4. Farland, William F., and MacInnis, A. J., Thymidine kinase activity: present in *Hymenolepis diminuta* (Cestoda) and *Moniliformis dubius* (Acanthocephala), but apparently lacking in *Ascaris lumbricoides* (Nematoda). *J. Parasitol. 64*, 564-565 (1978).
5. Fioravanti, C. F., and MacInnis, A. J., Metabolic indices for evaluating the *in vitro* maintenance of *Hymenolepis diminuta* in the presence and absence of various additives. *J. Parasitol. 62*, 741-748 (1976).
6. Insler, G. D. and Roberts, L. S., Developmental physiology of cestodes. XV. A system for testing parasite growth factors *in vitro*. *J. Exp. Zool. 211*: in press. (1980a).
7. Insler, G. D., and Roberts, L. S., Developmental physiology of cestodes. XV. Effects of certain excretory products on the incorporation of H^3-thymidine into DNA of *Hymenolepis diminuta*. *J. Exp. Zool. 211*: in press (1980b).
8. Kilejian, A., and MacInnis, A. J., Density distribution of DNA from parasitic helminths with special reference to *Ascaris lumbricoides*. *Rice Univ. Studies 62*, 161-174 (1976).
9. MacInnis, A. J., and Voge, M., "Experiments and Techniques in Parasitology". W. H. Freeman Co., San Francisco, (1970).
10. Meinke, W., Goldstein, D. A., and Hall, M. R., Rapid isolation of mouse DNA from cells in tissue culture. *Analyt. Biochem. 58*, 82-88 (1974).
11. Mettrick, D. F., and Cannon, C. E., Changes in the chemical composition of *Hymenolepis diminuta* (Cestoda, Cyclophyllidea) during prepatent development within the rat intestine. *Parasitology 61*, 229-243 (1970).
12. Parker, R. D., and MacInnis, A. J., *Hymenolepis diminuta*: isolation, purification, and reconstruction *in vitro* of a cell-free system for protein synthesis. *Exp. Parasitol. 41*, 2-16 (1977).
13. Pappas, P. W., Uglem, G. L., and Read, C. P., Ribonuclease activity associated with intact *Hymenolepis diminuta*. *J. Parasitol. 59*, 824-828

(1973).
14. Searcy, D. G., Techniques for DNA hybridization *in vitro* using nonradioactive DNA and DNA made radioactive by neutron activation, alkylation with radioactive alkylating agents, and by exchange with ^3H_2O. *Biochim. Biophys. Acta 166*, 360-370 (1968).
15. Searcy, D. G., and MacInnis, A. J., Measurements by DNA renaturation of the genetic basis of parasitic reduction. *Evolution 24*, 796-806 (1970).
16. Simmons, J. E., Buteau, G. H., MacInnis, A. J., and Kilejian, A., Characterization and hybridization of DNAs of gyrocotylidean parasites of chimaeroid fishes. *Int. J. Parasitol. 2*, 273-278 (1972).
17. Tanaka, R. D., Lukacs, J., Kim, R., and Kebo, D., MacInnis, A. J., Isolation of DNA from *Schistosoma mansoni* and studies on mode of action of anti-schistosomal drugs. Submitted to *J. Molec. Biochem. Parasitol.* (1980).

ENERGY METABOLISM OF
ADULT *HYMENOLEPIS DIMINUTA*

Carmen F. Fioravanti

Department of Biological Sciences
Bowling Green State University
Bowling Green, Ohio

Howard J. Saz

Department of Biology
University of Notre Dame
Notre Dame, Indiana

I. INTRODUCTION

The ability of adult parasitic helminths to consume available O_2 is well established (von Brand 1973). However, in all of the parasites examined, regardless of developmental stage, none of them appears to be capable of catabolizing glucose completely to CO_2 and H_2O. Organic end-products accumulate from glucose catabolism under either aerobic or anerobic atmospheres (Saz and Bueding 1966; Saz 1969, 1970; Fairbairn 1970; von Brand 1973). Thus, the parasitic helminths characteristically differ from numerous other multicellular systems in that the worms exhibit limitations with respect to their terminal respiratory mechanisms. Such limitations, in turn, present the question as to the physiological involvement of O_2 in the energetics of many of these worms.

It is now evident, that while some of the adult helminths display a required aerobic component to their energy generating metabolisms (e.g. *Litomosoides carinii* and *Nippostrongylus brasiliensis* (Bueding 1949a; Wang and Saz 1974; Roberts and Fairbairn 1965; D. Saz et al. 1971)) many others are considered microaerophillic or anaerobic in this regard [e.g. *Schistosoma mansoni*, *Dipetalonema viteae*, *Brugia pahangi* and *Ascaris lumbricoides* (Bueding 1950; Wang and Saz 1974; Saz 1971, 1972)]. It should be realized that some helminths which require small amounts of O_2 for normal development may utilize this gas for reactions not involving energy metabolism. For example, *S. mansoni* requires small quantities of O_2 for normal egg development, presumably for tanning of the egg employing phenol oxidase (Schiller et al. 1975). Similarly, *A. lumbricoides* requires O_2 for the formation of hydroxyproline which, in turn, is required for cuticle synthesis (Fujimoto and Prockop 1969). As will be detailed below, adult *Hymenolepis diminuta* logically falls within that category of helminths whose energy generating mechanisms appear to be essentially anaerobic. In this respect, *H. diminuta* metabolically resembles adult *A. lumbricoides* which serves as a model for the understanding of anaerobic energy generation resulting from the accumulation of succinate (or products derived from succinate). Based on this similarity, a general summary of ascarid energy metabolism is presented initially, followed by a more detailed discussion of *H. diminuta* metabolism.

II. ANAEROBIC ENERGY METABOLISM OF ADULT *ASCARIS LUMBRICOIDES*: A MODEL SYSTEM

Physiologically, the process of energy generation in adult *A. lumbricoides* appears to be primarily, if not completely, anaerobic (Bueding 1949b; Fairbairn 1957, 1970; Saz and Bueding 1966; Saz 1969). The dissimilation of carbohydrate by this nematode results in the accumulation of succinate and a variety of volatile fatty acid end-products (Saz and Bueding 1966). The nematode possesses very low levels of cytochrome oxidase activity, which is of questionable significance, and the tricarboxylic acid cycle system has been reported to be inoperative as an energy generating sequence (Kmetec and Bueding 1961; Ward and Fairbairn 1970).

The pathway for glucose catabolism, resulting in anaerobic energy generation and succinate formation by A. *lumbricoides* muscle, has been elucidated by Saz and Lescure (1969) and is summarized in Fig. 1. In ascarid muscle, glucose is catabolized, *via* the Embden-Meyerhof sequence, to phosphoenolpyruvate (PEP). Since the activity of pyruvate kinase is minimal in ascarid muscle (Bueding and Saz 1968), the further utilization of PEP requires CO_2 fixation. The fixation of CO_2 is catalyzed by means of phosphoenolpyruvate carboxykinase which acts physiologically in the direction of oxalacetate (OAA) formation. OAA, in turn, is reduced to malate, by soluble malate dehydrogenase, with the concomitant regeneration of cytoplasmic NAD^+.

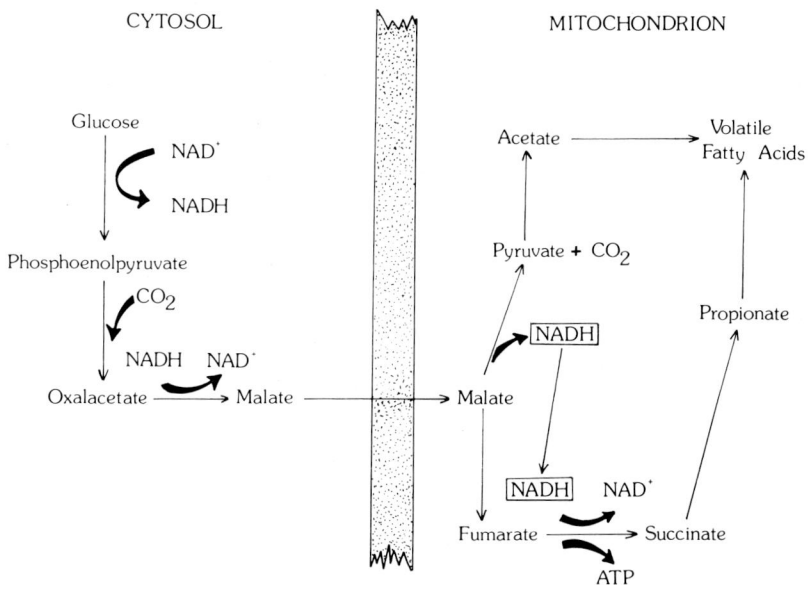

Fig. 1. *Carbohydrate dissimilation in muscle of adult Ascaris lumbricoides.*

Cytoplasmic malate then serves as the substrate for the ascarid mitochondrion. Upon entering the organelle, malate undergoes an anaerobic dismutation (oxidation/reduction) reaction. Half of the malate is oxidized to pyruvate and CO_2, by the action of the mitochondrial, NAD^+ linked "malic" enzyme (malate dehydrogenase, decarboxylating), resulting in the generation of intramitochondrial NADH. The remaining malate is dehydrated to form fumarate as catalyzed by mitochondrial fumarase. The fumarate thus formed, rather than oxygen, then serves as the terminal acceptor for the ascarid electron transport mechanism. The dismutation reaction is completed with the reduction of fumarate to succinate *via* the NADH coupled fumarate reductase system. Of paramount significance is the fact that the reduction of fumarate to succinate results in an anaerobic, electron transport associated, Site I phosphorylation (Kmetec and Bueding 1961; Seidman and Entner 1961; Saz 1971). In support of this malate dependent, electron transport mediated, anaerobic generation of ATP, Saz (1971) determined that the P/malate ratio for *A. lumbricoides* mitochondria is approximately 0.5, as would be calculated from the proposed pathway. In addition, balance studies of products arising from the mitochondrial utilization of malate also agree with the proposed dismutation sequence.

The products of the malate dismutation (i.e. succinate and pyruvate) are utilized by *A. lumbricoides* muscle as precursors for the anaerobic formation of the volatile fatty acid end-products (Saz and Vidrine 1959; Saz and Weil 1960, 1962; Saz and Lescure 1969). Although similarities do exist, definite differences are clearly demonstrable between β-oxidation and the *Ascaris* mechanism for the synthesis of the C_4 through C_6 acids (Ward and Fairbairn 1970; Suarez de Mata *et al.* 1977).

The mitochondria of *A. lumbricoides* muscle are morphologically similar to the corresponding organelles of free-living multicellular systems (Kmetec *et al.* 1962; Rew and Saz 1974). Like these other systems, they contain circular DNA molecules with a contour length approximating 5.0 microns (Carter *et al.* 1972). Nevertheless, it is obvious that both biochemically and physiologically the ascarid organelles appear remarkably different from those of most multicellular free-living systems. This is particularly true with respect to electron transport and the intramitochondrial metabolism of malate.

Kmetec and Bueding (1961) isolated a particulate fraction from *A. lumbricoides* muscle which contains both NADH oxidase and succinoxidase activities. Employing this preparation, it has been demonstrated that: (1) the ascarid electron transport system includes several flavoprotein carriers; (2) the NADH dehydrogenase and succinate dehydrogenase portions of this system are independent of each other, but (3) the aerobic utilization of NADH and succinate occur *via* the same terminal oxidase; (4) the aerobic activity of this terminal oxidase is stimulated by Mn^{++} ion and is dependent upon oxygen tension forming H_2O_2 (indicating flavin involvement); (5) succinate oxidation is insensitive to cyanide (as well as azide and antimycin A (Bueding 1963)), and (6) a cytochrome b like pigment may participate in this system but cytochrome c and cytochrome oxidase involvement appear to be minimal. Most important and in accord with the succinate forming metabolism of *A. lumbricoides* (Fig. 1), the particulate preparation of Kmetec and Bueding (1961) was able to catalyze not only a rapid, but also a complete anaerobic, NADH dependent reduction of fumarate to succinate. Presumably, the reduction of fumarate to succinate involves the ascarid succinate dehydrogenase acting physiologically as a fumarate reductase. With respect to this consideration, it is significant that malonate markedly inhibits the ascarid, malate dependent, anaerobic, mitochondrial phosphorylation (Saz 1971). In contrast to the mammalian electron transport system, the ascarid system couples with rhodoquinone rather than ubiquinone (Sato *et al.* 1972).

The data of Kmetec and Bueding (1961) indicate that in *A. lumbricoides* the aerobic utilization of either NADH or succinate results in the accumulation of toxic H_2O_2. As pointed out by Saz and Bueding (1966), the non-physiological nature of H_2O_2 formation is emphasized by the fact that *A. lumbricoides* is deficient in catalase activity. These data, in conjunction with information concerning the malate dismutation, ATP formation and succinate accumulation (Saz 1971) point to the primarily anaerobic character of energy generation in this system. Accordingly, aerobic phosphorylation by the ascarid system, if at all present, would appear to be of minor physiological impact.

Several reports have implied that O_2 requiring oxidative phosphorylation occurs in *Ascaris*. The validity and physiological significance of these reports remain to be evaluated. Chin and Bueding (1954) reported a very low rate of oxidative phosphorylation in a particulate preparation from *A. lumbricoides* muscle. When this preparation was supplied with exogenous NAD^+ and pyruvate, a slow oxidative phosphorylation was observable yet such activity could be accounted for *via* a Site I coupled generation of ATP (Chin and Bueding 1954; Bueding 1963). In addition, succinate utilization by the ascarid system was found either to inhibit oxidative phosphorylation or to support only minimally such activity (Chin and Bueding 1954; Rathbone 1955; Seidman and Entner 1961; Saz 1971). On the other hand, Fisherová and Kubištová (1968) suggested that malate utilization by the ascarid system, under aerobic conditions resulted in an increased phosphorylation over that observed anaerobically. However, Saz (1971) reported subsequently that the degree of net phosphorylation, resulting from the aerobic utilization of malate, by *A. lumbricoides* mitochondria, did not differ significantly from the net phosphorylation observed when malate was utilized anaerobically. More recently, Cheah (1974) reported that succinate, α-glycerophosphate and ascorbate plus N, N, N', N',-tetramethyl-p-phenylenediamine (TMPD) fostered presumed oxidative phosphorylation in *A. lumbricoides* mitochondria. Unfortunately, in these studies the assays for phosphorylation were indirect and based upon O_2 uptake measurements in the presence of ADP. A direct measurement of phosphorylation was not determined. In this context, it is of interest to note the importance of measuring net phosphorylation directly when considering substrate induced O_2 uptake by mitochondrial preparations and relating this uptake to phosphorylation. Sottibandhu and Palmer (1975), employing Jerusalem artichoke mitochondria, reported an NAD^+ linked, electron transport associated, substrate induced O_2 uptake which is enhanced by the addition of adenyl nucleotides (ADP, AMP) even though the mitochondrial phosphorylation system is uncoupled with p-trifluromethyoxyphenylhydrozone (FCCP). Thus, it is often incorrect to assume the equivalence of all tissues with mammalian tissues.

In recent years, the presence of cytochromes of the b type as well as cytochromes c, c_1 and low concentrations of a and a_3 have been reported for the ascarid system employing spectral methods (Kikuchi et al. 1959; Kikuchi and Ban 1961; Chance and Parsons 1963; Lee and Chance 1968; Cheah and Chance 1970; Cheah 1975; Cheah 1976 a,b). Both cytochrome c_{550} and a unique cytochrome b_{560} have been purified from *A. lumbricoides* muscle (Hill et al. 1971; Cheah 1973, 1976b). However, in light of the low activity of the terminal oxidase (Oya et al. 1965; Chance and Parsons 1963; Cheah and Chance 1970; Kmetec and Bueding 1961), and in light of what is known of the metabolism of *A. lumbricoides*, the physiological significance of the cytochrome oxidase in the energetics of the nematode remains obscure. Which of the cytochromes, if any, serves a required physiological function in substrate utilization and phosphorylation in adult *A. lumbricoides* remains to be determined. Whether any of the cytochromes represent a "carry over" from an earlier larval stage might be considered. It is of interest that a number of strictly anaerobic bacteria contain a primitive electron transport system with cytochrome b that is linked to the reduction of fumarate. These include *Clostridium thermoaceticum, Cl. formicoaceticum* (Gottwald et al. 1975), *Vibrio succinogenes* (Jacobs and Wolin 1963), *Desulfovibrio gigas* (Hatchikian and LeGall 1972), *Bacteroides* sp. (Rizza et al. 1968; Macy et al. 1978) and others. Therefore, the presence of cytochromes do not necessarily preclude that the organisms are indeed anaerobic.

Cheah (1975, 1976a) presented spectral evidence concerning the presence of a cytochrome of the b type, cytochrome o, in the ascarid system. It was suggested that cytochrome o serves as a terminal oxidase which would be cyanide and antimycin A insensitive and is linked to H_2O_2 formation (Cheah 1976b). In other systems, (i.e. adult *Moniezia expansa* and *Fasciola hepatica*) it has been suggested that cytochrome o may play a role in the reduction of fumarate to succinate (Cheah 1972; Cheah and Pritchard 1975). Again, as in the case of other cytochromes, the physiological role of cytochrome o in *A. lumbricoides* electron transport is not clear and requires further investigation. Certainly the presence of this cytochrome does not constitute evidence for its physiological involvement in ascarid energy metabolism.

The ascarid "malic" enzyme couples optimally with NAD^+ (Saz and Hubbard 1957; Fodge *et al.* 1972; Landsperger and Harris 1976) and allows for the production of intramitochondrial reducing equivalents in the form of NADH which, in turn, is required for succinate formation (Saz and Lescure 1969). Rew and Saz (1974) examined the localization of a number of enzymes in *Ascaris* mitochondria. Unlike other systems, both the "malic" enzyme and fumarase reside predominantly in the intermembrane space of the ascarid organelle. This would indicate that physiologically malate need only traverse the outer mitochondrial membrane (OM) whereupon malate would undergo oxidative decarboxylation forming NADH in the intermembrane space compartment. As in other mitochondrial systems, both the Mg^{++} dependent ATPase and succinate deyhdrogenase of *A. lumbricoides* are components of the inner mitochondrial membrane (IM) which, on negative staining, exhibits typical ATPase particles (elementary bodies; "lollipops"). Moreover, the rates of NADH or succinate dependent reduction of ferricyanide, by intact and disrupted ascarid organelles, support the supposition that NADH dehydrogenase and succinate dehydrogenase are oriented towards the matrix side of the IM as is assumed to be the case in mammalian tissues (Köhler 1976). It would appear probable, therefore, that fumarate reduction and the associated phosphorylation occur on the matrix side of the ascarid IM. If this is the case, then a mechanism would be required for the transfer of reducing equivalents from the intermembrane space NADH to the matrix NAD^+ to form matrix NADH so that mitochondrial electron transport and phosphorylation would take place. This would be necessary since the IM is impermeable to NADH. Fioravanti and Saz (1976) demonstrated an NADH → NAD^+ pyridine nucleotide transhydrogenase activity in

Ascaris mitochondria which may fulfill this required translocating function. This transhydrogenase activity catalyzes the following reaction:

$$NADH + NAD^+ \rightarrow NAD^+ + NADH$$

Although at first glance this may suggest a "nonsense" reaction, if a membrane is placed between the two sides of the reaction, it becomes a possible means of translocating hydride ions. The NADH → NAD$^+$ transhydrogenation reaction was essentially the only transhydrogenase activity detected and was found to be associated primarily with the ascarid IM fraction. Thus, an enzymatic mechanism, which might provide for the transmembrane movement of reducing equivalents and subsequent fumarate reduction, is apparent in the ascarid system (Fig. 2). In accord with this supposition, intact *A. lumbricoides* mitochondria are capable of utilizing reducing equivalents from exogenously supplied ^{14}C-NADH for anaerobic phosphorylation without significant accumulation of label within the mitochondria (Köhler and Saz 1976). These data support the concept that the translocation of reducing equivalents is occurring without the permeation of the pyridine nucleotide into the matrix compartment (Fig. 2). What appears to be the NADH → NAD$^+$ transhydrogenase has been solubilized from the *A. lumbricoides* IM, purified to apparent homogeneity and has been shown to possess both the transhydrogenase and dihydrolipoyl dehydrogenase activities (R. Komuniecki and Saz, in preparation). Therefore, whether or not this transhydrogenase activity functions physiologically remains to be determined.

With the above summary of anaerobic energy generation in the *A. lumbricoides* system as a model, consideration now can be given to the energy metabolism of adult *H. diminuta*.

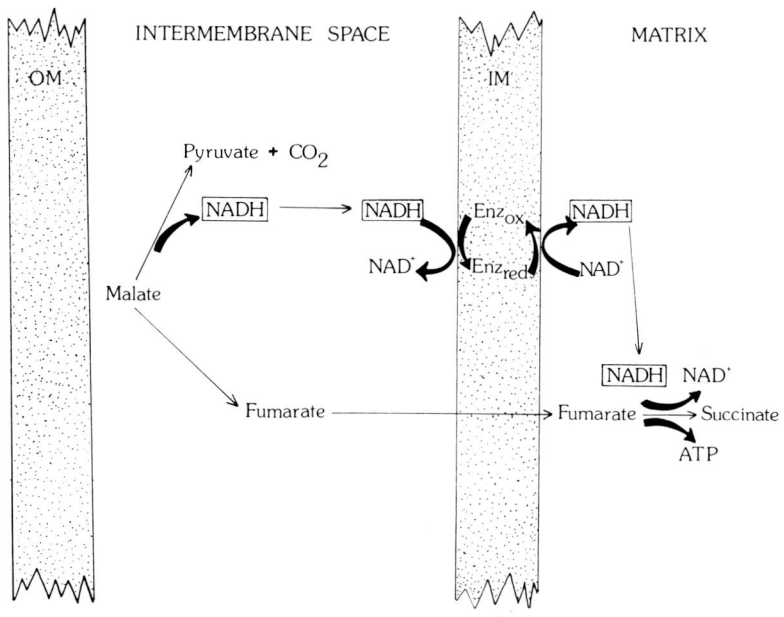

Fig. 2. Proposed mechanisms for the intramitochondrial utilization of malate by adult Ascaris lumbricoides.

III. CARBOHYDRATE CATABOLISM BY ADULT HYMENOLEPIS DIMINUTA

A. General Comments

In terms of the utilization of carbohydrate and the concomitant generation of energy, adult *Hymenolepis diminuta* to a large degree simulates adult *A. lumbricoides*. The fermentative nature of *H. diminuta* is reflected in the finding that although this cestode will consume O_2 when available (O_2 uptake being related to O_2 tension), the rate of assimilation of O_2 at best can account only for less than 5% of the total amount of glucose utilized if it is at all involved in glycolysis (Read 1956; Read and Simmons 1963). That glycolysis occurs in *H. diminuta* was determined by Read (1951, 1952a) who demonstrated the glycolytic formation of lactate by cell-free preparations of the cestode. The presence in this worm of a number of the required enzymes of the glycolytic sequence also was reported. Initially, lactate was considered to be the major product of glucose fermentation by *H. diminuta* (Read 1956). However, further investigation revealed that glucose dissimilation by adult *H. diminuta* results primarily in the accumulation of three fermentation acids, *viz*, succinate, acetate and lactate (Fairbairn *et al.* 1961). Of these fermentation acids, succinate is the major product (Fairbairn *et al.* 1961; Watts and Fairbairn 1974). Thus, *H. diminuta* is one of many representatives of the parasitic worms forming succinate from the dissimilation of carbohydrate (Table I). Alanine may also accumulate from glucose dissimilation and is thought to arise *via* the transamination of pyruvate (Prescott and Campbell 1965; Hochachka and Mustafa 1972).

TABLE I. *Representative Helminths Forming Succinate or Products Which May Arise from Succinate (after Saz 1972).*

NEMATODES	CESTODES
Ascaris lumbricoides	*Hymenolepis diminuta*
Heterakis gallinae	*Moniezia expansa*
Trichinella spiralis (larvae)	*Echinococcus granulosus*
Trichuris vulpis	*Echinococcus granulosus* (cysts)
Syphacia muris	*Taenia taeniaeformis*
Dictyocaulus viviparus	*Taenia taeniaeformis* (larvae)
	Spirometra mansonoides
	Spirometra mansonoides (spargana)

TREMATODES	ACANTHOCEPHALA
Fasciola hepatica	*Moniliformis dubius*
Paragonimus westermani	

The anaerobic nature of carbohydrate utilization by *H. diminuta* is indicated further by the findings of Scheibel and Saz (1966). Lactate and acetate accumulation by *H. diminuta* are unaffected by the presence or absence of O_2. Succinate accumulation is inhibited by an aerobic atmosphere, apparently reflecting an inhibition of succinate formation by O_2. In addition, by employing suitably labelled ^{14}C-glucose and assessing CO_2 evolution, it was found that a quantitatively significant energy generating tricarboxylic acid cycle (as well as a pentose shunt) was absent in *H. diminuta*. Accordingly, Ward and Fairbairn (1970), utilizing enzymatic assays, confirmed that adult *H. diminuta* does not have a functional tricarboxylic acid cycle. Although the presence of cytochrome oxidase in *H. diminuta* was suggested by measuring O_2 utilization employing ascorbate and cytochrome c (Read 1952b) or ascorbate plus TMPD (Rahaman and Meisner 1973), no cytochrome oxidase activity was detected in isolated mitochondria when the more specific assay procedure of measuring the direct oxidation of reduced cytochrome c was employed (Scheibel *et al.* 1968).

Possibly the strongest data which indicate the anaerobic nature of *H. diminuta* are derived from *in vitro* cultivation experiments. Applying earlier biochemical information, Schiller (1965) established that *H. diminuta* can be cultivated from excysted cysticercoid to ovigerous adult in an atmosphere of 97% N_2 - 3% CO_2. Oncospheres produced by these cultivated cestodes were infective as determined by the development to infective cysticercoids in the beetle host (Schiller 1965). Roberts and Mong (1969), employing Schiller's modifications and carefully excluding air as much as possible, found that 6-day-old *H. diminuta* can be cultivated *in vitro* under an atmosphere of 95% N_2 - 5% CO_2 for 12 days with the production of viable eggs yielding infective cysticercoids. The addition of O_2 to this gas phase (1, 5, and 20%) was without stimulatory effect on the *in vitro* development of the cestode. Further work on the cultivation of *H. diminuta* (Turton 1974) and the maintenance of this cestode (Fioravanti and MacInnis 1976) in an atmosphere of 95% N_2 - 5% CO_2 continues to attest to the anaerobic nature of *H. diminuta*. Interestingly, Voge *et al.* (1976) found with *H. diminuta*, that the axenic, *in vitro* development of hatched oncospheres to the cysticercoid stage was more rapid in an atmosphere of 100% nitrogen than in air. The presence of 95% N_2- 5 CO_2 or 95% N_2- 5% O_2 gave results like those found with 100% nitrogen which, in turn, would suggest that CO_2 does not affect the development of *H. diminuta* cysticercoids, but higher levels of O_2 inhibit the rate of development.

It is of further interest to note that Watts and Fairbairn (1974) determined that 6-day-old *H. diminuta* accumulate fermentation acids in the ratio of 0.9 succinate: 0.6 acetate: 1.0 lactate while 14-day-old worms produce fermentation acids in the ratio of 5.0 succinate: 2.5 acetate: 1.0 lactate. The data of Watts and Fairbairn (1974), in conjunction with the findings of Voge *et al.* (1976), present the possibility in *H. diminuta* of a developmental transition in the cestode towards a succinate forming metabolism.

Cestodes other than *H. diminuta* also appear to require anaerobiosis for successful cultivation. Seidel and Voge (1975) succeeded in growing cysticercoids of *Hymenolepis nana* axenically *in vitro*, from oncospheres hatched *in vitro* to fully developed organisms infective for mice. A gas phase of 95% N_2- 5% CO_2 was essential for normal development. Employing the same atmosphere, Schiller (Personal communication) obtained partial development of *Taenia crassiceps*.

B. *Carbon Dioxide Fixation*

The studies of Fairbairn *et al.* (1961) established clearly the essential involvement of carbohydrate catabolism in the overall metabolic economy of *H. diminuta*. In addition, it was demonstrated that *H. diminuta* requires CO_2 for both the effective fermentation of carbohydrate and anaerobic glycogen synthesis. These authors proposed that the key role of CO_2, in the processes of fermentation and glycogenesis in *H. diminuta*, may be related to the formation of fumarate which, in turn, could be reduced to succinate with the concomitant oxidation of glycolytically generated reduced pyridine nucleotide as was described previously for adult *A*.

lumbricoides. Kilejian (1963) also reported the need for CO_2 in the process of anaerobic glycogenesis in *H. diminuta*, and Read (1967) found that both glucose uptake and glycogen synthesis by *H. diminuta* are stimulated by 5% CO_2 in cominbation with either nitrogen or air.

With respect to CO_2 involvement in *H. diminuta* metabolism, Prescott and Campbell (1965) found that this adult cestode, when subjected to either aerobic or anaerobic conditions, incorporated $^{14}CO_2$ (from $NaH^{14}CO_3$) primarily into a fraction containing both succinate and fumarate thereby suggesting CO_2 fixation. Investigation of possible CO_2 fixing enzymatic activities in the cestode demonstrated a lack of both pyruvate carboxylase and propionyl-CoA carboxylase. However, a soluble phosphoenolpyruvate carboxykinase (PEP carboxykinase) was found which operated both in the direction of oxalacetate formation (CO_2 fixation) and phosphoenolpyruvate (PEP) formation (decarboxylation). It was suggested that the activity of PEP carboxykinase, in the direction of CO_2 fixation, could be coupled to malate accumulation *via* a malate dehydrogenase. Thus, the possibility of CO_2 fixation giving rise to malate, and the subsequent utilization of malate by the *H. diminuta* system in the formation of fumarate and succinate, was presented. In addition, the presence of a "malic" enzyme in *H. diminuta* was described by Prescott and Campbell (1965) (see Section IV, A).

Scheibel and Saz (1966) investigated the pathway for the anaerobic accumulation of succinate from the catabolism of glucose in *H. diminuta* by incubating the cestode with various species of ^{14}C-glucose and determining the labelling patterns in the carboxyl and methylene carbons of accumulated succinate. In essence, Scheibel and Saz (1966) demonstrated that isotope from glucose carbons 1, 2, and 6 gives rise to the methylene carbons of succinate while glucose carbons 3 and 4 serve as precursors for the carboxyl carbons of succinate. These labelling patterns are consistent with the consideration that glucose is catabolized to a C_3 acid (PEP) *via* the Embden-Meyerhof pathway followed by fixation of CO_2 into the C_3 acid producing succinate. In accord with these data, it was demonstrated further that the anaerobic incorporation of $^{14}CO_2$ from $NaH^{14}CO_3$ resulted primarily in labelling of the carboxyl carbons of succinate as would be predicted by CO_2 fixation into a C_3 acid.

The physiological occurrence of CO_2 fixation at the level of PEP in *H. diminuta* is supported by the data of Bueding and Saz (1968). Both pyruvate kinase (PK) and PEP carboxykinase (PEPCK) were found to be soluble components in adult *H. diminuta* and in a comparison of the activities of PK and PEPCK (measured in the direction of CO_2 fixation) the ratio of PK/PEPCK gave a mean value of 0.18 (Bueding and Saz 1968). Such a ratio reflects the predominance of CO_2 fixation and succinate formation by the adult cestode. Furthermore, Bueding and Saz (1968) demonstrated a very active, soluble malate dehydrogenase in *H. diminuta* which could account for the rapid reduction of oxalacetate, arising from CO_2 fixation, to form malate with the required concomitant regeneration of cytoplasmic NAD^+. Malate then could act in succinate formation (Bueding and Saz 1968).

Recently, Carter and Fairbairn (1975) reported on the cold lability of *H. diminuta* PK. In a comparison of the activities of both PK and PEPCK, derived from the soluble fraction of 21-day-old *H. diminuta* (excluding hexacanths), the ratio of PK/PEPCK, based on the data of Carter and Fairbairn (1975), was 0.28 which was similar to the earlier findings and which would still favor CO_2 fixation. In addition, the PK of *H. diminuta* exists as five isozymic variants, one of which appears in the adult stage of the worm. Although all isozymes were inhibited by ATP and Ca^{++} (none were affected by alanine), four of the isozymes were allosterically activated by fructose-1,6-diphosphate (FDP). The "adult" isozyme of *H. diminuta* was found to be insensitive to FDP thereby suggesting a developmental sequence in PK formation which may reflect also a change in the metabolism towards increased succinate accumulation in adult worms. The findings of Moon *et al.* (1977) were, in most respects, in agreement with the earlier findings with the additional suggestion of the possibility that HCO_3^- and/or CO_2 concentration may exert a control on the PK-PEPCK branchpoint of *H. diminuta* by inhibiting PK catalysis while activating PEPCK activity which, in turn, would foster succinate accumulation.

The presence of soluble lactate dehydrogenase (LDH), in adult *H. diminuta* was reported (Bueding and Saz 1968). Subsequently, Burke *et al.* (1972) found only one form of LDH in crude extracts of adult *H. diminuta* employing electrophoresis and isoelectric focusing. The purified preparation contained only one form of the enzyme which formed an abortive ternary complex with pyruvate and NAD^+, suggesting regulatory control of LDH based on cytoplasmic NAD^+ concentration. These findings would indicate metabolic control which tends to promote succinate formation. Walkey and Fairbairn (1973), utilizing isoelectric focusing, also found primarily one form of LDH in prepatent *H. diminuta* and in the anteriors of adult worms, while a different form of the enzyme predominated in eggs and cysticercoids. Logan *et al.* (1977) reported, on the basis of starch-gel electrophoresis, that two isozymes of LDH exist in adult *H. diminuta*, one of which is associated with ovarian tissue. These findings suggest that in different developmental stages of the cestode a different form(s) of LDH predominates which may be related to a metabolic transition allowing for succinate formation.

The experimental evidence indicates that, as with adult *A. lumbricoides*, adult *H. diminuta* engages in CO_2 fixation at the level of PEP, thereby permitting cytoplasmic malate formation, the regeneration of glycolytically required NAD^+ and subsequent succinate accumulation. Evidence is becoming increasingly apparent which suggests developmental and regulatory controls in the *H. diminuta* system which act to potentiate the succinate forming pathway in the adult worm.

IV. THE ANAEROBIC MITOCHONDRIAL METABOLISM OF ADULT *HYMENOLEPIS DIMINUTA*

Although differing somewhat from corresponding organelles of free-living multicellular systems (in terms of mitochondrial size and longitudinal arrangement of cristae), the mitochondria of adult H. *diminuta* bear many morphological similarities to those of aerobic systems. They exhibit "lollipop" (ATPase) elementary particles associated with the inner mitochondrial membrane (Harlow and Byram 1971) and they contain circular DNA of a contour length approximating 5.0 microns (Carter *et al*. 1972). However, unlike other systems, but similar to adult A. *lumbricoides*, the mitochondria of H. *diminuta* appear to be essentially anaerobic employing malate as the substrate for an electron transport associated, net generation of ATP.

A. *The Intramitochondrial Utilization of Malate*

In accord with the proposed physiological need for CO_2 fixation by adult H. *diminuta*, Scheibel *et al*. (1968) demonstrated that under anaerobic conditions, CO_2 is required by the cestode for the maintenance of ATP levels and for the incorporation of ^{32}P into ATP. Moreover, Scheibel *et al*. (1968) reported that isolated mitochondria, derived from adult H. *diminuta*, engage in a ^{32}P-ATP exchange reaction which is electron transport associated. These data, in conjunction with the information discussed above indicated malate could serve as the anaerobic substrate for a mitochondrial, electron transport associated, phosphorylation leading to the accumulation of succinate as postulated for the A. *lumbricoides* system (Saz 1971).

Further evidence in support of a malate dependent anaerobic phosphorylation in adult H. *diminuta* mitochondria was reported by Saz *et al*. (1972). These investigators found that isolated mitochondria from the cestode catalyze a malate dependent, electron transport associated, net incorporation of ^{32}P into ATP. This mitochondrial phosphorylation was found to be enhanced by fluoride (an inhibitor of ATPase) while malonate significantly inhibited the net ^{32}P esterification, thereby supporting the concept that a fumarate reductase system was involved. In addition, known inhibitors of electron transport associated phosphorylation (i.e. 2,4-dinitrophenol, carbonyl cyanide m-chlorophenylhydrozone, rotenone and oligomycin) markedly inhibited malate dependent phosphorylation by the mitochondria.

It was found that the *H. diminuta* "malic" enzyme was associated with a particulate fraction and required Mn^{++} for activity (as does the ascarid enzyme). However, in contrast with the *Ascaris* enzyme, *H. diminuta* "malic" enzyme has an absolute specificity for the pyridine nucleotide, $NADP^+$ (Prescott and Campbell 1965; Saz *et al.* 1972). The mitochondrial localization of *H. diminuta* "malic" enzyme was demonstrated by Li *et al.* (1972) who purified the "malic" enzyme to homogeneity (molecular weight approximately 120,000). The presence of the mitochondrial "malic" enzyme in the *H. diminuta* system indicates, by analogy with *A. lumbricoides*, that a mechanism is present for the generation of intramitochondrial reducing equivalents for electron transport. The additional finding of fumarase activity in cell-free preparations and in mitochondria of *H. diminuta* (Read 1953; Fioravanti and Saz, unpublished) would allow for the operation of the reductive leg of the malate dismutation *via* fumarate reductase.

The mitochondrial, NAD^+ linked malate dehydrogenase (MDH) might be considered as a source of reducing equivalents in the *H. diminuta* system rather than the "malic" enzyme. This would not appear likely, however, since NADH accumulation by this enzyme requires the formation of oxalacetate which would have to be removed rapidly by decarboxylation to form pyruvate; a process which does not appear to take place rapidly. Furthermore, as noted by Saz *et al.* (1972), the equilibrium of *H. diminuta* MDH significantly favors the formation of malate. Thus, it would be expected that the *H. diminuta*, mitochondrial "malic" enzyme would allow for the formation of pyruvate, CO_2 and reducing equivalents in the form of NADPH. Watts and Fairbairn (1974) reported on the presence of a mitochondrial pyruvate dehydrogenase activity which would account for the accumulation of acetate from pyruvate by adult *H. diminuta*.

In a comparison of the ascarid system and adult *H. diminuta*, one striking difference is evident. In the cestode's mitochondrial system, reducing equivalents are generated in the form of NADPH rather than NADH. This, in turn, indicates that reducing equivalents, needed for the electron transport dependent generation of ATP by *H. diminuta*, are derived initially from NADPH.

Mitochondria, from adult *H. diminuta*, exhibit a NADH coupled fumarate reductase activity (Scheibel et al. 1968). Sonicated mitochondria catalyze the oxidation of NADH which presumably reflects the activity of an NADH oxidase (Table II; after Fioravanti and Saz 1975). Apparently, NADPH is oxidized by this preparation at a rate which is lower than that found when NADH is the substrate. However, in the presence of exogenously added

TABLE II. Mitochondrial Fumarate Reductase Activity of Adult Hymenolepis diminuta.

Substrate	Addition	Activity
		n moles/min/mg[a]
NADH	None	12.7
NADPH	None	3.4
NADH	Fumarate	68.2
NADPH	Fumarate	3.2

[a]*Activity is expressed per mg mitochondrial protein.*

Sonically disrupted mitochondria were prepared essentially as reported by Fioravanti and Saz (1976) in the presence of EDTA. 0.19 mg mitochondrial protein were employed. Assays were performed in air by following the disappearance of reduced pyridine nucleotide at 340 nm. Assays consisted of enzyme, 5.0 mg bovine serum albumin and the following in μmoles: Tris-HCl (pH 7.5), 100; NADH or NADPH, 0.24; and where indicated disodium fumarate, 0.6. Total assay volumes were 1.0 ml.

fumarate, the rate of NADH oxidation is increased approximately 5.0 fold over that observed in the absence of the dicarboxylic acid acceptor. On the other hand, the rate of oxidation of NADPH remains essentially unaltered by the presence of fumarate (Table II). These data suggest that the *H. diminuta* fumarate reductase exhibits a specificity for NADH as the pyridine nucleotide hydride donor. It is clear also, that the utilization of NADH is significantly stimulated by fumarate despite the presence of oxygen. Fumarate, therefore, appears to be the preferred terminal acceptor in this system. Rotenone, the Site I inhibitor, significantly inhibits (84%) the *H. diminuta* system, thereby making evident the coupling of electron transport to the reduction of fumarate by adult *H. diminuta* (Table III).

The apparent specificity of the *H. diminuta* fumarate reductase for NADH presents a dilemma with respect to the utilization of intramitochondrial reducing equivalents. If reducing equivalents are generated by the "malic" enzyme reaction in the form of NADPH, a mechanism for the transfer of hydride ions from NADPH to NAD^+ producing NADH would be required by *H. diminuta* in order that electron transport associated activities could proceed and terminate with the reduction of fumarate to succinate. This dilemma was resolved by Saz *et al.* (1972) who demonstrated a mitochondrial pyridine nucleotide transhydrogenase in adult *H. diminuta* mitochondria which apparently could fulfill the required hydride ion transfer from NADPH to NAD^+. The mitochondria were found to catalyze the following reaction:

$$NADPH + AcPyAD^+ \rightarrow NADP^+ + AcPyADH.$$

The use of the acetylpyridine derivative of NAD^+ ($AcPyAD^+$) in this reaction allowed for the specific evaluation of pyridine nucleotide reduction, since AcPyADH absorbs light at a wavelength of 375 nm whereas NADH and NADPH both absorb at 340 nm.

B. *Mitochondrial Transhydrogenases*

Employing the appropriate acetylpyridine

nucleotide derivative, the *H. diminuta* mitochondrial NADPH → NAD$^+$ transhydrogenation reaction appeared to be reversible, i.e., the enzymatic reduction of the acetylpyridine derivative of NADP$^+$ was demonstrable employing NADH as the reductant (Fioravanti and Saz 1976). Both the mitochondrial NADPH → NAD$^+$ and NADH → NADP$^+$ reactions were found to be membrane bound. The NADH forming reaction (NADPH → NAD$^+$)

TABLE III. *Effects of Rotenone on the Mitochondrial Fumarate Reductase Activity of Adult Hymenolepis diminuta.*

Substrate	Addition(s)	Activity
		n moles/min/mg^a
NADH	None	12.7
NADH	Fumarate	68.2
NADH	Fumarate plus Rotenone (5×10^{-7}M)	10.9

^{a}*Activity expressed per mg mitochondrial protein. Protein concentration and assay conditions were as described in Table II.*

proceeds at approximately 5.0 times the rate of the NADPH forming reaction (NADH → NADP$^+$) under the assay conditions employed. This more rapid transhydrogenation to form NADH tends to support the physiological role of this reaction in the generation of NADH for fumarate reductase activity. Moreover, by enzymatic coupling to other systems (i.e. exogenous NADP$^+$-specific isocitrate dehydrogenase for the NADPH → NAD$^+$ reaction and exogenous NADPH-specific glutathione reductase for the NADH → NADP$^+$ reaction) Fioravanti and Saz (1976) demonstrated that these reactions are catalyzed by the *H. diminuta* disrupted organelles when the physiological pyridine nucleotides act as hydride ion acceptors rather than the acetylpyridine derivatives. Therefore, the reduction of the appropriate acetylpyridine nucleotide derivative again reflects a physiological reaction.

The NADPH → NAD$^+$ reaction can be differentiated from the NADH → NADP$^+$ reaction of adult *H. diminuta* based on sensitivity to ethylenediaminetetraacetate (EDTA), phosphate and adenylates. The presence of EDTA significantly inhibits the NADH → NADP$^+$ ("reverse") reaction while the NADPH → NAD$^+$ ("forward") reaction is unaffected by this chelating agent. Extensive dialysis affects neither the NADPH → NAD$^+$ reaction nor the NADH → NADP$^+$ activity. The inhibition by EDTA suggests that the latter activity is disrupted by the presence of the chelator either by the interaction of this agent with a tightly bound divalent cation required for activity or perhaps by a direct effect on the enzyme. As with EDTA, the presence of phosphate in the assay system inhibited only the NADH → NADP$^+$ "reverse" reaction.

In other systems, the activity of the NADPH → NAD$^+$ transhydrogenase, acting in the direction of NADPH formation, is positively modified by 2'AMP (bacterial) or ATP (the bacterial or mammalian energy-linked transhydrogenation) (Kaplan 1970; Rydström 1977). In contrast, 2'AMP and ATP (as well as AMP and ADP) were found to inhibit significantly the corresponding *H. diminuta* "reverse" NADH → NADP+ reaction. The adenylates had no effect upon the forward, NADH forming, reaction (Fioravanti and Saz 1976). These data concerning adenylate inhibition, in conjunction with the information relating to EDTA and phosphate inhibition, suggest a complexity (perhaps conformational modification) to this *H. diminuta* transhydrogenase system. Since inhibition by the adenylates was not specific, the possible physiological role(s) of the observed inhibition awaits further investigation. However, it would appear that unlike bacterial systems, 2'AMP does not act to modify positively the cestode's transhydrogenase. Moreover, the data would suggest that unlike other transhydrogenase systems, the *H. diminuta* transhydrogenase is not energy-linked.

The physiological interaction of the mitochondrial NADPH → NAD$^+$ transhydrogenase, with the electron transport associated fumarate reductase of adult *H. diminuta* mitochondria, is suggested in Table IV (Fioravanti and Saz, unpublished data).

TABLE IV. Effects of NAD^+ on the Oxidation of NADPH by Adult Hymenolepis diminuta Mitochondria.

Substrate	Addition(s)	Activity
		n moles/min/mg^a
NADPH	None	3.4
NADPH	NAD^+	8.9
NADPH	Fumarate	3.2
NADPH	Fumarate plus NAD^+	13.3

^{a}*Activity expressed per mg mitochondrial protein.*

Protein concentration and assay conditions were as described in Table II. Where indicated, 0.60 μmoles NAD^+ were contained in the 1.0 ml assay system.

These data point out once again that disrupted *H. diminuta* mitochondria, under aerobic conditions, oxidize exogenously supplied NADPH and this oxidation is not altered markedly by the presence of fumarate. However, it is evident that NADPH oxidation, in the absence of fumarate, is increased approximately 3.0 fold when NAD^+ is added to the reaction vessel. Of significance is the finding that NADPH utilization, in the presence of fumarate, is increased markedly (approximately 4.0 fold) when the system is supplied with NAD^+. These data indicate that a transhydrogenase mediated hydride transfer to NAD^+ allows for the oxidation of NADPH *via* an NADH oxidase or, in the presence of fumarate *via* an NADH coupled fumarate reductase. In addition these data suggest the possibility that NADPH oxidation, in the absence of added NAD^+, may be due to a transhydrogenase mediated interaction, under limiting conditions, with endogenous NAD^+ contained in the *H. diminuta* preparation.

An additional transhydrogenase activity has been described in *H. diminuta* mitochondria which, as described for *A. lumbricoides* (Section II), catalyzes a hydride transfer from NADH to NAD^+ (Fioravanti and Saz 1976). This hydride transfer was readily demonstrable, employing disrupted *H. diminuta* mitochondria, when the acetylpyridine nucleotide derivative of NAD^+ was used as the hydride acceptor according to the following reaction scheme:

$$NADH + AcPyAD^+ \rightarrow NAD^+ \rightarrow AcPyADH.$$

Interestingly, this active NADH → NAD^+ transhydrogenase reaction has been shown to be independent of the NADPH → NAD^+ transhydrogenase in *H. diminuta*. In an attempt to elucidate possible physiological roles for this enzyme in *H. diminuta*, mitochondria were fractionated according to Sottocasa *et al.* (1967) and the intramitochondrial localization of both the NADPH → NAD^+ and NADH → NAD^+ transhydrogenating systems were examined (Fioravanti and Saz 1976). Within the confines of the experimental procedure, the data demonstrate that, as with the *A. lumbricoides* transhydrogenation reaction, both the *H. diminuta* NADPH → NAD^+ and NADH → NAD^+ transhydrogenases were recovered in the mitochondrial inner membrane (IM) fraction (Table V).

In light of the postulated role of the IM bound NADH → NAD^+ transhydrogenase activity of adult *A. lumbricoides* (Fig. 2), the possibility is made evident that either or both IM bound transhydrogenations, catalyzed by *H. diminuta* mitochondria, may function in the translocation of reducing equivalents. With respect to the *H. diminuta* NADPH → NAD^+ transhydrogenase, preliminary evidence suggests that this enzyme may not function in the same transmembrane fashion as put forth for the ascarid NADH → NAD^+ activity (Fioravanti and Saz 1976). Such a consideration is based on the localization of the *H. diminuta* "malic" enzyme. Within the limitations of the fractionation technique, the majority ($\sim61\%$)

TABLE V. Mitochondrial Localization of NADPH → NAD$^+$ and NADH→NAD$^+$ Transhydrogenations of Adult Hymenolepis diminuta (after Fioravanti and Saz 1976).

Fraction	Transhydrogenation					
	NADPH → NAD$^+$			NADH → NAD$^+$		
	Activity		Recovery	Activity		Recovery
	units[a]		%	units[a]		%
Disrupted Mitochondria	0.118		100	2.22		100
Outer Membrane	0		0	.01		0.5
Intermembrane Space	0		0	0		0
Matrix	0.008		7	0.07		3
Inner Membrane	0.063		53	1.61		73

[a]Units (micromoles/min) express total activity in each fraction derived from the total mitochondrial fraction. Methods were as described by Fioravanti and Saz (1976).

of the "malic" enzyme activity of *H. diminuta* mitochondria is confined to the IM plus matrix fraction (Fioravanti and Saz, unpublished observation). This being the case, it would appear that physiologically, reducing equivalents are generated within the matrix compartment of *H. diminuta* and the IM bound NADPH → NAD$^+$ transhydrogenase engages in hydride transfer on the matrix side of the IM. Of course, such a consideration does not preclude an associated transmembrane proton flux which could operate in conjunction with the NADPH → NAD$^+$ transhydrogenase reaction. These considerations require further investigations. In terms of the NADH → NAD$^+$ transhydrogenation reaction of *H. diminuta* mitochondria, the physiological need, if there is such a need, is not clear.

The evidence presented concerning the NADPH → NAD$^+$ transhydrogenase indicates that, unlike a number of other systems, a physiological function can be assigned readily to this enzyme. The NADPH → NAD$^+$ transhydrogenase would serve a vital function in linking mitochondrial malate utilization with the anaerobic, electron transport associated generation of ATP *via* the *H. diminuta* fumarate reductase.

C. *Electron Transport*

There appears to be little doubt that the major energy generating electron transport system in *H. diminuta* is capable of functioning anaerobically. This is particularly true in this cestode which is best cultivated through the adult stage anaerobically (Schiller 1965; Roberts and Mong 1969). In spite of this, *H. diminuta*, like all other parasitic helminths examined, will consume O_2 particularly at high pO_2. In recent years, considerable effort has been spent in trying to elucidate the nature and the physiological function of this capability. Whether or not this O_2 uptake is of importance to the parasite and whether or not it is involved in the energy generation system remains to be determined. Certainly the worm can develop without it.

The mitochondrial electron transport system of adult *H. diminuta* appears similar to that of *A. lumbricoides* and supports a malate dependent generation of energy without the need for oxygen

(Saz et al. 1972). As noted above (Section IV, A), the cestode's anaerobic generation of ATP is disrupted by classical electron transport uncouplers. Moreover, the anaerobic generation of ATP, by *H. diminuta* mitochondria, is insensitive to antimycin A but is markedly inhibited by rotenone thereby indicating a Site I phosphorylation (Saz et al. 1972).

Read (1952b) reported on a succinate dependent O_2 consumption, catalyzed by *H. diminuta* cell-free preparations, which was stimulated by methylene blue, did not exhibit cyanide (KCN) sensitivity and was inhibited by malonate. On the other hand, Saz et al. (1972) demonstrated that malonate significantly inhibits the anaerobic, malate dependent phosphorylation of *H. diminuta*, making evident the operation of an electron transport coupled fumarate reductase (exhibiting an apparent specificity for NADH (Table II), which would account for the accumulation of succinate. Presumably, the cestode's fumarate reductase represents a flavin containing succinate dehydrogenase acting physiologically in the direction of fumarate reduction, although the possibility that these activities are catalyzed by two independent proteins can not be ruled out.

The mitochondria of adult *H. diminuta* display both NADH oxidase (Rahaman and Meisner 1973; Fioravanti and Saz 1975; Tables II and III) and succinoxidase activities (Read 1952b; Rahaman and Meisner 1973). It has been reported that NADH stimulated O_2 uptake, by the cestode's mitochondria, is sensitive to rotenone while succinate oxidation is unaffected by this inhibitor (Rahaman and Meisner 1973). However, in a consideration of the terminal oxidation mechanism involved in the aerobic utilization of these, as well as other substrates, a degree of caution must be exercised in the evaluation of the data accumulated, particularly since a coupling of these oxidations to phosphorylation has not been established.

Utilizing *H. diminuta* cell-free preparations, Read (1952b) reported, that in the presence of succinate, a cytochrome c stimulated O_2 consumption was observable (which was approximately 1/3 of that noted with methylene blue) and this O_2 consumption was inhibited by KCN. Interestingly, the stimulatory response to cytochrome c was essentially lost upon aging of the sample at 5°C for 30-36 hr (Read 1952b). In addition, based on O_2 utilization, Read (1952b) reported an α-glycerophosphate dehydrogenase activity in these cell-free preparations in the presence of cytochrome c. Rahaman and Meisner (1973) using measurement of O_2 utilization by isolated *H. diminuta* mitochondria, reported that (a) succinate oxidation was inhibited by antimycin and KCN, (b) α-glycerophosphate oxidation was sensitive to antimycin and KCN, and (c) malate plus pyruvate oxidation was stimulated by the addition of ADP and this stimulation was enhanced by the presence of cytochrome c. One explanation of these findings would be to evoke the presence of a classical cytochrome oxidase system in *H. diminuta*. Evidence at this point, however, is indirect and circumstantial.

By use of cell-free preparations derived from adult *H. diminuta*, Read (1952b) reported on the presence of cytochrome oxidase, based on O_2 consumption, in the presence of added ascorbate and cytochrome c. Rahaman and Meisner (1973) also presented data on the presence of a KCN sensitive cytochrome oxidase activity in mitochondria of *H. diminuta*, by assessing O_2 utilization in the presence of added ascorbate plus TMPD. Furthermore, Robinson and Bogitsh (1976), on the basis of cytochemical evidence derived from the oxidation of 3,3'-diaminobenzidine (DAB), reported on the presence, in *H. diminuta* mitochondria, of a cytochrome oxidase-like activity which exhibited both azide and KCN sensitivity. With respect to cytochemical observations of cytochrome oxidase-like activity in *H. diminuta*, employing DAB, Lumsden *et al.* (1969) made clear the caution that must be exercised in the interpretation of results. However, despite these reports suggesting the activity of a significant cytochrome oxidase being operative in the *H. diminuta* system, serious doubt is placed on these findings when a more specific assay system is employed in the assessment of this activity. Scheibel *et al.* (1968) found, using a more specific assay procedure *viz.*, the direct oxidation of exogenously added reduced cytochrome c, that isolated adult *H. diminuta* mitochondria do not display a detectable cytochrome oxidase activity. Thus, whether or not there is a quantitatively significant cytochrome oxidase activity in the cestode and if so, its possible physiological impact on the metabolic economy of adult *H. diminuta*, remains questionable.

Rahaman and Meisner (1973) presented data on the uptake of oxygen, by isolated *H. diminuta* mitochondria, in the presence of α-glycerophosphate, malate and malate in combination with pyruvate, glutamate or α-ketoglutarate. The combinations of malate with glutamate and α-ketoglutarate resulted in less O_2 uptake than with malate alone while the combination of pyruvate and malate increased only slightly the O_2 uptake over that observed with malate (5.8 *vs*. 6.7 nmoles O_2/min/mg mitochondrial protein). These investigators also reported on the stimulation of O_2 consumption by ADP when α-glycerophosphate, succinate or malate plus pyruvate served as substrate for the cestode's mitochondria. Although ADP/O ratios were calculated by Rahaman and Meisner (1973), no determination of a net, aerobic or anaerobic ATP generation was made. Based on their calculations, Rahaman and Meisner (1973) reported a rather high apparent Km (267 µM) for the mitochondrial nucleotide translocase of *H. diminuta*. Furthermore, these investigators found that atractyloside (an inhibitor of mitochondrial ADP-ATP translocase) effectively inhibited the ADP stimulated oxidation of malate plus pyruvate. This, of course, would be expected based on the operation of a Site I phosphorylation. In the absence of evidence concerning net ATP generation, data concerning O_2 uptake becomes less meaningful. In general, the ADP/O ratios determined by Rahaman and Meisner (1973) were low. Moreover, as noted in Section II, consideration of ADP/O ratios must be interpreted cautiously particularly since Sottibandhu and Palmer (1975) were able to demonstrate an enhancement of NAD^+ linked, substrate induced, electron transport associated O_2 consumption by adenylates (ADP and AMP) in plant mitochondria that were uncoupled with FCCP.

Concerning the apparent presence of an α-glycerophosphate dehydrogenase, it is of interest to note the findings of Weinbach (1972) who reported the presence of non-heme iron in mitochondria of

H. diminuta. Employing electron paramagnetic resonance with α-glycerophosphate as substrate, the characteristic presence of reduced non-heme iron in the cestode's organelles was demonstrated. However, in all of these evaluations of α-glycerophosphate oxidations, no evidence was presented concerning any associated generation of ATP which would be required to establish physiological import in energy metabolism.

Data have been presented concerning peroxidase activity, in *H. diminuta* mitochondria by use of cytochemical techniques employing DAB (Threadgold *et al*. 1968; Lumsden *et al*. 1969; Robinson and Bogitsh 1976). Again, Lumsden *et al*. (1969) pointed to the need for careful interpretation using DAB as substrate and the interaction of non-specific systems which would exhibit apparent peroxidatic activity. Thus, a possible physiological role for peroxidase activity in the metabolism of *H. diminuta* must await further experimentation.

In many respects the electron transport system of adult *H. diminuta* appears to simulate the ascarid system. *H. diminuta* exhibits a physiologically functional fumarate reductase system which couples to a Site I, anaerobic phosphorylation. Both NADH oxidase and succinoxidase activities are apparent, yet whether these systems contribute to additional ATP generation has not been determined. Although a degree of oxidative phosphorylation is conceivable, in conjunction with cytochrome involvement, this would not appear to contribute significantly to the energy generating sequence in light of the rate of succinate formation and the apparent requirement for anaerobic cultivation. The presence of non-heme iron is indicated in *H. diminuta*. Although α-glycerophosphate dehydrogenase is present in *H. diminuta* mitochondria, its role in possible ATP generation has not been determined. Certainly, the need for malate dependent, electron transport associated, anaerobic ATP generation and succinate formation becomes even more evident since some uncouplers, including some anticestodal agents (e.g., chorosalicylamide and desaspidin) act to disrupt this phosphorylation in adult *H. diminuta* mitochondria (Saz *et al*. 1972).

V. METABOLIC SCHEME FOR CARBOHYDRATE DISSIMILATION AND ENERGY GENERATION BY ADULT *HYMENOLEPIS DIMINUTA*

Based on the data presented, the metabolic pathway for carbohydrate dependent energy generation by adult *H. diminuta* is given in Fig. 3. As with *A. lumbricoides* muscle, glucose is dissimilated to the level of phosphoenolpyruvate (PEP) by means of the Embden-Meyerhof metabolic pathway. At this point, adult *H. diminuta* deviates somewhat from the ascarid model in that PEP is metabolized *via* pyruvate kinase and lactate dehydrogenase thereby accounting for lactate accumulation with concomitant oxidation of glycolytically generated NADH. The possibility of alanine formation by transamination of pyruvate was discussed in Section III, A. At the PEP branchpoint, the favored reaction in the mature adult is apparently CO_2 fixation. This is accomplished by a soluble PEP carboxykinase thereby forming oxalacetate (OAA). The presence of an active malate dehydrogenase allows for the rapid conversion of OAA to malate with the oxidation of reduced pyridine nucleotide which acts to replenish glycolytically required NAD^+. Malate, thus formed, serves as the substrate for the anaerobically functioning mitochondria. Intramitochondrially, malate undergoes a dismutation reaction. One half of the malate is oxidized *via* the mitochondrial, $NADP^+$ linked "malic" enzyme, producing pyruvate, CO_2 and, unlike *A. lumbricoides*, reducing equivalents in the form of NADPH. H_2O is removed from the remaining malate as catalyzed by fumarase to form fumarate. Evidence suggests that the "malic" enzyme of *H. diminuta* may be primarily a matrix component. Since the fumarate reductase of *H. diminuta* appears specific for NADH, a transhydrogenation from NADPH to NAD^+ forming NADH, required for the completion of the dismutation, would be vital. This would appear to be accomplished by means of a mitochondrial pyridine nucleotide transhydrogenase. With the formation of intramitochondrial NADH, the malate dismutation is completed by the reduction of fumarate to succinate *via* fumarate reductase. Most importantly, this reduction of the terminal acceptor, fumarate, to succinate is the basis of an anaerobic, electron transport associated, net generation of ATP

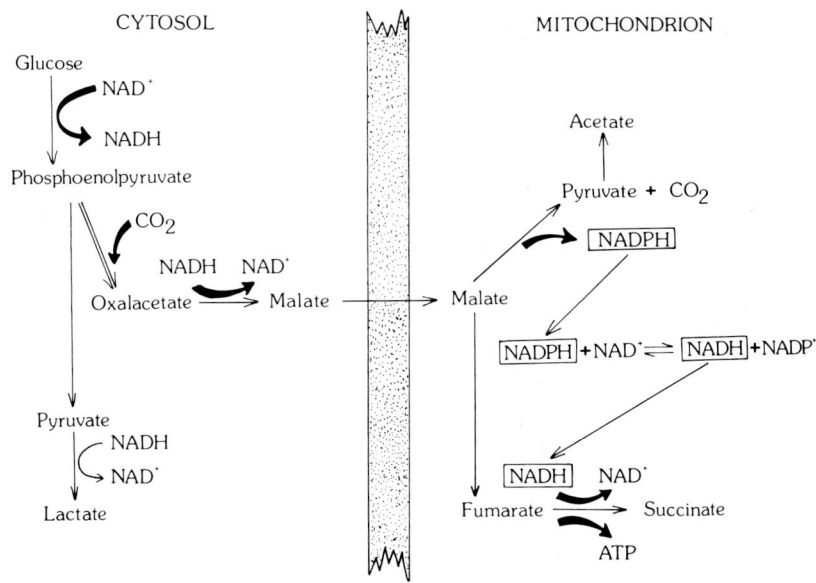

Fig. 3. Carbohydrate dissimilation by adult Hymenolepis diminuta.

via a Site I phosphorylation. Thus, like *A. lumbricoides*, fumarate rather than oxygen acts as the physiological acceptor for the cestode's electron transport system thereby accounting for the accumulation of succinate as a major end-product. The further metabolism of pyruvate, presumably catalyzed by pyruvate dehydrogenase, would account for the formation of acetate by the *H. diminuta* system. However, very little is known of the mechanism responsible for this anaerobic oxidative decarboxylation. Although the possibility of ATP generation being associated with acetate formation is apparent, no information is available on this point.

VI. CONCLUSIONS

The essentially anaerobic nature of energy production by adult *H. diminuta* is made evident both on the basis of biochemical evidence and *in vitro* cultivation studies. The adult cestode's energy producing pathways revolve about the formation of succinate and lactate as major fermentation products. Both of these are anaerobic end-products since a functional tricarboxylic acid cycle is apparently absent. Quantitatively, even acetate formation remains constant in air or anaerobically. The anaerobic nature of *H. diminuta* does not preclude entirely the presence of enzymatic activities which are normally associated, in other systems, with aerobic metabolism. However, in light of what is known of the metabolism of adult *H. diminuta*, the physiological importance of these "alternate" activities would appear minimal in terms of energy generation. Indeed, evidence suggests both developmental and regulatory controls in *H. diminuta* which would tend to potentiate the succinate forming pathways.

The energy generating metabolic pathways in *H. diminuta* differ significantly from corresponding sequences found in the host. Such differences might be made use of chemotherapeutically by allowing for the evaluation of potentially vulnerable sites and the development of agents which would act specifically against these sites in the parasite (e.g., anthelmintic disruption of electron transport). In addition, it is becoming increasingly clear that, aside from numerous parasitic helminths, free-living multicellular systems also engage in similar metabolic events (i.e., succinate accumulation) as found in *H. diminuta* and *A. lumbricoides*. This appears to be the case for many free-living invertebrates which are subject to periods of low oxygen tensions in their life cycles (e.g., molluscs) (Hammen 1966; Stokes and Awapara 1968; Lutz and Rhoads 1977) as well as for diving vertebrates (Hochachka *et al.* 1975). Interestingly, Wilson and Cascarano (1970) reported that mammalian heart, when made anoxic, would appear to catalyze a generation of ATP which is fumarate dependent. It is possible then, that further studies with the *H. diminuta* system will aid not only in the development and evolution of chemotherapeutic agents, but also in establishing the necessary biochemical information for evaluating anaerobic energy generation in free-living, multicellular systems.

ACKNOWLEDGMENTS

The research cited in this article was made possible by grants AI-02587, AI-05379 and AI-09483 from the National Institutes of Health and by grant No. 41148 from the National Science Foundation. C. F. gratefully acknowledges funds, made available for the writing of this article, from the Department of Biological Sciences, Bowling Green State University.

REFERENCES

1. Bueding, E., Studies on the metabolism of the filarial worm, *Litomosoides carinii*. J. Exptl. Med. *89*, 107-130 (1949a).
2. Bueding, E., Metabolism of parasitic helmenths. Physiological Reviews *29*, 195-218 (1949b).
3. Bueding, E., Carbohydrate metabolism of *Schistosoma mansoni*. J. Gen. Physiol. *33*, 475-495 (1950).
4. Bueding, E., Electron transport and fermentations in *Ascaris lumbricoides*. In: "Control Mechanisms in Respiration and Fermentation" (B. Wright, ed.) Chapter 8, pp. 167-176. The Ronald Press, New York, (1963).
5. Bueding, E., and Saz, H. J., Pyruvate kinase and phosphoenolpyruvate carboxykinase activities of *Ascaris* muscle, *Hymenolepis diminuta* and *Schistosoma mansoni*. Comp. Biochem. Physiol. *24*, 511-518 (1968).
6. Burke, W. F., Gracy, R. W., and Harris, B. G., Studies on enzymes from parasitic helminths. III. Purification and properties of lactate dehydrogenase from the tapeworm, *Hymenolepis diminuta*. Comp. Biochem. Physiol. *43B*, 345-359 (1972).
7. Carter, C. E., and Fairbairn, D., Multienzymic nature of pyruvate kinase during development of *Hymenolepis diminuta* (Cestoda). J. Exptl. Zool. *194*, 439-448 (1975).
8. Carter, C. E., Wells, J. R., and MacInnis, A. J., DNA from anaerobic adult *Ascaris lumbricoides* and *Hymenolepis diminuta* mitochondria isolated by zonal centrifugation. Biochim. Biophys. Acta *262*, 135-144 (1972).
9. Chance, B., and Parsons, D. F., Cytochrome

function in relation to inner membrane structure of mitochondria. *Science 142*, 1176-1179 (1963).
10. Cheah, K. S., Cytochromes in *Ascaris* and *Monieza*. In: "Comparative Biochemistry of Parasites" (H. van den Bossche, ed.), pp. 417-432. Academic Press, New York, (1972).
11. Cheah, K. S., Purification and properties of *Ascaris* cytochrome b$_{560}$. *J. Biol. Chem. 248*, 4101-4105 (1973).
12. Cheah, K. S., Oxidative phosphorylation in *Ascaris* muscle mitochondria. *Comp. Biochem. Physiol. 47B*, 237-242 (1974).
13. Cheah, K. S., Properties of *Ascaris* muscle mitochondria. 1. Cytochromes. *Biochim. Biophys. Acta 387*, 107-114 (1975).
14. Cheah, K. S., Electron transport system of *Ascaris* muscle mitochondria. In: "Biochemistry of Parasites and Host-Parasite Relationships" (H. van den Bossche, ed.), pp. 133-143. Elsevier/North-Holland Biomedical Press, Amsterdam, (1976a).
15. Cheah, K. S., *Ascaris lumbricoides* cytochrome b-560. In: "Biochemistry of Parasites and Host-Parasite Relationships" (H. van den Bossche, ed. ed.), pp. 145-150. Elsevier/North-Holland Biomedical Press, Amsterdam, (1976b).
16. Cheah, K. S., and Chance, B., The oxidase systems of *Ascaris* muscle mitochondria. *Biochim. Biophys. Acta 223*, 55-60 (1970).
17. Cheah, K. S., and Prichard, R. K., The electron transport systems of *Fasciola hepatica* mitochondria. *Int. J. Parasitol. 5*, 183-186 (1975).
18. Chin, C., and Bueding, E., Occurrence of oxidative phosphorylation in the muscle of *Ascaris lumbricoides*. *Biochim. Biophys. Acta 13*, 331-337 (1954).
19. Fairbairn, D., The biochemistry of *Ascaris*. *Exptl. Parasitol. 6*, 491-554 (1957).
20. Fairbairn, D., Biochemical adaptation and loss of genetic capacity in helminth parasites. *Biological Reviews 45*, 29-72 (1970).
21. Fairbairn, D., Wertheim, G., Harpur, R. P., and Schiller, E. L., Biochemistry of normal and irradiated strains of *Hymenolepis diminuta*. *Exptl. Parasitol. 11*, 248-263 (1961).
22. Fioravanti, C. F., and MacInnis, A. J., Metabolic indices for evaluating the *in vitro* maintenance of *Hymenolepis diminuta* in the presence and absence of various additives. *J.*

Parasitol. 62, 741-748 (1976).
23. Fioravanti, C. F., and Saz, H. J., Localization and possible physiological role of NADPH:NAD$^+$ transhydrogenase in *Hymenolepis diminuta*. Program and Abstracts. 50th Ann. Meet. Amer. Soc. Parasitol., 96 (1975).
24. Fioravanti, C. F., and Saz, H. J., Pyridine nucleotide transhydrogenases of parasitic helminths. *Arch. Biochem. Biophys. 175*, 21-30 (1976).
25. Fischerova, H., and Kubistova, J., *Ascaris lumbricoides*: Extraglycolytic phosphorylation in intact muscle. *Exptl. Parasitol. 23*, 244-253 (1968).
26. Fodge, D. W., Gracy, R. W., and Harris, B. G., Studies on enzymes from parasitic helminths. I. Purification and physical properties of malic enzyme from the muscle tissue of *Ascaris suum*. *Biochim. Biophys. Acta 268*, 271-284 (1972).
27. Fujimoto, D., and Prockop, D. J., Protocollagen proline hydroxylase from *Ascaris lumbricoides*. *J. Biol. Chem. 244*, 205-210 (1969).
28. Gottwald, M., Andrusen, J. R., LeGall, J., and Ljungdahl, L. G., Presence of cytochrome and menaquinone in *Clostridium formicoaceticum* and *Clostridium thermoaceticum*. *J. Bacteriol. 122*, 325-328 (1975).
29. Hammen, C. S., Carbon dioxide fixation in marine invertebrates. V. Rate and pathway in the oyster. *Comp. Biochem. Physiol. 17*, 289-296 (1966).
30. Harlow, D. R., and Byram, J. E., Isolation and morphology of the mitochondrion of the cestode, *Hymenolepis diminuta*. *J. Parasitol. 57*, 559-565 (1971).
31. Hatchikian, E. C., and LeGall, J., Evidence for the presence of a b-type cytochrome in the sulfate-reducing bacterium *Desulfovibrio gigas* and its role in the reduction of fumarate by molecular hydrogen. *Biochim. Biophys. Acta 267*, 479-484 (1972).
32. Hill, G. C., Perkowski, C. A., and Mathewson, N. W., Purification and properties of cytochrome c_{550} from *Ascaris lumbricoides* var. *suum*. *Biochim. Biophys. Acta 236*, 242-245 (1971).
33. Hochachka, P. W., and Mustafa, T., Invertebrate facultative anaerobiosis. *Science 178*, 1056-1060 (1972).
34. Hochachka, P. W., Owen, R. G., Allen, J. F.,

and Whitlow, G. C., Multiple end products of anaerobiosis in diving vertebrates. *Comp. Biochem. Physiol. 50B*, 17-22 (1975).
35. Jacobs, N. J., and Wolin, M. J., Electron-transport system of *Vibrio succinogenes*. I. Enzymes and cytochromes of the electron transport system. *Biochim. Biophys. Acta 69*, 18-28 (1963).
36. Kaplan, N. O., Pyridine nucleotide transhydrogenase. The Harvey Lectures (Series 66), pp. 105-133 (1970.
37. Kikuchi, G., and Ban, S., Cytochromes in the particulate preparation of the *Ascaris lumbricoides* muscle. *Biochim. Biophys. Acta 51*, 387-389 (1961).
38. Kikuchi, G., Ramirez, J., and Guzman Barron, E. S., Electron transport system in *Ascaris lumbricoides*. *Biochim. Biophys. Acta 36*, 335-342 (1959).
39. Kilejian, A., The effect of carbon dioxide on glycogenesis in *Moniliformis dubius* (Acanthocephala). *J. Parasitol. 49*, 862-863 (1963).
40. Kmetec, E., and Bueding, E., Succinic and reduced diphosphopyridine nucleotide oxidase systems of *Ascaris* muscle. *J. Biol. Chem. 236*, 584-591 (1961).
41. Kmetec, E., Miller, J. H., and Swartzwelder, J. C., Isolation and structure of mitochondria from *Ascaris lumbricoides* muscle. *Exptl. Parasitol. 12*, 184-191 (1962).
42. Kohler, P., Hydrogen transport in the muscle mitochondria of *Ascaris suum*. In:"Biochemistry of Parasites and Host-Parasite Relationships" (H. van den Bossche, ed.), pp. 125-132. Elsevier/North-Holland Biomedical Press, Amsterdam, (1976).
43. Kohler, P., and Saz, H. J., Demonstration and possible function of NADH:NAD^+ transhydrogenase from *Ascaris* muscle mitochondria. *J. Biol. Chem. 251*, 2217-2225 (1976).
44. Landsperger, W. J., and Harris, B. G., NAD^+-malic enzyme. Regulatory properties of the enzyme from *Ascaris suum*. *J. Biol. Chem. 251*, 3599-3602 (1976).
45. Lee, Il, and Chance, B., Activation of malate-linked reductions of NAD and flavoproteins in *Ascaris* muscle mitochondria by phosphate. *Biochem. Biophys. Res. Comm. 32*, 547-553 (1968).

46. Li, T., Gracy, R. W., and Harris, B. G., Studies on enzymes from parasitic helminths. II. Purification and properties of malic enzyme from the tapeworm, *Hymenolepis diminuta*. *Arch. Biochem. Biophys.* 150, 397-405 (1972).
47. Logan, J., Ubelaker, J. E., and Vrijenhoek, R. C., Isozymes of L (+) LDH in *Hymenolepis diminuta*. *Comp. Biochem. Physiol.* 57B, 51-53 (1977).
48. Lumsden, R. D., Oaks, J. A., and Mills, R. R., Mitochondrial oxidation of diaminobenzidine and its relationship to the cytochemical localization of tapeworm peroxidase. *J. Parasitol.* 55, 1119-1133 (1969).
49. Lutz, R. A., and Rhoads, D. C., Anaerobiosis and a theory of growth line formation. *Science* 198, 1222-1227 (1977).
50. Macy, J. M., Ljungdahl, L. G., and Gottschalk, G., Pathway of succinate and propionate formation in *Bacteroides fragilis*. *J. Bacteriol.* 134, 84-91 (1978).
51. Moon, T. W., Mustafa, T., Hulbert, W. C., Podesta, R. B., and Mettrick, D. F., The phosphoenol-pyruvate branchpoint in adult *Hymenolepis diminuta* (Cestoda): A study of pyruvate kinase and phosphoenol-pyruvate carboxykinase. *J. Exptl. Zool.* 200, 325-336 (1977).
52. Oya, H., Kikuchi, G., Bando, T., and Hayashi, H., Muscle tricarboxylic acid cycle in *Ascaris lumbricoides* var. *suis*. *Exptl. Parasitol.* 17, 229-240 (1965).
53. Prescott, L. M., and Campbell, J. W., Phosphoenolpyruvate carboxylase activity and glycogenesis in the flatworm, *Hymenolepis diminuta*. *Comp. Biochem. Physiol.* 14, 491-511 (1965).
54. Rahaman, R., and Meisner, H., Respiratory studies with mitochondria from the rat tapeworm *Hymenolepis diminuta*. *Int. J. Biochem.* 4, 153-162 (1973).
55. Rathbone, L., Oxidative metabolism in *Ascaris lumbricoides* from the pig. *Biochem. J.* 61, 574-579 (1955).
56. Read, C. P., Anaerobic glycolysis in fortified cell-free homogenates of tapeworm tissue. *Proc. Soc. Exptl. Med. Biol.* 76, 861-863 (1951).
57. Read, C. P., Studies on the enzymes and intermediate products of carbohydrate degradation in the cestode, *Hymenolepis diminuta*. *Exptl. Parasitol.* 1, 1-18 (1952a).

58. Read, C. P., Contributions to cestode enzymology. I. The cytochrome system and succinic dehydrogenase in *Hymenolepis diminuta*. *Exptl. Parasitol.* *1*, 353-362 (1952b).
59. Read, C. P., Contributions to cestode enzymology. II. Some anaerobic dehydrogenases in *Hymenolepis diminuta*. *Exptl. Parasitol.* *2*, 311-347 (1953).
60. Read, C. P., Carbohydrate metabolism of *Hymenolepis diminuta*. *Exptl. Parasitol.* *5*, 325-344 (1956).
61. Read, C. P., Carbohydrate metabolism in *Hymenolepis* (Cestoda). *J. Parasitol.* *53*, 1023-1029 (1967).
62. Read, C. P., and Simmons, J. E., Biochemistry and physiology of tapeworms. *Physiological Reviews* *46*, 263-305 (1963).
63. Rew, R. W., and Saz, H. J., Enzyme localization in the anaerobic mitochondria of *Ascaris lumbricoides*. *J. Cell. Biol.* *63*, 125-135 (1974).
64. Rizza, V., Sinclair, P. R., White, D. C., and Cuorant, P. R., Electron transport of the protoheme requiring anaerobe *Bacteroides melaninogenicus*. *J. Bacteriol.* *96*, 665-671 (1968).
65. Roberts, L. S., and Fairbairn, D., Metabolic studies on adult *Nippostrongylus brasiliensis* (Nematoda: Trichostrongyloidea). *J. Parasitol.* *51*, 129-138 (1965).
66. Roberts, L. S., and Mong, F. N., Developmental physiology of cestodes. IV. *In vitro* development of *Hymenolepis diminuta* in presence and absence of oxygen. *Exptl. Parasitol.* *26*, 166-174 (1969).
67. Robinson, J. M., and Bogitsh, B. J., Cytochemical localization of peroxidase activity in the mitochondria of *Hymenolepis diminuta*. *J. Parasitol.* *62*, 761-765 (1976).
68. Rydström, J., Energy-linked nicotinamide nucleotide transhydrogenases. *Biochim. Biophys. Acta* *463*, 155-184 (1977).
69. Sato, M., Yamada, K., and Ozawa, H., Rhodoquinone specificity in the reactivation of succinoxidase activity of acetone-extracted *Ascaris* mitochondria. *Biochem. Biophys. Res. Comm.* *46*, 578-582 (1972).
70. Saz, D. K., Bonner, T. P., Karlin, M., and Saz, H. J., Biochemical observations on adult *Nippostrongylus brasiliensis*. *J. Parasitol.* *57*, 1159-1162 (1971).

71. Saz, H. J., Carbohydrate and energy metabolism of nematodes and acanthocephala. *In* "Chemical Zoology" (M. Florkin, ed.), Vol. 3, pp. 329-360. Academic Press, New York, (1969).
72. Saz, H. J., Comparative energy metabolisms of some parasitic helminths. *J. Parasitol. 56*, 634-642 (1970).
73. Saz, H. J., Anaerobic phosphorylation in *Ascaris* mitochondria and the effects of anthelmintics. *Comp. Biochem. Physiol. 39B*, 627-637 (1971).
74. Saz, H. J., Comparative biochemistry of carbohydrates in nematodes and cestodes. *In* "Comparative Biochemistry of Parasites" (H. van den Bossche, ed.), pp. 33-47. Academic Press, New York, (1972).
75. Saz, H. J., Berta, J., and Kowalski, J., Transhydrogenase and anaerobic phosphorylation in *Hymenolepis diminuta* mitochondria. *Comp. Biochem. Physiol. 43B*, 725-732 (1972).
76. Saz, H. J., and Bueding, E., Relationships between anthelmintic effects and biochemical and physiological mechanisms. *Pharmacological Reviews 18*, 971-984 (1966).
77. Saz, H. J., and Hubbard, J. A., The oxidative decarboxylation of malate by *Ascaris lumbricoides*. *J. Biol. Chem. 225*, 921-933 (1957).
78. Saz, H. J., and Lescure, O. L., The functions of phosphoenolpyruvate carboxykinase and malic enzyme in the anaerobic formation of succinate by *Ascaris lumbricoides*. *Comp. Biochem. Physiol. 30*, 49-60 (1969).
79. Saz, H. J., and Vidrine, A., The mechanism of formation of succinate and propionate by *Ascaris lumbricoides* muscle. *J. Biol. Chem. 234*, 2001-2005 (1959).
80. Saz, H. J., and Weil, A., The mechanism of the formation of α-methylbutyrate from carbohydrate by *Ascaris lumbricoides* muscle. *J. Biol. Chem. 235*, 914-918 (1960).
81. Saz, H. J., and Weil, A., Pathway of formation of α-methylvalerate by *Ascaris lumbricoides*. *J. Biol. Chem. 237*, 2053-2056 (1962).
82. Scheibel, L. W., and Saz, H. J., The pathway for anaerobic carbohydrate dissimilation in *Hymenolepis diminuta*. *Comp. Biochem. Physiol. 18*, 151-162 (1966).

83. Scheibel, L. W., Saz, H. J., and Bueding, E., The anaerobic incorporation of ^{32}P into adenosine triphosphate by Hymenolepis diminuta. J. Biol. Chem. 243, 2229-2235 (1968).
84. Schiller, E. L., A simplified method for the in vitro cultivation of the rat tapeworm, Hymenolepis diminuta. J. Parasitol. 51, 516-518 (1965).
85. Schiller, E. L., Bueding, E., Turner, V. M., and Fisher, J., Aerobic and anaerobic carbohydrate metabolism and egg production of Schistosoma mansoni in vitro. J. Parasitol. 61, 385-389 (1975).
86. Seidel, J. S., and Voge, M., Axenic development of cysticercoids of Hymenolepis nana. J. Parasitol. 61, 861-864 (1975).
87. Seidman, I., and Entner, N., Oxidative enzymes and their role in phosphorylation in sarcosomes of adult Ascaris lumbricoides. J. Biol. Chem. 236, 915-919 (1961).
88. Sottibandhu, R., and Palmer, J. M., The activation of non-phosphorylating electron transport by adenine nucleotides in Jerusalem artichoke (Helianthus tuberosus) mitochondria. Biochem. J. 152, 637-645 (1975).
89. Sottocasa, G. L., Kuylenstierna, B., Ernster, L., and Bergstrand, A., An electron-transport system associated with the outer membrane of liver mitochondria. A biochemical and morphological study. J. Cell. Biol. 32, 415-438 (1967).
90. Stokes, T. M., and Awapara, J., Alanine and succinate as end-products of glucose degradation in the clam Rangia cuneata. Comp. Biochem. Physiol. 25, 883-892 (1968).
91. Suarez de Mata, Z., Saz, H. J., and Pasto, D. J., 2-methylacetoacetate reductase and possible propionyl coenzyme A condensing activity in branched chain volatile fatty acid synthesis by Ascaris lumbricoides. J. Biol. Chem. 252, 4215-4224 (1977).
92. Threadgold, L. T., Arme, C., and Read, C. P., Ultrastructural localization of a peroxidase in the tapeworm, Hymenolepis diminuta. J. Parasitol. 54, 802-807 (1968).
93. Turton, J. A., In vitro cultivation of Hymenolepis diminuta: Effect of antibiotics on the growth of three-day-old worms removed from the rat. Exptl. Parasitol. 36, 62-69 (1974).

94. Voge, M., Jaffe, J., Bruckner, D. A, and Meymarian, E., Synergistic growth promoting action of L-cysteine and nitrogen upon *Hymenolepis diminuta* cysticercoids *in vitro*. J. Parasitol. 62, 951-954 (1976).
95. von Brand, T., "Biochemistry of Parasites". Chapter 3, pp. 89-170. Academic Press, New York, (1973).
96. Walkey, M., and Fairbairn, D., L (+)-Lactate dehydrogenase from *Hymenolepis diminuta* (Cestoda). J. Exptl. Zool. 183, 365-374 (1973).
97. Wang, E. J., and Saz, H. J., Comparative biochemical studies of *Litomosoides carinii*, *Dipetalonema viteae* and *Brugia pahangi* adults. J. Parasitol. 60, 316-321 (1974).
98. Ward, C. W., and Fairbairn, D., Enzymes of beta-oxidation and the tricarboxylic acid cycle in adult *Hymenolepis diminuta* (Cestoda) and *Ascaris lumbricoides* (Nematoda). J. Parasitol. 56, 1009-1012 (1970).
99. Watts, S. D. M., and Fairbairn, D., Anaerobic excretion of fermentation acids by *Hymenolepis diminuta* during development in the definitive host. J. Parasitol. 60, 621-625 (1974).
100. Weinbach, E. C., Role of non-heme iron in cestode respiration. In "Comparative Biochemistry of Parasites" (H. van den Bossche, ed.), pp. 433-444. Academic Press, New York, (1972).
101. Wilson, M. A., and Cascarano, J., The energy-yielding oxidation of NADH by fumarate in submitochondrial particles of rat tissues. Biochim. Biophys. Acta 216, 54-62 (1970).

CONCEPTS OF MEMBRANE BIOLOGY IN
HYMENOLEPIS DIMINUTA

Ron B. Podesta

Department of Zoology
University of Toronto
Toronto, Ontario

I. INTRODUCTION

The biology of cell membranes is without doubt one of the most integrative studies in modern biology in terms of the basic sciences such as physics, mathematics and chemistry that have been brought together to formulate not only basic membrane theory but to develop the technology required to examine structure and function. This is clearly indicated in the several recent textbooks devoted solely to the study of biological membranes (Cereijido and Rotunno 1970; Nystrom 1973; Christensen 1975; Kotyk and Janacek 1975), and the numerous publications, monographs and symposia devoted each year to aspects of membrane biology. It can be safely assumed that membrane biology will play a central role in future paradigms in modern biology.

However, it is unfortunate that within the almost overwhelming documentation of membrane biology, the rightful place belonging to the epithelial syncytium of *Hymenolepis diminuta* as a model system has not been widely recognized. This is due, in part, to the rather narrow approach given the study of membrane transport in this species, and to the "C. P. Read Principle": that is, research on parasites has historically been published only in journals devoted to parasites and read only by parasitologists - to the detriment of both parasitologists and biologists.

The present article, therefore, is not designed to review in detail all the research involving membrane transport in *H. diminuta* and other helminths. This task has been accomplished in several recent reviews (Mettrick and Podesta 1974; Arme 1975, 1976; Pappas and Read 1975; Podesta 1978a). In keeping with the August Krogh Principle (Krebs 1975) the epithelial syncytium of *H. diminuta* has been 'designed' for the comparative physiologist to examine a number of membrane functions of broad application to membrane biology. As an epithelial layer, the epithelial syncytium represents one extreme membrane system within a continuum of epithelia with tight or leaky junctions and represents an extreme application of electrical and metabolic coupling between cells in an epithelial field. Moreover, why the parasitic flatworms evolved the very specialized structure of the epithelial syncytium is a fundamental question which has only recently been approached (Podesta 1978a) and which leads to a number of fascinating questions of a seminal nature concerning the structure and function of epithelial tissues. It is these concepts which I will explore in the present review with the hope of stimulating further research. Unfortunately, application of these concepts to the epithelial syncytium is only beginning so that I am forced to allude primarily to studies using tissues other than those of flatworms and to my own research that is in progress or only recently published. However, since my contribution to this monograph was to deal with concepts, this approach may be permissible.

II. MEMBRANE TRANSPORT

Investigations of membrane transport in *Hymenolepis diminuta* have demonstrated a remarkable diversity of functions which may be attributed to the external body covering of this organism. Since this parasite lacks a mouth and alimentary canal, all nutrient uptake must occur across the body surface. Thus, it was recognized that *H. diminuta* could serve a useful role in studies of membrane transport (Read *et al.* 1963). Ultrastructural studies soon thereafter established that, in keeping with an absorptive surface, the outward-facing membrane of

H. diminuta was a brush border surface. Subsequent studies have shown that this brush border surface may accomplish a number of vital functions including (for references see reviews by Lumsden 1975 a,b; Podesta 1980a): 1) it is a site of catalytic activity containing enzymes of both host and parasite origin; 2) it is a possible site for volume regulation; 3) it is a site of molecular and ion transport containing specific agencies for the transport of hexose sugars, amino acids, vitamins, purines, pyrimidines, nucleosides, lipids and cations; 4) it serves a protective function, binding bile acids, components of the host's immune reaction to the presence of the parasite and contains a surface coat which contains inhibitors of host digestive enzymes; and 5) it may, as will be discussed later in this review, serve as a site of information and metabolite transfer.

However, the results from previous studies have been concerned with and interpreted only in terms of the brush border membrane and transfer of non-electrolytes across this single barrier. Only recently has it been recognized that the syncytium overlying the tissue of *H. diminuta* is essentially an epithelial layer with two membranes in series (Podesta *et al.* 1977 a,b; Podesta 1980b). Once this is recognized, a number of other interesting possibilities concerning the structure and functional relationships of the epithelial syncytium of *H. diminuta* are revealed. In the following discussion I will first establish the theoretical basis of transepithelial transport and second, discuss some of the practical limitations of using *H. diminuta* as an experimental tool for studying transepithelial transport. Finally, the main thrust of transport studies using *H. diminuta* - establishing the validity of the gradient hypothesis as a means of active nonelectrolyte transport - will be considered.

A. *The Hymenolepis diminuta Model*

   1. An Epithelial Syncytium. The two-membrane model of Koefoed-Johnson and Ussing (1958) has provided the framework upon which most of the modern concepts of transepithelial transport of solutes and water are based. The two-membrane hypothesis assumes the presence of two membranes in series, each acting independent of the other, with the outward-facing membrane behaving similar to a Na^+-electrode and the inward-facing membrane behaving like a K^+-electrode. The transepithelial electrical potential difference was considered as the sum of the Na^+ and K^+ diffusion potentials arising from the different permeabilities of the two membranes. The two-membrane hypothesis therefore originated the concept of a polarized epithelial cell having asymmetric membrane functions characterizing the limiting membranes. However, the concept of functional as well as morphological polarization was not fully appreciated until Schultz and Zalusky (1964) confined the ouabain-sensitive site of transepithelial Na^+ and hexose sugar transport to the inward-facing membrane of the mammalian intestinal epithelial cell. Subsequent examination of a variety of epithelia confirmed the functional asymmetry of the inward- and outward-facing membranes in terms of their biochemical composition and transport functions (see Podesta 1980a). This suggests that functional polarization of the membranes allows the epithelial cell to regulate not only its own internal environment, a characteristic of non-polarized cells, but also the internal milieu. The latter is accomplished by vectorial transport of solutes and water from one side of the epithelial cell to the other as a consequence of the asymmetric properties of the two membranes.

Although the two-membrane model has been altered and made more complex on several occasions to meet new challenges (see Podesta 1980a), it would appear that the epithelial syncytium of *H. diminuta* was specifically 'designed' to test the validity of the two membrane hypothesis in its original form. For example, a major challenge to the two-membrane model was the discovery of two parallel routes of ion flow across some epithelial tissues. In addition to the transcellular route across the inward- and outward-facing membranes of the epithelial cells, it was shown that substantial ion flow occurs through the paracellular or shunt pathway via the tight junctions and lateral extracellular spaces between the epithelial cells. In fact, it is the resistance of the shunt pathway to ion flow which determines the magnitude of the transepithelial chemical and electrical potential gradients. However, this complicating feature of cellular epithelia is not a consideration with the acellular epithelial syncytium of *H. diminuta* which lacks the morphological prerequisites of an extracellular shunt pathway. The outward-facing brush border of the epithelial syncytium is uninterrupted by tight junctions and there is no contact between the outward-facing and inward-facing membranes. This does not, however, rule out the presence of trans-syncytial pathways of low resistance as low resistance pathways have been postulated for the transcellular route in cellular epithelia by Ussing (1975). Further, the epithelial syncytium appears ideally suited for examining transcellular low resistant pathways should they exist and their role in the interdependence of the inward- and outward-facing membranes of the epithelial layer as demonstrated by Finn (1976). The transport function of the epithelial syncytium of *H. diminuta* should be adequately predicted on the basis of the two-membrane model and, if not, it provides a model system to explore alternatives to the two-membrane hypothesis in an epithelial layer that is not complicated by an extracellular shunt pathway.

However, it is not sufficient simply to consider the epithelial syncytium of *H. diminuta* as an epithelial layer based on structure alone. As mentioned above, the functional asymmetry or polarization is an essential feature for a transporting epithelial layer to accomplish its major function - transepithelial transport. Since previous studies have examined the permeability properties of only the brush border membrane (see Pappas and Read 1975; Podesta 1978a), we have concentrated on exploring functional asymmetry in the syncytium of *H. diminuta* (Podesta *et al.* 1977 a,b; Podesta 1980b in preparation). For example, most previous studies have demonstrated that Na^+-coupled nonelectrolyte transport in *H. diminuta* and other helminths is not inhibited by ouabain (see Pappas and Read 1975; Podesta 1978a). However, using tissue slices of *H. diminuta*, a tissue preparation in which ouabain has access to the inward-facing membrane of the epithelial syncytium via the exposed tissue extracellular space, we have shown that uptake of glucose, galactose, alanine and other Na^+-sensitive amino acids is inhibited by ouabain. Hence, we have established functional asymmetry at least with respect to the site of ouabain sensitivity (Podesta *et al.* 1977b; Lussier *et al.* 1978). More recently I have been able to demonstrate a similar asymmetry with respect to the hexose and Na^+ permeabilities in the outward- and inward-facing membranes of the epithelial syncytium of *H. diminuta* (Podesta 1980b). According to these studies, galactose transport across the outward-facing membrane is Na^+-coupled and inhibited by ouabain whereas galactose influx and efflux across the inward-facing membrane is not sensitive to Na^+, is not inhibited by ouabain and has a different stereospecificity. Similarly, Na^+ influx across the brush border was a saturable function of extracellular Na^+, was insensitive to ouabain, inhibited by amiloride and was increased as a saturable function of external galactose or glucose. However, the influx and efflux that Na^+ across the inward-facing membrane were markedly depressed by ouabain, and were insensitive to amiloride. However, there are technical difficulties which must be considered in the interpretation of these results. These methodological limitations of using tissue slices are discussed in the next section of this review.

2. *Experimental Limitations.* With most transporting epithelial tissues, it is possible to mount the epithelial layer as a flat sheet between two chambers containing fluids of known composition. This allows the experimentor to measure the influx and efflux permeabilities and kinetics of both the inward- and outward-facing membranes, the unidirectional and net transepithelial transfer of solute, and the transmural electrical potential difference as outlined by Ussing and Zehran (1951) and more recently by Naftalin and Curran (1974). However, since *H. diminuta* does not contain a body cavity, it is not possible to mount the epithelial syncytium as a flat sheet separating two Ussing chambers. The electrical and ionic potential profile across the syncytium will therefore have to rely on the use of ion-sensitive and potential microelectrodes. Determination of transport properties of the epithelial syncytium will be more difficult. To overcome these problems, some recent methods have been devised whereby information concerning the fluxes across the inward-facing and outward-facing membranes and the syncytial transport pools may be estimated using tissue slices (Podesta *et al.* 1977 a,b; Podesta

1977 a,b,c; 1980 b,c). These studies consist of three experimental designs, including flux determinations of the *exocircum*, *bicircum*, *endocircum* and *contracircum* type, isotope equilibration experiments used to determine solute transport pools, and compartmental analyses, used to determine the number, size and rate constants of tissue compartments.

For experimental purposes, it is convenient to consider *H. diminuta* as a series of compartments separated by membranes whose permeability properties are of primary interest, as shown in Table I. In this table, [M], [S], [P], [E] are the concentrations of test solute in the incubation medium, syncytial intracellular compartment, parenchymal intracellular compartment and parenchymal extracellular compartment, respectively, and J represents the flux across the membrane(s) separating the compartments. The superscripts o and i refer to the outward-facing brush border and the inward-facing membrane of the epithelial syncytium while p represents the membranes of the cells underlying the syncytium. The subscripts refer to the direction of solute flow across the membranes separating the various compartments. Normally, S and P are treated as a single homogeneous intracellular compartment, although by analyzing the transport pools and *contracircum* experiments, a certain degree of separation between S and P may be achieved (see Podesta 1977c, 1978b). Separation of the extracellular and intracellular compartments can be accomplished either by using a nonabsorbable marker and tissue slices (see Podesta 1977 a-c) or by compartmental analysis (see Podesta 1980 a,b). The number of compartments can be increased to include the calcareous corpuscles in the case of tissue Ca^{++} (Podesta 1980c).

The transport pools represent the amount of tissue solute that equilibrates with radiolabelled test solute that originates from solute entering only across the outward-facing brush border (MTP, mucosal transport pool), across the outward-facing brush border and through membranes exposed to E using tissue slices (TTP, total transport pool), or only across the membranes exposed to the parenchymal extracellular space (PTP, parenchymal transport pool) using tissue slices in which J_{ms}^o and J_{sm}^o have been inhibited (Podesta 1977c; 1980b).

TABLE I. *Experimental Model of Hymenolepis diminuta:
Tissue Compartments, Membranes and Experiments.*

$$[M] \xrightleftharpoons[J^o_{sm}]{J^o_{ms}} [S] \xrightleftharpoons[J^i_{es}]{J^i_{se}} [E] \xrightleftharpoons[J^p_{pe}]{J^p_{ep}} [P]$$

Experiment	Influx	Efflux	Transport Pools
1. Exocircum	J^o_{ms}	J^o_{sm}	MTP
2. Bicircum	$J^o_{ms} + J^i_{es} + J^p_{ep}$	$J^o_{sm} + J^i_{se} + J^p_{pe}$	TTP
3. Endocircum	$J^i_{es} + J^p_{ep}$	$J^i_{se} + J^p_{pe}$	PTP
4. (2–3)	J^o_{ms}	J^o_{sm}	MTP
5. Contracircum	J^i_{es}	J^i_{se}	MTP

Historically, the *exocircum* experiments have been the only method used to examine solute fluxes across the epithelial syncytium of *H. diminuta* (see Pappas and Read 1975; Podesta 1980a). Using this type of experiment the initial rate influx kinetics across the outward-facing brush border membrane have been obtained for a wide variety of nonelectrolytes utilizing whole *H. diminuta* or different strobilar regions of the parasites. Although less common, efflux kinetics ($J\overset{o}{s}m$) have been determined for the outward-facing membrane using some test solutes assuming steady-state conditions, first order kinetics and the absence of metabolic sinks. The latter assumptions, however, have generally not been critically evaluated. Only recently has the *exocircum* experiment been used to determine the mucosal transport pool (Podesta *et al.* 1977b; Podesta 1977c).

Tissue slices are used to obtain transport parameters in the *bicircum* experiments. This type of preparation is not useful by itself since M = E and test solute can enter or exit the intracellular compartment by traversing the outward-facing brush border membrane or the membranes in contact with the extracellular fluid which is exposed to the incubation medium in tissue slices. However, if transport across the brush border membrane is inhibited, then the remaining fluxes must represent a hybrid of $J\overset{p}{e}s$ and $J\overset{p}{e}p$ for influx and $J\overset{i}{s}e$ and $J\overset{o}{p}o$ for efflux. This type of experiment I will refer to as *endocircum*. Inhibition of brush border transport will depend on the test solute used but can generally be accomplished in two ways. First, brush border fluxes can be irreversibly inhibited prior to preparing the tissue slices. After washing away the excess inhibitor, tissue slices can be prepared followed by the transport studies. This procedure has been used successfully using $HgCl_2$ as inhibitor and galactose or Na^+ as the test solute (Podesta *et al.* 1977 a,b; Podesta 1977c, 1980b). Second, in the case of an asymmetric inhibitor of Na^+ transport, $J\overset{o}{m}s$ can be inhibited with amiloride which does not affect Jes or Jep. However, since the effect of amiloride is reversible, it must be included in the incubation medium containing the tissue slices during the flux experiment. This procedure has been used to examine ion and hexose transport in *H. diminuta* (Podesta 1980 b,d).

Initial rate kinetics determined with the *endocircum* experiments will reflect the transport properties of parenchymal tissue membranes since, according to the time required for E to become uniformly labelled with a nonabsorbable marker ($t_{\frac{1}{2}}$ 3.6-5.1 min; Podesta 1977a), very little radiolabelled solute will enter the epithelial syncytium. Steady state kinetic determinations in *endocircum* experiments will, however, represent a hybrid of the parenchymal cell and inward-facing syncytial membranes. The major advantage of the *bicircum* and *endocircum* experiments is that their difference will estimate $J_{ms}^{°}$, $J_{sm}^{°}$ and MTP using tissue slices where the parenchymal extracellular space is exposed to the incubation medium. This is important, for example, when studying the effect of ouabain on $J_{ms}^{°}$ since this inhibitor must be exposed to the inward-facing syncytial membrane necessitating the use of tissue slices (see Podesta *et al.* 1977b; Podesta 1977c).

The above experiments do not give an accurate estimation of the fluxes which occur across the inward-facing membrane of the epithelial syncytium (Jse and Jes). We have therefore attempted the *contracircum* type of experiment to obtain estimates of these fluxes. While isolating brush border preparations for enzyme determinations, it was found that a brief (<20 sec) exposure of *H. diminuta* to detergent removes the brush border but leaves the inward-facing membrane of the epithelial syncytium intact and covered by a layer of cytoplasmic components (Rahman, M.S., pers. comm.). Therefore, using the parasites with the brush border removed should theoretically lead to an evaluation of Jse and Jes. Preliminary results indicate that the permeability properties of the inward-facing membrane of the epithelial syncytium of *H. diminuta* do not differ significantly from the membranes of the underlying parenchymal tissue. Moreover, removal of the syncytial cytoplasm with detergents in the *contracircum* type of experiment leads to a more accurate determination of MTP. The mucosal transport pool of Na^+ estimates by the *contracircum* experiment is less than half of that determined by the *exocircum* or (*bicircum* - *endocircum*) experiments, confirming my suspicions concerning previous estimates of the mucosal Na^+ transport pool (Podesta 1977c).

Another approach to studying the transport properties of *H. diminuta* is to determine the amount of solute in tissue compartments and the rate constants for the compartments using compartmental analysis (see Jacquez 1972). For example, Fisher and Read (1971) followed the efflux of radiosodium from the tissues of *Calliobothrium verticillatum*. Treating their results by compartmental analysis indicates that this species has two tissue Na^+ compartments, each constituting approximately 50% of total tissue Na^+. They obtained a 'fast' Na^+ compartment with a half time ($t_{\frac{1}{2}}$) of approximately 4.6 min and a slower pool with a $t_{\frac{1}{2}}$ of 23 min. Ouabain did not alter the 'slow' pool but the $t_{\frac{1}{2}}$ for the 'fast' Na^+ pool was decreased to 14 min. Two tissue Na^+ pools have also been discerned in *H. diminuta* using compartmental analysis, one containing 158 mmoles Na^+ per Kg dry wt ($t_{\frac{1}{2}}$ 16.4 min) and a second pool of 122 mmoles/Kg dry wt ($t_{\frac{1}{2}}$ 47.6 min) (Podesta 1980b). The larger fast pool was considered extracellular due to the similar $t_{\frac{1}{2}}$ obtained for an extracellular marker substance (PEG : $t_{\frac{1}{2}}$ 14.1 min). The smaller 'slow' pool was similar to K^+ ($t_{\frac{1}{2}}$ 44.1 min) indicating that this Na^+ compartment was intracellular. In contrast to the results for *C. verticillatum*, ouabain decreased the size and $t_{\frac{1}{2}}$ for the intracellular Na^+ pool while increasing the size and $t_{\frac{1}{2}}$ for the intracellular pool of tissue Na^+. Glucose, amiloride and Na^+ substitutions altered the two Na^+ pools in *H. diminuta* in accordance with the predictions of the two-membrane hypothesis (Podesta 1980b).

In the experiments discussed above, the extracellular compartment or 'membrane' compartment represented by the unstirred water layer over the brush border membrane surface of *H. diminuta* has not been considered. It is assumed that correction for the unstirred diffusion barrier is routine in initial rate kinetic studies. This is necessary since it can result in large over-estimations of Jms and, conversely, underestimations of Jsm (Podesta *et al.* 1977a). Moreover, the initial rate kinetics of a carrier mediated transport system or a diffusional process will be markedly altered by the thickness of the unstirred layer (Podesta 1977b). This problem will not be as serious in steady state kinetic studies.

B. *Coupled Transport Systems*

The majority of studies dealing with membrane transport in *H. diminuta* have concentrated on initial rate kinetics, accumulation and stereospecificity of carrier mediated transport systems for a variety of nonelectrolytes in the outward-facing brush border membrane. Moreover, a major emphasis in these studies has been given to the dependency of the transport systems on extracellular Na^+ concentrations. The transport agencies which appear to depend on the concentration of Na^+ in the bathing medium include those for glucose, amino acids sharing the A transport agency, glycerol, uridine and thymidine (see Podesta 1980a). It has therefore been suggested that these solutes are not transported across the brush border by primary active transport coupled directly to the flow of metabolic energy, but are accumulated by secondary active transport coupled to the electrochemical gradient of Na^+ across the brush border membrane. In the discussion below, I will first outline those results which are consistent with the gradient hypothesis and second, I will deal with those results which are inconsistent with the gradient hypothesis. The latter observations will then be interpreted in terms of an alternative to the gradient hypothesis - a convective-coupling hypothesis. Third, a consideration will be made of osmotically induced fluxes across the brush border and how these fluxes modify the interpretation of both the ion-gradient and convective-coupling hypothesis.

1. *Gradient-Hypothesis*. The ion-gradient hypothesis assumes that a carrier catalyzes a reversible reaction whose asymmetry is maintained by the asymmetric distribution of ions (Na^+ and K^+) between the cell and the extracellular fluid. The active transport of nonelectrolyte is driven by the electrochemical potential gradient of ions in such a way that the two fluxes concerned (Na^+ and nonelectrolyte in animal cells or H^+ and nonelectrolytes in microorganisms, mitochondria and chloroblasts), are energetically coupled to each other by cotransport, presumably through the formation of a ternary complex between membrane carrier, nonelectrolyte and co-ion at a fixed stoichiometry. This concept that ion gradients may provide energy for accumulation of

nonelectrolytes was developed originally into the Na^+-gradient hypothesis by Crane (1962) and Schultz and Curran (1970), based on the following three basic observations. First, with reference to transporting epithelia, nonelectrolyte transport across the brush border was dependent upon the concentration of Na^+ in the fluid bathing the brush border. Second, addition of nonelectrolyte to the bathing fluid accelerated Na^+ influx with a fixed stoichiometry. Third, inhibition of Na^+ influx across the brush border with ouabain (which inhibits the Na^+-pump located in the inward-facing membrane), also inhibited nonelectrolyte transport across the brush border. Although the ion-gradient hypothesis has been modified on several occasions in order to incorporate new information, it still remains an attractive and widely accepted hypothesis (see Podesta 1980a).

Unfortunately, studies dealing with the epithelial syncytium of *H. diminuta* have not, until recently (see below), advanced beyond the stage of making the first two of the three basic observations mentioned above. On this basis the accumulation of a number of nonelectrolytes by *H. diminuta* has been interpreted in terms of the Na^+-gradient hypothesis (see Pappas and Read 1975; Podesta 1980a). This has been done without knowledge concerning trans-syncytial fluxes across both limiting membranes, ion electrochemical potential profiles across the syncytium, Na^+ transport mechanisms and the location of the Na^+-pump (Na^+, K^+-Mg^{++} dependent ATPase). For example, external Na^+ is required for glucose uptake and accumulation by *H. diminuta* and external glucose causes two Na^+ ions to cross the brush border for every glucose molecule absorbed (Pappas and Hansen 1977). However, the third basic observation - that inhibition of Na^+ transport with ouabain inhibits glucose uptake - was not succesfully established since whole *H. diminuta* and hence, only the brush border membrane, were exposed to ouabain (see Pappas and Read 1975). As mentioned previously this is a clear indication in previous studies of the lack of insight into the nature of the epithelial syncytium since, according to the asymmetry inherent in the two-membrane model, only ouabain exposed to the inward-facing membrane of the epithelial syncytium would be expected to inhibit Na^+ and glucose influx across the outward-facing brush border. Fortunately, more recent studies have confirmed the third basic observation by demonstrating that Na^+ and hexose influx across the brush border are indeed inhibited by ouabain using tissue slices, in which ouabain has access to the inward-facing membrane of the epithelial syncytium (Podesta *et al.* 1977b; Podesta 1977c, 1980b).

More recently, a number of detailed observations have been made concerning hexose transport across the epithelial syncytium of *H. diminuta* which are also consistent with the prediction of the ion-gradient hypothesis. These results are summarized in Table II and are taken from Podesta (1977c, 1980b; in preparation). The ratio of radiolabelled galactose entering the tissue via the brush border to radiogalactose entering via the exposed extracellular space indicated that under control conditions, 5-6 times as much galactose enters through the brush border than via the extracellular space using tissue slices. The asymmetry of influx and efflux permeabilities across the brush border is clearly indicated by their ratio in which influx is favored by a factor of 11.9. This asymmetry is even more remarkable since, under steady state conditions, the intracellular concentration of galactose exceeds the medium concentration by a factor of approximately five (Podesta *et al.* 1977 a,b; Podesta 1977c, 1980b). The asymmetric properties of the inward- and outward-facing membranes of the epithelial syncytium are also evident in Table II. The influx permeability across the inward-facing membrane was much less than across the brush border and the flux asymmetry favors influx across the brush border and efflux, although only slightly, across the inward-facing membrane. The results for the inward-facing membrane were obtained using *endocircum* (Podesta 1977c, 1980b) and *contracircum* (Podesta, in preparation) experiments. The mucosal Na^+ transport pool, determined using the *contracircum* experiments, was only 24.5 mmoles/Kg dry wt. which is less than half of that determined under similar conditions using the *bicircum* and *endocircum* experiments reported previously (Podesta 1977c, 1980b). With the exception of the efflux permeabilities across the brush border membrane which will be considered later, the results using Na^+-free and ouabain incubation

TABLE II. *Summary of Steady-State Influx and Efflux Permeabilities of Outward-Facing and Inward-Facing Membranes of Epithelial Syncytium in Hymenolepis diminuta*

Treatment	$^{14}C_m/^{14}C_e$	Permeabilities ($P = \mu moles/cm^2/h/mM$)						Na^+MTP
		Galactose (5 mM)						
		J^o_{ms}	J^o_{sm}	J^o_{ms}/J^o_{sm}	J^i_{se}	J^i_{es}	J^i_{se}/J^i_{es}	mmoles/Kg dry wt.
Control	5.64	0.692	0.058	11.9	0.198	0.174	1.1	24.5
Na-free	0.24	0.182	0.166	1.1	0.209	0.162	1.3	7.8
Ouabain	0.66	0.304	0.282	1.1	0.195	0.181	1.1	51.2

procedures were entirely consistent with the predictions of the gradient hypothesis. These include the decrease in the $^{14}Cm/^{14}Ce$ ratio, the decreased influx permeability of the brush border and the expected changes in the amount of Na^+ in the syncytium (MTP). The absence of an effect of ouabain and Na^+-depletion on the influx-efflux permeability of the inward-facing membrane is another case of asymmetry which is consistent with both the two-membrane and ion-gradient hypotheses. On the basis of these results and those published previously, dealing with Crane's (1962) three basic observations (see Pappas and Read 1975; Podesta 1980a), the ion-gradient hypothesis would appear to be an adequate explanation for the mechanism of hexose absorption across the epithelial syncytium of *H. diminuta*. However, there are a number of observations which are not consistent with the gradient hypothesis. The inconsistencies are dealt with below and are used to develop a convective-coupling hypothesis as an alternative to the ion-gradient hypothesis.

2. Coupling via Convective Transport. A stoichiometry of 2 for the ratio of glucose-stimulated Na^+ influx and glucose influx has been determined for *Calliobothrium verticillatum* and *Hymenolepis diminuta* in similar publications by Pappas and Read (1972a) and Read *et al.* (1974), respectively. In both species, the Na^+-dependent glucose uptake is a J_{max} system, that is, external Na^+ affects the maximum velocity of glucose influx but has little effect on the Michaelean constant, K_t (see Geck and Heinz 1976). In both instances, model carrier agencies for glucose influx were postulated with three binding sites for Na^+, the important difference being that the coupling coefficients in *H. diminuta* decreased to unity as external Na^+ was raised to 50 mM. The latter observation made it necessary to postulate 'activating' and 'nonactivating' sites for Na^+ binding, with the 'nonactivating' sites having the highest affinity for Na^+ and therefore being saturated at very low external Na^+ concentrations. Since the 'nonactivating' site does not activate glucose translocation and since it would be completely saturated at higher physiological concentrations of Na^+ where the stoichiometry of Na^+ and glucose uptake is close to unity, one is led to the conclusion that glucose influx is independent of Na^+ when external Na^+ concentrations exceed 50 mM. Only at Na^+ concentrations less than this would Na^+ be necessary to activate glucose influx giving rise to the coupling coefficients of 2 or more. It is surprising, therefore, that Read et al. (1974) and Pappas and Read (1975) considered these results as being consistent with Crane's Na^+-gradient hypothesis. In other animal cells, different Na^+ : amino acid stoichiometries have been observed depending on the chemical structure of the amino acid (Christensen 1972). In these systems the composition of the transported complex was always the same but the exchange probability of Na^+ and amino acid at the two surfaces of the membrane is different. This allows net transport of labelled Na^+ to take place without net transport of amino acid. In the green alga, *Chlorella vulgaris*, evidence has been obtained that the stoichiometry of protons per carrier is the same for all glucose analogues, but some analogues initiate the translocation of carrier-proton complex without themselves becoming translocated, so that protons are transported in excess of the sugar transported (Gruneberg and Komor 1976). The explanations proposed above for differing stoichiometries in other cells appear to offer a more fruitful avenue of enquiry for explaining the results of Read et al. (1974).

In contrast to the results of Read et al. (1974), Uglem (1976) has suggested a stoichiometric relationship between glucose-stimulated Na^+ influx and glucose influx of unity for *H. diminuta* bathed in low Na^+ solutions (10 mM), with the added feature that for every Na^+ entering a Na^+ is translocated in the opposite direction. The Na^+-exchange was thought to be related to the ability of the worms to absorb glucose coupled to an electrically neutral ion exchange, although it must be emphasized that Na^+ efflux would be enhanced in these studies due to the low ambient Na^+ concentrations used. Furthermore, nonelectrogenic ion-coupled glucose uptake by *H. diminuta* is clearly inconsistent with the results of Uglem (1976) and those of others (e.g. Podesta 1977c) showing that glucose promotes an increase in tissue Na^+ without any compensating change in tissue K^+. Membrane depolarization is a common feature associated with Na^+-dependent nonelectrolyte uptake in other cells and tissues (see Hoshi et al. 1976).

The main purpose of the study by Uglem (1976) was to demonstrate that apparent glucose-independent Na^+ uptake recorded by Pappas and Read (1972a) and Read et al. (1974) was due to a glucose leak into an unstirred layer where it would stimulate Na^+ influx. Support for this hypothesis was based on a 30% inhibition of glucose-independent Na^+ influx by phlorizin, a potent inhibitor of glucose uptake. However, if glucose leakage was responsible for glucose-independent Na^+ uptake, phlorizin should also increase efflux of Na^+ since this would prevent recapture of Na^+ exiting the worm through the unstirred layer. However, Uglem (1976) found that phlorizin inhibited Na^+ efflux, therefore contradicting his original hypothesis. There is no reason to suspect that Na^+ uptake cannot take place by means other than coupled nonelectrolyte-Na^+ influx. For example, CO_2 is a potent stimulator of Na^+ uptake in *H. diminuta* and a wide variety of other cells and tissues (see Podesta and Mettrick 1974, 1975, 1976, 1977 a,b; Podesta 1980d).

A number of other observations on hexose uptake by tapeworms are also inconsistent with the gradient hypothesis. According to this hypothesis, external glucose, which increases intracellular concentrations of Na^+ (Podesta 1977c), should increase Na^+ efflux but, except for the results of Uglem (1976), external glucose and galactose do not alter Na^+ efflux in *C. verticillatum* (Pappas and Read 1972a) or *H. diminuta* (Podesta 1977c). Also, in Table 4 of Pappas and Read (1972a), glucose continued to be accumulated against a chemical potential when the Na^+ gradient was reversed (external Na^+ 20 mM, tissue Na^+ 200 mM). Read et al.(1974) also observed glucose influx when the gradient of Na^+ was reversed, at least with respect to the data presented on the Na^+-glucose coupling ratios. Another consistent feature of the tapeworm studies is that glucose uptake by worms following a Na^+-free incubation is not immediately reversible (see Podesta et al. 1977b). Preincubation in Na^+-free conditions depletes the amount of Na^+ in the epithelial syncytium of *H. diminuta* from 31 to 2 mmoles Kg dry wt^{-1} (Podesta 1977c), so when the worms are then placed in a fluid containing physiological Na^+ concentrations, the trans-brush border gradient for Na^+ is larger than normal. If the chemical potential difference for Na^+ provides the energy to drive glucose accumulation, then one would expect an enhanced influx under the above conditions. However, Read et al. (1974) found that it takes a minimum of 10 min in a Na^+-containing fluid before glucose uptake even approaches control values following incubation in a Na^+-free fluid (see Podesta et al. 1977b). It is unlikely that this delay is due to diffusion of Na^+ from the bulk fluid being delayed by an unstirred layer as vigorous stirring does not reduce the time for glucose uptake to become fully reversible in Na^+-containing fluids following incubation in a Na^+-free fluid (Podesta, unpublished).

It also takes at least 10 min (Podesta et al. 1977b) and as long as 15-30 min (Pappas and Read 1972a; Pappas et al. 1973, 1974; Read et al. 1974) preincubation in Na^+-free fluids before an effect of Na^+-replacement can be observed to inhibit glucose influx in tapeworms. If, as predicted by the gradient hypothesis, Na^+ external to the brush border is the only site involved in the effect of Na^+ on glucose influx, Na^+-replacement should have a rapid effect on glucose uptake even considering the effects of an unstirred layer (Podesta 1980a).

Currently, the strongest evidence against the ion-gradient hypothesis in epithelial tissues are the observations made on rabbit ileum by Naftalin and coworkers (Naftalin and Curran 1974; Naftalin and Holman 1974, 1975; Holman and Naftalin 1975; Simmons and Naftalin 1976 a,b). Their diffusive-convective model of galactose transport was prompted originally by the increased exit permeability of the brush border membrane to galactose as tissue Na^+ concentrations were increased. Compare for example, the efflux permeabilities of the outward-facing brush border of *H. diminuta* when incubated in Na^+-free fluids and with ouabain (Table II). Ouabain, which increases cellular Na^+ concentrations, would be expected on the basis of the ion-gradient hypothesis to increase the efflux permeability of the brush border. The results for *H. diminuta* are consistent with the predictions when the parasites are bathed in a solution containing ouabain (Table II). Conversely, if cellular Na^+ concentrations are reduced by incubating *H. diminuta* in solutions depleted of Na^+, the ion-gradient hypothesis would predict a decreased efflux permeability of the brush border to galactose.

In this case, the results were not consistent with
the predictions as galactose efflux permeability
across the brush border of H. diminuta was increased
during the Na^+-free incubations. On the basis of
results similar to those in Table II for H. diminuta,
Naftalin and co-workers suggested that galactose
transport was correlated more closely with intracellular Na^+ concentrations (hence, Na^+-pump activity),
than the gradient of Na^+ across the brush border as
predicted by the ion-gradient hypothesis. This is
clearly demonstrated in Table III. As intracellular

TABLE III. *Summary of Brush Border Influx and Efflux Galactose Permeabilities as a Function of Na^+-Pump Activity in the Epithelial Syncytium of Hymenolepis diminuta.*

		Galactose (5mM)		
	$[Na^+]i$	Permeabilties ($\mu moles/cm^2/hr/$ mm)		
Incubation	(mM)	J^o_{ms}	J^o_{sm}	J^o_{ms}/J^o_{sm}
Na^+ 0 mM	2.4	0.182	0.166	1.1
50 mM	39.1	0.460	0.107	4.3
100 mM	51.5	0.555	0.091	6.1
140 mM	57.3	0.692	0.058	11.9
Ouabain	87.2	0.304	0.282	1.1

Na^+ is increased, there occurred an increase in
galactose influx permeability. Moreover, when the
Na^+-pump activity is inhibited by ouabain, galactose
influx is increased even though intracellular Na^+
is elevated. Therefore, assuming that Na^+-pump activity is proportional to intracellular concentrations
of Na^+, the influx and efflux permeabilities of the
brush border to galactose were correlated with Na^+-pump activity and this correlation occurs in both
the rabbit ileum and the epithelial syncytium of H.
diminuta.

In order to couple Na^+-pump activity located in the inward-facing membrane of the epithelial layer, to galactose transport across the brush border, Naftalin and co-workers reflected on the possibility that the well-known relation between transepithelial Na^+ and water transport may be important. According to the standing-gradient osmotic flow hypothesis of water transport across epithelial tissues (see Diamond 1971), Na^+ is pumped across the inward-facing membrane into the lateral extracellular spaces separating the epithelial cells. This results in an osmotic gradient between extracellular channels separating the cells and the fluid bathing outward-facing brush border membrane. Water then flows from the mucosal fluid bathing the brush border into the lateral extracellular channels. Coupling between water and galactose transport across the brush border could then be achieved by convection; that is, galactose may be entrained in a stream of fluid traversing the brush border through narrow channels, the ultimate driving force being the Na^+-pump located in the inward-facing membrane of the epithelial cells. Accordingly, coupling between Na^+ and galactose transport is achieved indirectly through convective transport or solvent drag of galactose across the brush border. This would be compatible with most of the results consistent with the ion-gradient hypothesis as well as with the inverse relation between the efflux and influx permeability of the brush border to galactose as intracellular Na^+ is increased. The convective-coupling hypothesis would similarly account for the absence of hexose-stimulated efflux of Na^+ across the brush border mentioned previously, the stimulated efflux being a necessary consequence of the ion-gradient hypothesis. Both observations can be explained on the basis of fluid flowing through narrow channels in the brush border stimulated by Na^+-pump activity. The inward flow of water through the channels would hinder efflux through the channels as intracellular Na^+ is increased by increasing extracellular Na^+, in the first case dealing with galactose efflux permeability and by increasing extracellular galactose, in the second case dealing with Na^+ efflux permeabilities.

It is not surprising that the results for *H. diminuta* in Tables II and III may offer stronger support for Naftalin's convective-coupling hypothesis than the results using the rabbit ileum where there may be some confusion concerning the route of transepithelial water transport. The convective-coupling hypothesis requires that water traverses the brush border membrane whereas there is substantial evidence that regulation of volume flow across epithelia is controlled by the shunt pathway (Hill 1975, 1977). However, this will not be a complicating factor with *H. diminuta* as all water transport across the epithelial syncytium must occur across the brush border. The difficulty of establishing the validity of the convective-coupling hypothesis as a mechanism of nonelectrolyte active transport by *H. diminuta* is the paucity of information regarding water transport in this organism. Studies conducted *in vivo* indicated that water flux in *H. diminuta* could be interpreted in terms of the local osmotic gradient hypothesis provided a fluid circuit is present across the inward-facing membrane to account for the increased solute/water flux ratios as net Na^+ influx is increased in response to extracellular glucose and/or carbon dioxide (Podesta and Mettrick 1975). However, these studies have not been confirmed on the basis of ultrastructural localization of the extracellular channels responsible for the coupling of ion and water flows, or on the basis of *in vitro* investigations. Nevertheless, it should be possible to test the convective-coupling hypothesis in *H. diminuta* following galactose fluxes across the brush border when the direction and volume of water flow across the brush border is altered in anisotonic incubations. The results and implications of this test are discussed below.

3. *Coupling Mechanisms and Volume Regulation.* An increased in net water influx in *H. diminuta* incubated in a hypotonic fluid should increase the convective influx permeability and decrease the efflux permeability of the brush border to galactose if the convective-coupling hypothesis is valid. Conversely, net water efflux in response to a hypertonic incubation should increase efflux and decrease the influx permeability of the outward-facing brush border. However, the results shown in Table IV (Podesta 1980b; Lussier *et al.* 1978) indicate that just the opposite of the predicted effects occurred as the influx permeability was decreased and the efflux permeability increased in response to hypotonic incubations while hypertonicity increased the

TABLE IV. *Summary of Alanine and Galactose Fluxes Across the Brush Border of Hymenolepis diminuta in Response to Anisotonic Incubation.*

Incubation Medium		Permeabilities ($\mu moles/cm^2/h/mM$)					
		Galactose			Alanine		
Tonicity	Na	J^o_{ms}	J^o_{sm}	J^o_{ms}/J^o_{sm}	J^o_{ms}	J^o_{sm}	J^o_{ms}/J^o_{sm}
(mOsm)	(mM)						
250	90	0.394	0.185	2.1	0.316	0.438	0.7
300	90	0.563	0.083	6.8	0.574	0.064	9.0
300	140	0.692	0.058	11.9	0.739	0.041	18.0
350	140	0.741	0.043	17.2	0.781	0.023	34.0

influx and decreased the efflux permeabilities of the brush border to galactose and alanine. I will outline below why incubations in anistonic fluids are not good tests for the convective-coupling hypothesis even though certain aspects of these studies are, indeed, consistent with the diffusive-convective model.

When cell volume is increased due to hypoosmotic swelling, cell volume is regulated back toward normal in virtually all animal cells (Schmidt-Nielsen 1975; Hoffmann 1977). Hypoosmotic cell volume regulation is usually achieved by an increased membrane permeability resulting in an increased passive efflux of K^+ (but Na^+ permeability is not altered) and small organic molecules such as the nonessential amino acids (Hoffmann and Hendil 1976; Hoffmann 1977). *H. diminuta* is an osmoconformer capable of volume regulation in hypotonic fluids and since the total amount of change in tissue ions cannot account for the dilution of tissue fluids, small organic molecules must also play a role in the regulatory volume decrease observed in this organism (Podesta 1980a). It is not surprising, therefore, to find an increased efflux permeability of the brush border of *H. diminuta* to alanine during hypotonic incubations (Table IV), although it is unusual to find a similar response for galactose fluxes during hypoosmotic stress (is the latter an adaptive consequence of these parasites living in a nutrient rich environment?). However, the osmotically induced change in brush border permeability would have to be asymmetrical to explain the decreased influx permeability to both alanine and galactose. Although evidence in this respect is lacking, it is a possibility that requires examination in view of the well-known structural and functional asymmetric properties of biological membranes. The main point concerning the convective-coupling hypothesis is that it was assumed only the volume and direction of water flow across the brush border would be altered in anisotonic incubations and not membrane permeability. This assumption is no longer tenable.

Animal cells are generally less capable of volume regulation in hypertonic media (Schmidt-Nielsen 1975) and again, *H. diminuta* is no exception (Podesta 1977a). However, the influx and efflux permeabilities of the brush border to galactose and alanine (Table IV) are unusual in the sense that there is no known mechanism to account for an increased influx permeability and decreased efflux permeability against the direction of net osmotically induced water flow and opposed to concentration gradients. In most cells, membrane permeability to Na^+ (but not K^+) is increased during the regulatory volume increase in hypertonic extracellular fluids (Schmidt-Nielsen 1975). This may explain the increased amount and concentration of tissue Na^+ of *H. diminuta* incubated in hypertonic fluids (Podesta 1977a). These results may, therefore, be consistent with the convective-coupling hypothesis since an increase in cellular Na^+ would increase the activity of the Na^+-pump located in the inward-facing membrane of the epithelial syncytium. However, this assumes that the routes of water transport across the brush border are different for Na^+-stimulated water transport and osmotically induced water transport.

It is important to consider, however, that the convective-coupling hypothesis related galactose uptake to Na^+-pump activity. There is now substantial evidence which indicates that the mechanism of cell volume regulation is independent of the Na^+-pump activity which is responsible for transepithelial Na^+-sensitive nonelectrolyte transport in *H. diminuta* (Podesta 1977c) and other tissues (Schmidt-Nielsen 1975; Macknight *et al.* 1975; Hoffmann 1977). The flux permeabilities reported in Table IV are osmotically induced fluxes and may not have any relation to Na^+-pump activity. Therefore, osmotically induced fluxes cannot be used as evidence in support of or in contradistinction of the diffusive-convective model or the ion-gradient hypothesis. Nevertheless, in an organism such as *H. diminuta*, osmotically induced fluxes may be of physiological importance. This parasite may encounter an environment of widely fluctuating osmotic characteristics depending on the type of food eaten by its host and the position of the parasites in the postprandial intestine (see Mettrick and Podesta 1974). Moreover, the osmotic characteristics of the tissue fluids in *H. diminuta* will also fluctuate widely in response to environmental levels of carbon dioxide (Podesta *et al.* 1976). Therefore, osmotically induced changes in membrane permeability must be considered in the overall adaptation of this parasite to its intestinal environment.

III. MEMBRANE BIOLOGY

A. Evolutionary Aspects of the Epithelial Syncytium

Why did *Hymenolepis diminuta* and other parasitic flatworms sacrifice the cellular arrangement of their tegument, a feature characteristic of free-living platyhelminths (see Lumsden 1975 a,b), for the acellular epithelial syncytium? In order to gain some insight into this problem, it is necessary to ask the following. First, what advantage has the syncytium over a cellular epithelial layer with respect to ion fluxes between the organism and its environment? Second, does the syncytium allow for better metabolic and electrical cooperation within the field of the epithelial sheet? Third, are electrical signals transferred directly from the environment to the subepithelial neuromuscular system by electrotonic coupling to the epithelial syncytium? Fourth, is the syncytium adaptive in the sense that tight junctional regions exposed at the surface of the parasite, should they have been retained along with a cellular epithelial layer, would be more susceptible to attack and breakdown by the actions of digestive enzymes, bile acids or components of the host's immune system?

1. Transepithelial Electrochemical Potential Gradients. As mentioned previously, the two-membrane model of transporting epithelia has been made more complex by the discovery of permeable tight junctions and the role of the tight junctions in determining the transepithelial resistance and electrical potential differences (see Erlij 1976). With the advent of cable theory, it became obvious that in some epithelia the sum of the resistances of the outward-facing and inward-facing membranes was much higher than the transepithelial resistance. This implied that somewhere in the epithelial layer there occurred pathways of low resistance to the flow of ions (Frömter and Diamond 1972; Ussing *et al.* 1974;

Diamond 1974; Ussing 1975; Erlij 1976). Two lines of evidence indicated that the low resistance pathways in some epithelia coincided with tight junctions. First, the urinary bladder of *Necturus* was mapped for sites of low resistance to current flow and it was demonstrated that the regions of low resistance coincided with the regions of cell contact (Frömter 1972). Second, a striking parallelism was found between the ability of lanthanum to penetrate tight junctions and transepithelial resistance (Erlij 1976). Epithelia have since been categorized as those having 'leaky' cell junctions and those having 'tight' cell junctions; the former correlating with epithelia having low transmural electrical resistance and potential differences while the latter are characteristic of epithelia with larger resistances and electrical potential differences. Accordingly, the variation in the tightness of epithelial tissues leads to two major conclusions. First large ion concentration gradients can be maintained only in 'tight' epithelia. For example, the maximum concentration ratio compatible with active transport is only 12 in the 'leaky' rabbit ileum but is 600 in the 'tight' urinary bladder of the toad (see Erlij 1976). Second, physiological control of transepithelial ion and water transport can be accomplished not only by regulating the permeability properties of the epithelial membranes, but also by altering the resistance of the tight junctions. Osmotic gradients (Erlij 1976) and choleragen (Powell 1974) are two instances where transepithelial fluxes and electrical properties are altered at least in part by their action on the resistance of the shunt pathway.

Although it has not been shown experimentally, the epithelial syncytium of *H. diminuta* can be considered on the above basis to be an extreme case of a 'tight' epithelial layer since it lacks the morphological prerequisites of a shunt pathway. It should, therefore, be capable of maintaining large ion and electrical potential gradients, at least equivalent to those of other 'tight' epithelia such as the amphibian skin and urinary bladder. However, is this the major adaptive feature of the epithelial syncytium for which *H. diminuta* sacrificed a cellular arrangement of its surface epithelial layer? It is evident from the previous discussion of other transporting epithelia, that the major advantage of a 'tight' epithelial layer involves its capacity to maintain larger concentration gradients and, therefore, 'tight' epithelia are more likely to serve an osmoregulatory role. Although recent evidence has indicated that *H. diminuta* volume regulates and has some control over the quantity of tissue ions, and that this regulation is probably confined to the epithelial syncytium (Podesta 1977c), it is unlikely that this aspect of the syncytium is its major adaptive feature. *H. diminuta* inhabits a fluid which is essentially isosmotic with its tissue fluids and therefore osmotic stress is not likely to be of major importance to the adult parasites. Moreover, the free-living platyhelminths have far more severe osmoregulatory problems and yet have retained the cellular arrangement of their surface epithelial layer.

More recently, Augustus *et al.* (1977) have concluded from studies on the electrical and permeability properties of the rabbit submaxillary main duct epithelium that the only criterion establishing whether an epithelium is 'tight' or 'leaky' is the conductance ratio of the cellular and extracellular route. Electrical resistance alone is not sufficient to discriminate between 'tight' and 'leaky' epithelia since, as in the rabbit submaxillary duct, the resistance of the cell membranes can be very low and, combined with 'tight' cell junctions, produces an epithelial layer with a low transepithelial resistance (characteristic of 'leaky' epithelia) but larger electrical gradients and low permeability (characteristic of 'tight' epithelia). This means that the epithelial syncytium of *H. diminuta* cannot be considered 'tight' based solely on the absence of an extracellular shunt pathway. Whether it is 'tight' or 'leaky' will depend on the resistance and permeability properties of the inward- and outward-facing membranes. However, that the epithelial syncytium of *H. diminuta* is 'tight' can be considered reasonably secure based on preliminary experiments indicating a transepithelial potential of (58-92 mV) which is comparable to other 'tight' epithelia (Podesta, unpublished).

Another aspect of the two-membrane model that is presently under discussion is the assumption that the two series membranes behave independently. More recent evidence has indicated that the independence assumption is no longer tenable (Reuss and Finn 1975; Finn 1976). The potentials measured across the outward-facing and inward-facing membranes of the toad urinary bladder epithelial cells changed simultaneously when the composition of the fluid bathing the outward-facing membrane was changed or amiloride added. The dependence of the membrane potential across the inward-facing membrane on the changes produced at the opposite pole of the cell could not be explained by the presence of low resistance extracellular shunt, changes in the resistance of the shunt pathway or by changes in intracellular ion concentrations mediated by diffusion. These results suggested that there is some kind of signal that electrically couples one membrane to the other (Reuss and Finn 1975; Finn 1976). Remarkably, Ussing (1975) has recently demonstrated that fast intracellular ion transport in frog skin may occur via the endoplasmic reticulum. Similar conclusions have been made with respect to ion transport in chloride cells of fish gills (see Potts 1977). It is possible, therefore, that electrical coupling of the inward- and outward-facing membranes of epithelia may be modulated by the endoplasmic reticulum. However, the independence assumption and, if present, the mechanism of electrical signals between the two membranes, is an area where the epithelial syncytium of *H. diminuta* may be obviously and profitably explored since, in this membrane system, there is no plasma membrane contact between the outward and inward membranes.

2. Electrotonic Coupling and Cytoplasmic Resistance. The classic paper of Loewenstein and Kanno (1964) on ionic coupling or electrotonic coupling through gap junctions between the epithelial cells of *Drosophila* salivary gland, renewed interest in this form of intercellular communication in a wide variety of differentiated tissues (see reviews by Bennett 1973; Goldfarb *et al.* 1974; Revel 1974; Loewenstein 1973, 1974, 1975; Gilula and Epstein 1976; Caveney 1976; Larsen 1977). Intercellular communication by exchange of ions and low molecular weight compounds across gap junctions has led to a number of exciting implications with respect to excitability-coupling between excitable cells, metabolic cooperation, cellular differentiation and the spatial patterning of cell types and organization in various tissues (Caveney 1976). Moreover, it appears that control of electrotonic coupling between cells can be achieved by altering the permeability of the junctional regions in response to changing intracellular concentrations of Ca^{++} (Deleze and Loewenstein 1976; Rose and Loewenstein 1976). It has also been suggested that gap junctions may be aggregates of cell membrane hormone receptors, the permeability of which will be controlled by the specific hormones involved (Larsen 1977). The presence of gap junctions, their electrical properties and the demonstration that they are permeable to molecules at least as large as nucleotides (Pitts and Simms 1977), implies that the cell can no longer be considered a biochemical and physiological unit isolated by a plasma membrane. Instead, the functional unit may be the functional syncytium formed by cells in contact through gap junctions.

In the previous section, the epithelial syncytium of *H. diminuta* was considered as an extreme example of a 'tight' epithelium due to the absence of 'tight' junctions and associated lateral extracellular shunt pathways. It is this same feature - the absence of membrane contact between the outward- and inward-facing membranes - which makes the syncytium an extreme example of coupling within the field of the epithelial layer. The epithelial syncytium of *H. diminuta* is, therefore, a morphological syncytium and, by association, a functional syncytium since lateral molecular and ionic diffusion is assured by a continuous layer of cytoplasm. However, the problem remains as to why the parasites did not simply retain a cellular epithelial layer similar to their free-living ancestors and couple the cells through gap junctions. Moreover, in the absence of gap junctions, has *H. diminuta* sacrificed control over cooperation within the morphological and functional syncytium?

Insight into the first problem may be gained by examining a unique environmental factor. *H. diminuta* inhabits the fluid in the small intestine of rats which periodically contains high levels of CO_2 resulting in considerable acidification of the parasite's tissue fluids (Podesta 1980d; Podesta *et al.*

1976). In response to increased levels of ambient CO_2, *H. diminuta* mobilizes the carbonate and phosphate buffer components in small inorganic concretions distributed widely in the parasite's tissues. Since the buffer components are present in the concretions as Ca^{++} precipitates, there also occurs a shift of corpuscular Ca^{++} into the soft tissues in response to increased ambient levels of CO_2 (Podesta 1980c). More important, intracellular Ca^{++} is raised by 22-27% of control intracellular Ca^{++} pools. Moreover, the increase in environmental CO_2 and tissue Ca^{++} concentrations occurs in the postprandial intestine during which time the parasites are most active (see Mettrick and Podesta 1974). Since cell communication through gap junctions may be inhibited by local Ca^{++} concentrations above or below a certain optimal level (Loewenstein 1975; Gilula and Epstein 1976), it would appear advantageous if *H. diminuta* could circumvent the Ca^{++} control of communication in the epithelial layer during periods in which it is exposed to high levels of CO_2. One way to achieve this, although extreme, would be to develop a system of communication and cooperation in the epithelial layer which did not depend on the permeability of gap junctions. In this sense, a morphological syncytium may be considered adaptive given the unique circumstances of high ambient levels of CO_2 and the ensuing responses of *H. diminuta* to minimize tissue acidification.

However, does *H. diminuta* have any control over the lateral transport of ions and molecules in the epithelial syncytium? Cable studies on nerve axons or muscle fibers and dielectric measurements on suspensions of cells, have indicated that the electrical resistivity of cytoplasm of most cells is 2-10 times the resistivity of the extracellular fluid (Foster *et al.* 1976; Zeuthen 1977 a,b). The higher cytoplasmic resistivity suggests low ionic mobility in the cells, perhaps indicating a higher degree of ion binding or water structure in the cytoplasm (Foster *et al.* 1976; Zeuthen 1977 a,b; Ling *et al.* 1973; Lev and Armstrong 1975). Moreover, cytoplasmic resistivity, ionic activity and ion binding may vary in different regions of the cell and may be altered by the action of drugs, hormones, Ca^{++} and metabolic products (Zeuthen 1977 a,b; Ling and Ochsenfeld 1973; Lev and Armstrong 1975). However, studies of electrotonic coupling between cells in response to Ca^{++} (Rose and Loewenstein 1976) or hormones (Caveney 1976; Larsen 1977) are interpreted as changes only in the permeability properties of the gap junctions. However, one may ask whether coupling can be controlled by altering cytoplasmic resistance. Can Ca^{++} levels, hormones, drugs and other factors alter the resistance of the cytoplasm to the lateral movements of ions and molecules in an epithelial layer? Obviously, these are problems for which the epithelial syncytium was 'designed' to investigate. It should be possible to examine cytoplasmic resistance over large areas without plasma membrane interference and regions of cell contact. In this sense, studies on the epithelial syncytium may have considerable impact on a ubiquitous and fundamental concept of membrane biology - the physical state of the cytoplasm.

3. Information Transfer by the Epithelial Syncytium. A number of sensory receptors in the epithelial syncytium of parasitic flatworms have been revealed by ultrastructural studies (see Webb and Davey 1974, 1975). For the most part, the function of these sensory receptors remains unknown but some are thought to be chemoreceptors while others are probably mechanoreceptors. Another mechanism of information transfer which has not been considered previously in parasitic flatworms, but which is responsible for propagation of action potentials in the excitable epithelia of coelenterates (see Kass-Simon 1980), is transfer of electrical signals along and across the syncytium to the underlying muscle cells via electrotonic junctions. Although Koopowitz (1975) argued that a conducting epithelium or a muscle syncytium could not explain the conduction of action potentials recorded extracellularly on the surface of a free-living polyclad, it is apparent from a reexamination of the numerous published electron micrographs of the surface of *H. diminuta* and other parasitic flatworms (see Lumsden 1975 a,b for references) that there occur many regions of junctional cell contact between the cells underlying the epithelial cyncytium. Some of these junctions occur between muscle cells while others involve muscle cells and the inward-facing membrane of the epithelial syncytium. That the latter regions of cell contact may be electrotonic can only be supported by circumstantial evidence. Ambient CO_2 causes an increased flow of fluid in the protonephridial canals of *H. diminuta* by stimulating rhythmic waves of muscle contraction along the length of the parasites (Webster 1971). However, when the brush border of *H. diminuta* has been removed, as in the *contracircum* experiments described previously, the parasites are completely immobile and unresponsive to increased ambient CO_2 (Podesta, unpublished). Since, in the *contracircum* experiments, only the brush border of the epithelial syncytium has been removed, it would appear that there is a relationship between CO_2-stimulated muscle contraction and the brush border. There are a number of responses of *H. diminuta* to increased ambient CO_2 including increased influx of Na^+ across the brush border (Podesta and Mettrick 1975, 1976; Podesta 1980d), increased H^+ secretion (Podesta and Mettrick 1976; Podesta 1980d) and an increase in intracellular Ca^{++} (Podesta 1980c). As evidenced by numerous studies on other types of cells, each of these responses could be accompanied by a depolarization of the brush border membrane of the epithelial syncytium. Recent microelectrode observations have indicated a depolarization of the brush border of 50-60 mV in response to an increase in ambient CO_2 (Podesta, unpublished), although it is not yet certain what ion fluxes are involved. However, the major problem with hypothesizing electrotonic coupling between the syncytium and the underlying cells is coupling an electrical event at the brush border with one occurring across the inward-facing membrane of the syncytium. As discussed previously with reference to the independence assumption of the two membrane hypothesis, electrical coupling between the two series membranes can be accomplished by some mechanism of fast intracellular transport. However, the evidence presented above for a correlation between CO_2-stimulated muscle contraction and the brush border is circumstantial and is not sufficient to establish with any certainty electrotonic coupling between the epithelial syncytium and underlying muscle cells. Although other explanations have not been ruled out, excitability and electrotonic coupling between the syncytium and underlying cells should be considered as a possible feature of the epithelial syncytium that deserves further study.

4. *Adaptation of Syncytium to Digestive, Detergent and Immunological Attack.* Another possible adaptive feature of the epithelial syncytium relates to several unique aspects of the parasitic habitat.

Invariably, endoparasites are exposed to and have had to contend with the host's immune response and, in the intestinal habitat occupied by *H. diminuta*, the host's digestive enzymes and the detergent activity of bile acids. A number of recent studies have demonstrated that immunoglobulin (Befus 1977), digestive enzymes (Pappas and Read 1972 b,c; Ruff and Read 1973), and bile acids (Surgan and Roberts 1976) are bound to and, in most cases, inactivated by the outward-facing brush border membrane of *H. diminuta*. The binding and inactivation of these environmental chemical factors is thought to be a property of the glycocalyx or some other surface property of the microvilli on the surface of the parasites. Since the brush border of the syncytium is not interrupted by tight junctions and since an exposed tight junctional region of a cellular epithelial layer would presumably not have the protective function associated with the glycocalyx, making it more susceptible to immunological, detergent or digestive attack, it is not unreasonable to speculate that this would be a major adaptive feature leading to the development of the epithelial syncytium in the endoparasitic platyhelminths. The correlation between endoparasitism and the surface epithelial syncytium tends to support this hypothesis. However, the major challenge to present and future generations of parasitologists is to develop the means by which to test this hypothesis.

IV. SUMMARY AND CONCLUSIONS

Krebs (1975) recently discussed the importance in comparative physiology of the August Krogh Principle - that for most physiological problems there exists an animal, because of its unique design, upon which the problem can be most conveniently studied. Classic examples include the transmission of nerve impulses by squid axons, permeability of red cells and giant algal cells, circulatory dynamics in turtles, fertilization of sea urchin eggs, and so on through a long list of 'model' tissues. It is the role of comparative physiologists to first, discover and choose favorable animal models in which to explore certain physiological concepts, and second, to examine other animal models to ascertain the general applicability of the concept. In this sense, C.P. Read and his colleagues (see Pappas and Read 1975) first suggested and investigated the usefulness of cestodes in studies of membrane transport. They are responsible for recognizing that the surface of cestodes, which lack oral and alimentary systems, was adapted for nutrient uptake and resembled the vertebrate gut in having an outward-facing brush border membrane. Subsequent studies by Read and co-workers (see Pappas and Read 1975) established the remarkable similarity in terms of permeability and transport functions of the brush border membrane of cestodes and the mammalian small intestine. However, unlike studies concerned with mammalian gut and other epithelial tissues, parasitologists did not venture beyond the brush border membrane and therefore failed to recognize that they were dealing with an epithelial layer. As concluded in the present review, recognition of this fact leads to a number of exciting features of the cestode epithelial model which are of general interest and applicability to studies of epithelial physiology.

First, the epithelial syncytium of *H. diminuta* is of obvious importance as a model tissue to test the validity of the two-membrane model of transporting epithelia. In its original form, this model adequately described the electrical properties of most epithelia studied and predicted vectorial ion and molecular transport across epithelia as a consequence of the asymmetric permeability properties of the outward-facing and inward-facing membranes of epithelial layers. Since extracellular shunt pathways for transepithelial ion flow, which are absent in *H. diminuta* were not considered in the original two-membrane model, it should be a precise description of the morphological and functional properties of the epithelial syncytium of *H. diminuta* (see Section IIA). Recent studies have confirmed the validity of the two-membrane model with respect to ion and sugar fluxes across the epithelial syncytium (see Section IIB). Since the epithelial syncytium is uninterrupted by tight junctions and associated paracellular pathways, it is a model system in which the properties and regulation of the transcellular pathway of epithelial transport can be investigated in isolation (see Section IIIA1). Moreover, in the absence of plasma membrane contact between the outward- and inward-facing membrane, the validity of the independence assumption can be examined profitably using the epithelial syncytium (see Section IIIA1). If the independence assumption is found to be untenable, as in other epithelia, then the mechanisms of electrical signalling between the two membranes should be more easily revealed using this model tissue. It is not too late, therefore, for studies using the cestode epithelial syncytium to contribute significantly to the general theory of transport across epithelial tissues.

Second, the absence of membrane barriers to the lateral movement of solutes within the epithelial syncytium also leads to a number of exciting, but still speculative, possible properties of this tissue. Metabolic cooperation within the surface epithelial layer of *H. diminuta* is an obvious consequence of it being a morphological as well as a functional syncytium (see Section IIIA2). In view of recent studies on cytoplasmic resistance, however, control of lateral movement in the syncytium may be found in altered resistance of the cytoplasm. This is an attractive problem with the epithelial syncytium which is a large sheet of cytoplasm in which resistance measurements could be made without interference from membrane barriers. Since cytoplasmic resistance remains an area of controversy in cell biology the epithelial syncytium of *H. diminuta* is of obvious importance in this respect (see Section IIIA2). Electrical coupling between the syncytium and muscle cells underlying the epithelial syncytium through gap junctions is also a possible function of the epithelial layer which deserves attention (see Section IIIA3).

Third, in any discussion of the advantages of a syncytial over a cellular epithelial layer in *H. diminuta* it is necessary to consider that the syncytium appears to be an adaptation to parasitism in the platyhelminths (see Section IIIA4). The syncytial structure may, therefore, have developed as a barrier protecting the parasite against the several unique environmental factors encountered in the parasitic habitat, including digestive enzymes, bile salts and immunoglobulins. It has been shown that each of the latter factors are bound to, and presumably inactivated, by some as yet unidentified component of the brush border surface of *H. diminuta*. Although evidence is completely lacking, it is possible that exposed tight junctional regions, should *H. diminuta* have retained a cellular epithelial layer, would be more susceptible to attack by digestive enzymes, bile acids and antibodies since tight junctions would not have the same surface binding properties of the brush border. Testing this assumption on a system which represents the end result of an evolutionary selection process represents a considerable challenge.

A number of other aspects of membrane biology in *H. diminuta* have not been considered in the present review but are no less demanding of investigation. Of major importance are the effects on transport of immunoglobulin bindings to the brush border surface (see Befus and Podesta 1976) and the ionic and membrane events accompanying excitability in neural and neuromuscular tissues (see Podesta 1978a). Virtually no attention has been given the membrane physiology of sensory receptors (see Webb and Davey 1974, 1975) or inexcitable, nonpolarized parenchymal tissues (see Podesta 1980a). Another area which has been overlooked is the role of membrane surface properties in the differentiation of parenchymal cells into male and female genitalia in individual parasites. These, and other problems discussed above, point to a very promising future for studies of membrane biology in *H. diminuta*.

REFERENCES

1. Arme, C., Tapeworm-host interactions. *In* "Symbiosis", *Symp. Soc. Exp. Biol.* 29, pp. 505-532 (1975).
2. Arme, C., Feeding. *In* "Ecological Aspects of Parasitology" (C. R. Kennedy, ed.), pp. 76-97. North-Holland, Amsterdam, (1976).
3. Augustus, J., Bijman, J., van Os, C. H., and Slegers, J. F. G., High conductance in an epithelial membrane not due to extracellular shunting. *Nature, Lond.* 268, 657-658 (1977).

4. Befus, A. D., *Hymenolepis diminuta* and *H. microstoma*: Mouse immunoglobulins binding to the tegumental surface. *Exp. Parasitol. 41*, 242-251 (1977).
5. Befus, A. D., and Podesta, R. B., Intestine. In "Ecological Aspects of Parasitology" (C. R. Kennedy, ed.), pp. 303-325. North-Holland, Amsterdam, (1976).
6. Bennett, M. V. L., Function of electrotonic junctions in embryonic and adult tissues. *Fed. Proc. Soc. Fedn. Am. Socs. Exp. Biol. 32*, 65-75 (1973).
7. Caveney, S., The insect epidermis: a functional syncytium. In "The Insect Integument" (H. R. Hepburn, ed.), pp. 259-274. Elsevier, Amsterdam, (1976).
8. Cereijido, M., and Rotunno, C. A., "Introduction to the Study of Biological Membranes". Gordon and Breach, N.Y., (1970).
9. Christensen, H. N., Does the stoichiometry of coupling necessarily reveal the composition of the ternary complex? In "Na-linked Transport of Organic Solutes" (E. Heinz, ed.), pp. 161-165. Springer-Verlag, New York, (1972).
10. Christensen, H. N., "Biological Transport". W. A. Benjamin, London, (1975).
11. Crane, R. K., Hypothesis for mechanism of intestinal active transport of sugars. *Fedn. Proc. Fedn. Amer. Socs. Exp. Biol. 21*, 891-895 (1962).
12. Deleze, J., and Loewenstein, W. R., Permeability of a cell junction during intracellular injection of divalent cations. *J. Membrane Biol. 28*, 71-86 (1976).
13. Diamond, J. M., Standing-gradient model of fluid transport in epithelia. *Fedn. Proc. Fedn. Am. Socs. Exp. Biol. 30*, 6-13 (1971).
14. Diamond, J. M., Tight and leaky junctions of epithelia. *Fedn. Proc. Fedn. Am. Socs. Exp. Biol. 33*, 2220-2224 (1974).
15. Erlij, F., Solute transport across isolated epithelia. *Kidney Int. 9*, 76-87 (1976).
16. Finn, A. L., Changing concepts of transepithelial sodium transport. *Physiol. Rev. 56*, 453-464 (1976).
17. Fisher, F. M., and Read, C. P., Transport of sugars in the tapeworm *Calliobothrium verticillatum*. *Biol. Bull. 140*, 46-62 (1971).

18. Frömter, E., The route of passive ion movement through the epithelium of *Necturus* gallbladder. *J. Membrane Biol.* 8, 259-301 (1972).
19. Frömter, E., and Diamond, J., Route of passive ion permeation in epithelia. *Nature, Lond.* 235, 9-13 (1972).
20. Geck, P., and Heinz, E., Coupling in secondary transport. *Biochim. Biophys. Acta* 443, 49-53 (1976).
21. Gilula, N. B., and Epstein, M. L., Cell-to-cell communication, gap junctions and calcium. *Sym. Soc. Exp. Biol.* 30, 257-272 (1976).
22. Goldfarb, P. S. G., Slack, C., Subaksharpe, J. H., and Wright, E. D., Metabolic cooperation between cells in tissue culture. *Sym. Soc. Exp. Biol.* 28, 463-473 (1974).
23. Grüneberg, A., and Komor, E., Different proton-sugar stoichiometries for the uptake of glucose analogues by *Chlorella vulgaris*. *Biochim. Biophys. Acta* 448, 133-142 (1976).
24. Hill, A. E., Solute-solvent coupling in epithelia: a critical examination of the standing gradient osmotic flow theory. *Proc. R. Soc. Lond. B 190*, 99-114 (1975).
25. Hill, A. E., General mechanisms of salt-water coupling in epithelia. *In:* "Transport of Ions and Water in Animals" (B. L. Gupta, R. B. Moreton, J. L. Oschman, and B. J. Wall, eds.), pp. 183-214. Academic Press, New York and London, (1977).
26. Hoffmann, E. K., Control of cell volume. *In:* "Transport of Ions and Water in Animals" (B. L. Gupta, R. B. Moreton, J. L. Oschman, and B. J. Wall, eds), pp. 285-332. Academic Press, New York and London, (1977).
27. Hoffmann, E. K., and Hendil, K. B., The role of amino acids and taurine in isosmotic intracellular regulation in Ehrlich Ascites mouse tumour cells. *J. Comp. Physiol.* 108, 279-286 (1976).
28. Holman, G. D., and Naftalin, R. J., Galactose transport across the serosal border of rabbit ileum and its role in intracellular accumulation. *Biochim. Biophys. Acta* 382, 230-245 (1975).
29. Hoshi, T., Sudo, K., and Suzuki, Y., Characteristics of changes in the intracellular potential associated with transport of neutral, dibasic and acidic amino acids in *Triturus*

proximal tubule. *Biochim. Biophys. Acta 448*, 492-504 (1976).
30. Jacquez, J. A., "Compartmental Analysis in Biology and Medicine." Elsevier, Amsterdam, (1972).
31. Kass-Simon, G., Aspects of coelenterate membrane physiology. *In:* "Membrane Physiology of Invertebrate Organisms" (R. B. Podesta, ed.). Marcel Dekker Inc., New York, (1980).
32. Koefoed-Johnson, U., and Ussing, H. H., The nature of the frog skin potential. *Acta Physiol. Scand. 42*, 298-308 (1958).
33. Koopowitz, H., Electrophysiology of the peripheral nerve net in the polyclad flatworm *Freemania litoricola*. *J. Exp. Biol. 62*, 469-479 (1975).
34. Kotyk, A., and Janacek, K., "Cell Membrane Transport." Plenum, New York and London, (1975).
35. Krebs, H. A., The August Krogh Principle: "For many problems there is an animal on which it can be most conveniently studied." *J. Exp. Zool. 194*, 221-226 (1975).
36. Larsen, W. J., Gap junctions and hormone action. *In:* "Transport of Ions and Water in Animals" (B. L. Gupta, R. B. Moreton, J. L. Oschman, and B. J. Wall, eds.), pp. 333-362. Academic Press, New York and London, (1977).
37. Lev, A. A., and Armstrong, W. McD., Ionic activities in cells. *Current Topics in Membranes and Transport 6*, 59-123 (1975).
38. Ling, G. N., and Ochsenfeld, M. M., Control of cooperative adsorption of solutes and water in living cells by hormones, drugs, and metabolic products. *Ann. N.Y. Acad. Sci. 204*, 325-336 (1973).
39. Loewenstein, W. R., Membrane junctions in growth and differentiation. *Fedn. Proc. Fedn. Am. Soc. Exp. Biol. 32*, 60-64 (1973).
40. Loewenstein, W. R., Cellular communication by permeable membrane junctions. *Hospital Practice 9*, 113-122 (1974).
41. Loewenstein, W. R., Permeable junctions. *Cold Spring Harbor Sym. Quant. Biol. 40*, 49-63 (1975).

42. Loewenstein, W. R., and Kanno, Y., Studies on an epithelial (gland) cell junction. I. Modification of surface membrane permeability. *J. Cell Biol.* 22, 565-575 (1964).
43. Lumsden, R. D., Surface ultrastructure and cytochemistry of parasitic helminths. *Exp. Parasitol.* 32, 267-339 (1975a).
44. Lumsden, R. D., The tapeworm tegument: a model system for studies on membrane structure and function in host-parasite relationships. *Trans. Amer. Micro. Soc.* 94, 501-507 (1975b).
45. Lussier, P. E., Podesta, R. B., and Mettrick, D. F., *Hymenolepis diminuta*: Na^+-dependent and Na^+-independent components of neutral amino acid transport. *J. Parasitol.* (submitted).
46. MacKnight, A. D. C., Civan, M. M., and Leaf, A., Some effects of ouabain on cellular ions and water in epithelial cells of toad urinary bladder. *J. Membrane Biol.* 20, 387-401 (1975).
47. Mettrick, D. F., and Podesta, R. B., Ecological and physiological aspects of helminth-host interactions in the mammalian gastrointestinal canal. *Adv. Parasitol.* 12, 183-278 (1974).
48. Naftalin, R., and Curran, P. F., Galactose transport in rabbit ileum. *J. Membrane Biol.* 16, 257-278 (1974).
49. Naftalin, R. J., and Holman, G. D., The role of Na as a determinant of the asymmetric permeability of rabbit ileal brush border to D-galactose. *Biochim. Biophys. Acta* 383, 453-470 (1974).
50. Naftalin, R. J., and Holman, G. D., The effects of removal of sodium ions from the mucosal solution on sugar absorption by rabbit ileum. *Biochim. Biophys. Acta* 419, 385-390 (1976).
51. Hystrom, R. A., "Membrane Physiology." Prentice-Hall, New Jersey, (1973).
52. Pappas, P. W., and Hansen, B. D., Chloride-sensitive glucose transport in *Hymenolepis diminuta*. *J. Parasitol.* 63, 800-804 (1977).
53. Pappas, P. W., and Read, C. P., Sodium and glucose fluxes across the brush border of a flatworm (*Calliobothrium verticillatum*, Cestoda). *J. Comp. Physiol.* 81, 215-228 (1972a).
54. Pappas, P. W., and Read, C. P., Trypsin inactivation by intact *Hymenolepis diminuta*. *J. Parasitol.* 58, 864-871 (1972b).

55. Pappas, P. W., and Read, C. P., Inactivation of α- and β-chymotrypsin by intact *Hymenolepis diminuta* (Cestoda). *Biol. Bull. 143*, 605-616 (1972c).
56. Pappas, P. W., and Read, C. P., Membrane transport in helminth parasites: a review. *Exp. Parasitol. 37*, 469-530 (1975).
57. Pappas, P. W., Uglem, G. L., and Read, C. P., *Taenia crassiceps*: absorption of hexoses and partial characterization of Na^+-dependent glucose absorption by larvae. *Exp. Parasitol. 33*, 127-137 (1973).
58. Pappas, P. W., Uglem, G. L., and Read, C. P., Anion and cation requirements for glucose and methionine accumulation by *Hymenolepis diminuta* (Cestoda). *Biol. Bull. 146*, 56-66 (1974).
59. Pitts, J. D., and Simms, J. W., Permeability of junctions between animal cells. *Exp. cell Res. 104*, 153-163 (1977).
60. Podesta, R. B., *Hymenolepis diminuta*: marker distribution volumes of tissues and mucosal extracellular spaces. *Exp. Parasitol. 42*, 289-299 (1977a).
61. Podesta, R. B., *Hymenolepis diminuta*: unstirred water layers and effects on active and passive transport kinetics. *Exp. Parasitol. 43*, 12-24 (1977b).
62. Podesta, R. B., *Hymenolepis diminuta*: electrolyte transport pools of tissues and metabolic inhibitors. *Exp. Parasitol. 43*, 295-306 (1977c).
63. Podesta, R. B., Membrane physiology of helminths. *In* "Membrane Physiology of Invertebrate Organisms" (R. B. Podesta, ed.). Marcel Dekker, Inc., New York, (1980a).
64. Podesta, R. B., Na^+ and galactose transport across the membrane of an epithelial syncytium. *Biochim. Biophys. Acta* (1980b).
65. Podesta, R. B., Displacement of tissue Ca^{++} pools and Ca^{++} secretion stimulated by pH and CO_2 in a parasitic flatworm. *Comp. Biochem. Physiol.* (1980c).
66. Podesta, R. B., Characterization *in vitro* of $H^+ : Na^+$ exchange in response to ambient CO_2 in a parasitic flatworm (*Hymenolepis diminuta*). *Can. J. Zool.* (1980d).

67. Podesta, R. B., and Mettrick, D. F., The effect of bicarbonate and acidification on water and electrolyte absorption by the intestine of normal and infected (*Hymenolepis diminuta*: Cestoda) rats. *Am. J. Dig. Dis. 19*, 725-735 (1974).
68. Podesta, R. B., and Mettrick, D. F., *Hymenolepis diminuta*: acidification and bicarbonate absorption in the rat intestine. *Exp. Parasitol. 37*, 1-14 (1975).
69. Podesta, R. B., and Mettrick, D. F., The interrelationships between the *in situ* fluxes of water, electrolytes and glucose by *Hymenolepis diminuta*. *Int. J. Parasitol. 6*, 163-172 (1976).
70. Podesta, R. B., and Mettrick, D. F., HCO_3 transport in rat jejunum: relationship to NaCl and H_2O transport *in vivo*. *Am. J. Physiol. 232*, E63-E68 (1977a).
71. Podesta, R. B., and Mettrick, D. F., $\overline{HCO_3}$ and H^+ secretion in rat ileum *in vivo*. *Am. J. Physiol. 232*, E62-E68 (1977b).
72. Podesta, R. B., Evans, W. S., and Stallard, H. E., *Hymenolepis diminuta* and *Hymenolepis microstoma*: effect of ouabain on active nonelectrolyte uptake across the epithelial syncytium. *Exp. Parasitol. 43*, 25-38 (1977b).
73. Podesta, R. B., Mustafa, T., Moon, T. W., Hulbert, W. C., and Mettrick, D. F., Anaerobes in an aerobic environment: role of CO_2 in energy metabolism of *Hymenolepis diminuta*. In: "Biochemistry of Parasites and Host-Parasite Relationships" (H. Van den Bossche, ed.), pp. 81-88. Elsevier/North-Holland, Amsterdam, (1976).
74. Podesta, R. B., Stallard, H. E., Evans, W. S., Lussier, P. E., Jackson, D. J., and Mettrick, D. F., *Hymenolepis diminuta*: determination of unidirectional uptake rates for nonelectrolytes across the surface epithelial membrane. *Exp. Parasitol. 42*, 300-317 (1977a).
75. Potts, W. T. W., Fish gills. In: "Transport of Ions and Water in Animals" (B. L. Gupta, R. B. Moreton, J. L. Oschman and B. J. Wall, eds.), pp. 453-480. Academic Press, New York and London, (1977).
76. Powell, D. W., Intestinal conductance and permselectivity changes with theophylline and choleragen. *Am. J. Physiol. 227*, 1436-1443 (1974).

77. Read, C. P., Rothman, A. H., and Simmons, J. E., Studies on membrane transport, with special reference to parasite-host integration. *Ann. N.Y. Acad. Sci. 113*, 154-205 (1963).
78. Read, C. P., Stewart, G. L., and Pappas, P. W., Glucose and sodium fluxes across the brush border of *Hymenolepis diminuta* (Cestoda). *Biol. Bull. 147*, 146-162 (1974).
79. Reuss, L., and Finn, A. L., Dependence of serosal membrane potential on mucosal membrane potential in toad urinary bladder. *Biophys. J. 15*, 71-75 (1975).
80. Revel, J. P., Contacts and junctions between cells. *Sym. Soc. exp. Biol. 28*, 447-459 (1974).
81. Rose, B., and Loewenstein, W. R., Permeability of a cell junction and the local cytoplasmic free ionized calcium concentration: a study with aequorin. *J. Membrane Biol. 28*, 87-119 (1976).
82. Ruff, M. D., and Read, C. P., Inhibition of pancreatic lipase by *Hymenolepis diminuta*. *J. Parasitol. 59*, 105-111 (1973).
83. Schmidt-Nielsen, B., Comparative physiology of cellular ion and volume regulation. *J. exp. Zool. 194*, 207-220 (1975).
84. Schultz, S. G., and Curran, P. F., Coupled transport of sodium and organic solutes. *Physiol. Rev. 50*, 637-718 (1970).
85. Schultz, S. G., and Zalusky, R., Ion transport in isolated rabbit ileum. I. Short circuit current and Na fluxes. *J. gen. Physiol. 47*, 567-584 (1964).
86. Simmons, N. L., and Naftalin, R. J., Factors affecting the compartmentalization of sodium within rabbit ileum *in vitro*. *Biochim. biophys. Acta 448*, 411-425 (1976a).
87. Simmons, N. L., and Naftalin, R. J., Bidirectional sodium ion movements via the paracellular and transcellular routes across short-circuited rabbit ileum. *Biochim. biophys. Acta 448*, 426-450 (1976b).
88. Surgan, M. H., and Roberts, L. S., Absorption of bile salts by the cestodes, *Hymenolepis diminuta* and *H. microstoma*. *J. Parasitol. 62*, 78-86 (1976).

89. Uglem, G. L., Evidence for a sodium ion exchange carrier linked with glucose transport across the brush border of a flatworm (*Hymenolepis diminuta*, Cestoda). *Biochim. Biophys. Acta* 443, 126-136 (1976).
90. Ussing, H. H., Epithelial transport phenomena. *In* "Intestinal Absorption and Malabsorption" (T. Z. Csaky, ed.), pp. 1-7. Raven Press, New York, (1975).
91. Ussing, H. H., and Zehran, K., Active transport of sodium as the source of electrical current in the short-circuited, isolated frog skin. *Acta Physiol. Scand.* 23, 110-127 (1951).
92. Ussing, H. H., Ehrlij, D., and Lassen, U., Transport pathways in biological membranes. *Ann. Rev. Physiol.* 36, 17-49 (1974).
93. Webb, R. A., and Davey, K. G., Ciliated sensory receptors of the unactivated metacestode of *Hymenolepis microstoma*. *Tiss. Cell* 6, 577-598 (1974).
94. Webb, R. A., and Davey, K. G., The gross anatomy and histology of the nervous system of the metacestode of *Hymenolepis microstoma*. *Can. J. Zool.* 53, 661-667 (1975).
95. Webster, L. A., The flow of fluid in the protonephridial canals of *Hymenolepis diminuta*. *Comp. Biochem. Physiol.* 39A, 785-793 (1971).
96. Zeuthen, T., Intracellular gradients of electrical potential in the epithelial cells of the *Necturus* gallbladder. *J. Membrane Biol.* 33, 281-309 (1977a).
97. Zeuthen, T., The vertebrate gall-bladder - the routes of ion transport. *In* "Transport of Ions and Water in Animals" (B. L. Gupta, R. B. Moreton, J. L. Oschman and B. J. Wall, eds.), pp. 511-540. Academic Press, New York and London, (1977b).

IMMUNITY AND *HYMENOLEPIS DIMINUTA*

C. A. Hopkins

Wellcome Laboratories for Experimental Parasitology
University of Glasgow
Glasgow, Scotland

I. HISTORICAL

The history of immunity to intestinal tapeworms essentially starts with Chandler (1939) who carried out a number of experiments with *H. diminuta* in rats as a result of which he concluded that adult worms do not evoke an immune response. Because these results fitted the climate of scientific thought at that time (the intestine was still considered to be outside the body), and because of Chandler's authority and standing in experimental parasitology, his conclusions were not to be challenged for a quarter of a century. [On the other hand, there was abundant evidence that larval stages of tapeworms living in the tissues were strongly immunogenic (reviewed by Weinmann 1970; Gemmell & MacNamara 1972; Gemmell 1976).]

Chandler, in his initial experiments, superimposed a secondary infection on a primary infection. To this day, it is not certain why the worms in the secondary infections were smaller, though it is customary to attribute the poor rate of growth, as Chandler did, to a 'crowding effect'. The possibility, however, that growth was stunted for immunological, rather than physiological, reasons was realized and Chandler decided to eliminate the primary worm infection before challenging, in order to determine whether the rats had acquired resistance. In retrospect, the methods used to remove the primary infection, laparotomy followed by lavaging the intestine with "a large amount of hot water", or the administration of carbon tetrachloride *per os*, were hardly likely to have left the intestine in a fit condition to respond to anything. In the event, both establishment and growth were appreciably less than would have been expected (from his earlier experiments) in untreated rats, but as the worms did no better in the control rats, which had received no primary infection than in the experimentals, Chandler concluded that no acquired immunity existed. Hence, the small size of worms in superinfections, i.e., secondary infections superimposed upon existing primary infections, was "due entirely to a crowding effect and not to immunity in the ordinary sense".

The isolation from immune defences of worms in the intestinal lumen was apparently further confirmed by several studies on *H. nana*, a worm which is exceptional in that both the larval stage (in the mucosa) and adult (in the lumen) can occur in the same animal. Heyneman (1962a) concluded that a larval infection of *H. nana* protects strongly against a second larval infection and has a weak protective effect against the adult, but an adult infection evokes no protective responses against a larval challenge. Similarly, there was evidence that some degree of immunity could be induced against adult *Echinococcus granulosus* by immunizing the host with larval stages (Gemmell 1962), but before 1966, there was no experimental evidence that adult tapeworms could induce a protective immune response. The epidemiological evidence that existed, e.g., the oft-reported observations that *Moniezia expansa* only occurred in lambs (reviewed by Weinmann 1970) and that *Cittotaenia* sp. was found only in the caecum of young rabbits (Boughton 1932), were attributed, possibly correctly, to physiologically mediated age-resistance rather than acquired immunity.

The turning point came when Weinmann (1966) made the critical observation that *H. diminuta* in mice had a short life, the longevity of which depended on the number of worms, "few survived 10 days in multiple (10 worm) infections or 12 days in single worm infections: none survived 15 days ...". He also observed that mice which had received three infections had no worms on day 7 following challenge with 10 cysticercoids, whereas the control mice had an average 5.9 worms. The immunological implication of these results now seems obvious, but they were so contrary to beliefs at the time that Weinmann wrote almost apologetically "lumen-dwelling worms can, *in time*, evoke changes ... sufficient to enhance resistance" (author's italics), "only a transitory immunity appeared to develop against lumen stages", and "a degree of resistance ... probably not surprising considering the tenuous existence of the worms in their abnormal hosts." These quotations are in no way meant to disparage Weinmann's (1964, 1966) work, to the contrary, they are quoted to show how strongly entrenched was the concept that lumen-dwelling worms were non-immunogenic, and hence, how crucial Weinmann's observations were.

Progress after 1966 should have been rapid, immunological 'know-how' was expanding rapidly and great interest had been aroused by the introduction of the first commercial vaccine ("Dictol", Allen & Hanbury, now Glaxo) against a parasitic worm (*Dictyocaulus viviparus*) following the work of Jarrett, Jennings, Martin, McIntyre, Mulligan, Sharp & Urquhart (reviewed by Poynter 1963). But as Weinmann (1970) wrote, work with cestodes lagged, probably because of the "greater economic and medical importance of other metazoans."

Since 1970, a considerable amount of work has been done on the *H. diminuta*/mouse system, which forms the bulk of this review and of our knowledge about the immunological rejection of adult tapeworms from the lumen of the small intestine. This is an extremely good model for laboratory experimentation because of the large amount that is known about the mouse immune mechanism, the availability of inbred strains and the ease with which *H. diminuta* can be maintained. However, it would be of far less value were it not that all the evidence that is accruing from other adult tapeworm/host complexes (*Raillietina cesticillus*/chicken: Gray 1973; *H. microstoma*/mouse: Tan & Jones 1968, Moss 1971, Howard 1977; *H. citelli*/ *Peromyscus maniculatus*: Wassom, DeWitt & Grundmann 1974; *H. citelli*/mouse: Hopkins & Stallard 1974; *H. diminuta*/rat reviewed by Chappell & Pike 1976b) suggests that most, if not all, tapeworms evoke an immune response. How they evade it is probably the most intriguing and important question facing cestodologists at the present time.

II. THE COURSE OF A PRIMARY INFECTION IN MICE

1. *Single Worm Infection*

In young (6-week-old) mice, over 90% of cysticercoids administered by stomach tube establish and grow (Hopkins, Subramanian & Stallard 1972a). It is not necessary to administer opium (Read & Voge 1954) or morphine (Weinmann 1966) at the time of infection. A large number of factors influence how long *H. diminuta* survives, but in general, the immune response appears first to affect growth about days 6-8 and to cause loss of worms from days 8-10 onwards, 90% rejection being reached sometimes as early as day 11, but in other cases not until day 16, or exceptionally, day 18. There is, however, ambiguity as Befus & Featherston (1974) have pointed out, by what different people take as time of rejection. They (Befus & Featherston) used the term to mean "the first day when <50% of the worms administered[1] were recovered (including only worms >0.1 mg)". This problem of how best to measure rejection is not an easy one to resolve as there are disadvantages to all methods. The difficulties are often not appreciated by nematode immunologists and hence bedevil communication. The four principal parameters used and their limitations are:

---

[1]*Here and elsewhere in this chapter, for brevity, animals are referred to as having an infection of x worms, when strictly it should be stated that x cysticercoids were administered. However, it is usual for at least 80-90% of administered cysticercoids to become established in rats, mice and hamsters, so the error introduced is small. In experiments where this may not have been the case, the number of cysticercoids administered (by stomach tube) is stated.*

1. *Total Number of Worms*. The major disadvantage of this method is that it does not distinguish between large and destrobilated worms. It is also very time consuming to determine and introduces a source of potential error - the difficulty of finding worms, often less than 1 mm in length, in the intestine.

2. *Number of Worms, Excluding Destrobilated Worms*. This is a better parameter, but it introduces subjective decisions, e.g., how to distinguish between a worm that has grown poorly - a 'runt', and a worm that has grown and destrobilated. This distinction is particularly difficult in secondary infections where worms show little growth.

3. *Mean Worm Weight*. This is usually useless. Adding the weights of worms weighing possibly 20-100 mg to those weighing less than 1 mg is a statistical horror and the mean weight obtained is totally misleading. The diligence of the observer in finding or failing to find small worms greatly affects the mean.

4. *Biomass*. The total weight of worms recovered from a group of mice. In most instances this is the most satisfactory parameter and it has the great advantage that it makes little difference whether destrobilated or small worms are missed (as their weight is minute) and it calls for no arbitrary decisions about when a worm should be counted as a worm or excluded as a 'destrobe'. There is one major disadvantage. Up to about day 16 p.i. (post infection) *H. diminuta* grows almost exponentially (in rats or immunosuppressed mice), approximately doubling its weight every day during the period days 6-14. This means that the biomass of worms recovered from a group of mice may continue to rise even though worms are being rejected, because growth in surviving worms can more than compensate for the weight of the worms lost.

2. Influence of Worm Number (= Worm Burden)

Befus (1975a, Fig. 1) found that the main loss of worms occurred on day 11 ± 1 in six-worm infections, whereas in single worm infections 50% loss did not occur until day 16. A similar pattern was observed by the writer with 1, 3, 6, 12 and 24 worm infections. Rejection, defined as first day on which only destrobilated worms remained in 90% of the mice, occurred on days 16, 14, 11, 10 and 9, respectively. Three points arise. There appears to be no low threshold below which rejection does not occur, as there is with *H. citelli* (Hopkins & Stallard 1974) and *H. microstoma* (Hopkins, Goodall & Zajac 1977), but although one *H. diminuta* evokes a response, "six-worm infections provide more predictable results" (Befus 1975a, p. 73). There is little point in using infections of more than 6-12 worms, as the response is not materially accelerated by larger numbers of worms and the minimum time for induction and rejection appears to be about 8 days. Andreassen (personal communication, 1977) using 100 cysticercoid infections found only destrobilated worms (or runts?) by day 5, but factors other than an immunologically mediated response may have been involved in so heavy an infection.

3. Influence of Age of Host

Befus & Featherston (1974) found mice <5 weeks old at time of infection took, on average, about 4 days longer to reject their worms than did mice 5-7 weeks old. This, as the authors point out, correlates well with many reports on the development of the gut-associated lymphoid tissue in mice. In the Peyer's patches, which may be the antigen trapping region of the small intestine (Parrott 1976, p. 8), considerable changes in the lymphocyte population occur with the appearance of the germinal centres in 4-5 week-old mice (Ferguson & Parrott 1972). This leads to a switch from a predominantly T-cell to a predominantly B-cell population. There is also a dramatic increase between 3 and 6 weeks after birth in the number of intraepithelial lymphocytes (Ferguson & Parrott 1972); cells which Parrott (1976) suggests are "effector T-cells".

As mice age, growth of worms frequently becomes poorer, for instance, the total dry weight of 9-day-old *H. diminuta* recovered from 10 mice, infected with three cysticercoids each when 5 or 7 weeks old, was 45 mg (27/30 worms recovered) and 42 mg (25/30 recovered) respectively, whereas sibling mice allowed to grow until 13 weeks and 19 weeks old before infection yielded only 10.6 mg (23/30 recovered) and 9.9 mg (24/30). (Approximately half of the total mass of the worms from the 10 older mice came in each case from a single mouse.) The situation is confused as the age effect is not consistent, occasionally good growth occurs in some older mice and vice versa. Undoubtedly this reflects interaction between several variables. Potentially, older mice should support better growth because of their larger carbohydrate intake, but the dominant variable is probably the development of the gut-associated lymphoid tissue depressing growth of the worms at an earlier stage and possibly the degree to which the immune system and its effector mechanisms, e.g., macrophages, polymorphs, mast cells, etc., are committed, at the time of the tapeworm infection to intercurrent infections elsewhere in the body. Until more is known about how the immune system does express itself, there is probably little to be gained in trying to measure the effect of age of the mouse on rejection. There is one other relevant observation; the effect of age is completely annulled by cortisone, worms grow as well in old as in young mice when cortisone is given and there is no rejection.

4. Influence of Strain of Mouse

Weinmann (1966) made the original observation on the rejection of *H. diminuta* using Swiss albino mice; Hopkins *et al.* (1972a) recorded rejection in 'CFLP' and 'Porton'. Isaak, Jacobson & Reed (1975), Bland (1976a) and Andreassen, Hindsbo & Ruitenberg (1978), respectively, found littermates (see Section V5) of BalbC (*nu/nu*), an unidentified *nu/nu* strain, and $B_{10}LP$ (*nu/nu*) rejected *H. diminuta*, and the writer has used C57, C3H, NIH, CBA and CD1 mice. All strains reject *H. diminuta*, but without simultaneous infections in different strains of mice in the same laboratory it is impossible to say whether there are differences.

5. Influence of Host Sex

There is little difference in the rate of growth and time of rejection of tapeworms in young, 6-8 week-old, male and female mice. In older mice, bigger differences have occasionally been observed, but these may have been due to stress associated with increased fighting among males.

6. Pregnancy and Lactation

There is no published information about the effect of pregnancy or lactation on the survival of *H. diminuta* and I am indebted to Dr. Peter Christie for a synopsis of his recent work in this field. The most obvious feature is that both pregnant and lactating mice often support enormous worms stretching the length of the small intestine, which weigh upwards of 200 mg dry weight. This is a similar size to worms growing in a cortisone-suppressed host (Section IV1). It is, however, wrong to assume this large size is solely due to modulation of the immune response. Hormonal changes lead to gut hypertrophy, greatly increased food intake (Elias & Dowling 1976) and almost certainly to an increase in the exocrino-enteric flow. All of these changes probably contribute to the faster growth of *H. diminuta* in pregnant and lactating mice compared with that in nulliparous mice. There is also the possibility of an effect on the tapeworm either directly by sex hormones or indirectly through changes in the gastro-intestinal hormones which are associated with hypertrophy of the intestine (Johnson 1976).

Apart from the worms growing more quickly, the rejection of *H. diminuta* is delayed by 4-5 days. In pregnant and lactating mice, growth slows 12-14 days p.i. and rejection occurs 14-20+ days p.i., whereas in nulliparous siblings, growth slows 7-9 days p.i. and rejection occurs 10-14 days p.i.

What causes the diminished response to *H. diminuta* by a lactating or pregnant mouse is unknown. Although the phenomenon of a weaker immunological response in pregnancy is well established (Anderson 1971; Stern 1975; Skowron-Cendrzak, Ptak, Bubak & Czarnik 1975), there is much controversy as to how it occurs (briefly reviewed with reference to the mouse, Rembiesa, Ptak & Bubak 1974), what is affected, and the extent to which different species of mammals respond in the same way. It is also well established that "during lactation, and sometimes during late pregnancy, the immune response of the host to its gastrointestinal nematodes is partially suppressed" (Connan 1976). [There is a paradox however, in that 'foetal immunologists' have in general emphasized the suppression of the immune response during pregnancy, associated, one assumes, with avoiding the rejection of the conceptus which is an allograft, whereas 'parasite-immunologists' have found the mother's immune response against parasites suppressed much more markedly during lactation.] Sensitization to *H. diminuta* occurs during pregnancy and lactation, i.e., a mouse which has had a primary *H. diminuta* infection (chemically terminated) while pregnant and/or lactating gives a secondary response when challenged after the end of lactation. It is the expression of the response, to either a primary or secondary infection, that is depressed. From many immunological investigations, it seems probable that it is T-cell, not B-cell, dependent functions which are particularly affected (Fabris 1973) which suggests that T-cells or T-cell dependent mechanisms are involved in the rejection of *H. diminuta* (Section V5).

III. SECONDARY INFECTION AND MEMORY

The single most important experiment which indicates that rejection is immunologically mediated is the demonstration of memory. From a practical point of view, establishment that memory not only exists but lasts for a considerably time is essential if an estimate is to be made of the potential value of a vaccine (Section IX).

Weinmann (1966) observed that mice, challenged 4 weeks after the third of three, one cysticercoid, *H. diminuta* immunizing infections given at 10 day intervals, were completely resistant to a 10 *H. diminuta* cysticercoid challenge infection (autopsied day 7 p.i.). Although he did not investigate the duration of memory in *H. diminuta*, he did observe that with *H. citelli* a single immunizing infection of 10 cysticercoids gave good protection against an homologous challenge 65 days later but protection had disappeared when the mice were challenged 181 days after the primary. Weinmann's results, when looked at in detail, suggest (i) fewer worms establish in secondary infections, (ii) worms that do establish grow less well, and (iii) based on one group of 10 mice only, that memory in mice to *H. citelli* is short lived.

Later investigations (Hopkins *et al.* 1972a) confirmed that a challenge infection given 22 days after the primary gave rise to severely stunted worms. However, although fewer worms were recovered from immunized, than from control mice, it was not clear whether this was due to fewer worms establishing, earlier rejection, or as Befus (1975a) suggested the greater difficulty of finding worms because of their small size in immunized mice. From evidence obtained by surgically transplanting worms into immunized mice (see below), it is almost certain that establishment is not affected. Whether rejection occurs more quickly is also doubtful, Befus (1975a) (to his surprise) could find no evidence that worms in a secondary infection were actually rejected more quickly than in a primary. There was, however, no doubt that growth ceased earlier in a secondary infection thereby giving severely stunted worms.

Duration of memory has been investigated in two ways by the writer. Mice which had received a five-worm immunizing infection at 6 weeks of age and a booster infection of three worms when 9-weeks-old followed by an anthelmintic at 11 weeks of age were found to remain highly resistant to a cysticercoid challenge infection up to the end of the experiments 4 months later. In another experiment, mice which had been immunized when 7-weeks-old with an infection of eight worms, received intra-duodenal transplants of a single 7-day-old worm from donor mice (Section VI). Nearly all surgically transplanted worms became established and, in naive mice, continued to grow during the ensuing 6 days; in immunized mice, worm growth stopped in 2-3 days and all worms were rejected by day 6. The experiment was continued, testing the mice at intervals for 6 months without showing any weakening in resistance. There appears no doubt, therefore, that real immunological memory is evoked, not just a transient change in reactivity of the intestine-wall and that memory persists for at least 6 months.

Another aspect of memory induction which has been looked at is the minimum duration of an infection necessary to evoke a secondary response to a challenge infection. This has turned out to be a surprisingly short time. A primary infection would normally grow for at least 7-10 days, survive for 9-15 days with worms reaching a length of 5-10 cm and having a dry weight of 1-10 mg. Such mice, when challenged on day 21, are strongly resistant but so are mice in which a three-worm infection has been terminated (by drugs) on day 3 p.i., by which time the cysticercoids have grown only into minute worms about 2 mm long, with a dry weight probably not exceeding 10 µg. It cannot, of course, be assumed that the termination of the infection on day 3 means the termination of antigenic stimulus. The point of interest is that the experiment shows how little tapeworm tissue is necessary to evoke a response and it gives some support to those workers who believe that it is the scolex (and/or neck) region that is of primary importance as the source of antigens (Section V1).

IV. IMMUNOSUPPRESSANTS

1. *Cortisone*

Using cortisone acetate, Hopkins, Subramanian & Stallard (1972b) reported 1.25 mg i.m. every 48 hours completely suppressed rejection up to day 18 and permitted worms to continue increasing in weight as they do in rats until maturity and egg loss commenced about day 17 by which time the worms were enormous, stretching from just behind the stomach into the caecum. This result has been repeatedly verified and it is now known that a regimen of 1 mg/mouse i.m. (or s.c.) thrice weekly will permit worms to continue growing at least until day 45 (Hopkins & Stallard 1976).

The effect of cortisone is also quantitative, if the dose given is reduced to half on day 20 p.i. (0.5 mg/thrice weekly instead of 1 mg), worms are still retained but decrease in size until a new (lower) weight plateau is reached (*ibid*, Fig. 2). One possible explanation is that at 1 mg/thrice weekly, the level of cortisone is sufficient to completely prevent damage by the immune response, but that 0.5 mg is effective for only part of the injection period. This could lead to worm growth being inhibited and worm weight decreasing until a new dynamic equilibrium is established between the reduced amount of growth and loss of proglottids and eggs.

Although quite a lot is known about the effect on the rejection of *H. diminuta* of different levels of cortisone and the effect of starting or stopping cortisone on different days post infection (*ibid*), it must be admitted that nothing is known about how cortisone has its effect. One may reasonably assume from its speed of action in inhibiting loss of badly damaged, i.e., destrobilated worms, that one function is to suppress the effector mechanism of the immune response, but as it is not known what damages a tapeworm and leads to its expulsion, one can only speculate on how cortisone prevents it. There are many possibilities mostly revolving around the well documented "profound suppressive effects (glucocorticoids have) on almost every step of the inflammatory process" (Kantor 1976). Cortisone alters the permeability of the intestine (Jarrett, Jarrett, Miller & Urquhart 1968), inhibits release of prostaglandins (Lewis & Piper 1975), inactivates complement (Gewurz, Wernick, Quie & Good 1965), stabilizes the lysosomal membrane and thereby inhibits release of lytic enzymes by polymorphs (Baggiolini 1972) and blocks activation of macrophages by lymphokines (Claman 1975). Apart from an immediate action on the effector mechanism, it is certain that cortisone will greatly affect the inductive pathway. Again, a very voluminous literature exists describing *inter alia*: lymphocytolytic effects - immature thymocytes seem particularly susceptible (Lance 1972, p. 200), lymphopaenia - possibly through death of cells but partly at least through divagation of lymphocytes from the circulation (Moorhead & Claman 1972), inhibition of B-cells (Cohen & Claman 1971), decreased response to phytomitogens (Fye, Moutsopoulos & Talal 1977), monocytopaenia (which can last for 14 days if 0.6g insoluble hydrocortisone acetate is injected (Thompson & Van Furth 1970)), inhibition of release of monocytes from the bone marrow (Thompson & Van Furth 1973) and very many other effects, any or all, of which could greatly impede either the induction of a humoral or a cell mediated response. Unfortunately, for many statements, one can find a contradictory one. This reflects the extreme complexity and variety of processes in the host that corticosteroids affect, the variety of glucocorticosteroids (and the products they are converted into following injection), and the great variation between mammals in their susceptibility to steroids. In general, rats and mice have lymphocytes which are extremely sensitive, hence cortisone injections lead to rapid death of lymphocytes (shown grossly by decrease in size of lymph nodes and spleen), whereas human and guinea pig lymphocytes are extremely resistant to glucocorticosteroids. Even within a species, there is probably considerable variation. Despite our lack of understanding as to how cortisone works (reviewed by Claman 1972, 1975; Berenbaun 1974), it remains the best tolerated and most effective suppressor of rejection by a mouse of *H. diminuta*.

2. *Cyclophosphamide*

Cyclophosphamide (Cy) has been used extensively as an immunosuppressant (Hill 1975). It is a cytostatic drug and hence is likely to be particularly effective against short-lived rapidly dividing B-cells. Histological examination of lymph nodes has confirmed this as, following Cy treatment, the B-cell areas are severely depleted, whereas there is little effect on the lymphocytes in the thymus dependent areas (Turk & Poulter 1972). Hopes that Cy would prove useful in distinguishing between humoral (antibody) and cellular (CMI) responses were not realised as both types of response involve rapid cell division and hence were suppressed when Cy was given after stimulating the response. Turk, Parker & Poulter (1972), however, noted that when Cy was given before antigen challenge, although antibody production was partially suppressed, the CMI response was strengthened and prolonged. In later work, Turk & Parker (1973) and Katz, Parker, Sommer & Turk (1974) showed that it was particularly the weak CMI responses (sometimes called Jones-Mote or cutaneous basophil hypersensitivity) that were enhanced by giving Cy before presenting the antigen to the sensitized animal. This enhancement they concluded was due to the Cy depleting not only the B-cells which would produce antibodies but B suppressor cells which would normally modulate a CMI response (see also Parker & Turk 1978).

The effect of Cy as an immunosuppressant is not entirely due to its cytolytic effect on dividing lymphocytes. Balow, Parrillo & Fauci (1977) have shown "cyclophosphamide can selectively suppress certain functional capabilities of lymphocytes independently of either cell death or depletion of lymphocyte subpopulations", and Winklestein (1973) suggested that CMI responses [in the expression of which macrophages are important - Mackaness (1970)] are inhibited at least in part by cyclophosphamide's action on the rapidly dividing monocytic precursors of macrophages in the bone marrow. The conclusion is that, as with cortisone, Cy affects many systems in the body with some processes, particularly those involving dividing cells being more sensitive than others. Irrespective of how Cy has its effect, some results are clear. For instance, there is acute lymphopaenia with a 97% decrease in circulating small lymphocytes at the nadir, 3 days after injecting a single dose of 300 mg kg^{-1} i.p. (Turk & Poulter 1972). Recovery to a normal level occurs in about 7 days.

As might be predicted, Cy prevents the rejection of *H. diminuta* by mice. Using a three worm infection in CFLP mice, the writer found a regimen of 150, 100, 75, 75 mg kg^{-1} of Cy, administered i.p. on days -1, +3, 7 and 11 of an infection, delayed rejection until about day 25. The untreated mice rejected their worms on day 12 ± 2. Although the mice receiving Cy were immunosuppressed throughout the duration of the primary infection in the controls, no tolerance was induced. This dose regimen is about the maximum amount that can be given to CFLP mice; it leads to massive loss in body-weight, over 20%, and some deaths. Clearly, the mice are severely stressed and results from such experiments are of very limited value. In the experiment quoted, it is impossible to say how long the effect of Cy persisted on the various parts of the immune system, whether any part of the rejection process commenced under Cy or when the immune system began as a whole to respond to the worms. However, as Cy remains active in the body for only a few hours (Hill 1975, p. 69), the drug could be of value in a single large dose (300 mg kg^{-1}), like whole-body irradiation (Section IV5), as a 'blanket' suppressor of the immune response. Following this, the value of specific groups of cells, recovered from naive and immune donor mice could be assessed by determining the effectiveness of such cells to restore the ability of Cy treated mice to reject worms.

From a wide range of experiments in which various regimens were tested, it was found that as the dose of Cy was reduced to a level at which it had little effect on mouse body-weight (e.g., 50 mg kg^{-1} every 4 days) so also did the effect of Cy on prolonging the survival of worms decrease. The best compromise between toxicity to the mouse and effectiveness in delaying rejection appears to be a regimen of about 300 mg kg^{-1} in total. Interpretation of the results is easier if the Cy is given either as two doses of 200 and 100 mg kg^{-1} 4 days apart or as a single dose of 250-300 mg kg^{-1}.

As Cy enhances instead of suppressing weak CMI responses (mediated by T-cells) when administered before antigen presentation, and bearing in mind that the rejection of tapeworms certainly involves T-cells (Section V5), it is of interest to know the effect of Cy given before a tapeworm infection. This has been studied using both a two dose regimen (200 mg kg^{-1} day -6 and 100 mg kg^{-1} day -2) and a single dose regimen of 250 mg kg^{-1} administered on one of the days, 2-10 days before infecting the mice. The effect is the same as giving Cy after infecting, i.e., in all the regimens used, rejection was suppressed, not enhanced, though Cy administered more than 4 days before infecting the mice with worms had a progressively less suppressive effect (as shown by comparing the weight of the worms recovered from groups of 10 mice on day 11 p.i.). In general, all results indicate that the effect of Cy on rejection is a quantitative one; the more Cy given, the more cells are killed, the greater the loss in body weight of the mouse, and the slower the recovery of the ability to respond to the worm.

3. Methotrexate

Methotrexate is another drug which was developed to inhibit division of malignant cells. It functions by linking to dihydrofolate reductase thereby preventing this enzyme reducing dihydrofolate to the active tetrahydrofolate. The latter is essential for purine and thymine synthesis, blocking of which stops nucleic acid synthesis. Part of methotrexate's immunosuppressive action presumably stems from the blocking of the cell multiplicative process which is essential after sensitization of a lymphocyte by contact with antigen.

Hopkins *et al.* (1972b) found 0.125 mg i.m. every 48 hours inhibited rejection and permitted worms to continue to grow until day 16; thereafter growth inhibition and worm loss occurred. As the authors remark, this was probably due to physiological changes in the intestine. By day 16, the methotrexate had profoundly affected cell division in the intestine wall and the whole intestine was clearly, both by smell and sight, abnormal.

4. Antilymphocyte Serum (ALS)

Antilymphocyte serum should be a good immunosuppressor since, unlike the other immunosuppressive agents, it is more specific to the immune system, rather than having a general metabolic effect which happens to affect rapidly dividing cells of the immune system more than most other tissues.

ALS (or ATS - antithymocytic serum - if it is prepared by raising an antiserum against thymus cells) has its main effect against T-lymphocyte mediated responses, i.e., CMI and certain humoral responses (de Sousa 1973). Many antibody responses, however, are not greatly affected. It has been extensively used to suppress graft rejection and for treatment of auto-immune diseases, like SLE (systemic lupus erythematosus).

Only one experiment investigating the effect of ALS (actually ATS) on the rejection of *H. diminuta* by mice has been reported (Hopkins *et al.* 1972b). In this experiment, ATS was administered subcutaneously on days -2, 0 and +5 post infection and rejection was delayed, but the results (2/10 large worms surviving on day 16) are not very impressive. Featherston (unpublished) carried out a much more extensive investigation and found no difference between a regimen in which ATS was administered on days -2, 0, 2, 5, 7 and 10, and another in which it was given only on days +2, 5, 7 and 10. In both cases, rejection occurred about day 20 compared with day 14 in the controls. This was a substantially shorter lived effect than had been anticipated as such a course of ATS would have been expected to greatly deplete the T-cell population. [In rats infected with 100 worms, Hindsbo & Andreassen (1976) observed a similar short delay in rejection, from day 10 in the controls to day 16 in the ATS-treated (Section VIII).]

In two other experiments differing only in minor details, no delay in rejection was observed. Such results might indicate that T-cells play only a small role in rejection (Section V5). More probably it indicates considerable variations in the potency of the ATS, and controls showing that the ATS was suppressing rejection of skin allografts would give one more confidence in interpreting the results.

5. *X-Irradiation*

Although irradiation by γ- or X-rays has long been used to suppress cell division in cancers and as an immunosuppressant, there is still no certain knowledge as to which subsets of lymphocytes are radiosensitive. Beverley (1977) in his review states "in general, humoral are more sensitive than cell-mediated responses .... because antibody forming cell precursors, B-cells, are more radiosensitive

than at least some T effector precursors", but
X-irradiation at higher doses certainly inhibits
CMI responses (Turk 1969, p. 91-94).

In mice, Bland (1976b) observed that sublethal
X-irradiation (600 rads) given on one of the following days: -1, 5, 7 or 8 p.i. with *H. diminuta* suppressed rejection up to day 12 and probably up to
day 14 (only one group killed on this day), but most
worms had been rejected by day 18. If irradiation
was not carried out until day 10 (at which time over
90% of the worms were still present in the mice)
rejections was not delayed, and over 50% of the
worms had been rejected by day 12 both in the controls and in mice irradiated on day 10. At first
sight, these results suggest there is a radiosensitive step operating up to and including day 8, but
thereafter the rejection process is irradiation
insensitive. This is almost certainly too facile
an interpretation. X-irradiation early in, or just
before, the infection probably interferes with the
multiplicative phase of induction, but it is not at
all certain whether X-irradiation as late as day 8 p.i.
(when immunoglobulins already coat the worm - Section V3) act by blocking lymphocyte multiplication.
The problem with this type of experiment is that
X-irradiation is such a sledge-hammer. Until more
is known about what cells are involved in rejection,
it is doubtful if much can be learned just by using
different doses of irradiation at different stages
in the infection.

X-irradiation (550 rads the day before infecting)
prevented naive CFLP mice from rejecting surgically
transplanted worms for about 12 days but had much
less effect on preventing rejection by immunized
mice (Hopkins & Zajac 1976). This result agrees
with the well established observation that X-irradiation is far more effective at inhibiting induction of a primary response than suppressing an
anamnestic (memory) response.

V. NATURE OF THE RESPONSE

1. Source of the Immunogen

The main point at issue is whether the antigens which elicit a protective response originate from the scolex or over the whole area of the tegument. The former idea tended to be favoured because, since uptake of intact proteins by the intestine was considered to end around weaning (Brambell 1970; Hemmings 1976), it followed that antigen uptake from worms in the lumen of adult hosts could occur only when the mucosa was damaged. However, it is now well established that protein uptake in immunologically significant amounts continues throughout life (reviewed by Bazin 1976, p. 44; Hemmings 1978). There is, therefore, no necessity for a tapeworm to have intimate contact with the lamina propria, as occurs with *Echinococcus granulosus* (reviewed by Smyth 1973), for there to be macromolecular uptake and hence there is less reason to believe the rostellar glands or the scolex to be the sole origin of the antigens (Smyth 1964, 1969). Andreassen *et al.* (1978), however, think that "the functional antigens are related to the scolex region". Their reason is that two worm infections were not rejected by their $B_{10}LP$ nu/nu mice although they grew to a bigger mass than that reached by five worm infections which were rejected. There are, however, other interpretations of such a result. For instance, the growth of individual worms in mice is similar in two and five worm infections during the first 7 days of an infection. There is, therefore, a much greater mass of tegument present during this period in a five, than in a two, worm infection. If we assume that this is the critical induction period, because after this the presence of IgA inhibits antigen uptake (Section V3), then a five worm infection could be more strongly antigenic by providing a greater mass of tegument than by providing more scoleces.

On the other hand, Christie (unpublished) found that if he surgically implanted 4-day-old worms (one per mouse) into the duodenum of naive mice, the worms were rejected in 10-13 days whereas 8-day-old donor worms were rejected in 8-10 days. This suggests that the mass of strobila is the critical factor, though it could be argued that the older worms were rejected more quickly because the scolex and neck of an 8-day-old worm is either more active as an immunogen or more susceptible to attack than are the scolex and neck of a 4-day-old worm. All that is certain is that a large mass of strobila is not essential as infections starting with cysticercoids and terminated with an anthelmintic after 72h, during which period the worms are little more than scolex and neck, are sufficient to immunize a mouse (Section III).

Nevertheless, in the absence of conclusive evidence either way, the writer favours the hypothesis that antigenic material is constantly released over the whole surface of the tegument. These molecules may arise from either the breakdown of the glycocalyx which it is known has a rapid turnover (Oaks & Lumsden 1971), or from secretory products. Such secretions are believed to function to protect the tegument from host enzyme attack (Pappas & Read 1972a, b) and to aid in the digestion of food in the immediate proximity of the uptake sites on the tegumentary membrane (reviewed by Pappas & Read 1975). The problem of the relative importance of the scolex and tegument as the source of antigens may ultimately be resolved by immunizing with different fractions from dead worms in the same way as experiments have shown the stichosome to be source of protective antigens in *Trichinella spiralis* (Despommier, Campbell & Blair 1977) and in *Trichuris muris* (Jenkins & Wakelin 1977). Alternatively, if medium in which *H. diminuta* have been cultured proves an effective source of antigens (Section IX), it may be possible to culture worms without a scolex as Smyth (1958) was able to do with fragments of *Schistocephalus solidus*.

2. Immunogen Uptake

Although macromolecular uptake by the gut is firmly established (reviewed by Hemmings 1978), how and where uptake occurs is a major problem being investigated at the present time. There is experimental evidence which suggests that the epithelium covering the 'dome' of Peyer's patches is an important region for uptake (Bockman & Cooper 1973) but macromolecular transport also occurs over the general intestinal epithelium (Walker, Isselbacher & Bloch 1972). The amount of protein taken up from the lumen is controversial, most figures quoted in the Ciba Symposium (1977, Discussion p. 356-60) are in the range 0.01% - 0.2%, but Hemmings (1978, p. 38) quotes an uptake of "at least 2%" of a dose of bovine serum albumen by adult rats. In general, if uptake is measured as the total amount of precipitable protein retaining the antigenicity of the parent macromolecule, i.e., including large breakdown products - usually of 20-50 thousand daltons, uptake of orally fed proteins is much higher than formerly believed (Hemmings & Williams 1978).

3. Antibody Induction and Function

The handling of the antigens within the body is an even more controversial topic which is beyond the scope of this chapter, but some brief mention of types of responses to intestinal antigens is necessary to form a framework into which the scraps of information about *H. diminuta* can be fitted (for a more detailed recent review see Befus & Podesta 1976).

1. IgA. In general, much recent work on the immunological response of the intestine has centred around the secretory IgA system (Bazin 1976; Lamm 1976; Cebra *et al.* 1977; Husband, Monie & Gowans 1977). There seems little doubt that the gut lies in a "cylinder" of lymphoid cells situated in the lamina propria and that over 80% of the immunoglobulin containing cells are IgA plasma cells. A lot of work has been done on the origin of these cells, most of which suggests they originate from B-cells with surface IgA situated in the follicular regions of Peyer's patches (Cebra *et al.* 1977, p. 8). There is also little doubt that the B-cells on sensitization by specific antigens in Peyer's patches leave the follicles and migrate via the lymph drainage ducts to the mesenteric lymph node. More controversial is whether further stimulation has to occur in the mesenteric lymph nodes (MLN). Husband *et al.* (1977, p. 35) describe how removal of the MLN in rats had little effect on the IgA response. Be that as it may, the blast cells pass from the MLN via the thoracic lymph duct into the blood and so back to the intestine at which point another controversy arises. Do the IgA blast cells 'home' preferentially to a specific region of the intestine; if so, is this induced by the presence of the antigen in the lamina propria causing extravasation of the IgA cells, or may the antigen cause IgA blast cells which have already left the venules to lose their mobility, accumulate in the tissues and complete transformation into plasma cells? Whatever the mechanism, IgA plasma cells collect to a density of over 350,000 mm^3 of lamina propria in man (quoted from Bazin 1976, p. 40) and produce the characteristic dimeric IgA molecule, which is then secreted into the lumen after bonding with another molecule, the secretory component (SC) produced by epithelial cells. Again, whether the IgA-SC molecule escapes into the lumen across the apical tight junction between epithelial cells or through the cytoplasm is controversial (for a discussion of the possible pathways, see Brandtzaeg & Baklien 1977), but it is the most abundant immunoglobulin in the intestine. It is natural, therefore, to ask whether production of IgA is evoked by *H. diminuta*, and if so, to consider what role it may play.

Befus (1975b, 1977) using immunofluorescent techniques, found that *H. diminuta* in mice became coated with IgA by day 9, though as he was careful to point out, there was no certain evidence that this was specific anti-worm IgA, as distinct from IgA produced in response to other intestinal antigens which had been nonspecifically adsorbed onto the polyanionic glycocalyx (Lumsden 1975). However, the timing of its appearance and evidence from other work (see below) suggests that it was specific anti-tapeworm antibody. But even the knowledge that the IgA is specific antibody tells one nothing about its role. Until recently, there was no evidence that IgA had an opsonic role comparable to IgG or M and there still is doubt as to how important this aspect of its function is. However, it has been demonstrated by a number of workers that polymorphonuclear leukocytes (PMN) have receptor sites for the Fc region of IgA and that aggregated IgA stimulates phagocytosis, or, if the aggregates are too large to be phagocytosed, the release of lysosomal enzymes (briefly reviewed by Speigelberg, Lawrence & Henson 1974). It has also been observed that the addition of IgA (recovered from patients with IgA myeloma) inhibits the chemotaxis of PMN - which have been stimulated by a variety of factors (Van Epps & Williams 1976) and suppresses the bacteriocidal action of PMN (Van Epps, Reed & Williams 1978). Presumably, these suppressive activities arise as a result of unaggregated or combined IgA blocking receptor sites on the PMN. There is then reason to believe that IgA may activate a protective response through PMN and it is also known that it can activate complement through the alternate pathway (Speigelberg & Götze 1972; Lachmann 1975; Müller-Eberhard 1976). However, the main role of IgA in the lumen of the intestine may be a quite different one. If, as seems proved, it is impossible to have an intestine completely impermeable to macromolecules, it may be essential to control uptake in some other way. Were this not done, the organism would be in danger of forming immune complexes involving IgM and IgG in the lamina propria which would activate various lytic systems and damage the surrounding tissues. There is evidence to show that rats fed orally a macromolecule (human serum albumin), produce specific IgA, detectable in the intestinal secretions and that the capacity to absorb that macromolecule thereafter is reduced (reviewed by André, André & Vaerman 1978). Assuming that this is a major role of secretory IgA, then its abundance in infected mice is not a measure of the mouse's attack on the tapeworm but rather a measure of the attack - by released antigens - of the tapeworm on the mouse. If this is the case, the presence of IgA on the surface of the tapeworm may have no significance as far as rejection is concerned. Alternatively, its presence may be more akin to an enhancing antibody, i.e., it may enhance the survival of the tapeworm by masking its 'foreign surface' with self (host) protein.

To summarize the position as far as IgA is concerned, both *H. diminuta* which is rejected and *H. microstoma* which is not rejected (in light infections), become coated about day 8/9 of a primary infection with IgA which is probably specific antibody, but there is no evidence whether the IgA is deleterious, neutral or beneficial to the tapeworm;

on balance probably not the first, in which case one must look to other immunoglobulins or defence mechanism as the source of the attack on tapeworms.

2. *IgE, Mast Cells and Anti-inflammatory Drugs*. Studies on cell traffic to the intestine of *H. diminuta* infected animals have only just started. Andreassen *et al*. (1978) reported that there was in mice a dramatic rise in intestinal mast cells (IMC) and globule leucocytes (GL) from none on day of infection to 12 IMC and 96 GL per villus crypt unit (VCU) on day 10, by which time, worm rejection was complete. These results raise several questions. One is whether it is justifiable to equate metachromatic staining cells, i.e., IMC and GL, of mice with metachromatic staining cells in rats. Recent work has raised doubt as to whether even connective tissue and intestinal mast cells in the same animal have a common "lineage and physiology" (Mayrhofer 1977, p. 171). Another doubt is whether all workers differentiate IMC from GL to the same degree. As originally defined, in rats "mature GL are IMC which have migrated intraepithelially and discharged their granule content" (Miller & Walshaw 1972; see also Miller, Murray & Jarrett 1968; Murray 1972). Accepting this as correct, although there is no direct evidence that granulated IMC in the lamina propria do migrate into the epithelium and become degranulated GL (Mayrhofer 1977, p. 220), there is still considerable difficulty in distinguishing with certainty the varying grades of maturing, mature and discharged IMC and GL and relative counts in different laboratories may vary extensively. Andreassen *et al*.'s (1978) figures, however, clearly demonstrate a considerable rise in toluidine blue positive cells (= IMC + GL) and a high ratio of GL to granulated IMC would normally be thought to indicate that the IMC, which had previously been stimulated to proliferate, were migrating, discharging and becoming degranulated GL. This response pattern was first associated with helminth rejection by Jarrett *et al*. (1968), who measured a rapid rise in GL (and granulated IMC) during the rejection of *Nippostrongylus brasiliensis* from rats. There is also marginal support for mast cell proliferation as a response to

intestinal tapeworm infections from the work of Gray (1976), who found a rise in IMC in fowl following primary and secondary infections with *Raillietina cesticillus*.

What role do the mast cells play? The usually accepted role is that by releasing pharmacologically active amines, notably histamine and 5-hydroxytryptamine (5HT) but other longer acting amines as well, they initiate an inflammatory response which, *inter alia*, increases vascular permeability and brings leucocytes and macromolecules from the blood into the area and, in the intestine, increases the permeability of the intestine wall. Barth *et al.* (1966) suggested that this inflammatory response created a "leak lesion" which permitted antibodies in the serum to cross the intestinal mucosa into the gut lumen. Since then, a considerable amount of work has supported the importance of mast cells in the worm rejection process, for example, the effectiveness of anti-inflammatory drugs in suppressing rejection (Murray, Smith, Waddell & Jarrett 1971). It is possibly important to note that much better suppression of rejection of *N. brasiliensis* from rats was obtained by these latter workers when both histamine and a 5HT antagonist was administered than with either separately.

Working with *H. diminuta* in mice, no significant slowing in rejection (measured both in terms of weight and number of worms) was obtained by the writer using promethazine (primarily an antihistamine), methysergide (primarily an anti-5HT), or cyproheptadine hydrochloride (effective both as an antihistamine and anti-5HT), although the experiments were all repeated at least once, each using several drug doses with groups of 10 mice killed on days 8, 9, 11, 12 and 14 post-infection. A negative result is always unsatisfactory and leaves doubts in the experimenter's mind, and it would be interesting to measure changes in serum CRP [type C polysaccharide reacting protein - a sensitive indicator of inflammation (Bodmer & Siboo 1977)] to discover whether there is evidence of an inflammatory response at the time of rejection. Andreassen *et al.*'s findings that $B_{10}LP$ *nu/nu* (athymic) mice reject *H. diminuta*, although they have no demonstrable intestinal mast cells, would give some support to the concept that rejection of tapeworms is not dependent on a mast cell mediated inflammatory response. It should also be noted that neither Goodall (1973) nor Turton, Williamson & Harris (1975) found evidence of IgE production associated with the rejection of *H. diminuta* from mouse and man, respectively. Again this is negative evidence but it must be concluded that the involvement of mast cells and IgE in the rejection of *H. diminuta* is far from proved.

3. IgM and Complement. The early occurrence of IgM, along with IgA on *H. diminuta* in mice presumably reflects the facts that IgM is usually produced before IgG in a response and equally importantly that IgM, like IgA, combines with a secretory component thereby aiding its passage across the mucosa into the intestinal lumen. Whether its role is the same as IgA is not known. IgM readily fixes and activates complement, which Befus (1977) found on the surface of *H. diminuta* but not on *H. microstoma* (which is not rejected in light infections). If one was dealing with a parasite in the tissue, this observation would immediately suggest the possibility of complement mediated lysis, but there is doubt whether complement remains active in the intestine. Nevertheless, the result is an interesting one which merits further investigation.

4. IgG. Specific antibody of both IgG_1 and IgG_2 subclasses are formed and almost certainly coat *H. diminuta* in the mouse (see Section V4) and this class of antibody is known to activate various lytic systems (Roitt 1977) but its role, if any, against *H. diminuta* is unknown.

4. Antibodies and Passive Protection

Coleman, Carty & Graziadei (1968), using a microcomplement fixation method, detected antibodies in the serum of *H. diminuta* infected rats. This was confirmed by Harris & Turton (1973) who, using the indirect fluorescent technique, showed that immunoglobulins appeared in the serum between days 7 and 14 p.i. Extending the work by use of short- (4h) and long-term (72h) PCA (passive cutaneous anaphylaxis) tests they claimed to demonstrate IgGa and IgE. These results need confirming as the rat serum was apparently not heated to destroy IgE before use for the 4h test, so it is possible the 4h positive PCA could have arisen from IgE. Befus (1977), as well as showing the appearance of IgA on the surface of *H. diminuta* in mice, found IgM present by day 9 pi. and IgG_1 and IgG_2 by day 11, and Choromanski (1978), using two worm infections in mice, found the sera had "highest titers" of agglutinating antibodies (to red blood cells coated with *H. diminuta* antigen) "between 7 and 10 days" pi., following which the titers decreased, then "increased from 13 days post infection." Although, therefore, knowledge of which classes of antibody are involved is still meagre, there is no reasonable doubt that antibodies are produced both by mice and rats in response to *H. diminuta* infections and that probably all the main classes, IgA, IgM, IgG and IgE, are involved. The fact that these antibodies have been shown in rats which do not reject *H. diminuta*, at least at low infections (Section VIII), is not surprising as the presence of antibodies in the serum has long been known to be a poor indicator of the ability of a host to reject helminths (reviewed by Ogilvie & Jones 1971; but note, reference to *H. diminuta* is a misquotation for *H. nana*). Apart from the fact that antibodies are definitely formed as a response to *H. diminuta*, the only other reasonably certain fact is that passive protection cannot be induced by serum transfer. Even three massive transfusions, each of 2 ml of hyperimmune serum (obtained from mice infected on days 0, 20 and 35, and bled at autopsy on day 45) failed to suppress the growth or accelerate the rejection of *H. diminuta* in the recipient mice. This experiment, using different numbers and times of infections in the donor mice has been repeated several times by workers in the writer's laboratory, always without success. Recently, Andreassen *et al.* (1978) have tried to passively protect athymic mice (Section V5) with serum from immunized normal littermates but without success. Such experiments have proved notoriously fickle and unreliable in the *Nippostrongylus brasiliensis*/rat system (reviewed by Ogilvie & Love 1974). Nevertheless, the experiments probably mean that if antibodies are involved in expulsion at all, they are only part of the mechanism. Even this conclusion, however, has to be hedged as the injection of antibodies parenterally does not mean they can necessarily enter the intestinal lumen (Section V3).

5. The Role of T-Cells

Isaak et al. (1975) using nude mice (congenitally athymic and hairless when homozygous for the mutant nu/nu, but with a normal thymus in the phenotypically indistinguishable hairy $nu/+$ or $+/+$ littermates) found that they were unable to reject either one or three worm primary infections of H. diminuta, whereas littermates had virtually completed rejection by day 14 p.i. The intravenous injection of thymus cells, or the grafting of neonatal thymus glands under each renal capsule, restored competency to the nudes both to respond to a thymus-dependent antigen (sheep red blood cells - SRBC) and to reject H. diminuta.

Similar results were obtained by Bland (1976a) who, using one worm infections, obtained 100% recovery of very large worms from all 16 nude mice killed between days 17-33 p.i., by which time rejection was complete in the 45 thymic littermates. Dependence of rejection on T-cells was further investigated by thymectomizing adult (inbred) NIH mice and destroying their mature T-cells with a lethal dose (850 rad) of X-rays, before reconstituting with syngeneic bone marrow cells and infecting with H. diminuta (Bland 1976b). Such animals were found to give only a weak response to a thymus-dependent antigen (SRBC) and be unable to reject H. diminuta. However, ambiguity arose in the interpretation of the experiment because sham operated, X-irradiated, reconstituted (control) mice, although giving a good humoral response to SRBC, had lost much of their ability to reject H. diminuta. The implication is that while thymus cells are necessary there is another radiation sensitive step.

The importance of T-cells in the rejection of H. diminuta appeared firmly established as it is in the rejection of Trichinella spiralis and several other intestinal nematodes (reviewed by Larsh & Weatherly 1974), until recently when Andreassen et al. (1978)

reported nude mice were able to reject *H. diminuta* between days 10-17 p.i., i.e., the very period when Bland's (1976a) littermates rejected. The immediate suspicion is that Andreassen *et al.*'s nudes were not wholly *nu/nu*, i.e., they had rudiments of thymus present (which Bland found in some of his *nu/nu* nudes), but neither lymphocyte transformation tests with PHA (phytohaemagglutinin - a stimulator of T-cells) nor skin grafts produced evidence for the presence of T-cells. Are these contradictory results explicable?

It should be noted that the strains of mice used by Isaak *et al.*, Andreassen *et al.* and Bland were all different - with the *nu/nu* gene bred into them. The littermates of Bland's *nu/nu* strain were relatively poor rejectors - 11-17 days, whereas in the strain used by Andreassen *et al.*, they were strong rejectors - all worms lost by day 10. [There is insufficient information to classify the BalbC used by Isaak *et al.*] A possible explanation is that T-cells help rejection but are not essential, hence the strong rejector mouse strain ($B_{10}LP$) used by Andreassen *et al.* expelled a strongly stimulating five worm infection even without a thymus but Bland's weak rejector mouse strain presented with a weakly stimulating single worm infection, was in most cases unable to reject the worm in the absence of T-cells. This interpretation is supported by Andreassen *et al.*'s statement "we observed that 1 and 2 worm infections are not expelled from (our) nude mice", i.e., even a strong rejector strain cannot reject a weakly stimulating infection without T-cells to amplify the response. If this interpretation is correct, the implication is that the actual effector response which brings about worm loss may be released by several mechanisms as with mast cell degranulation, complement activation, clotting and all the other essential homeostatic control mechanisms in the body. It is possibly quite wrong to search for a specific key antibody or cell type. A more profitable approach might be to discover what actually damages the worm. Once one knew that, it might be possible to work backwards and discover where it is synthesized, where stored, how released and the role of lymphokines from T-cells in these processes.

6. The Effector Arm

There is no good evidence as to what actually does the damage to the tapeworm. As has been discussed above, there is a suggestion that complement may be involved but as yet the evidence is extremely tenuous. Although to date no thorough search has been made, initial examination of the tegument of immune damaged tapeworms using a scanning electron microscope has failed to reveal the presence of any host cells in contact with the microvilli nor did Befus & Threadgold (1975) observe such cells when examining sections through damaged tegument. It seems unlikely therefore, that the damage is brought about by direct contact of macrophages, granulocytes, K-cells or any other cells, though this does not preclude the possibility that such cells enter the intestinal lumen and release nonspecific cell membrane lysing enzymes. Such a process seems improbable as it would be very haphazard but there is evidence of an enormous increase in β-phospholipase in the intestinal wall of mice infected with *Hymenolepis nana* (Ottolenghi 1973) and a 10-fold increase in peroxidase activity in lamina propria cells from rats infected with *T. spiralis* (Castro, Roy & Stockstill 1974). Whether a similar increase occurs in mice infected with *H. diminuta* and if so, whether it reaches the lumen, has never been investigated. There is also the possibility that the large number of globule leucocytes (Section V3 2) in the epithelium at the time of rejection (Andreassen *et al.* 1978) is indicative of massive amine discharge into the intestine. Bearing in mind the enormous amount of muscle tissue in a tapeworm such an amine wave might destroy the tapeworm's ability to combat peristalsis and lead to its expulsion. However, neither the injection of histamine and 5HT directly into the duodenum (by laparotomy), nor their administration orally, influence worm survival (Hopkins, unpublished).

Recently it has been claimed that certain of the prostaglandins (notably PGE) play a part in the rejection of *Nippostrongylus* from rats (Dineen & Kelly 1976), but 150 μg of PGE_2 injected intraduodenally into mice on day 5 of a two worm infection had no effect on the survival or growth of *H. diminuta* as determined by autopsy of the mice on day 8

of the infection. It has also been observed that
mesenteric lymph node cells taken from *H. diminuta*
infected mice at the time of worm rejection inhibit
the migration of macrophages (Choromanski 1978),
which suggests a cell-mediated response and lympho-
kine production is involved in rejection.

7. Destrobilation and Death

When *H. diminuta* is attacked by an immune response, the whole worm may be lost or the worm may
destrobilate. Whether all worms destrobilate before
being expelled has never been determined but destrobilation is certainly a common response. The longevity of the destrobilated scolex is also poorly
known (Section II4). Such scoleces, at least for a
time, appear to be suppressed rather than damaged
as they can regrow immediately on surgical transfer-
ence into a naive host (Hopkins *et al*. 1972a).

Examination of worms in a mouse about the time
destrobilation occurs shows that particularly in the
neck region large swollen opaque areas occur (Befus
& Threadgold 1975). Electron microscopic examination of the tegument in those dark areas shows the
distal cytoplasm of the tegumental cells to be
extremely dense though apparently no thinner (cf.
Befus & Threadgold 1975, Plate 2a and 3b). The
mitochondria appear abnormal and there is some lipid
accumulation, both characteristic of degenerative
changes. Because more of these darkened areas appear in multiple, more strongly rejected infections,
than in single worm infections and because dark
areas increase in number and severity prior to
rejection, it seems probable that they are induced
by the immune response. At least when first formed,
the dark areas readily disappear *in vitro*. Worms
can be recovered in a dreadful condition from mice
(see Befus & Threadgold 1975, Plate 1) yet after 30
minutes in balanced salt solution may appear unblem-
ished.

One of the most interesting problems about these
darkened areas is why do they occur predominantly in
the neck region? What is different about the neck
region? The obvious answer is that it is a region
of massive cell proliferation and tegument formation

and expansion. Putting these two facts together, a
reasonable hypothesis would be that newly formed
tegument is open to immune mediated attack, whereas
tegument on older proglottids and the scolex is less
easily damaged. Such a hypothesis fits with the
known facts of immune rejection. Destrobilation
occurs in the neck region and shed strobila can
often be found intact in the caecum with little
apparent damage and the scolex may persist for some
time. The scolex cannot regrow, however, unless
surgically transplanted into a naive host as the new
tissue would be rapidly destroyed. Dark areas are
also found on the neck of *H. diminuta* in rats but
disappear as the affected proglottids age and move
further down the strobila. This again would suggest
newly formed tegument in expanding proglottids is
susceptible to attack, but that in rats, the attack
is weaker and the tegument survives long enough
without severe damage occurring to reach the stage
of being relatively resistant. Although such resistance may arise from extrinsic causes such as the
absorption of IgA or other host protein, it is just
as likely to occur because of intrinsic changes in
the glycocalyx.

In summary, it is probable that the darkened
areas are an outward and visible sign of an immune
mediated response though their reported occurrence
on day 4 in a primary infection in mice (Befus &
Threadgold 1975) and frequent occurrence by day 6
in rats (Hopkins & Allen, unpublished) casts some
doubt on whether they are always a result of an
immune mediated response. Certainly these areas
deserve much more intensive study; how labile are
they, do they occur in the anterior region of other
tapeworms or even other species of *Hymenolepis?*

Another possible aspect of immunological damage
that has been examined is the ability of *H. diminuta*
as it approaches the stage at which it would be
rejected (days 7-11 p.i.) to transport small molecules across its tegument. Bland (1976b) examined
the uptake *in vitro* of 0.1 mM D-glucose, 0.1 mM
acetate ions and 2 mM L-methionine by worms recovered
from mice, cortisone treated mice, rats and cortisone treated rats. He found no significant difference in glucose transport but the "transport of
^{14}C-labelled L-methionine and sodium acetate was

shown to be less in *H. diminuta* from mice than in *H. diminuta* of equivalent weight from immunosuppressed mice or rats respectively". He concluded that the results indicated "specific depression of methionine and sodium acetate transport by an immune mediator in mice acting on tegumental transport loci of *H. diminuta*". The problem is that there are so many complicating factors. For example, 8-day-old worms from mice and rats cannot be directly compared because of weight difference. [Uptake per mg decreases as weight increases, but age is itself a parameter (Henderson 1977).] The addition of cortisone alters the physiological environment of the intestinal lumen in many ways, hence changes in metabolic uptake need not necessarily be related to the immunosuppressive function of cortisone. There is also the worry that if the critical damage is largely confined to the neck, even major changes in transport in this region would be masked by normal transport over the much larger area of undamaged tegument. Further investigations are justified but meaningful results may prove difficult to obtain.

VI. SURGICAL TRANSPLANTATION OF *H. DIMINUTA* BETWEEN HOSTS

One of the problems of investigating the immune response to *H. diminuta* is that it is difficult during the first 6 days of an infection commencing with cysticercoids, to recover and accurately measure worms. Length is a highly variable parameter in tapeworms and dry weight although ambiguous, requires sophisticated equipment for its determination as usually worms of this age weigh <0.1 mg. After day 6, worms in a primary infection (except sometimes in old mice - Section II3) are easier to recover and weigh but considerable variation occurs, particularly between experiments in the time when growth slows and rejection commences. Multi-worm infections help to reduce this variation (Befus 1975a) but make experiments very much more time consuming and introduce problems of inter-worm competition especially if the number of worms to establish varies in different mice.

To overcome these difficulties, Hopkins & Zajac (1976) transferred by laparotomy, single, relatively large (2-4 cm long and approximately 0.3 mg dry weight), 7- or 8-day-old *H. diminuta* from donor mice into the duodenum of recipient mice. The technique was highly successful, more than 90% of all worms transferred became established and transferred worms although reaching a very large size, 10-20 cm in length, were never rejected by naive mice in less than 7 days; in immune mice they were rejected in less than 5 days. In more recent work (Hopkins & Allen, unpublished) the distinction between the response by naive or immunized mice has become even more apparent in that growth stops in worms transferred into immunized mice on days 2 or 3 after transplantation whereas the weight of worms in naive mice continues to double daily for at least 6 days. This technique should permit very much quicker and more precise assay of the effect of blocking various known defence components, e.g., depleting complement with cobra venom (Lachmann 1975), degranulating or blocking mast cells with anti-inflammatory drugs, increasing intestinal permeability, anaphylactic shock (Barth *et al.* 1966), blockading, depleting or divagating macrophages, etc. Such experiments can be done starting with cysticercoid infections but mice, subjected to such drug treatments over the much longer period that is then necessary to allow significant growth in the controls, show many side effects which make the results of doubtful value. The technique should also prove of value for determining the importance of lymphoid cells, macrophages, eosinophils, serum, etc., derived from immunized mice to convey immunity to naive, isogeneic recipients. It has already proved an excellent method for demonstrating the persistence of memory in immunized mice (Section III).

An interesting point that has emerged is that *H. diminuta* surgically transplanted into immunized mice are rejected equally quickly whether they come from light infections in rats (in which they would have survived indefinitely - Section VIII) or from mice (in which they were on the point of rejection). The intestine of a mouse immunized with *H. diminuta* appears therefore to be completely inimical to the survival of *H. diminuta*, irrespective of the condition of the worm at transplant. It would be interesting to know whether this condition of the intestine is specific to challenge with *H. diminuta* of any age and from any host or whether it is nonspecific operating against other tapeworms, e.g., *H. citelli*.

The technique has also been used to determine whether the intestine of an immunized mouse lacks the signals which normally operate to locate *H. diminuta* in a particular position (see Arai, this volume). Worms were surgically implanted into the ileum of naive and immune mice. In both groups of animals, the donor worms migrated within 24 hours to their normal anterior position of attachment, 10-25% down the small intestine. There is no evidence therefore, that site selection stimuli are altered in an immune mouse. Worms only leave their normal position just before expulsion when presumably they have been damaged and are no longer capable of responding to the signals (but see anterior displacement of destrobilated worms in immune rats - Section VIII).

The disadvantage of the transplantation technique is the initial surgery which is necessary to bypass the stomach. Apart from the time involved, there is the inevitable shock and inflammatory response across the intestine wall against a worm or alternatively preempt the response by draining effector cells into the area of the duodenum where the incision was made. There is evidence (Hopkins & Zajac 1976, Fig. 4) that, in fact, laparotomy and intestinal incision delay a response by 24-48 hours. The obvious solution is to passage the worm through the stomach. This is normally not possible because the stomach acidity kills the worm. There is also a behavioral problem involved in that the worm appears to actively resist moving with peristalsis and so tends to move up to form a 'ball' in the cardiac region of the stomach, remaining there until rising acidity kills it. The problem is difficult but one feels that the judicious manipulation of acid production suppressors, antacids, and pyloric sphincter relaxors should make passage through the stomach possible and thereby obviate surgury.

VII. CROSS REACTION WITH OTHER INTESTINAL HELMINTHS

Several experiments have been carried out to determine the effect of a concurrent infection on the growth and survival of *H. diminuta*. The difficulty about these experiments is interpretation, a decrease in growth or establishment may result from a number of disparate causes other than an immunological response. For instance, the decreased rate of growth of *H. citelli* when in a concurrent infection with *H. diminuta* in hamsters was interpreted by Read & Phifer (1959) as due to competition for starch. Holmes (1961) considered the decrease in size of *H. diminuta* when rats were infected concurrently with the acanthocephalan *Moniliformis dubius* to be due to "competition, possibly for carbohydrates" (see Roberts, this volume).

Intercurrent infections with *H. diminuta* and *H. nana* have been studied fairly extensively but interpretation of the results is even more difficult in this case because *H. nana* has both a tissue and lumen-dwelling phase. Infections of *H. nana* initiated by administering eggs, develop for 4-5 days in the mucosa after which the cysticercoids that have formed escape into the intestinal lumen. Infections initiated by administering cysticercoids (grown in beetles) develop to adult worms in the gut lumen, but autoinfection, due to eggs either hatching directly or following coprophagy (Ghazal & Avery 1976), initiate a tissue phase after approximately 10 days. Heyneman (1962b) carried out a series of experiments "immunizing" mice with *H. nana* eggs and challenging after various periods with *H. diminuta*. He obtained over 80% reduction in the number of *H. diminuta* over 3 cm long in mice infected with *H. nana* compared with the non-immunized controls, a reduction he attributed to an immune cross reaction initiated by the tissue phase. [It was then (Heyneman 1962a) and still is, generally believed that the lumen stage of *H. nana* is non-immunogenic. The writer doubts this.]

As far as these experiments were concerned however, the poor establishment and/or growth of *H. diminuta* might equally have been due to an immune response initiated by the adult *H. nana* in the lumen, physiological disturbances of the gut associated with large concurrent *H. nana* populations or in those experiments where there were no controls and autopsy was not until days 20 or 32 of the *H. diminuta* infection, have arisen from an immune response initiated by *H. diminuta* itself. While, therefore, it is impossible to be certain of the sequence of events, Heyneman's experiments certainly demonstrated that *H. nana* has an effect on the development of *H. diminuta* and possibly hinted that an immune response once initiated could operate across the intestine wall on worms in the lumen.

In 1964, Weinmann tested the cross reactivity of a number of worms including *H. diminuta* with *H. nana*. These experiments are easier to interpret because the *H. nana* egg challenge was allowed to develop for only 90-94 hours before the mice were autopsied and the number of cysticercoids in the mucosal wall counted. Primary infections with the nematodes *Capillaria hepatica*, *Ascaris lumbricoides* and *Trichinella spiralis* given at various periods before challenging with *H. nana* eggs had little effect on the number of *H. nana* that developed, except for an infection of *T. spiralis* given 15 days before challenge (see below). Primary infections with the tapeworms *H. microstoma* and *H. citelli*, however, considerably reduced the number of cysticercoids found. This cast considerable doubt on the sacrosanct premise that the lumen-phase of tapeworms was non-immunogenic. Weinmann (1966) extended these experiments, confirmed the ability of an *H. citelli* infection to protect against *H. nana* and showed also that there was a dramatic decrease in the number of *H. nana* eggs to develop into cysticercoids in mice immunized with *H. diminuta*. (Immunization schedule: one cysticercoid every 10 days on three occasions, challenge 10 or 20 days after third *H. diminuta* infection.) In view of this strong immunogenicity of *H. diminuta* in the mouse, it would be interesting to repeat and extend Weinmann's earlier 1964 experiments using rats in which *H. diminuta* failed to protect against *H. nana*, though, as the author stressed, his conclusions were based on a single small experiment. If *H. diminuta* is ineffective in protecting rats against *H. nana* yet strongly protective in mice, the reason could well help explain why mice can reject all *H. diminuta* whereas rats can only reject 'heavy' infections (Section VIII).

Weinmann's (1966) experiments demonstrated another interesting point, that the immunity initiated in the mouse by *H. diminuta* in the lumen was effective in decreasing by 66% the size of *H. nana* adults. This was the first evidence that a tapeworm living in the lumen was able to stimulate an immune response which would operate against another lumen-dwelling tapeworm.

Recently, Hopkins, Goodall & Zajac (1977) studied the cross reaction between *H. diminuta* and *H. microstoma* in mice. This is an interesting combination as in the strain of mice used, *H. diminuta* is rejected rapidly (Section II) whereas *H. microstoma* is lost only slowly. It was found that *H. microstoma* and *H. diminuta* cross reacted, but of much greater interest was the fact that *H. microstoma* strongly protected the mouse against challenge by *H. diminuta* although the mouse was unable to reject the *microstoma*. (To avoid ambiguity due to concurrent infection, the *H. microstoma* was removed with 'Zanil' 4 days before infecting with *H. diminuta*.) In the reciprocal cross, a primary *H. diminuta* which was itself rejected, only weakly protected against challenge by *H. microstoma*. The level of protection measured by a decrease in worm weight (there is no diminution in number of worms to establish) was similar to that induced by a primary *H. microstoma* on a secondary *microstoma* infection (Howard 1976).

H. citelli has also been found to cross react with *H. diminuta*. Mice which had received an immunizing infection of two *H. diminuta* were challenged on day 24 (by which time all *H. diminuta* would have been rejected) with two *H. citelli* cysticercoids. The combined weight of the *H. citelli* recovered from groups of 10 immunized mice autopsied 16, 18 and 20 days after challenge was less than 25% that of the controls. The reciprocal cross, i.e., mice immunized with two *H. citelli* [which had to be removed with 'Zanil' as two worm infections are near or below the threshold at which rejection occurs (cf. Hopkins & Stallard 1974)] showed only a weak protection when challenged with one *H. diminuta*.

This lack of reciprocity is different from that between *H. diminuta* and *H. microstoma*. In the latter case as discussed above, the strongly antigenic *H. diminuta* failed to protect appreciably against *H. microstoma*, suggesting *H. microstoma* can evade the effector arm of the response. Against *H. citelli* however, the strongly immunogenic *H. diminuta* gives strong protection suggesting *H. citelli* is susceptible like *H. diminuta* to immune attack by the host and hence its long survival in a low level primary infection is due to weak stimulation of the immune response. This interpretation would explain why a primary two worm *H. citelli* infection had little effect on an *H. diminuta* infection. [Although this is a nice 'tidy' explanation of the facts observed, the writer is not totally convinced that *H. citelli* survives in low level infections because it is weakly immunogenic. The extraordinarily small amount of *H. diminuta* that needs to be present for just 3 days (Section III) in order to elicit a response makes it hard to believe that relatively enormous *H. citelli* survive because they are below an immunologically stimulating threshold.]

There is no evidence of specific cross immunity between *H. diminuta* or any other tapeworm and nematodes, but there is clear evidence of interaction. For instance, Hendrix, Kopia & Lattime (1975) reported that "approximately simultaneous infections" of *Nippostrongylus brasiliensis* and *H. diminuta* led to stunting and a posterior shift in position of attachment of *H. diminuta* and Morcock & Roberts (1976) obtained a similar result, administering 11 *H. diminuta* cysts on day 5 of the *N. brasiliensis* infection (see Roberts, this volume). When infection of the rats with *H. diminuta* was delayed until day 10 of the *Nippostrongylus* infection, no *H. diminuta* established (Hendrix *et al.*, *loc. cit.*). This suggests that the inflammatory response which occurs during the rejection of *N. brasiliensis* starting about day 10 (reviewed by Ogilvie & Jones 1971), was the cause. It is, of course, possible that the *H. diminuta* itself aggravates the inflammation by, for instance, releasing mast cell degranulators. Whatever the cause, there is evidence from other sources that *H. diminuta* is susceptible to an inflammatory response. Behnke, Bland & Wakelin (1977) found that in mice infected with *Trichinella spiralis* there was a

"profound effect" on the growth and survival of
H. diminuta. This effect was not due to immunological cross reaction as *H. diminuta* developed normally in mice which had been immunized with *T. spiralis* 19-21 days before challenging with *H. diminuta* (the intestinal phase of a primary *T. spiralis* infection is lost in 8-12 days in NIH mice, Wakelin & Lloyd 1976). Nor was the effect of the *T. spiralis* on *H. diminuta* likely to have been due to interspecific competition since *H. diminuta* was only affected in concurrent infections when the inflammatory phase of rejection was reached. *H. diminuta* was not affected if cortisone was given, which would *inter alia*, suppress the inflammatory response. These results of Behnke *et al.* support Weinmann's (1964) conclusions that the "intensive inflammation ... prominent during the second week of infection with *T. spiralis*" reduced the number and altered the distribution of *H. nana* cysticercoids which developed in mice following an egg infection given 15 days post infection with *T. spiralis* and that "there was no indication that an immune response was evoked".

A very different cross reaction occurs between *H. diminuta* and *Nematospiroides dubius*. In the presence of *N. dubius*, the survival of *H. diminuta* is considerably enhanced, for instance, on day 13 of an *H. diminuta* infection, 4 intact and 18 destrobilated worms, with a total dry weight of 6 mg, were recovered from 10 control mice, whereas the recovery from the experimental group, infected with *N. dubius* was 42 large *H. diminuta* with a total dry weight of 650 mg. This effect of *N. dubius* to enhance a concommitant infection, is not confined to *H. diminuta*; Behnke *et al.* (1977) found that the rejection of *T. spiralis* by mice was also suppressed by an *N. dubius* infection. It is probable that this diminished response is another aspect of the depression in the immune response to orally administered antigens which Shimp, Crandall & Crandall (1975) observed when they infected mice with *N. dubius* and is well worth further investigation.

VIII. SURVIVAL IN A RAT

In a rat, *H. diminuta* appears to have a longevity limited only by the life-span of its host. Indeed, Read (1967), by surgically transplanting worms every year into younger rats, maintained worms for 14 years; many times the rat's life-span. Equally, the writer found no sign of aging when he compared (i) the rate of regrowth following surgical insertion into the duodenum of rats of the scolex and an anterior part of the strobila cut from old and young worms, and (ii) the rate of methionine uptake *in vitro* by old (600-day-old) and young (14-day-old) worms cut to the same size (approximately that of a 9-day-old worm). Until recently, therefore, there was no reason to believe the rat developed any immune response to *H. diminuta*. Indeed, Roberts & Mong (1968) wrote with regard to their experiment in which they superimposed 10 secondary worms on rats already infected for 21 days with various primary infections (1-40 worms), that the effect of the primary on the growth of the secondary worms "can be regarded simply as an aspect of the crowding effect manifested in the presence of a pre-existing infection, ... not relevant to resistance". They concluded, "Whether or not the phenomenon of premunition occurs in human *Taenia* infections or those of any other lumen-dwelling cestode, available evidence makes its existence somewhat doubtful". As they wrote, experiments were already underway in various laboratories which were to prove their interpretation wrong. The unkind twist to the story is that Roberts & Mong calculated from their data the very levels of worms "58 ... primary worms required to give essentially complete protection against superinfection", by a crowding effect, which Hindsbo & Andreassen (1976) (see below) were later to show were strongly immunogenic.

In 1968, Coleman, Carty & Graziadei described how *H. diminuta* evoked an antibody response in rats showing that serum contained antibody which on combination with "cell-sap" antigens from *H. diminuta* (or *H. nana*) fixed complement. However, it was not until conclusive evidence of a protective immune response by mice was established that the ability of *H. diminuta* to survive in a rat became an interesting immunological problem. Harris & Turton (1973) confirmed that *H. diminuta* evoked antibody production (see Section V4) and suggested that the rat/*H. diminuta* system might be a valuable model for the study of the uptake of antigens across the 'mucous membranes'. They also considered the model an interesting one "for the emphasis and examination of the functional distinction between protective and non-protective responses". This raises the most fundamental issue in the host/parasite relationship between an adult tapeworm and its host:- does *H. diminuta* survive in the rat because it evokes only a non-protective response or does it survive because it evades the potentially protective response it evokes? The evidence is equivocal.

Chappell & Pike (1976a) observed that while there was no loss of worms up to day 85 from 5 worm infections there was a small loss from 15 worm infections (of doubtful statistical significance) and a considerable loss from 30 worm infections, a result which agrees with those of Harris & Turton (1973) who found no loss up to day 98 p.i. from 5 worm infections but a 60% loss from 25 cyst infections. Similarly, Hindsbo, Andreassen & Hesselberg (1974) reported that infections initiated with a hundred cysticercoids led to rapid loss of worms between 2 and 6 weeks p.i., and Hesselberg & Andreassen (1975) found that at autopsy 56 days p.i., no loss had occurred from 1, 2, 5 and 10 cysticercoid infections but that 21% and 35%, respectively, of worms from 12 and 20 cysticercoid infections had been lost. [The experiment is of particular value as SPF rats were used.] That spontaneous loss usually occurs in heavy infections is certain, but where infections are of a moderate number of worms (12-25) there is great variation in the number lost by different rats in an experiment, and hence the *mean* percentage losses quoted above are potentially misleading. In view of this variability, it is not surprising that Holmes (1961) found no significant loss occurred from a 20 cysticercoid infection in rats autopsied 8 weeks p.i. Chappell & Pike's (1976b) observation that hooded Lister rats (from a different supplier to those used in the earlier work, referred to above 1976a) failed to reject 50 worm infections, at least up to day 48 p.i., is more unexpected. Although loss of worms does not occur from light infections, worms by day 6 of such infections often have extensive dark areas forming on the neck region. As has been discussed (Section V7), these areas are believed to be the result of immune-mediated damage and the harbingers of destrobilation and death.

If then there is uncertainty about the threshold in number of worms above which loss occurs, there is even more uncertainty about the cause of loss. Earlier workers assumed the loss was a manifestation of the 'crowding effect', i.e., a vague physiological phenomenon attributed to various factors, particularly, in view of the critical dependence of adult *H. diminuta* on dietary carbohydrates (Read 1959), to insufficient carbohydrate to support heavy infections. [It has been known for years (Reid 1942) that a decrease in the diet leads to loss of *Raillietina cesticillus* from fowls.] Another physiological interpretation of the "crowding effect" is that site selection stimuli may become blurred and thus worms would become more widely distributed in the intestine (Hopkins 1970). Away from 'preferred regions', worms would almost certainly grow less well, giving rise to stunted worms and probably have a greater chance of being lost completely. Hindsbo *et al.* (1974), however, found that when cortisone was administered to a 100 worm infection, worm loss did not occur. This is not conclusive evidence that an immune response is involved, as cortisone has so many other effects (Section IV1 and Baxter & Forsham 1972), but Hindsbo *et al.* (1974) also found that worms were rejected more quickly from secondary than primary 100 worm infections. Again, it is possible to argue that a 100 worm primary infection causes sufficient damage to the intestine to affect the growth of the secondary infection especially when there is only a short interval between the expulsion of the primary and start of the secondary infection. More recently, however, Andreassen and his colleagues have shown that rats, which had received a 50 worm primary infection terminated after 7 weeks with 'Zanil' (I.C.I.), appeared to be strongly immune when challenged 6 weeks later with a 50 cysticercoid infection. The control rats contained 91±5% of the worms administered with a mean worm weight of 0.6 mg at autopsy on day 7 p.i., whereas the 'immunized' rats contained 65%, many of which were little more than scoleces, with a mean worm weight of 0.16 mg, a highly significant difference. There seems no doubt that given a sufficient challenge a rat will reject *H. diminuta* and the whole concept of "crowding effect" needs very careful re-appraisal. The rat/*H. diminuta* relationship is a fascinating one, a key aspect of which is the threshold at which the immune response becomes effective. Exactly how many worms are needed to evoke a measurable response has not been determined but the Danish workers have always found that a 50 or 100 worm infection stimulated a primary response and gives rise to a strong secondary response when the rats are challenged with 50 or 100 worms. When the primary infection is reduced to 5 worms (terminated with anthelmintics on day 21 and rats challenged with 50 worms on day 28), there was no reduction in the number of worms recovered on day 7 p.i. (96% in immune, 98% in the controls) but the mean weight (0.68 ± 0.30 mg) of the worms from the "immunized" rats was significantly less than that (1.04 ± 0.25 mg) of the worms in the control rats. There is also some evidence that the growth of a 5 worm challenge is reduced in rats previously immunized by a 50 worm infection. [In this case, the challenge was not by five cysticercoids but by five 6-day-old worms recovered from donor rats (see Section VII) and introduced into the duodenum of the immunized and naive control rats (Andreassen & Hopkins, unpublished). The impression is, therefore, that a threshold exists at about five worms above which a demonstrable anamnestic response is evoked.

This concept, that there is a threshold below which the worm either does not initiate a response or alternatively initiates so weak a response that the homeostatic powers of the worm can annul the attack, is not new but has been poorly explored. The situation is confused by many factors. The term 'threshold' is itself used in different senses, i.e. to describe the number of worms which remain after rejection has ceased (Jarrett & Urquhart 1971, referring to *N. brasiliensis* in rats); the number of worms below which there is no effect on worm growth (Dobson 1974, with reference to *Oesophagostomum columbianum* in sheep), the number of worms below which loss by rejection does not occur (Hopkins & Stallard 1974, referring to *H. citelli* in mice). Furthermore, age, sex, intercurrent infections, immunological history of the host, lactation, etc., as well as the method whereby the worms are administered, i.e., as a single dose or as trickle infections (Jenkins & Phillipson 1971) may all affect the threshold. It should also be stressed that sub-threshold primary infections, although not rejected, may be strongly immunogenic, as is the case with *Trichuris muris* (Wakelin 1973) and as appears to be the case with *H. diminuta* where a 5 worm infection although itself unaffected, strongly suppresses the growth and accelerates the loss of a superimposed 50 worm challenge (Andreassen, unpublished). It may be that all intestinal helminths stimulate an immune response but that the effective threshold level for rejection is reached only by large infections in a 'good host', whereas much lower levels are effective at inducing rejection in 'poor hosts'. If this is correct, the question posed is, why should the response be so much less effective in the rat (a good host) than in the mouse (a poor host): there is at present no answer.

As in a mouse, humoral antibodies are produced by a rat in response to infection with *H. diminuta* and immunoglobulins coat *H. diminuta* (Befus 1975b). It has also been observed that rejection of *H. diminuta* by rats is delayed by ALS (Section IV4) and that 'nude' rats (*nu/nu* - see Section V5 - on hooded Listers) fail to reject worms from a 100 worm infection, although the control rats expelled their worms between 15-29 days p.i. Normal apolysis (shedding of proglottids containing eggs) commenced in the 'nude' rats on day 23 p.i. and was still continuing on day 49. An autopsy on day 49 p.i. confirmed a heavy infection had persisted in a 'nude' but no worms remained in the normal 'thymic' control (Andreassen, personal communication).

One other aspect of the rat response which may turn out to be an important clue as to the nature of the immune response is the position of destrobilated worms. Both Andreassen and Hindsbo have observed that following the commencement of rejection in a primary and in a secondary infection, a large number of destrobilated worms are found far forward in the intestine, in the anterior 10 cm from the stomach. This is similar to the anterior migration of *Nippostrongylus brasiliensis* which occurs in the later stages of an infection (Alphey 1970).

IX. VACCINATION AGAINST ADULT CESTODES

Coleman *et al.* (1968) have shown that a crude worm homogenate of *H. nana* injected into mice evokes >99% protection against an *H. nana* egg challenge. However, it would be more relevant to the *H. diminuta* situation if it was known whether protection was evoked against an *H. nana* cysticercoid challenge. In general, arising largely from work with nematodes, many workers are sceptical about the value of extracts of dead worms for vaccination; as Ogilvie & Jones (1973, p. 114) wrote, "antigens concerned in immunity to nematodes and embryonic cestodes are released by actively metabolising worms from ducted glands and are probably enzymes". Nevertheless, using extracts of killed *T. spiralis* larvae Despommier, Campbell & Blair (1977) were able to protect mice and rats against *T. spiralis* and Wakelin and Selby (1973) protected mice against *Trichuris muris* using either whole worm homogenate or the oesophageal region only. The latter would contain the secretion rich stichosome cells from which in *T. spiralis* larvae, Despommier & Müller (1970, 1976) have separated functional, i.e., protective, antigens.

With regard to *H. diminuta* in the intestine, the investigator is faced with three main questions. First, is the extensive work with intestinal nematodes of relevance to tapeworms bearing in mind the utterly different host/parasite interface offered by the tapeworm tegument? Second, are the protective antigens which clearly are produced by live *H. diminuta* in the intestine, structural proteins sloughed off with the glycocalyx (for a review of the structure of the glycocalyx of *Fasciola*, much of which is probably applicable to tapeworms, see Threadgold 1976), tegumentary (enyzmic) secretions or substances escaping from specific areas such as the scolex (Section Vl)? Third, must the antigens be presented enterally? This area of cestode immunology has hardly been touched and in view of the amount that is known about immune responses in mice, the relative cheapness of mice and the availability of specific pathogen free and inbred strains, the mouse/*H. diminuta* system is a good laboratory model. In the first place, it would be interesting to establish whether whole-worm homogenates or stripped tegument (Oaks & Knowles 1974), administered parenterally or enterally, protect. Seddon (1931) claimed he protected sheep against *Moniezia expansa* by injecting ground up proglottids but Elowni, working in the writer's laboratory, failed to induce any protection by parenteral (subcutaneous) injection of an homogenate of *H. diminuta* ± FIA (Freund's incomplete adjuvant) nor did the intraperitoneal implantation of live immature and mature worms have any effect on the growth of 'challenge' worms subsequently implanted into the duodenum (see Section VI). The only parenteral procedure which gave any protection was the intra-peritoneal injection of 80 excysted cysticercoids repeated three times at weekly intervals. Even this procedure yielded results which were only just statistically significant. This failure to immunize by parenteral procedures is not surprising; parenteral vaccines against enteric diseases have been notoriously poor. What is surprising is how little interest until recently has been shown in oral immunization yet the fact that one can induce hypersensitivity by oral administration of proteins was experimentally demonstrated nearly 70 years ago (Wells & Osborne 1911). It is now abundantly established that extensive macromolecular uptake occurs across the ileum of adult rats (reviewed by Hemmings 1978) and that sensitization with a protein leads to a marked decrease in the amount of that specific protein which is subsequently absorbed (reviewed by André, André & Vaerman 1978). *A priori* it would appear that, as *H. diminuta* lives in the intestine and as it induces a strong long-lasting immunity (Section III), the logical approach to a vaccine is the presentation of the antigen(s) enterally. Problems such as denaturation of the protein in the stomach should easily be overcome (Section VI), but as yet the best that has been achieved by giving homogenates of *H. diminuta* orally to mice (six doses at 72h intervals) is a 35% reduction in size of challenge worms (Elowni, unpublished). There is also the problem that the amount of antigen that is needed to sensitized may in fact be very small (Section VI) so the administration of large (gram) quantities of homogenate in the hope that at least some of the important 'protective' antigens are included by inducing tolerance (cf. Andre, Vaerman & Heremans 1978) may be self-defeating. A more precise indication of the quantity of live tapeworm necessary to induce protection should be forthcoming from experiments by Christie, in which the ability of irradiated cysticercoids of *H. diminuta* to immunize mice is being assessed. [An irradiated cysticercoid excysts and the small worm survives but does not grow in the mouse intestine.] However, not only may the quantity of antigen presented by important but also its form. Ebersole & Molinari (1978) have shown that an antigen presented to a mucosal surface in a soluble form evokes a very different response to that evoked by the same antigen in a particulate form.

If extracts of dead worms fail, medium in which worms have been cultured may be effective as it is against the larval stages of *Taenia* spp. in the tissues (Rickard & Bell 1971; Heath 1976; Rickard & Adolph 1976; Rickard & Katiyar 1976; Rickard, White & Boddington 1976) and against egg production by *Echinococcus granulosus* in the intestines of dogs (Herd, Chappel & Biddell 1975). The field is certainly worthy of exploration, after all it is easier to vaccinate a pastoralist than his herd or a sheep dog than its flock.

X. CONCLUSIONS

The immunological model presented by a tapeworm stretching over much of the length of the small intestine and bombarding the host with foreign macromolecules, is of interest to a far wider range of scientists than are tapeworms. The basic problem of how it is that a tapeworm such as *H. diminuta* can survive in a light infection in a rat as long as the rat lives (Section VIII), yet be rejected within 9-14 days by a mouse (Section II), is central to our understanding of host specificity. So far, adult tapeworms in the intestine as distinct from larval stages in the tissues have received very little attention compared with intestinal nematodes. There are a number of reasons, e.g., the greater ease with which nematodes are maintained in the laboratory and their greater economic importance. It may be that the problem of how the gut keeps itself to itself can be unravelled completely from nematode studies, but there is no proof of this and cestodes do have certain advantages. One of these is that the interface between a tapeworm and its host lies on the surface of the tapeworm where all digestive/absorptive processes occur. A second advantage is that by worm standards, a lot is known about the fine structure (Lumsden 1975) and biochemical properties (Pappas & Read 1975) of this surface. A third and often not appreciated point is that some tapeworms, like *H. diminuta* and *H. citelli* have no hooks, only a transitory attachment to the villi and no tissue phase in the definitive host. Very few, if any, nematodes are confined throughout development to the intestinal lumen.

The position at present is that *Hymenolepis diminuta* undoubtedly evokes an immune response in mice which involves both antibody production (Section V4) and T-cells (Section V5). Immune responses are also evoked by *Raillietina cesticillus* in fowl and by *H. citelli* and *H. microstoma* in mice (see Introduction). The hypothesis may reasonably be advanced that all tapeworms evoke a response. If this is assumed to be true, the corollary is that to be successful, tapeworms must be able to avoid the immune response. Work on *H. diminuta* in a rat supports this. There is growing evidence that while the threshold at which rejection occurs is above five worms, infections of five worms evoke both concomitant protection against challenge and immunological memory (Section VIII). Whether all host specificity in mammals depends on the ability or failure of a worm to combat a host attack is not known. Probably this is overstating the importance of immunity but even if the 'composition of the bile salts', 'nature of the mucus secretion', the 'composition of the exocrino-enteric circulation', 'lack of correct site selection stimuli' and various other physiological factors which have been suggested as influencing the survival of the worm are important, ultimately a worm which has survived these physiological hazards must surely meet an immune response. What the antigens are that the worm releases, where they come from - desquamated tegument or secretions, where they are taken up, what cells are stimulated, where these cells develop, what the effector arm is, what part of the tapeworm is affected and what steps a tapeworm takes in a 'good host' to negate the attack, we do not know, but unlike a decade ago, we now realize that answers to such questions are essential if we are to understand host specificity.

REFERENCES

1. Alphey, T. J. W., Studies on the distribution and site location of *Nippostrongylus brasiliensis* within the small intestine of laboratory rats. *Parasitology 61*, 449-460 (1970).
2. Anderson, J. M., Transplantation - Nature's success. *Lancet II*, 1077-1082 (1971).
3. André, C., André, F., and Vaerman, J. P., Biological function of antigen - IgA antibody complexes: *in vivo* and *in vitro* interference with intestinal absorption and tolerogenic effect. In "Antigen Absorption by the Gut" (W. A. Hemmings, ed.), pp. 73-80. MTP Press Limited, Lancaster, (1978).
4. André, C., Vaerman, J. P., and Heremans, J. F., Oral immunization of rats with human serum albumin: interference with intestinal absorption and tolerogenic effect. In "Antigen Absorption by the Gut" (W. A. Hemmings, ed.), pp. 65-71. MTP Press Limited, Lancaster, (1978).
5. Andreassen, J., Hindsbo, O., and Ruitenberg, E. J., *Hymenolepis diminuta* infections in congenitally athymic (nude) mice: worm kinetics and intestinal histopathology. *Immunology 34*, 105-113 (1978).
6. Baggiolini, M., The enzymes of the granules of polymorphonuclear leukocytes and their functions. *Enzyme 13*, 132-160 (1972).
7. Balow, J. E., Parrillo, J. E., and Fauci, A. S., Characterization of the direct effects of cyclophosphamide on cell-mediate immunological responses. *Immunology 32*, 899-904 (1977).
8. Barth, E. E. E., Jarrett, W. F. H., and Urquhard, G. M., Studies on the mechanism of the self-cure reaction in rats infected with *Nippostrongylus brasiliensis*. *Immunology 10*, 459-464 (1966).

9. Baxter, J. D., and Forsham, P. H., Tissue effects of glucocorticoids. *Am. J. Med. 53*, 573-589 (1972).
10. Bazin, H., The secretory antibody system. *In* "Immunological Aspects of the Liver and Gastrointestinal Tract" (A. Ferguson and R. N. M. MacSween, eds.), pp. 33-82. MTP Press Limited, Lancaster, (1976).
11. Befus, A. D., Secondary infection of *Hymenolepis diminuta* in mice: effects of varying worm burdens in primary and secondary infections. *Parasitology 71*, 61-75 (1975a).
12. Befus, A. D., Intestinal immune responses of mice to the tapeworms *Hymenolepis diminuta* and *H. microstoma*. Ph.D. Thesis, University of Glasgow, (1975b).
13. Befus, A. D., *Hymenolepis diminuta* and *H. microstoma*: Mouse immunoglobulins binding to the tegumental surface. *Exp. Parasitol. 41*, 242-251 (1977).
14. Befus, A. D., and Featherston, D. W., Delayed rejection of single *Hymenolepis diminuta* in primary infections of young mice. *Parasitology 69*, 77-85 (1974).
15. Befus, A. D., and Podesta, R. B., Intestine. *In* "Ecological Aspects of Parasitology" (C. R. Kennedy, ed.), pp. 303-325. North-Holland Publishing Company, Amsterdam, (1976).
16. Befus, A. D., and Threadgold, L. T., Possible immunological damage to the tegument of *Hymenolepis diminuta* in mice and rats. *Parasitology 71*, 525-534 (1975).
17. Behnke, J. M., Bland, P. W., and Wakelin, D., Effect of the expulsion phase of *Trichinella spiralis* on *Hymenolepis diminuta* infection in mice. *Parasitology 75*, 79-88 (1977).
18. Berenbaum, M. C., Comparison of the mechanisms of action of immunosuppressive agents. *In* "Progress in Immunology II" (L. Brent and J. Holborow, eds.) Vol. 5, pp. 233-243. American Elsevier Publishing Company, Inc., New York, (1974).
19. Beverley, P. C. L., Lymphocyte heterogeneity. *In* "B and T Cells in Immune Recognition" (F. Loor and G. E. Roelants, eds.), pp. 35-37. John Wiley and Sons, London, (1977).

20. Bland, P. W., Immunity to *Hymenolepis diminuta*: unresponsiveness of the athymic nude mouse to infection. *Parasitology* 72, 93-97 (1976a).
21. Bland, P. W., The immune response of the mouse to the tapeworm *Hymenolepis diminuta*. Ph.D. Thesis, University of Glasgow, (1976b).
22. Bockman, D. E., and Cooper, M. D., Pinocytosis by epithelium associated with lymphoid follicles in the bursa of Fabricius, appendix, and Peyer's patches. An electron microscopic study. *Am. J. Anat.* 136, 455-477 (1973).
23. Bodmer, B., and Siboo, R., Isolation of mouse C-reactive protein from liver and serum. *J. Immunol.* 118, 1086-1089 (1977).
24. Boughton, R. V., The influence of helminth parasitism on the abundance of the snowshoe rabbit in Western Canada. *Can. J. Res.* 7, 524-547 (1932).
25. Brambell, F. W. R., "The Transmission of Passive Immunity from Mother to Young, Frontiers of Biology" Vol. 18. North-Holland, Amsterdam; American Elsevier, New York, (1970).
26. Brandtzaeg, P., and Baklien, K., Intestinal secretion of IgA and IgM: a hypothetical model. *In* "Immunology of the Gut, Ciba Foundation Symposium", pp. 77-113. Elsevier/Excerpta Medica/North-Holland, Amsterdam, (1977).
27. Castro, G. A., Roy, S. A., and Stockstill, R. D., *Trichinella spiralis*: Peroxidase activity in isolated cells from the rat intestine. *Exp. Parasitol.* 36, 307-315 (1974).
28. Cebra, J. J., Kamat, R., Gearhart, P., Robertson, S. M., and Tseng, J., The secretory IgA system of the gut. *In* "Immunology of the Gut, Ciba Foundation Symposium", pp. 5-28. Elsevier/Excerpta Medica/North-Holland, Amsterdam, (1977).
29. Chandler, A. C., The effects of number and age of worms on development of primary and secondary infections with *Hymenolepis diminuta* in rats, and an investigation into the true nature of "premunition" in tapeworm infections. *Am. J. Hyg.* 20(D), 105-114 (1939).
30. Chappell, L. H., and Pike, A. W., Loss of *Hymenolepis diminuta* from the rat. *Int. J. Parasitol.* 6, 333-339 (1976a).

31. Chappell, L. H., and Pike, A. W., Interactions between *Hymenolepis diminuta* and the rat. In "Proceedings of the Second International Symposium on the Biochemistry of Parasites and Host-Parasite Relationships" (H. Van den Bossche, ed.), pp. 379-384. Elsevier/North-Holland Biomedical Press, Amsterdam, (1976b).
32. Choromanski, L., The influence of cyclophosphamide on the development of *Hymenolepis diminuta* in mice. *Short Communications Fourth Int. Cong. Parasitol. E*, 32-33 (1978).
33. Ciba Foundation Symposium, Immunology of the Gut. Elsevier/Excerpta Medica/North-Holland, Amsterdam, (1977).
34. Claman, H. N., Corticosteroids and lymphoid cells. *New England J. Med. 287*, 388-397 (1972).
35. Claman, H. N., How corticosteroids work. *J. Allergy & Clin. Immunol. 55*, 145-151 (1975).
36. Cohen, J. J., and Claman, H. N., Thymus-marrow immunocompetence. V. Hydrocortisone-resistant cells and processes in the hemolytic antibody response of mice. *J. Exp. Med. 133*, 1026-1034 (1971).
37. Coleman, R. M., Carty, J. M., and Graziadei, W. D., Immunogenicity and phylogenetic relationship of tapeworm antigens produced by *Hymenolepis nana* and *Hymenolepis diminuta*. *Immunology 15*, 297-304 (1968).
38. Connan, R. M., Effect of lactation on the immune response to gastrointestinal nematodes. *Vet. Rec. 99*, 476-477 (1976).
39. de Sousa, M. A. B., Ecology of thymus dependency. In "Contemporary Topics in Immunobiology" (A. J. S. Davies and R. L. Carter, eds.) Vol. 2, pp. 119-136. Plenum Press, New York, (1973).
40. Despommier, D., and Müller, M., Functional antigens of *Trichinella spiralis*. Proceedings of the Second International Congress of Parasitology, Washington, D.C. *J. Parasitol. 56*, No. 4, Section II, Part 1, 76 (1970).
41. Despommier, D. D., and Müller, M., The stichosome and its secretion granules in the mature muscle larva of *Trichinella spiralis*. *J. Parasitol. 62*, 775-785 (1976).
42. Despommier, D. D., Campbell, W. C., and Blair, L. S., The *in vivo* and *in vitro* analysis of immunity to *Trichinella spiralis* in mice and rats. *Parasitology 74*, 109-119 (1977).

43. Dineen, J. K., and Kelly, J. D., Levels of prostaglandins in the small intestine of rats during primary and secondary infection with *Nippostrongylus brasiliensis*. *Int. Arch. of Allergy and Applied Immunol.* 51, 429-440 (1976).
44. Dobson, C., Studies on the immunity of sheep to *Oesophagostomum columbianum*: effects of different and successive doses of larvae on worm burdens, worm growth and fecundity. *Parasitology* 68, 313-322 (1974).
45. Ebersole, J. L., and Molinari, J. A., The induction of salivary antibodies by topical sensitization with particulate and soluble bacterial immunogens. *Immunology* 34, 969-979 (1978).
46. Elias, E., and Dowling, R. H., The mechanism for small-bowel adaptation in lactating rats. *Clinical Sci. and Mol. Med.* 51, 427-433 (1976).
47. Van Epps, D. E., and Williams, R. C., Suppression of leukocyte chemotaxis by human IgA myeloma components. *J. Exp. Med.* 144, 1227-1242 (1976).
48. Van Epps, D. E., Reed, K., and Williams, R. C., Suppression of human PMN bactericidal activity by human IgA paraproteins. *Cell. Immunol.* 36, 363-376 (1978).
49. Fabris, N., Immunological reactivity during pregnancy in the mouse. *Experientia* 29/5, 610-612 (1973).
50. Ferguson, A., and Parrott, D. M. V., The effect of antigen deprivation on thymus-dependent and thymus-independent lymphocytes in the small intestine of the mouse. *Clin. Exp. Immunol.* 12, 477-488 (1972).
51. Fye, K. H., Moutsopoulos, H., and Talal, N., B and T lymphocytes in autoimmunity. *In* "B and T Cells in Immune Recognition" (F. Loor and G. E. Roelants, eds.), pp. 355-376. John Wiley and Sons, London, (1977).
52. Gemmell, M. A., Natural and acquired immunity factors interfering with development during the rapid growth phase of *Echinococcus granulosus* in dogs. *Immunology* 5, 496-503 (1962).
53. Gemmell, M. A., Immunology and regulation of the cestode zoonoses. *In* "Immunology of Parasitic Infections" (S. Cohen and E. H. Sadun, eds.), pp. 333-358. Blackwell Scientific Publications, Oxford, (1976).

54. Gemmell, M. A., and MacNamara, F. N., Immune response to tissue parasites. II. Cestodes. In "Immunity to Animal Parasites" (E. J. L. Soulsby, ed.), pp. 235-272. Academic Press, New York, (1972).
55. Gewurz, H., Wernick, P. R., Quie, P. G., and Good, R. A., Effects of hydrocortisone succinate on the complement system. *Nature 208*, 755-757 (1965).
56. Ghazal, A. M., and Avery, R. A., Observations on coprophagy and the transmission of *Hymenolepis nana* infections in mice. *Parasitology 73*, 39-45 (1976).
57. Goodall, R. I., Studies on the growth, location specificity and immunobiology of some hymenolepid tapeworms. Ph.D. Thesis, University of Glasgow, (1973).
58. Gray, J. S., Studies on host resistance to secondary infections of *Raillietina cesticillus* (Molin 1858) in the fowl. *Parasitology 67*, 375-382 (1973).
59. Gray, J. S., The cellular response of the fowl small intestine to primary and secondary infections of the cestode *Raillietina cesticillus* (Molin). *Parasitology 73*, 189-204 (1976).
60. Harris, W. G., and Turton, J. A., Antibody response to tapeworm (*Hymenolepis diminuta*) in the rat. *Nature, London 246*, 521-522 (1973).
61. Heath, D. D., Resistance to *Taenia pisiformis* larvae in rabbits: Immunization against infection using non-living antigens from *in vitro* culture. *Int. J. Parasitol. 6*, 19-24 (1976).
62. Hemmings, W. A., "Maternofoetal Transmission of Immunoglobulins". Cambridge University Press, Cambridge, (1976).
63. Hemmings, W. A., The transmission of high molecular weight breakdown products of protein across the gut of suckling and adult rats. In "Antigen Absorption by the Gut" (W. A. Hemmings, ed.), pp. 37-47. MTP Press Limited, Lancaster, (1978).
64. Hemmings, W. A., and Williams, E. W., Transport of large breakdown products of dietary protein through the gut wall. *Gut 19*, 715-723 (1978).
65. Henderson, D., The effect of worm age, weight and number in the infection on the absorption of glucose by *Hymenolepis diminuta*. *Parasitology 75*, 277-284 (1977).

66. Hendrix, S., Kopia, G., and Lattime, E., Effects of concurrent infection with *Nippostrongylus brasiliensis* upon *Hymenolepis diminuta* in the rat small intestine. *Prog. Abst. Am. Soc. Parasitol. Fiftieth Ann. Meet.*, No. 241, 101 (1975).
67. Herd, R. P., Chappel, R. J., and Biddell, D., Immunization of dogs against *Echinococcus granulosus* using worm secretory antigens. *Int. J. Parasitol. 5*, 395-399 (1975).
68. Hesselberg, C. A., and Andreassen, J., Some influences of population density on *Hymenolepis diminuta* in rats. *Parasitology 71*, 517-523 (1975).
69. Heyneman, D., Studies on helminth immunity: I. Comparison between lumenal and tissue phases of infection in the white mouse by *Hymenolepis nana* (Cestoda: Hymenolepididae). *Am. J. Trop. Med. Hyg. 11*, 46-63 (1962a).
70. Heyneman, D., Studies on helminth immunity. II. Influence of *Hymenolepis nana* (Cestoda: Hymenolepididae) in dual infections with *H. diminuta* in white mice and rats. *Exp. Parasitol. 12*, 7-18 (1962b).
71. Hill, D. L., "A Review of Cyclophosphamide". Charles Thomas, Illinois, (1975).
72. Hindsbo, O., and Andreassen, J., Immunity to *Hymenolepis diminuta* in the rat: effects of ATS treatment. *Parasitology 73*, xxx (1976).
73. Hindsbo, O., Andreassen, J., and Hesselberg, C. A., Immunity to *Hymenolepis diminuta* in the rat. Proceedings of the Scandinavian Society for Parasitology. *Norwegian J. Zool. 23*, 197 (1974).
74. Holmes, J. C., Effects of concurrent infections on *Hymenolepis diminuta* (Cestoda) and *Moniliformis dubius* (Acanthocephala). I. General effects and comparison with crowding. *J. Parasitol. 47*, 209-216 (1961).
75. Hopkins, C. A., Location-specificity in adult tapeworms with special reference to *Hymenolepis diminuta*. *Proc. Second Int. Cong. Parasitol.*, Washington, D.C. *J. Parasitol. 56*, No. 4, Section II, Part 3, 561-564 (1970).
76. Hopkins, C. A., Goodall, R. I., and Zajac, A., The longevity of *Hymenolepis microstoma* in mice and its immunological cross reaction with *H. diminuta*. *Parasitology 74*, 175-183 (1977).

77. Hopkins, C. A., and Stallard, H. E., Immunity to intestinal tapeworms: the rejection of *Hymenolepis citelli* by mice. *Parasitology 69*, 63-76 (1974).
78. Hopkins, C. A., and Stallard, H. E., The effect of cortisone on the survival of *Hymenolepis diminuta* in mice. *Rice Univ. Studies 62*, No. 4, 145-159 (1976).
79. Hopkins, C. A., Subramanian, G., and Stallard, H., The development of *Hymenolepis diminuta* in primary and secondary infections in mice. *Parasitology 64*, 401-412 (1972a).
80. Hopkins, C. A., Subramanian, G., and Stallard, H., The effect of immunosuppressants on the development of *Hymenolepis diminuta* in mice. *Parasitology 65*, 111-120 (1972b).
81. Hopkins, C. A., and Zajac, A., Transplantation of *Hymenolepis diminuta* into naive, immune and irradiated mice. *Parasitology 73*, 73-81 (1976).
82. Howard, R. J., The growth of secondary infections of *Hymenolepis microstoma* in mice: the effect of various primary infection regimes. *Parasitology 72*, 317-323 (1976).
83. Howard, R. J., *Hymenolepis microstoma*: a change in susceptibility to resistance with increasing age of the parasite. *Parasitology 75*, 241-249 (1977).
84. Husband, A. J., Monie, H. J., and Gowans, J. L., The natural history of the cells producing IgA in the gut. *In:* "Immunology of the Gut, Ciba Foundation Symposium", pp. 29-54. Elsevier/Excerpta Medica/North-Holland, Amsterdam, (1977).
85. Isaak, D. A., Jacobson, R. H., Reed, N. D., Thymus dependence of tapeworm (*Hymenolepis diminuta*) elimination from mice. *Inf. and Immun. 12*, 1478-1479 (1975).
86. Jarrett, E. E. E., and Urquhart, G. M., The immune response to nematode infections. *Int. Rev. Trop. Med. 4*, 53-96 (1971).
87. Jarrett, W. F. H., Jarrett, E. E. E., Miller H. R. P., and Urquhart, G. M., Quantitative studies on the mechanism of self-cure in *Nippostrongylus brasiliensis* infections. *Proc. Third Int. Conf. World Assoc. Adv. Vet. Parasitol. In:* "The Reaction of the Host in Parasitism" (E. J. L. Soulsby, ed.), pp. 191-198. Elwert Universitäts und Verlagsbuchhandlung, Marburg/Lahn, (1968).

88. Jenkins, D. C., and Phillipson, R. F., The kinetics of repeated low-level infections of *Nippostrongylus brasiliensis* in the laboratory rat. *Parasitology 62*, 457-465 (1971).
89. Jenkins, S. N., and Wakelin, D., The source and nature of some functional antigens of *Trichuris muris*. *Parasitology 74*, 153-161 (1977).
90. Johnson, L. R., Progress in gastroenterology: the trophic action of gastrointestinal hormones. *Gastroenterology 70*, 278-288 (1976).
91. Kantor, T. G., Anti-inflammatory drugs. *In* "Textbook of Immunopathology" (P. A. Miescher and H. J. Müller-Eberhard, eds.) Vol. 1, pp. 329-342. Grune and Stratton, New York, (1976).
92. Katz, S. I., Parker, D., Sommer, G., and Turk, J. L., Suppressor cells in normal immunisation as a basic homeostatic phenomenon. *Nature 248*, 612-614 (1974).
93. Lachmann, P. J., Complement. *In* "Clinical Aspects of Immunology" (P. G. H. Gell, R. R. A. Coombs and P. J. Lachmann, eds.), pp. 323-364. Blackwell Scientific Publications, Oxford, (1975).
94. Lamm, M. E., Cellular aspects of immunoglobulin A. *Adv. Immunol. 22*, 223-290 (1976).
95. Lance, E. M., Immunosuppression, *In* "Clinical Immunobiology" (F. H. Bach and R. A. Good, eds.) Vol. I, pp. 193-218. Academic Press, New York, (1972).
96. Larsh, J. E. Jr., and Weatherly, N. F., Cell-mediated immunity in certain parasitic infections. *Current Topics Microbiol. Immunol. 67*, 113-137 (1974).
97. Lewis, G. P., and Piper, P. J., Inhibition of release of prostaglandins as an explanation of some of the actions of anti-inflammatory corticosteroids. *Nature 254*, 308-311 (1975).
98. Lumsden, R. D., Surface ultrastructure and cytochemistry of parasitic helminths. *Exp. Parasitol. 37*, 267-339 (1975).
99. Mackaness, G. B., The monocyte in cellular immunity. *Seminars Hematology 7*, 172-184 (1970).

100. Mayrhofer, G., "Immunology of the Gut, Ciba Foundation Symposium". Elsevier/Excerpta Medica/North-Holland, Amsterdam, (1977).
101. Miller, H. R. P., and Walshaw, R., Immune reactions in mucous membranes. IV. Histochemistry of intestinal mast cells during helminth expulsion in the rat. *Am. J. Pathol.* 69, 195-206 (1972).
102. Miller, H. R. P., Murray, M., and Jarrett, W. F. H., Globule leukocytes and mast cells. In "The Reaction of the Host to Parasitism", *Proc. Third Int. Conf. World Assoc. Adv. Vet. Parasitol.* (E. J. L. Soulsby, ed.), pp. 198-210. N.G. Elwert Universitäts- und Verlagsbuchhandlung, Marburg/Lahn, (1968).
103. Moorhead, J. W., and Claman, H. N., Thymus-derived lymphocytes and hydrocortisone: identification of subsets of theta-bearing cells and redistribution of bone marrow. *Cell. Immunol.* 5, 74-86 (1972).
104. Morcock, R. E., and Roberts, L. S., Concurrent infections of *Hymenolepis diminuta* and *Nippostrongylus brasiliensis*: Effects of host diets deficient in protein. *Prog. Abst. Am. Soc. Parasitol. Fifty-First Ann. Meet.*, No. 109, 49 (1976).
105. Moss, G. D., The nature of the immune response of the mouse to the bile duct cestode *Hymenolepis microstoma*. *Parasitology* 62, 285-294 (1971).
106. Müller-Eberhard, H. J., The serum complement system. In "Textbook of Immunopathology" (P. A. Miescher and H. J. Müller-Eberhard, eds.) Vol. 1, pp. 45-73. Grune and Stratton, New York, (1976).
107. Murray, M., Immediate hypersensitivity effector mechanisms. II. *In vivo* reactions. In "Immunity to Animal Parasites" (E. J. L. Soulsby, ed.), pp. 155-190. Academic Press, New York, (1972).
108. Murray, M., Smith, W. D., Waddell, A. H., and Jarrett, W. F. H., *Nippostrongylus brasiliensis*: Histamine and 5-hydroxytryptamine inhibition and worm expulsion. *Exp. Parasitol.* 30, 58-63 (1971).

109. Oaks, J. A., and Knowles, W., Isolation and partial characterization of fractions derived from the tegument of *Hymenolepis diminuta*. *Prog. Abst. Am. Soc. Parasitol. Forty-Ninth Ann. Meet.*, No. 84, 37 (1974).
110. Oaks, J. A., and Lumsden, R. D., Cytological studies on the absorptive surfaces of cestodes. V. Incorporation of carbohydrate-containing macromolecules into tegument membranes. *J. Parasitol. 57*, 1256-1268 (1971).
111. Ogilvie, B. M., and Jones, V. E., *Nippostrongylus brasiliensis*: A review of immunity and the host/parasite relationship in the rat. *Exp. Parasitol. 29*, 138-177 (1971).
112. Ogilvie, B. M., and Jones, V. E., Immunity in the parasitic relationship between helminths and hosts. *Progress in Allergy 17*, 93-144 (1973).
113. Ogilvie, B. M., and Love, R. J., Cooperation between antibodies and cells in immunity to a nematode parasite. *Transplantation Review 19*, 147-168 (1974).
114. Ottolenghi, A., High phospholipase content of intestines of mice infected with *Hymenolepis nana*. *Lipids 8*, 426-428 (1973).
115. Pappas, P., and Read, C., Trypsin inactivation by intact *Hymenolepis diminuta*. *J. Parasitol. 58*, 864-871 (1972a).
116. Pappas, P., and Read, C., Inactivation of α- and β-chymotrypsin by intact *Hymenolepis diminuta*. *Biol. Bull. 143*, 605-616 (1972b).
117. Pappas, P. W., and Read, C. P., Membrane transport in helminth parasites: A review. *Exp. Parasitol. 37*, 469-530 (1975).
118. Parker, D., and Turk, J. L., The effect of cyclophosphamide pretreatment on B-cell stimulation: dissociation of action on homocytotropic antibody and other B-cell functions. *Immunology 34*, 115-121 (1978).
119. Parrott, D. M., The gut-associated lymphoid tissues and gastrointestinal immunity. *In* "Immunological Aspects of the Liver and Gastrointestinal Tract" (A. Ferguson and R. N. M. MacSween, eds.), pp. 1-32. MTP Press Limited, Lancaster, (1976).
120. Poynter, D., Parasitic bronchitis. *Adv. Parasitol. 1*, 179-212 (1963).

121. Read, C. P., The role of carbohydrates in the biology of cestodes. VIII. Some conclusions and hypotheses. *Exp. Parasitol. 8*, 365-382 (1959).
122. Read, C. P., Longevity of the tapeworm, *Hymenolepis diminuta*. *J. Parasitol. 53*, 1055-1056 (1967).
123. Read, C. P., and Phifer, K., The role of carbohydrates in the biology of cestodes. VII. Interactions between individual tapeworms of the same and different species. *Exp. Parasitol. 8*, 46-50 (1959).
124. Read, C. P., and Voge, M., The size attained by *Hymenolepis diminuta* in different host species. *J. Parasitol. 40*, 88-89 (1954).
125. Reid, W. M., Certain nutritional requirements of the fowl cestode *Raillietina cesticillus* (Molin) as demonstrated by short periods of starvation of the host. *J. Parasitol. 28*, 319-340 (1942).
126. Rembiesa, R., Ptak, W., and Bubak, M., The immunosuppressive effects of mouse placental steroids. *Experientia 30*, 82-83 (1974).
127. Rickard, M. D., and Adolph, A. J., Vaccination of calves against *Taenia saginata* infection using a "parasite-free" vaccine. *Vet. Parasitol. 1*, 389-392 (1976).
128. Rickard, M. D., and Bell, K. J., Successful vaccination of lambs against infection with *Taenia ovis* using antigens produced during *in vitro* cultivation of the larval stages. *Res. Vet. Sci. 12*, 401-402 (1971).
129. Rickard, M. D., and Katiyar, J. C., Partial purification of antigens collected during *in vitro* cultivation of the larval stages of *Taenia pisiformis*. *Parasitology 72*, 269-279 (1976).
130. Rickard, M. D., White, J. B., and Boddington, E. B., Vaccination of lambs against infection with *Taenia ovis*. *Aust. Vet. J. 52*, 209-214 (1976).
131. Roberts, L. S., and Mong, F. N., Developmental physiology of cestodes. III. Development of *Hymenolepis diminuta* in superinfections. *J. Parasitol. 54*, 55-62 (1968).
132. Roitt, I. M., "Essential Immunology". 3rd edition. Blackwell Scientific Publications, Oxford, (1977).

133. Seddon, H. R., The development in sheep of immunity to *Moniezia expansa*. *Ann. Trop. Med. Parasitol.* 25, 431-435 (1931).
134. Shimp, R. G., Crandall, R. B., and Crandall, C. A., *Heligmosomoides polygyrus* (= *Nematospiroides dubius*): Suppression of antibody response to orally administered sheep erythrocytes in infected mice. *Exp. Parasitol.* 38, 257-269 (1975).
135. Skowron-Cendrzak, A., Ptak, W., Bubak, M., and Czarnik, Z., Non-specific decrease of cell-mediated immunity in female mice during syngeneic and allogeneic pregnancy. *Folia Biologica* (Prague) 21(1), 70-74 (1975).
136. Smyth, J. D., Cultivation and development of larval cestode fragments *in vitro*. *Nature, London* 181, 1119-1122 (1958).
137. Smyth, J. D., Observations on the scolex of *Echinococcus granulosus*, with special reference to the occurrence and cytochemistry of secretory cells in the rostellum. *Parasitology* 54, 515-526 (1964).
138. Smyth, J. D., Parasites as biological models. *Parasitology* 59, 73-91 (1969).
139. Smyth, J. D., Some interface phenomena in parasitic protozoa and platyhelminths. *Can. J. Zool.* 51, 367-377 (1973).
140. Spiegelberg, H. L., and Götze, O., Conversion of C3 proactivator and activation of the alternate pathway of complement activation by different classes and subclasses of human immunoglobulins. *Fed. Proc.* 31, 655 (1972).
141. Spiegelberg, H. L., Lawrence, D. A., and Henson, P., Cytophilic properties of IgA to human neutrophils. In "Advances in Experimental Medicine and Biology, The Immunoglobulin A system" (J. Mestecky and A. R. Lawton, eds.) Vol. 45, pp. 67-74. Plenum Press, London, (1974).
142. Stern, C. M., Fetomaternal relationships. In "The Immune System" (M. J. Hobart and I. McConnell, eds.), pp. 308-316. Blackwell Scientific Publications, Oxford, (1975).
143. Tan, B. D., and Jones, A. W., Resistance of mice to reinfection with the bile duct cestode, *Hymenolepis microstoma*. *Exp. Parasitol.* 22, 250-255 (1968).

144. Thompson, J., and Van Furth, R., The effect of glucocorticosteroids on the kinetics of mononuclear phagocytes. *J. Exp. Med. 131*, 429-442 (1970).
145. Thompson, J., and Van Furth, R., The effect of glucocorticosteroids on the proliferation and kinetics of promonocytes and monocytes of the bone marrow. *J. Exp. Med. 137*, 10-21 (1973).
146. Threadgold, L. T., *Fasciola hepatica*: ultrastructure and histochemistry of the glycocalyx of the tegument. *Exp. Parasitol. 39*, 119-134 (1976).
147. Turk, J. L., "Immunology in Clinical Medicine". William Heinemann Medical Books Ltd., London, (1969).
148. Turk, J. L., and Parker, D., Further studies on B-lymphocyte suppression in delayed hypersensitivity, indicating a possible mechanism for Jones-Mote hypersensitivity. *Immunology 24*, 751-758 (1973).
149. Turk, J. L., and Poulter, L. W., Selective depletion of lymphoid tissue by cyclophosphamide. *Clin. Exp. Immunol. 10*, 285-296 (1972).
150. Turk, J. L., Parker, D., and Poulter, L. W., Functional aspects of the selective depletion of lymphoid tissue by cyclophosphamide. *Immunology 23*, 493-501 (1972).
151. Turton, J. A., Williamson, J. R., and Harris, W. G., Haematological and immunological responses to the tapeworm *Hymenolepis diminuta* in man. *Tropenmed. Parasitol. 26*, 196-200 (1975).
152. Wakelin, D., The stimulation of immunity to *Trichuris muris* in mice exposed to low-level infections. *Parasitology 66*, 181-189 (1973).
153. Wakelin, D., and Lloyd, M., Immunity to primary and challenge infections of *Trichinella spiralis* in mice: a re-examination of conventional parameters. *Parasitology 72*, 173-182 (1976).
154. Wakelin, D., and Selby, G. R., Functional antigens of *Trichuris muris*. The stimulation of immunity by vaccination of mice with somatic antigen preparations. *Int. J. Parasitol. 3*, 711-715 (1973).
155. Walker, W. A., Isselbacher, K. J., and Bloch, K. J., Intestinal uptake of macromolecules: effect of oral immunization. *Science 177*, 608 (1972).

156. Wassom, D. L., DeWitt, C. W., and Grundmann, A. W., Immunity to *Hymenolepis citelli* by *Peromyscus maniculatus*: genetic control and ecological implications. *J. Parasitol. 60*, 47-52 (1974).
157. Weinmann, C. J., Host resistance to *Hymenolepis nana*. II. Specificity of resistance to reinfection in the direct cycle. *Exp. Parasitol. 15*, 514-526 (1964).
158. Weinmann, C. J., Immunity mechanisms in cestode infections. *In* "Biology of Parasites" (E. J. L. Soulsby, ed.), pp. 301-320. Academic Press, New York, (1966).
159. Weinmann, C. J., Cestodes and Acanthocephala. *In* "Immunity to Parasitic Animals" (G. J. Jackson, R. Herman and I. Singer, eds.) Vol. 2, pp. 1021-1059. Appleton-Century-Crofts, New York, (1970).
160. Wells, H. G., and Osborne, T. B., The biological reactions of the vegetable proteins. I. Anaphylaxis. *J. Inf. Dis. 8*, 66-124 (1911).
161. Winkelstein, A., Mechanisms of immunosuppression: effects of cyclophosphamide on cellular immunity. *Blood 41*, 273-284 (1973).

MIGRATORY ACTIVITY AND RELATED PHENOMENA IN *HYMENOLEPIS DIMINUTA*

Hisao P. Arai

Department of Biology, University of Calgary
Calgary, Alberta, Canada

I. INTRODUCTION

Periodic activity, recurring on roughly a 24-hr interval is a well known phenomenon which is widespread throughout the animal kingdom. These rhythms (variously referred to as diurnal, circadian, or diel) were well documented by Harker (1958). In his excellent review on circadian and other rhythms of parasites, Hawking (1975) identified the migration of intestinal worms as one of the four patterns of circadian rhythms exhibited by parasitic animals. Crompton's (1973) extensive review entitled "The sites occupied by some parasitic helminths in the alimentary tract of vertebrates" is not only important for his treatment of the subject but also for his position on and explanation of the terms: *site*, *emigration*, and *migration*. He supports his preference for the term *site* since "the word is simpler than 'location', it avoids confusion with a parasite's posture which might be implied by the use of the term 'position' and it reduces the misuse of the term 'niche', which has an important ecological meaning...." He defined *emigration* to describe a change of site without a return journey, and reserves the use of *migration* to movements involving a regular phase of coming and going between sites or within a site.

The literature dealing directly with observations

on migratory activity of helminths in the alimentary tract of vertebrates is relatively small, and that dealing with *Hymenolepis diminuta* is smaller still. Those observations of importance which impinge on the topic under review is voluminous and cannot be considered in any detail in this review. However, reference to other chapters of this volume should yield information of relevance.

A type of activity, perhaps more accurately, emigratory activity of helminths, has been competently documented and summarized in reviews such as those of Ulmer (1971), Crompton (1973), and Holmes (1973). The phrases: site-finding behaviour, location-specificity, site-seeking, and site-selection have been used by these and other authors to denote a predilection of helminths for establishment in specific sites in the host. Although these phenomena are based primarily on observations during early ontogenetic development of worms in the definitive host, other studies involving surgical transplantation of worms, have indicated that similar activity in adult stages (Goodchild 1958; Bråten and Hopkins 1969) does occur.

II. SITE-SELECTION IN *H. DIMINUTA*

The initial observations of site-selection in *H. diminuta* in its early stages of development in the rat's intestine have frequently been attributed to Chandler (1939) who stated that "The worms usually make their original attachment 40 centimeters or more behind the stomach, but most of them move forward between the seventh and tenth days." Presumably this conclusion is based on information obtained from his studies on the growth rate of *H. diminuta* in the rat host. However, the evidence presented does not provide sufficient details to confirm his contention nor is it adequate (in light of current knowledge) to determine whether or not he was observing emigratory or migratory activity.

Perhaps the best early evidence for site selection in developing *H. diminuta* is presented by Goodchild and Harrison (1961). In their study, they showed that, at various intervals over a 4 to

120 h period, the young worms are located anteriorly soon after entry into the small intestine of the rat and at the end of this period (i.e. 120 h), "36 of 53 (68%) were found from 25 to 28 cm behind the stomach." Mettrick and Dunkley (1969) reported that both the scoleces and biomass of 3- and 5-day-old worms were concentrated in the second quarter of the intestine, with the mean scolex attachment point for 5-day-old worms at 39% of the total intestinal length behind the pyloric sphincter. Turton (1971), who also studied the distributional pattern of *H. diminuta* in the rat intestine during the early development of the strobilate stage, supplemented the observations of Goodchild and Harrison (*loc. cit.*). He found a distribution encompassing some 35% of the length of the intestine from 10% to the 45% position, with mean points of 25.9% (16 h), 26.9% (day 3) and 29.5% (day 6). The evidence presented by the authors cited immediately above, varies in detail, but does confirm the view that *H. diminuta*, soon after excysting, shows a propensity for localizing in relatively restricted sites along the length of the rat intestine.

Another aspect of site-selecting activity of *H. diminuta* was initially demonstrated by Goodchild (1958) who reported that "regardless of the site of implantation in the small intestine adult tapeworms succeeded in crawling forward or backward to reach their normal position, with the scolex usually 5 to 30 cm behind the pyloric valve." Although he reported that the growth of tapeworms transfaunated into the small intestine of rats was rather rapid, worms implanted into the large intestine did not survive or, at least, were not recovered at autopsy. Bråten and Hopkins (1969), in a refinement of Goodchild's (*loc. cit.*) experiments, have verified the site-selecting behaviour of *H. diminuta* in their elaborate transfaunation studies. They showed that 6 1/2- and 7 1/2-day-old worms surgically implanted into the small intestine of recipient rats some 3 cm posterior to the stomach emigrated posteriorly and those inserted some 5 cm anterior to the ileocecal junction emigrated anteriorly. In another experiment designed to assess the rate of movement of 6 1/2- to 7 1/2-day-old worms implanted near the cecum, they found that: within 13 h most worms had moved anteriorly almost half the length of the intestine; by 19 h some worms had reached the anterior third of the small intestine, although the majority of the worms still lay in the 40-50% region; by 24 h some of the worms had reached the 15-30% region. At 29 h a segregation of the worms into two discrete groups was noted, one group distributed anterior to 35%, and the other group not advancing further than the region reached in the 13-14 h period. They correlated the distributional patterns observed at 24 and 29 h with differences in weight of the worms at the time of transfer into the recipient host. (This brief summary represents only a minor portion of evidence presented by the latter authors. The reader is urged to consult the original work, not only for the wealth of information, but also for the variety of research possibilities suggested by their studies.)

The effects of concurrent infection (with *Moniliformis dubius*) on site-selection in *H. diminuta* was clearly illustrated by Holmes (1961, Fig. 1). In single-species infections, the majority of the tapeworms were attached in the anterior third of the rat intestine; however, when the hosts were infected concurrently with 5 *H. diminuta* cysticercoids and 10 *M. dubius* cystacanths, the tapeworms were displaced posteriorly into the mid-third of the gut. The acanthocephalans, on the other hand, were not affected appreciably in their intraintestinal distribution. Employing the same materials and procedures, Holmes (1962) examined the distribution of these worms in hamsters. In contrast to the results obtained from rats (i.e. the posteriad displacement of *H. diminuta* by *M. dubius*), he did not obtain evidence of any alteration in the distribution of either of the two species of parasites. In a different set of experiments to assess intraspecific effects, Holmes (1961, Figs. 2 and 3) showed that increasing the numbers of tapeworms in single-species infections tended to extend the ranges in distribution of *H. diminuta*: 40% of the anterior intestine in 5-worm infections; 50% of the anterior gut in 10-worm infections; and nearly 70% of the anterior portion of the gut in 20-worm infections.

III. EMIGRATIONAL AND MIGRATIONAL ACTIVITIES OF
    H. DIMINUTA

As mentioned above, the first observations on an anteriad movement during the growth of *H. diminuta* in the rat gut were recorded by Chandler (1939). A number of subsequent workers (e.g. Goodchild and Harrison 1961; Holmes 1962; Bråten and Hopkins 1969; Cannon and Mettrick 1970; Evans and Wickham 1971; Bailey 1971 and Turton 1971) have amplified on his observations and have demonstrated similar activity. We (Chappell *et al.* 1970), examining distributional patterns of worms 5-14 days of age, concluded that three distinct patterns of activity were distinguishable, i.e. an anteriad migration within the first 20 in of the intestine from a.m. to p.m. on days 5, 6, and 7; followed on day 8 by a period when no activity is apparent; which in turn, is followed by a reversal of the first pattern involving the entire intestine on all subsequent days of experimentation. Our conclusions were tested by Tanaka and MacInnis (1975) who modified the procedure to emphasize the absolute age of the worms and stomach emptying time of the rat hosts. Based on their results, they concluded that "*H. diminuta* exhibited two concurrent migrations: an age-dependent forward migration (Chandler 1939) and a circadian migration (Read and Kilejian 1969)." They summarized their findings of the forward and diel patterns of activity as a "continuous, oscillating sine wave, slowly moving forward, then stopping the forward migration but continuing to oscillate, the amplitude of the oscillations being approximately 10% of the gut's length." They attribute the initial pattern of activity described by Chappell *et. al* (1970) "to be an anomaly resulting from the method whereby both the age and size of the worms were assumed to be uniform throughout the 24 hr test period."

IV. MIGRATION OF *H. DIMINUTA* IN ALTERED ENVIROMENTS

Although there is a relatively substantial body of literature dealing with the effects of altered feeding regimes and modified diets of hosts on such aspects as growth, development and fecundity of *H. diminuta*, there is a paucity of reports on the effects of these procedures on migratory activity of this tapeworm.

Perhaps the first suggestion that this behavior is related to ingestion of food by the host was made by Read and Kilejian (1969) who reported that short periods of host starvation delayed anteriad migration and that a temporal displacement by some 10 h of the feeding period of the host altered the migratory behavior by a commensurate period of time. At nearly the same time, Hopkins (1969) noted a change in the position of tapeworms in the rat intestine following a host meal and questioned whether this change could be correlated to the time intervals after a normal meal. These observations were extended by Bailey (1971) who noted that migration was not exhibited by worms in starved rats and by Evans and Wickham (1971) who reported an inhibition of cestode migration in hosts which were starved for 10 h; the latter authors also reported a reduction in the number of worms (as measured by weight) migrating in hosts from which food was withheld for 5.5 h.

Chappell *et al.* (1970) carried out experiments to determine the effects upon worm migration of various diets administered to the rat host. These effects were measured in terms of worm wet-weight distributions in the rat intestine at three periods during the day. Worms harboured by rats fed experimental diets of low-starch for 2 days and high-starch for 2 days did not migrate; on the other hand, worms on a high-starch diet for a single day migrated from the anterior intestine to the posterior intestine during host fasting. Migration was also observed in worms on a high-protein diet administered for a single day. However, the migrations shown by by these worms in hosts on the latter two diets did differ from control worms in that they did not show a subsequent anteriad shift of tissue into the anterior intestinal segment of the host between 0830 and 1200 h. A fifth diet was clearly unsatisfactory since rats refused to eat the mixture of corn oil and alphacel which was provided. In those experiments in which the cestodes did not migrate, the bulk of worm tissue was located in the anterior 20 in. of the rat intestine, irrespective of the time of day.

Mettrick (1971) investigated the influences of the quality and quantity of host dietary factors on migrational response of *H. diminuta*. The dietary constituents which he tested included: glucose, dextrin, galactose, olive oil, and a mixture containing 17 amino acids and ammonia. An initial anteriad movement of worm biomass and scoleces were noted for each of the carbohydrate diets, as well as for the one with olive oil. The tapeworms responded to the amino acid diet by only a posteriad movement 1 h after feeding before returning to a position close to the original distribution. Quantitatively, the movements of biomass and scoleces were delayed in hosts that were fed 3 g glucose in contrast to those fed 1 g quantities. The observations on the effects of glucose diets on migration of the worms confirm Mettrick's (1971) earlier results and were again re-confirmed by Mettrick (1972).

Using rats fasted for 20-24 h and harbouring 5-worm, 14-day-old *H. diminuta* infections, Mead (1976) applied a method (Mead and Roberts 1972) to alter the glucose gradient of the rat's small intestine. By feeding rats (via a stomach tube) a meal of soluble starch, he obtained small amounts of glucose in the anterior and middle thirds of the small intestine and greater quantities in the posterior third, i.e. in contrast to rats which obtained starch through meal feeding. A posteriad migration was noted as the glucose content of the middle and distal segments increased. However, 2 h post-feeding, the tapeworms had moved anteriorly, although glucose was still present in the posterior third and absent in the anterior two-thirds of the gut. After 3 h, the distribution of the tapeworms was similar to that prior to feeding by intubation.

V. MIGRATION IN ALTERNATIVE HOST SPECIES

Using rats, hamsters, and mice for comparative purposes, Turton (1971) examined the distribution of *H. diminuta* in the intestine of these hosts during the first 3 weeks of infection. In rats, he noted an initial attachment of scoleces about a mean of 26% along the length of the small intestine, followed by an anteriad movement after about day 6. By day 21, the worms exhibited a distribution with a mean attachment position about 13% of the length of the small intestine from the pylorus. In the hamster, the mean initial attachment (after 16 h) was at 50% with the anteriad movement occurring after day 2. This movement progressed incrementally so that by day 21, the mean point of scolex attachment was at 11.7%. In mice, the distributions at 16 h, 3 and 6 days were 31.9, 28.1 and 31.6%, respectively. From day 9 until the infections were lost by day 21, the worms were widely dispersed in the host gut and did not display a discrete distributional pattern.

In contrast to Turton's (*loc. cit.*) protocol where he examined the positions of the worms at the same time each day over the 21-day interval, we, in this laboratory, at 4 h intervals examined the pattern of movement of worm biomass over a 24 h period, starting at 0900 on day 11 pi. Although multivariate analysis of variance for the proportions of wet-weights of *H. diminuta* in the first two segments (thirds) of the intestine were not significantly different, we noted that the proportion of worm tissue in the proximal third of the intestine decreased to a minimum at 0100 and 0500 hrs and then increased between 0500 and 0900 hrs. There were corresponding changes in the proportion of tissue in the distal third of the intestine: from 2100 to 0500 hrs, the proportion of tissue increased and from 0500 and 0900 hrs it decreased. The proportion of tissue in the middle third of the gut remained fairly constant throughout the testing period. Although these data suggest a diel migratory pattern involving a posteriad movement from 2100 to 0100 hrs and an anteriad movement from 0500 to 0900, it should be emphasized that these movements were not statistically significant.

VI. MIGRATION OF *HYMENOLEPIS DIMINUTA* IN SINGLE AND MULTIPLE WORM INFECTIONS

Using a design to test effects of worm number and age on migratory behavior, Read and Kilejian (1969) examined worm movement in rats harboring infections of 10 worms, 14-days-old; 10 worms, 21-days-old; 1 worm, 14-days-old; and 30 worms, 10-days-old. They concluded that, within the limits of the conditions tested, migratory behavior of *H. diminuta* appears to be independent of age and worm burden.

The influence of population density of tapeworms on the position of the worms in the rat gut was assessed by Hesselberg and Andreassen (1975). Reporting on the position of worms between 0800 and 1000 hrs, they noted that in 1, 2, or 5 worm infections, the mean position of the worms were significantly anterior to the mean position of the worms in heavier (10, 12, 20 worm) infections. In addition to the differences in mean positions, worms in the heavier infections showed a greater dispersion about the mean.

VII. MIGRATION OF OTHER SPECIES OF *HYMENOLEPIS*

Subsequent to the early observations of Joyeux and Kobozieff (1927) on the distribution of *Hymenolepis microstoma* in the definitive host, the studies of Dvorak *et. al.* (1961) appear to be the first to document the chronology of site selection in this species of cestode. The latter authors indicated that the tapeworms exhibit a random wandering in the upper 25% of the mouse intestine during the first 24 h pi, before becoming more localized in the next 24 h. They also found that the worms begin establishing themselves in the bile duct within 96 h, that those which have remained in the duodenum start to show a more dispersed distribution, and that those which have not reached the bile duct after 144 h do not become established.

Litchford (1963) provided evidence that the laboratory rat and hamsters can also serve as hosts for *H. microstoma* and that site selection by this tapeworm in these hosts is similar to that observed in mice, although the number of adult worms remaining attached to the wall of the duodenum increased from mouse to hamster to rat. He also noted that in the latter host, duodenal attachment by the worms was markedly greater in older (i.e. 23-day-old vs. 34-day-old) rats.

De Rycke (1966) confirmed the results of Dvorak *et al.* (*loc. cit.*) on the establishment of *H. microstoma* in its early stages in the mouse; however, De Rycke's data appear to indicate that these worms can become established in the host, although they have not reached the bile duct within 144 h.

Using three strains of rats, Goodall (1972)

reported that an average of 60% of the cysticercoids became established in weanling rats, in contrast to only 10% in rats over 10 weeks old. Movement of the worms into or near the bile duct was noted on days 4, 5, and 6 pi. Of the 35% of worms which remained attached to the duodenum, most failed to develop and after 9 (± 2) days, destrobilated before being lost from the host.

In their publication entitled "Migratory behavior of *Hymenolepis microstoma*", Cooreman and De Rycke (1972) presented their evidence for site selection by *H. microstoma* in mice. Examining the distribution soon after administering 20-100 cysticercoids *per os*, they found that these worms pass rapidly through the alimentary tract so that by 1.5 h pi, a distribution of individuals to a point some 30-35 cm posterior to the pylorus can be noted. The authors attribute this random distribution of worms during the first 24 h to differences in individual rates of excystation and in ability for attachment to the intestinal wall. The recovery of greater percentages of worms in progressively anterior sites during days 1-8 is interpreted by Cooreman and De Rycke (*loc. cit.*) as an anteriad movement of the parasites. They concluded that entrance of the cestodes into the bile duct is initiated on day 5 pi and is virtually completed on day 8. To confirm the view that an anteriad movement does occur during ontogeny of *H. microstoma*, these same worker designed an imaginative experiment where cysticercoids, excysted *in vitro*, were implanted at 5 cm intervals along the length of the mouse gut. Although no worms were recovered from portions of the intestine posterior to a point 25 cm from the pylorus and some posterior relocation was noted initially, the anterior shift of worm tissue with time is quite evident. The results of this specific experiment also confirmed the chronology of movement of these worms from the duodenum into the bile duct.

In studies conducted primarily to assess the histopathological response of mice to *H. microstoma*, Pappas and Mayer (1976) transplanted the anterior 2 mm section of 21-day-old worms into the small intestine approximately 5 cm posterior to the duodenal papilla. On day 1 pi the transplanted worms were still in the small intestine but the anteriad movement of the worms had begun; on day 2 pi, however, the worms had entered the bile duct, i.e. some three days earlier than any time recorded previously.

Another aspect of site selection in *H. microstoma* was investigated by Lang (1967) in determining whether *Fasciola hepatica* would establish and mature in the bile ducts of mice harbouring 5-worm infections of the tapeworm; he also investigated the effects of concurrent infection on both parasites. In mice where the 25-day-old cestodes were challenged with two *F. hepatica* metacercariae, the tapeworms after 60 days of co-habitation were found attached in the duodenum, at the junction of the common bile duct, and in the distal 2 or 3 mm of the bile duct. Although the total weight of *H. microstoma* tissue per mouse from the concurrent infections was significantly less than that for the single-species infection, the average weight per tapeworm was similar in the two groups. From these results, Lang (*loc. cit.*) concluded that "Apparently, *F. hepatica* caused *H. microstoma* to move from its optimum attachment site, which resulted in re-attachment in less favorable location and (caused) a decrease in the number of tapeworms."

In this laboratory, we examined single worm infections of *H. citelli* and *H. peromysci* in hamsters for evidence of diel migration. Data for *H. citelli* were collected from samples comprised from four hosts between 0900 hrs on day 11 and 0900 hrs on day 12 pi. The distribution of tissue in the anterior, middle, and posterior thirds (each about 10 cm in length) of the intestine was determined. Although examinations were made at 4 h intervals during the test period, no worm tissue was present in the posterior third of the gut at any time of the day. As shown in Figure 1, from 0900 to about 2100 (day 11 pi), the bulk of *H. citelli* tissue was located in the middle third of the intestine. The only statistically significant shift in tissue occurred soon after 2100 resulting in an increase in tissue in the anterior segment with a commensurate decrease of tissue in the middle third. A diel migration is not indicated, however, since *H. citelli* did not assume a more posterior position by 0900 hrs on day 12. These results are very similar to those obtained by Arai and Chappell (unpublished) using 5- and 10-worm infections, also in hamsters.

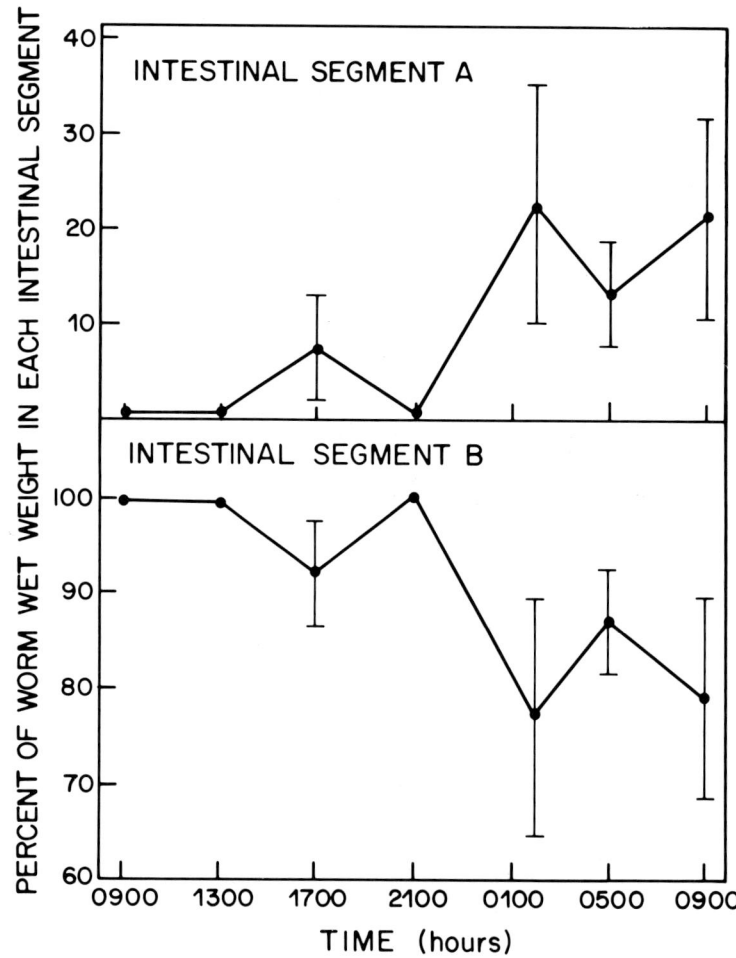

Figure 1. The distribution of H. citelli in the intestine from 0900 h on day 11 to 0900 h on day 12 pi. The vertical bars represent standard errors.

Applying the same protocol and using the same methods, we have also determined the distribution of *H. peromysci* in the hamster gut between 0900 h on day 15 and 0900 h on day 16 pi. Differing from *H. diminuta* and *H. citelli* in hamsters, *H. peromysci* appears to restrict itself to the posterior two-thirds of the hamster's gut (Fig. 2), i.e. no tapeworm tissue was recovered from the anterior third of the gut at any time during the period of examination. Although a relocation of tissue did occur, treatment of the data using analysis of variance did not indicate shifts which were statistically significant.

Although no statistically significant movement of tissue was noted between 0900 hrs on day 11 and 0900 hrs on day 12 pi, Figure 3 is included to illustrate the distributional patterns of *H. diminuta* at 4 h intervals during the testing period.

The majority of the various hypotheses, stated or implied, concerning site-selection in the definitive host has been restricted primarily to a "concept" of an optimal site for growth and development of the worm. However, what constitutes an optimal site has not been determined with any degree of definition. In spite of this lack, the evidence now available confirms the fact that *H. diminuta*, like many other helminths, is capable of site-selection. The subsequent relocation of the worms during early ontogeny of the strobilate stage has been attributed to the changing requirements of the tapeworms during this period (see Mettrick and Podesta 1974). However, since this relocation has been observed in the majority of the cases at or about 6-8 days pi, the question remains whether this anteriad shift in position is an integral part of site-selecting behavior or is merely representing the initiation of the diel migratory response noted in older worms.

For interpretations and commentaries on diel migration of *H. diminuta*, the reader is referred to the excellent reviews of the subject by Holmes (1973) and Mettrick and Podesta (1974). From these reviews, it is obvious that most early authors have taken Read and Kilejian's (1969) lead and have attempted to assess a variety of nutritional factors as cues for "triggering" migratory activity. Others have

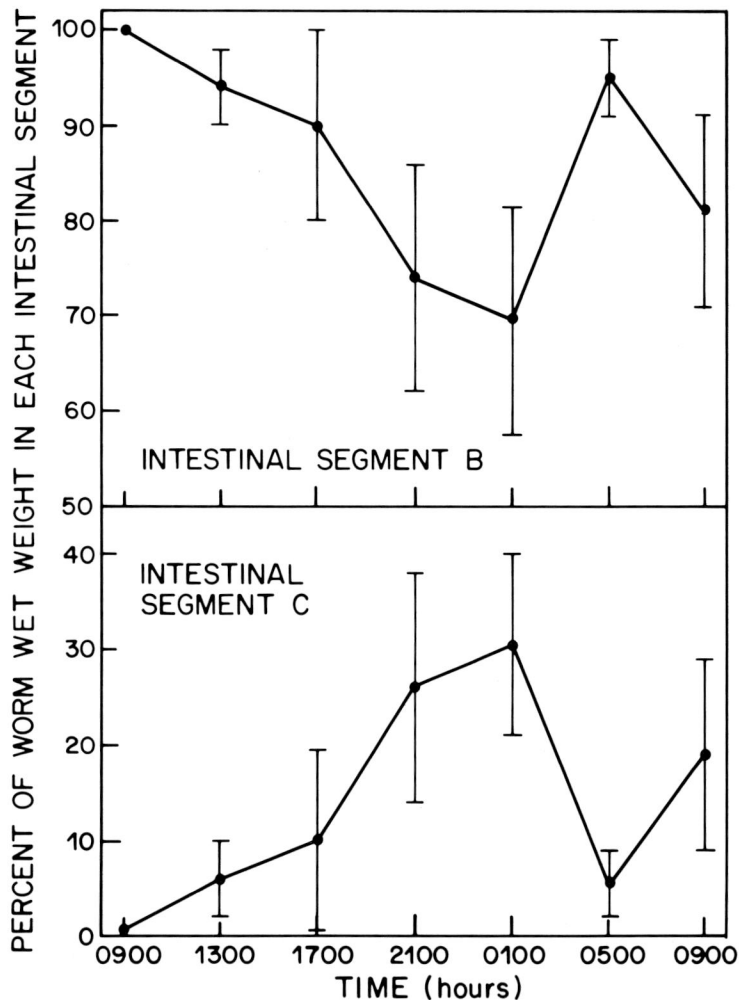

Figure 2. The distribution of H. peromysci in the intestine from 0900 h on day 15 to 0900 h on day 16 pi. The vertical bars represent standard errors.

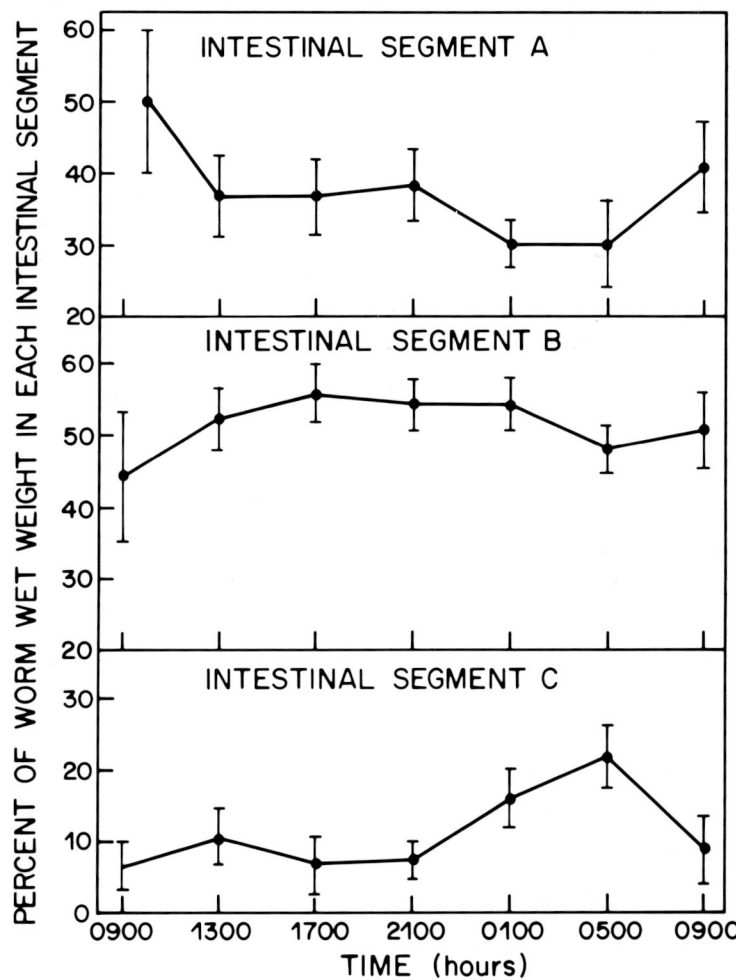

Figure 3. The distribution of H. diminuta in the intestine from 0900 h on day 11 to 0900 h on day 12 pi. The vertical bars represent standard errors.

hypothesized environmental gradients and optimal sites as bases for diel migration; these views also emphasized nutritional requirements as stimulating influences for this behavioral response. Still others (e.g. Hopkins 1970), stressed the need for a consideration of the perceptive abilities of the worm in terms of stimuli and, as well, changes in the environmental cues.

The view that *H. diminuta* has the ability to respond to a variety of environmental stimuli has been expressed by Hopkins and Allen (1979). Their results from surgically altered tapeworms, appear to support the contention that the tapeworm is able to monitor information about its immediate environment over the entire strobila and that the tapeworm is able to integrate this information to the extent that a migratory pattern is developed. This orientation to possible answers on migratory behavior is quite appealing, especially when one reads a statement by Wilson and Schiller (1969) that "Such apparently purposeful alignment [juxtapositioning of sexually mature proglottids *in vitro*] suggest that these worms respond to reproductive stimuli, and the relatively intense enzymatic activity around the genital atrium of *H. diminuta* implies that neurosecretory cells and chemoreceptors occurring in this area may be responsible for production and recognition of such stimuli."

Additional avenues of research were indicated by Mettrick (1973); his presentation of an elaborate and well-conceived model of possible host-parasite interactions clearly indicates the multiplicity of factors and the dynamic equilibria which must be considered in any subsequent assessment of site-selection and migratory behavior of *H. diminuta*.

VIII. DISCUSSION

It is clear from the evidence discussed above that the tapeworm and its host represents a complex, integrated and dynamic association consisting of a multitude of ecological, physiological and biochemical factors. For this reason, it appears that answers to questions involving site-selection and diel migration in *H. diminuta* cannot be found by manipulation of only one or a few aspects of the interaction between the parasite and its host.

Although the bulk of the experimentation does not deal directly with site-selection or migratory behavior *per se*, studies on the rat intestine as an environment for *H. diminuta* (see Mettrick, this volume) and helminth-host interactions in the mammalian gastrointestinal tract (e.g. Podesta and Mettrick 1973, 1974a, 1974b, 1974c, 1975, 1976a, 1976b, 1976c, 1977) have provided ample suggestions for further research. In addition, the work of Castro *et. al.* (1976), reporting on the course of infection with *H. diminuta* in rats shifted from enteral to total parenteral nutrition, should be considered carefully for the actual role that exogenous (enteral) food plays in determining migratory activity. The observation that *H. diminuta* destrobilates and restrobilates under total parenteral nutrition is evidence that the requirements for growth and development of the worm are available from the exocrinoenteric circulation of the host.

Insight into the role of environmental stimuli, particularly in site-selection, has been furnished by Hopkins and Allen (1979). Their results provide evidence that *H. diminuta* can and does monitor environmental stimuli, but little is known of these cues. A review of the neuroanatomy of *H. diminuta*, suggesting the possible roles of the nervous system of these tapeworms is presented by Lumsden and Specian (this volume). Further studies of this nature should add invaluable information on the sensory capabilities of these worms.

The report by Kearn (1973) of an endogenous circadian rhythm in a monogenean trematode, *Entobdella soleae* and that of Page *et. al.* (1977) on a diurnal periodicity of uridine uptake by *H. diminuta* should raise questions as to the integrative capacity of flatworm nervous systems. Perhaps the assessment recorded by Webb and Davey (1975) that "The gross anatomy of the nervous system of cestodes is remarkably complex, and therefore, statements suggesting that parasites have simple nervous systems or that cestodes have suffered secondary simplification may be discarded." best summarizes the need for further examination and experimentation on this aspect of the biology of these tapeworms.

Another area which requires attention but not treated in any systematic fashion is the need for standardization of the biological materials used in assessing factors influencing site-selection and the development of the migratory pattern of *H. diminuta*. It is rather common knowledge that "stocks" of *H. diminuta* differ from one laboratory to another and that a high degree of variability exists, even in a given stock. Compounding the difficulties in attempting to compare results derived from sources such as these, is the variability which exists in the so-called "rat host". Read and Voge (1954) clearly indicated the relative responses in terms of growth of *H. diminuta* in various species of hosts and in two strains of rats. The appreciable differences noted even within a single strain of laboratory rats might be explained by the observations of Teitelbaum and Campbell (1958) who, investigating ingestion patterns in hyperphagic and normal rats, noted that the intake of solid food varied: in the amount eaten daily, in the average meal size, in the number of meals per day, and in the rate of ingestion. By adding the difference in the protocols used by various workers, it is not difficult to ascribe the discrepancies in results and differences in interpretation which are prevalent in the literature, to the inherent biological variability of *H. diminuta* and its host(s).

Perhaps the oft-quoted remark that we have come a long way but we still have a long way to go, is the most appropriate description of the state of the art in this aspect of the biology of *H. diminuta*.

REFERENCES

1. Bailey, G. N. A. *Hymenolepis diminuta:* circadian rhythm in movement and body length in the rat. *Exp. Parasitol.* 29, 285-291 (1971).
2. Bråten, T., and Hopkins, C.A., The migration of *Hymenolepis diminuta* in the rat's intestine during normal development and following surgical transplantation. *Parasitology* 59, 891-905 (1969).

3. Cannon, C. E., and Mettrick, D. F., Changes in the distribution of *Hymenolepis diminuta* (Cestoda: Cyclophyllidea) within the rat intestine during prepatent development. *Can. J. Zool.* 48, 761-769 (1970).
4. Castro, G. A., Johnson, L. R., Copeland, E. M., and Dudrick, S. J., Course of infection with enteric parasites in hosts shifted from enteral to total parenteral nutrition. *J. Parasitol.* 62, 353-359 (1976).
5. Chandler, A. C., The effects of numbers and age of worms on development of primary and secondary infections with *Hymenolepis diminuta* in rats, and an investigation into the true nature of "premunition" in tapeworm infections. *Am. J. Hyg.* 29D, 105-114 (1939).
6. Chappell, L. G., Arai, H. P., Dike, S. C., and Read, C. P., Circadian migration of *Hymenolepis* (Cestoda) in the intestine. I. Observations on *H. diminuta* in the rat. *Comp. Biochem. Physiol.* 34, 34-46 (1970).
7. Cooreman, I., and De Rycke, P. H., Migratory behavior of *Hymenolepis microstoma*. *Z. Parasitenk.* 39, 269-276 (1972).
8. Crompton, D. W. T., The sites occupied by some parasitic helminths in the alimentary tract of vertebrates. *Biol. Rev.* 48, 27-83 (1973).
9. De Rycke, P. H., Development of the cestode *Hymenolepis microstoma* in *Mus musculus*. *Z. Parasitenk.* 27, 350-354 (1966).
10. Dvorak, J. A., Jones, A. W., and Kuhlman, H. H., Studies on the biology of *Hymenolepis microstoma* (Dujardin, 1845). *J. Parasitol.* 47, 833-838 (1961).
11. Evans, D. S., and Wickham, M. G., The migratory behavior of *Hymenolepis diminuta* in rats. *Proc. West Virginia Acad. Sci.* 43, 99-102 (1971).
12. Goodall, R. I., The growth of *Hymenolepis microstoma* in the laboratory rat. *Parasitology* 65, 137-142 (1972).
13. Goodchild, C. G., Transfaunation and repair of damage in the rat tapeworm, *Hymenolepis diminuta*. *J. Parasitol.* 44, 345-351 (1958).
14. Goodchild, C. G., and Harrison, D. L., The growth of the rat tapeworm, *Hymenolepis diminuta*, during the first five days in the final host. *J. Parasitol.* 47, 819-829 (1961).
15. Harker, J. E., Diurnal rhythms in the animal

kingdom. *Biol. Rev.* *33*, 1-52 (1958).
16. Hawking. F., Circadian and other rhythms of parasites. *In:* "Advances in Parasitology" (B. Dawes, ed.), Vol. 13, pp. 123-216 (1975).
17. Hesselberg, C. A., and Andreassen, J., Some influence of population density on *Hymenolepis diminuta* in rats. *Parasitology* *71*, 517-523 (1975).
18. Holmes, J. C., Effects of concurrent infections on *Hymenolepis diminuta* (Cestoda) and *Moniliformis dubius* (Acanthocephala). I. General effects and comparison with crowding. *J. Parasitol.* *47*, 209-216
19. Homes, J. C., Effects of concurrent infections on *Hymenolepis diminuta* (Cestoda) and *Moniliformis dubius* (Acanthocephala). III. Effect on hamsters. *J. Parasitol.* *48*, 97-100 (1962).
20. Holmes, J. C., Site selection by parasitic helminths: interspecific interactions, site segregations, and their importance to the development of helminth communities. *Can. J. Zool.* *51*, 333-347 (1962).
21. Hopkins, C. A., Location-specificity in adult tapeworms with special reference to *Hymenolepis diminuta*. *J. Parasitol.* *56(4:II:3)*, 561-564 (1970a).
22. Hopkins, C. A., Diurnal movement of *Hymenolepis diminuta* in the rat. *Parasitology* *60*, 255-271 (1970b).
23. Hopkins, C. A., and Allen. L. M., *Hymenolepis diminuta*: the role of the tail in determining the position of the worm in the intestine of the rat. *Parasitology* *79*, 401-409 (1979).
24. Joyeux, Ch., and Kobozieff, N. I., Recherches sur l'*Hymenolepis microstoma* (Dujardin, 1845). *Comp. Rend. Soc. Biol.* *97*, 12-13 (1927).
25. Kearn, G. C., An endogenous circadian rhythm in the monogenean skin parasite *Entobdella soleae*, and its relationship to the activity rhythm of the host (*Solea solea*). *Parasitology* *66*, 101-122 (1973).
26. Lang, B. Z., *Fasciola hepatica* and *Hymenolepis microstoma* in the laboratory mouse. *J. Parasitol.* *53*, 213-214 (1967).
27. Litchford, R. G., Observations on *Hymenolepis microstoma* in three laboratory hosts: *Mesocricetus auratus*, *Mus musculus* and *Rattus norvegicus*. *J. Parasitol.* *49*, 403-410 (1963).

28. Mead, R. W., Effect of abnormal intestinal glucose distribution on the migration of *Hymenolepis diminuta*. *J. Parasitol. 62*, 328-329 (1976).
29. Mead, R. W., and Roberts, L. S., Intestinal digestion and absorption of starch in the intact rat: effects of cestode (*Hymenolepis diminuta*) infection. *Comp. Biochem. Physiol. 41A*, 749-760 (1972).
30. Mettrick, D. F., Effect of host dietary constituents on intestinal pH and migrational behavior of the rat tapeworm *Hymenolepis diminuta*. *Can. J. Zool. 49*, 1513-1525 (1971).
31. Mettrick, D. F., Changes in the distribution and chemical composition of *Hymenolepis diminuta*, and the intestinal nutritional gradients of uninfected and parasitized rats following a glucose meal. *J. Helminthol. 46*, 407-429 (1972).
32. Mettrick, D. G., Competition for ingested nutrient between the tapeworm *Hymenolepis diminuta* and the rat host. *Can. J. Publ. Hlth. 64(Monog. Suppl.)*, 70-82 (1973).
33. Mettrick, D. F., and Dunkley, L. C., Variation in the size and position of *Hymenolepis diminuta* (Cestoda: Cyclophyllidea) within the rat intestine. *Can. J. Zool. 47*, 1091-1101 (1969).
34. Mettrick, D. F., and Podesta, R. B., Ecological and physiological aspects of helminth-host interactions in the mammalian gastrointestinal canal. *In:* "Advances in Parasitology" (B. Dawes, ed.), Vol. 12, pp. 183-278. Academic Press, New York & London (1974).
35. Page, C. R. III, MacInnis, A. J., and Griffith, L. M., Diurnal periodicity of uridine uptake by *Hymenolepis diminuta*. *J. Parasitol. 63*, 91-95.
36. Pappas, P. W., and Mayer, L. P., The effect of transplanted *Hymenolepis microstoma*, the mouse bile duct tapeworm, on CF-1 mice. *J. Parasitol. 62*, 329-332 (1976).
37. Podesta, R. B., and Mettrick, D. F., Pathophysiology of cestode infections: movements of water and electrolytes in the rat jejunum infected with the tapeworm, *Hymenolepis diminuta*. *The Physiologist. 16*, 424 (1973).
38. Podesta, R. B., and Mettrick, D. F., Pathophysiology of cestode infections: effect of

Hymenolepis diminuta on oxygen tensions, pH, and gastrointestinal function. *Int. J. Parasitol.* 4, 277-292 (1974a).

39. Podesta, R. B., and Mettrick, D. F., Components of glucose transport in the host-parasite system, *Hymenolepis diminuta* (Cestoda) and the rat intestine. *Can. J. Physiol. Pharmacol.* 52, 183-197 (1974b).
40. Podesta, R. B, and Mettrick, D. F., The effect of bicarbonate and acidification on water and electrolyte absorption by the intestine of normal and infected (*Hymenolepis diminuta*: Cestoda) rats. *Am. J. Digest. Dis. New Ser.* 19, 725-735 (1974c).
41. Podesta, R. B., and Mettrick, D. F., *Hymenolepis diminuta*: acidification and bicarbonate absorption in the rat intestine. *Exp. Parasitol.* 37, 1-14 (1975).
42. Podesta, R. B., and Mettrick, D. F., Pathophysiology and compensatory mechanisms in a compatible host-parasite system. *Can. J. Zool.* 54, 694-703 (1976a).
43. Podesta, R. B., and Mettrick, D. F., Permeability alterations in the diseased small intestine. *In:* "Biochemistry of Parasites and Host-Parasite Relationships" (H. Van Den Bossche, ed.), pp. 373-377. North-Holland Publishing Co., Amsterdam, The Netherlands. (1976b).
44. Podesta, R. B., and Mettrick, D. F., The interrelationships between the in situ fluxes of water, electrolytes and glucose by *Hymenolepis diminuta*. *Int. J. Parasitol.* 6, 163-172 (1976c).
45. Podesta, R. B., and Mettrick, D. F., Permeability changes in the parasitized (*Hymenolepis diminuta:* Cestoda) rat intestine. *Comp. Biochem. Physiol.* 57A, 265-274 (1977).
46. Read, C. P., and Kilejian, A. Z., Circadian migratory behavior of a cestode symbiote in the rat host. *J. Parasitol.* 55, 574-578 (1969).
47. Read, C. P., and Voge, M. , The size attained by *Hymenolepis diminuta* in different host species. *J. Parasitol.* 40, 88-89 (1954).
48. Tanaka, R. D., and MacInnis, A. J., An explanation of the apparent reversal of the circadian migration by *Hymenolepis diminuta* (Cestoda) in the rat. *J. Parasitol.* 61, 271-180 (1975).

49. Teitelbaum, P., and Campbell, B. A., Ingestion patterns in hyperphagic and normal rats. *J. Comp. Physiol. Psychol. 51*, 135-141 (1958).
50. Turton, J. A., Distribution and growth of *Hymenolepis diminuta* in the rat, hamster and mouse. *Z. Parasitenk. 37*, 315-329 (1971).
51. Ulmer, M. J., Site-finding behavior in helminths in intermediate and definitive hosts. *In:* "Ecology and Physiology of Parasites" (A. M. Fallis, ed.), pp. 123-160. University of Toronto Press, Toronto, Ontario.
52. Webb, R. A., and Davey, K. G., The gross anatomy and histology of the nervous system of the metacestode of *Hymenolepis microstoma*. *Can. J. Zool. 53*, 661-667 (1975).
53. Wilson, V. C. L., and Schiller, E. L., The neuroanatomy of *Hymenolepis diminuta* and *H. nana*. *J. Parasitol. 55*, 261-170 (1969).

CHEMOTHERAPY OF HYMENOLEPIASIS

Hugo Van den Bossche

Laboratory of Comparative Biochemistry
Janssen Pharmaceutica - Research Laboratories
B 2340 Beerse - Belgium

I. INTRODUCTION

As noted elsewhere in this volume, *Hymenolepis diminuta* is a common parasite of rodents and other mammals, including man. The tapeworm is practically cosmopolitan in its geographical distribution and human infections are being reported with increasing frequency (see Burt, this volume).

Although some gastro-intestinal complaints such as anorexia, nausea, vomiting, abdominal pain, and diarrhea may be associated with human infection by *H. diminuta*, many cases are apparently asymptomatic (Turner 1975). One case reported by Luney (1934) where 40 worms were passed by a 19-month-old child after treatment seems to support the latter observation. Gross symptoms were similarly lacking in non-human hosts infected with *H. diminuta* although more recent results (documented elsewhere in this work) indicate that pathology at the physiological and biochemical levels are apparent.

Due, perhaps, to the recent nature of this evidence for pathology, very little interest has been generated in the treatment of *H. diminuta* among practioners of human and veterinary medicine. For this reason and possibly to facilitate studies on *H. diminuta*, this review of the variety of pharmaceuticals used in the treatment of a wide variety of tapeworms is presented.

CLASSES OF ANTITAPEWORM DRUGS

In general drugs used in cestode diseases can be divided in four classes: herbal preparations; inorganic - and metallorganic compounds; antibiotics; and synthetic organic compounds.

II. HERBAL PREPARATIONS

The vegetable kingdom was the first medicine chest. Barks, berries, blossoms, leaves, roots and seeds from all kind of plants have been used by the medicine men of all civilizations (Haynes 1946). Examples are given below.

A. *Phloroglucinol compounds*

1. *Oleoresin of Aspidium.* Powdered rhizomes (subterranean root stems of plants) of *Dryopteris filix-mas* and extracts of the plants, have been used as anthelmintics for millenniums (Rüneberg 1963). It appears that the ancient Greeks already knew the substance and it is mentioned as a potent anthelmintic in the writings of many ancient and medieval authorities (Rüneberg 1963). The dried rhizome and stipes of the male fern is called aspidium. For several decades, oleoresin of aspidium was the standard preparation against *Diphyllobothrium latum* (Bylund et al. 1977). However, extracts of the male fern contain a toxic component for the host and must be used with caution. Male fern probably interferes with the uptake of bilirubin into the liver cells (Manson-Bahr 1972). Oleoresin of aspidium when given undiluted, causes nausea, vomiting and bloody diarrhea. In advanced pregnancy it may cause abortion. It is thought that the mechanism of aspidium's anthelmintic activity is due to a paralyzing effect on the muscle of the parasite (Rollo 1965).

Several pure substances with an anthelmintic effect have been isolated from the crude extract. All these substances are chemically closely related and can be characterized as phlorobutyrophenone derivatives (Penttilä and Sundman 1962, 1963). It is of interest to note that Bowden *et al.* (1965) tried to synthesize phloroglucinol derivatives. They found that one, diacetylphloroglucinol, (I; the structural formulas are given at the end of the chapter) has an appreciable activity *in vitro* against *H. nana*.

Blakemore *et al.* (1964) prepared extracts, oils and some individual compounds from the fern *D. filix-mas* and from the related fern *D. dilatata*. The latter is reported to be a more effective taeniafuge (Rosendahl 1911). In *D. dilatata* activity against *H. nana* is concentrated mainly in aspidin (II), phloropyrone and aspidinol (III) (Blakemore *et al.* 1964). The major phloroglucinol compounds in *D. filix-mas* appeared as flavaspidic acid (IV) and aspidinol. Flavaspidic acid is somewhat less active than aspidin both *in vitro* and *in vivo*. The two substances were slightly active against *H. nana* in mice at 100 mg/kg; aspidinol was inactive. At 200 mg/kg, flavaspidic acid and aspidin showed activities varying between 75 and 100%.

Another phloroglucinol derivative, desaspidin (V), was isolated by Aebi *et al.* (1957) from the Finnish broad buckler fern, *D. austrica*. Desaspidin is *in vivo* more potent that either aspidin or flavaspidic acid (Blakemore *et al.* 1964). According to Scheibel (1973) desaspidin is still in use in the U.S.A. and it still seems to be one of the drugs of choice for *Diphyllobothrium latum* in Finland (Bylund *et al.* 1977).

Rüneberg (1962, 1963) studied the effect of desaspidin, ortho-desaspidin (VI), flavaspidic acid, nor-flavaspidic acid (VII) and desaspidinol (VIII) on respiration and oxidative phosphorylation in rat liver mitochondria. All these phlorobutyrophenone derivatives uncouple oxidative phosphorylation. Desaspidin and ortho-desaspidin show maximum activity at 2-4 µM, the other substances in concentrations of 16-64 µM.

Scheibel *et al.* (1968) demonstrated that desaspidin inhibits both the anaerobic incorporation of ^{32}P into ATP by intact *H. diminuta* and the ^{32}P-ATP exchange in mitochondria of this tapeworm. The authors also demonstrated that 2,4-dinitrophenol

(DNP) affects the ^{32}P-ATP exchange reaction and incorporation of ^{32}P into ATP in *H. diminuta*. A similar effect of substituted phenols on the anaerobic phosphorylation system in *Ascaris suum* mitochondria was observed (Van den Bossche 1972b). Thus, in many aspects the action of desaspidin resembles that of DNP, the well known uncoupler of oxidative phosphorylation in mammalian mitochondria.

These studies suggest that the anthelmintic effect of desaspidin may, at least partly, be due to interference with ATP production. The studies of Saz and his collaborators demonstrate some similarity between the mitochondrial phosphorylation systems in cestodes and nematodes (Saz 1972a, b). In spite of these similarities this anticestodal agent is specific for tapeworms. A permeability barrier is indicated to explain the failure of desaspidin to affect intact *A. suum* (Saz 1972b).

2. *Kamala*. Kamala consists of glandular and fasciculate hairs covering the fruits of spoonwood, *Mallotus philippinensis* (Euphorbiaceae) (The Pharmacopoeia of Japan 1971). *Mallotus* is found in the Philippines, India, China and Australia. Rotterlin (IX) and isorotterlin are active compounds of kamala (de Carneri and Vita 1973). This naturally occurring taeniacide also contains the phloroglucinol structure.

Deworming with 0.4 g kamala per kg body weight in food was effective against hymenolepidids in ducks. This compound was well tolerated by the 70,000 ducks treated (Mineev 1964). For prophylaxis 25 mg/kg of kamala was added to the food of 25,000 ducks for 40 days. The weight gain over 40 days was on the average 230 g greater in birds receiving kamala than in controls (Mineev 1964).

The extracts of powdered spoonwood was also active against *H. nana* and *H. diminuta in vitro* and in rats (Srivastava *et al.* 1967). *In vitro*, kamala also affects *Moniezia expansa* but not *Ascaris lumbricoides* nor *Fasciolopsis buski* (Srivastava *et al.* 1967).

The ED_{50} of kamala in mice infected experimentally with *H. nana*, varied from 0.24 to 0.34 g/kg body weight; the LD_{50} was 0.96 g/kg (Nurtaeva 1972; Krotov et al. 1973).

Dikshit and Lalit (1970) treated 65 children, infected with *H. nana*, with kamala at 1 or 2 g twice daily for 2 days and cured 96% after a single course. The drug was well tolerated and the authors believe that the drug is active against the cysticercoids in the intestinal villi as well as against the adults in the lumen of the intestine.

Like aspidium (Rollo 1965) kamala (Nurtaeva 1972) seems to interfere with the smooth muscles of the host and the muscle system of the parasites.

B. *Other Natural Anthelmintics*

1. *Chenopodium oil.* *Chenopodium graveolens* (Epazote del Zorrillo), *C. foetidum*, *C. ambrosioides* (Yapotzote, Epazote) have been used in Mexico for anthelmintic purposes (Maximino Martinez 1969; Diaz 1976a, b). In the U.S.A. *C. ambrosioides* var. *anthelminticum* (American wormseed plant) is a common plant from which the extracted oil has been used for the treatment of intestinal verminous parasitosis and was introduced in Europe in 1881 (Watkins 1958). The active constituent, a terpenic peroxide, ascaridol (X), is present to the extent of 45-70% (Watkins 1958). The oil is highly toxic *in vitro* for *Ascaris* (Cavier 1973) and *H. nana* (Sen and Hawking 1960a). *In vitro*, chenopodium oil first causes a rise in muscle tonus, then paralysis and death of *Ascaris* (Cavier 1973). This oil was widely used for the removal of ascarids from pigs (Watkins 1958; Cavier 1973). In man, it was found effective against *Ascaris* and *Ancylostoma* (Cavier 1973).

Although it is an effective ascaricide, it is no longer used because of its high toxicity. It exerts very marked toxic actions on the human nervous system e.g. ataxia, vertigo, hallucinations, deafness and blindness and it produces marked gastrointestinal disturbances (del Castillo 1969).

2. *Arecoline.* The alkaloid, arecoline (XI), is the principle constituent of the seeds of the betel-nut *Areca catechu* L. a palm cultivated in

the Far-East and East-India. It has been used in the form of a variety of salts as an effective taenicidal agent particularly for dogs (Watkins 1958); de Carneri and Vita 1973).

Mineev (1964) found arecoline hydrobromide at 5 mg/kg body weight in food effective against hymenolepidids in ducks. For prophylaxis against hymenolepidids 1 mg arecoline per kg was added to the food of 25-day-old ducklings. The weight gain over 40 days was on the average 210 g greater in birds receiving arecoline than in controls (Mineev 1964). A comparison of arecoline (1 : 2,000 solution, 1 ml/kg body weight i.e., 0.5 mg/kg) with kamala, male fern extract (both administered as a bolus of 0.5 g/duck) and turpentine (1 ml/kg in milk) showed that arecoline of those tested was the most effective against *Drepanotaenia* in geese and *Hymenolepis* in ducks (Zakhryalov and Gorodovich 1971).

Arecoline frequently causes vomiting. It causes violent peristaltic movements and an outpouring of mucous secretion. Its taenicidal action may therefore be purely mechanical in that it causes the tapeworm to become detached and hence expelled from the host (Watkins 1958).

3. Pelletierines. The Egyptian papyrus (Papyrus Ebers), dating from about 1550 B.C. and discovered by Georg Moritz Ebers in 1872, described a worm, probably the beef tapeworm, *Taenia saginata*, as pathogenic in man, and prescribed infusion of the bark of the pomegranate tree (*Punica granatum* L.) for its evacuation. One to 3% of the bark of the roots of the pomegranate consists of four alkaloids i.e. pelletierine (XII), methylpelletierine, isopelletierine, and pseudopelletierine (Maximino Martinez 1969). Pelletierine is believed to be active against *Taenia* spp. but it seems ineffective against *H. nana* (de Carneri and Vita 1973).

In the early sixties much work was done to prove that the extracts of the root bark of *P. granatum*, did not contain pelletierine [3-(2'-piperidyl) propanol] but isopelletierine i.e. 1-(2'-piperidyl) propanone-2 (Gilman and Marion 1961). Van Noordwijk *et al.* (1963) showed that synthetic 3-(2-piperidyl) propanol possesses no paralysing effect on the liver fluke *in vitro* whereas isopelletierine has anthelmintic activity.

The four alkaloids are toxic and pelletierine even in therapeutic doses, can cause headache, diarrhea, vomiting, vertigo (Maximino Martinez 1969; de Carneri and Vita 1973).

4. Diospyrol. The unripe berries of an Ebenacea common in Thailand, *Diospyros mollis*, and known as "Maklua" are used in popular medicine for the treatment of ancylostomiasis (Cavier 1973; Sadun and Vajrathiza 1954). The anthelmintic activity seems to be due to diospyrol (XIII) i.e. 1, 1', 8, 8'-tetrahydroxy-6, 6'-dimethyl-2, 2'-binaphthalene (Sen *et al.* 1974). Diospyrol, given orally to mice with mixed experimental infections of *Nematospiroides dubius* and *H. nana*, completely eliminated *H. nana* at a single dose of 100 mg/kg (Sen *et al.* 1974). One dose of 500 mg/kg expelled 80% of *N. dubius* while 2 or 3 such daily doses expelled 97%. The compound was well tolerated by a range of laboratory animals (Sen *et al.* 1974) and by man (Cavier 1973).

5. Cucurbita (Pumpkin seeds). For thousands of years the home of herbal medicine was China. One of that country's most successful herb remedies comes from ground pumpkin seeds (Aikman 1974). The seeds have proved effective in treating schistosomiasis (Aikman 1974) and the taeniafugal properties of pumpkin seeds have been known for centuries (Davis 1973). In Mexico, minced seeds from *Cucurbita pepo* (calabazas) have been used in the treatment of *Ascaris* and *Taenia* (Maximino Martinez 1969). Herzig (1946) found in the seeds of *C. pepo* and *C. moschata* a sulfur-containing protein (27% in Spring) and demonstrated anthelmintic activity in the aqueous extracts.

The seeds of *C. moschata* contain 3-amino-3-carboxy pyrrolidin (XIV) which may be responsible for the anthelmintic activity (de Carneri and Vita 1973).

In vivo experiments with *Hymenolepis* spp. in rats showed that aqueous, alcoholic and ethereal extracts of *C. maxima* seeds had a similar cestocidal activity (Srivastava and Singh 1967). Kymographic studies indicated a decrease in movement leading to temporary paralysis (Srivastava and Singh 1967).

Junod (1964) tested 150 *T. saginata* patients with an extract of the seeds. The dose was 30 ml of extract (from 500 g seeds). Oral treatment cured 85%. In 9 cases in which the drug was given by duodenal tube, all were cured. Success was obtained in all patients treated via an intragastric tube.

Post-treatment purgation is necessary (Davis 1973). Toxicity of the extracts is minimal (de Carneri and Vita 1973). However, standardization is difficult due to the great variability of activity according to the origin (Junod 1964).

III. METALLORGANIC AND INORGANIC COMPOUNDS

A. *Tin Compounds*

Tin was used as a vermifuge in the days of Theophrastus Bombastus von Hohenheim better known as Paracelsus (1493-1541).

Hymenolepis carioca, parasitic in the small intestines of the fowl, were 100% removed by tin sulfate, -oxalate and -phosphate given at 1 to 1.25 g/kg. Tin oxalate proved very toxic at 1.25 g/kg resulting in 50% mortality of the fowl (Kumar *et al.* 1974).

Preparations based on mixtures of metallic tin with its oxide and chloride, e.g. the tablet preparation called cestodin, were used successfully against tapeworm infections (Hirte 1951; Kuhls 1953). Pawlowski (1970) reviewed the results of treatment of 1203 patients with various tin preparations e.g. cestodin, stannotean, tenitosse. According to the author the efficacy depends on metallic tin and tin oxide and not necessarily on tin chloride. In 325 hospitalized patients and 145 ambulant patients infected with *T. saginata*, Pawlowski (1970) claimed cure rates of about 85%.

The frequency of side effects was slightly lower than after acridine derivatives (Sect. IV, A) but much higher than after niclosamide (Sect. IV, E,

1) (Brown 1969). The variable frequency of side effects such as vomiting, nausea, abdominal pain or cramps, diarrhea, fever, anorexia and tinnitus limit the value of tin preparations (Davis 1973).

B. *Antimonials*

Cavier et al. (1974) studied the anthelmintic properties of antimony complexes of 8-oxyquinolines. The complexes, XV and XVI, were comparable to niclosamide in controlling *H. nana* infestation in mice. One oral dose of 200 mg/kg cured more than 90% of the infected mice.

The trivalent organic antimonials, such as stibophen (XVII) have been employed for the chemotherapy of schistosomas and filarial infections (for reviews see Katz 1977; Hawking 1966). These antimonials have been of great help in elucidating schistosomal glycolysis. Evidence indicates that the mode of action of these drugs against schistosomes is associated with their effect on the worm's phosphofructokinase (PFK) which is the limiting enzyme of the schistosomes's glycolytic pathway (Mansour and Bueding 1954; Bueding and Mansour 1957; Bueding and Fisher 1966; Bueding 1972; Coles 1973). *H. diminuta* also exhibited PFK activities which were susceptible to inhibition by stibophen (Saz and Dunbar 1975). Important is the finding that the parasite PFK is considerably more sensitive to inhibition with the trivalent antimonials than the corresponding mammalian enzyme (Bueding and Mansour 1957; Saz and Dunbar 1975).

IV. ANTIBIOTICS

A. *Paromomycin (XVIII)*

Paromomycin (Humatin), an antibiotic related to streptomycin, was isolated in 1959 from a strain of *Streptomyces rimosus*. Paromomycin sulfate was marginally effective against *H. nana* at dietary levels of 0.5% or with doses of 2 g/kg/day by gavage in mice (Waitz et al. 1966). It was ineffective against *H. diminuta* at 200 mg/kg for 4 days in rats (Waitz et al. 1966). In the same study it was found to be effective against *Hydatigera taeniaeformis* infections in cats. Daily doses of 50 or 200 mg/kg for 5 days cured most the cats.

Ulivelli (1968) treated 208 infections with *T. saginata*, 32 cases of *T. solium* and 8 cases of *H. nana*: the overall efficacy was 98-100%. Doses of 20-30 mg/kg/day divided into 4 parts for 4 consecutive days were given. Wittner and Tanowitz (1971) treated 13 patients with *H. nana* infection. Twelve were cured, 10 by the single 4 g dose, and 2 out of 3 by the administration of 45 mg/kg of body weight over a period of 5 days. The requirement for this rather high dose for *H. nana* in the single-dose regimen is believed to be related to the low absorption of the antibiotic and the inaccessibility to the cysticercoids deep within the mucosa of the villi (Wittner and Tanowitz 1971).

The treatment is normally well tolerated (Ulivelli 1968). Side-effects are mostly transient and not intense (Botero 1970). Diarrhea and abdominal pain are the most frequent complaints. Since nausea and vomiting were also present in some patients it is advisable to use antiemetics, especially in patients infected with *T. solium*, in order to minimize the possibility of cysticercosis, which is possible when proglottids or eggs are regurgitated to the stomach (Botero 1970).

The mode of action is unknown. Since neither the scolex nor intact segments are usually found it has been suggested that the action against *Taenia* may be by changing the ultrastructure of the tegumental membrane of the cestode (Garin *et al*. 1970) or by modification of the intestinal flora creating an unfavorable environment for the metabolism of the parasite as suggested by Ulivelli (1964, 1967). Both effects would make the parasite susceptible to the host's digestive mechanisms (Garin *et al*. 1970; Ulivelli 1964, 1967).

B.   *Axenomycins*

Axenomycins A, B and D from *Streptomyces lisandri* showed high anthelmintic activity *in vitro* against *Rhabditis macrocerca*, *S. mansoni* and *H. nana*

(Bianchi et al. 1974). The activities of axenomycin D against *H. nana*, *Taenia pisiformis*, *Dipylidium caninum* and *Diphyllobothrium* spp. in dogs and *M. expansa*, *M. benedeni* and *Avitellina centripunctata* in lambs were studied in experimentally and naturally infected animals (Della Bruna et al. 1973). Worm reduction rates after a single oral dose of 5-10 mg axenomycin D/kg were 90-100%. This macrolide antibiotic isolated from the fermentation broth of *S. lisandri* was well tolerated by the oral route. Axenomycin D should be further evaluated.

V. SYNTHETIC ORGANIC COMPOUNDS

A. *Acridine dyes*

1. *Mepacrine* (XIX). Mepacrine (quinacrine, atabrine, atebrin), introduced in 1935 as an antimalarial (Peters 1970), was first used by Neghme (1939) for treatment of *T. saginata* and *T. solium* infections. Culbertson (1940) found that this acridine dye was active against *H. nana* in mice. Mepacrine was also found to be a potent drug against *H. nana* infections in men (Neghme and Faiguenbaum 1947). However, Beaver and Sodeman (1952) noted that the compound often fails to eradicate the infection completely. Similar results were obtained more recently by El-Masry et al. (1974). Twelve out of 20 patients infected with *H. nana* were ova-free 2 weeks after treatment with mepacrine at a single dose of 15 mg/kg; 5 weeks after treatment the cure rate had fallen to 3. This seems to indicate that the drug is active against the adult stage but less active or inactive against the cysticercoids in the walls of the small intestine.

According to Kean and Hoskins (1976) mepacrine, preferably by duodenal tube instillation, is still reserved for patients with *T. solium* and when niclosamide fails to rid the patient of *T. saginata*, *D. latum* or *H. nana*.

The mode of action of mepacrine against cestodes is unknown. Using fluorescence microscopy of frozen sections of *T. saginata*, Saikkonen and Mustakallio (1963) observed that mepacrine concentrated in the radial musculature of the scolex more efficiently than in other muscular elements. This resulted in a loosening and expulsion of the whole motile worm. Mepacrine inhibited the uptake of glucose by *H. diminuta in vitro* (Madsen 1972). Incorporation of ^{14}C-glucose into glycogen was inhibited to a much greater extent than could be accounted for by the inhibition of absorption. In the absence of exogenous glucose, mepacrine appeared to stimulate slightly the catabolism of glycogen. With exogenous glucose, succinate excretion usually decreased, while lactate nearly always increased. In the absence of exogenous glucose, excretion of both acids usually increased. The level of ATP in *H. diminuta* decreased as the cure progressed *in vivo*. This fact, together with the observed stimulation of the metabolism, suggests that mepacrine may uncouple energy metabolism, but the results obtained by Madsen (1972) gave no indications of the site or mode of this uncoupling.

2. *Acranil*. The acridine derivative known as acranil (XX) is of interest because of its noteworthy effectiveness against the cestodes *T. saginata* (Beier 1965) and *H. nana* (Marinoni and Sperzani 1966). Apparently acranil treatment affects the neuromuscular system of *T. saginata* inducing an increased motility followed by paralysis (Beier 1965).

3. *Acriflavine*. Acriflavine (XXI) was found by Sen and Hawking (1960b) to have some activity against *H. nana*. The commercial product consists of a mixture of 3, 6-diaminoacridine dihydrochloride (proflavine XXIa) and 3, 6-diamino-10-methylacridinium chloride (XXIb).

Acriflavine, which had a good activity against trypanosomes and is a good antiseptic, is a highly toxic compound (Steck 1971). Therefore acriflavine and other acridine derivatives may be considered rather as interesting investigational probes than as drug having practical value. In fact, the mode of action studies have yielded much valuable information about nucleic acid structure and function (for review see Newton 1976).

B. *Benzimidazoles*

In the last 17 years several benzimidazole compounds have been introduced as anthelmintics. It began with the development of thiabendazole of which the anthelmintic properties were first reported in 1961 (Brown *et al.* 1961). The anthelmintic efficiency and safety margin found in this benzimidazole was the start for the development of a great number of highly potent and safe broad-spectrum anthelmintics.

1. *Thiabendazole*. Thiabendazole (XXII), the first of the so-called broad-spectrum anthelmintics, is a tasteless, rapidly absorbed, metabolized and excreted benzimidazole, introduced for the treatment of intestinal nematodes and trichinosis in veterinary and human medicine (Merck Sharp and Dohme 1968; Tocco 1964, 1965; Gibson 1964; Stone *et al.* 1964; McManus *et al.* 1966; Dunlop 1967; Douglas and Baker 1968; Davis 1973; Wilson *et al.* 1973; Davis *et al.* 1976; Kean and Hoskins 1976).

Only limited success was claimed when thiabendazole at a dose of 1.25 g twice daily for 3 days was used in the treatment of taeniasis (Salunkhe 1966).

Four out of 20 patients with *H. nana* were ova-free 2 weeks after treatment with thiabendazole at 25 mg/kg twice daily for 2 days (El-Masry *et al.* 1974). Five weeks after treatment the cure rate had fallen to one. However, much better results were obtained by Taffs (1975, 1976). Anthelmintic action against artificial *Hymenolepis* infections was assessed by continuously feeding a medicated diet to mice from the 14th day of infection for periods of 5 to 18 days. Complete removal of *H. nana* was obtained after 14 days medication. Taffs' studies showed that thiabendazole at the 0.3% level is a safe and effective anthelmintic for the treatment of *H. nana* in mice. It has been shown that thiabendazole affects the fumarate reductase system in *Haemonchus contortus*, *F. hepatica* and *H. diminuta* (Prichard 1970, 1973, 1974; Malkin and Camacho 1972; Romanowski *et al.* 1975; Coles 1977).

In vitro, *Nippostrongylus brasiliensis*, *Fasciola hepatica* and *H. diminuta* concentrate thiabendazole respectively 60, 2.8 and 2.4 times (Coles and Briscoe, mentioned by Coles 1977). The high concentration of thiabendazole found in *N. brasiliensis* reflects the sensitivity of this nematode to the anthelmintic (Coles 1977). *N. brasiliensis* is an aerobic metabolising organism (Saz *et al.* 1971) in which until now no fumarate reductase activity has been found (Coles 1977). Therefore it can be suggested that thiabendazole either affects sensitive helminths in different ways or its inhibitory effect on the fumarate reductase is not involved in the antiworm activity. However, the fact that in many parasitic stages of nematodes and cestodes (for reviews see: Saz 1972a, Barrett 1976a, b, von Brand 1973) and *F. hepatica* (Van Vugt 1977) the fumarate reductase is an essential component of carbohydrate metabolism makes the latter assumption difficult to retain.

Side effects may occur 3 or 4 hours after ingestion of the drug and include anorexia, diarrhea, dizziness, nausea and vomiting. Rarely bradycardia, drowsiness, hypotension, pruritus and xanthopsia may occur (Gilles 1976).

2. *Cambendazole*. Cambendazole (XXIII) has been found to be effective against a wide variety of nematodes parasitising cattle (Stoye *et al.* 1971; Benz 1971a, b, 1973), horse (Bello *et al.* 1973), sheep (Egerton and Campbell 1970) and swine (Hoff *et al.* 1970; Egerton *et al.* 1970; Taffs 1971).

Campbell *et al.* (1975) found that cambendazole, given intraperitoneally to mice harboring secondary metacestode infections of *Taenia crassiceps*, was partially active at 500 mg/kg body weight. It also has some activity against *T. hydatigena* in dogs (Gemmell *et al.* 1977b) and seems to reduce the viability of the cysticerci of *T. saginata* in cattle (Campbell and Blair 1974). Cambendazole also showed marked action against *M. expansa* (Gibbs and Gupta 1972; Kates *et al.* 1973) and *Thysanosoma actinioides* (Allen 1973) in sheep.

Although no studies on the effects of cambendazole on *Hymenolepis* were found, this benzimidazole derivative was included in order to be able to summarise important studies on the effects of cambendazole on the regulatory metabolism in cestodes (Rahman and Bryant 1977). Anaerobically and aerobically, and in the presence of glucose, cambendazole inhibits glucose uptake and increases glycogen utilisation in the anterior portion of *M. expansa*. Anaerobically it reduces succinate production by inhibiting fumarate reductase and phosphoenolpyruvate carboxykinase activities and increases lactate production. The drug diminishes ATP synthesis and decreases the concentration of total nucleotides in the parasite within 30 min under anaerobic and aerobic conditions. These effects are also observed in *Moniezia* collected from sheep treated with cambendazole (Bryant *et al.* 1976). It is of interest to note that *in vitro* the cambendazole effects are less pronounced aerobically than anaerobically. This may be consistent with the authors' idea that "a significant effect of the anthelmintics is on the phosphoenolpyruvate-succinate pathway, which is less important aerobically (Rahman and Bryant 1977).

3. *Parbendazole*. Parbendazole (XXIV), synthesized in 1966 (Actor *et al.* 1967) has been reported to be an effective anthelmintic against gastrointestinal parasites of cattle, goats, mice, sheep and swine (Brody and Elwards 1971; Theodorides *et al.* 1968a, b; Nurtaeva 1973; Daněk *et al.* 1970; Chang and Wescott 1969; Gibson and Parfitt 1971; Bennett 1968).

Parbendazole at 15 mg/kg body weight was found to have a destrobilation effect on *M. expansa* in sheep but this action is obviously of limited value since no significant action against scoleces was found (Kates *et al.* 1971).

Brody and Elward (1971) found that 1000 ppm of the drug in the diet of mice for 18 days exhibited nearly 100% activity against *H. nana*. This benzimidazole carbamate at 0.05% of the diet completely eliminated *H. nana* from mice treated continously for 7 days from the 14th day after infection (Kunkle and and Theordorides 1971). Its activity against *H. microstoma* was lower i.e. 57.3%, even at 0.1% only 55.1% reduction of the *H. microstoma* burden in the biliary system was observed (Kunkle and Theodorides 1971).

4. Oxibendazole. If a methylene group in the butyl portion of parbendazole is replaced by an oxygen atom oxibendazole (XXV) is obtained. This benzimidazole carbamate is active against a great number of gastrointestinal parasites (Theodorides *et al.* 1973, 1976a; Kates *et al.* 1975; Nawalinski and Theodorides 1976). It is of interest to note that oxibendazole at 500 mg/kg (injected intraperitoneally) was partially, but significantly, active against *T. crassiceps* in mice whereas the parent compound, parbendazole, was inactive at the same dosage (Campbell *et al.* 1975).

Two weeks after infection with *H. nana* mice were fed diets, containing 0.025 and 0.05% oxibendazole, for 7 days. The worm burden was reduced by 89 to 100% (Theodorides *et al.* 1973) thus resembling the activity of parbendazole (Kunkle and Theodorides 1971).

5. Albendazole. A benzimidazole derivative active against nematodes and cestodes, as well as trematodes was recently obtained by Smith-Kline and French researchers, by substitution of the benzimidazole nucleus in the 5-position by propylthio (Theodorides *et al.* 1976b). Albendazole (XXVI) is, as most other benzimidazole derivatives, insoluble in water (Theodorides *et al.* 1976b). Activities in cattle and sheep, swine, chicken, horses and dogs, have been reported against the common gastrointestinal nematodes as well as *F. hepatica* in sheep (Theodorides *et al.* 1976b, c, d; Knight and Colglazier 1977; Herlich 1977; Benz and Ernst 1977).

It is of interest to note that the replacement of an oxygen atom (oxibendazole XXV) by a sulfur atom (albendazole XXVI) resulted in a marked enlargement of the spectrum of activity. In experiments with sheep and cattle artificially infected with larvae of lung nematodes of the genus *Dictyocaulus*, a single oral dose of 5 mg albendazole/kg eliminated 84-100% of the worms (Theodorides *et al.* 1976b). Oxibendazole was found to be inactive against *Dictyocaulus* (Kates *et al.* 1975).

In sheep naturally infected with *Moniezia*, an oral dose of 10 mg/kg of albenzadole was 100% active against these tapeworms (Theodorides *et al.* 1976b).

Knowledge on the difference in the uptake, distribution and metabolism of these alkyl benzimidazole 2 yl carbamates within hosts and helminths would be of great help for the development of compounds with different biological spectra.

6. *Mebendazole.* An impoŕtant advance in the treatment of parasitic helminths was obtained when the butyl group of parbendazole was replaced by a benzoyl group (Brugmans *et al.* 1971). Mebendazole (XXVII) has been proved effective against most gastrointestinal helminths in human and veterinary medicine (Brugmans *et al.* 1971; Chaia *et al.* 1971, 1972; Banerjee *et al.* 1972; Chavarria *et al.* 1973; Vandepitte *et al.* 1973a, b; Chanco *et al.* 1973; Bekhti 1974; Partono *et al.* 1974; Goldsmid 1974; Aguilar *et al.* 1976; Nagalingam *et al.* 1976; Walker and Knight 1972; Grevel and Eckert 1973). Mebendazole is able to kill the encysted phase of *Trichinella spiralis* (Thienpont *et al.* 1974a; Martinez-Fernandez and Rodriguez-Coabiero 1976; Spaldonová *et al.* 1976; Fernando and Denham 1976; Sonnet and Thienpont 1977). It is presently considered the anthelmintic of choice for the treatment of intestinal capillariasis (Singson *et al.* 1975).

The effect of mebendazole on the development of *H. diminuta* in its intermediate host, the flour beetle *Tribolium confusum* has been studied by Evans and Novak (1976). Feed mixtures composed of 0.005-20.0 g of mebendazole in 10 g of flour were given to *T. confusum* parasitized by *H. diminuta* from day 1 to day 9 post infection. Retarded cysticercoid development, lowered incidence of infection, and reductions in the number of cysticercoids recovered per beetle were produced by drug levels of 0.1, 1.0 and 10 g respectively. However, none of the drug concentrations tested produced 100% mortality.

Ten mg mebendazole per kg body weight given for 5 dayş to geese was 80% effective against *Hymenolepis* sp. (Červenka *et al.* 1975). No tapeworms (*H. lanceolata* and *H. setigera*) were found in geese examined after receiving 30 mg mebendazole/kg body weight/day in the feed for one week (Enigk *et al.* 1973).

Mice artificially infected with *H. nana* were orally treated with mebendazole 28 days after infection (Janssen Pharmaceutica report 1972). When the animals were treated with 10 mg/kg (b.i.d.) for 5 consecutive days no worms could be found in 6 out of 9 mice.

Biagi *et al.* (1974) found that 100 mg mebendazole given orally twice daily for 3 days cured 12 out of 24 patients infected with *Hymenolepis*.

Encouraging results were obtained by Chavarria *et al.* (1977). According to these authors, mebendazole has a taenicidal action against *T. solium* infections in man. The optimum effective dose of mebendazole appears to be 300 mg twice daily for 3 days.

Mebendazole has been found to be effective against experimental *Cysticercus fasciolaris* (Thienpont *et al.* 1974b), tetrathyridia of *Mesocestoides corti* (Heath *et al.* 1975; Eckert and Pohlenz 1976), cysticerci of *Taenia crassiceps* (Campbell *et al.* 1974) and *T. pisiformis* (Heath *et al.* 1975). *Echinococcus granulosus* cysts (Heath and Chevis 1974; Heath *et al.* 1975; Kammerer and Judge 1976; Kovalenko, I. I. *et al.* 1976; Pawlowski *et al.* 1976) and against the larval stage of *E. multilocularis* (Eckert and Pohlenz 1976; Campbell *et al.* 1974; Krotov *et al.* 1974b, 1976). Based on these animal experiments and on preliminary information (Goodman 1976; Bekhti *et al.* 1977; Ludin *et al.* 1977) mebendazole can be considered as an adjunct to surgery in humans suffering from hydatidosis.

Mebendazole affects *in vitro* and *in vivo* the glucose uptake by nematodes (Van den Bossche 1972a, 1976; Van den Bossche and De Nollin 1973; De Nollin and Van den Bossche 1973). In *C. fasciolaris* 30 and 64% inhibition of glucose uptake *in vivo* was found after the mice had been fed, for respectively 24 and 48 h, a medicated feed containing 250 ppm of mebendazole (Van den Bossche 1976). Rahman and Bryant (1977) found that anaerobic incubation of *M. expansa* in the presence of glucose resulted in a decreased glucose uptake and increased glycogen utilisation. Glycogen levels also decreased in the scoleces of *M. expansa* removed from sheep 6 hours after oral treatment with 10 mg/kg body weight (Rahman *et al.*

1977). Mebendazole also reduced the glycogen content of nematodes (Van den Bossche 1972a, 1976) and that of *C. fasciolaris* (Van den Bossche 1976). A marked decrease was observed in the glycogen content of *H. nana* from mice, killed 24 hours after the second of two doses of mebendazole (50 mg/kg) given 12 hours apart (Van den Bossche 1972a). McCracken (mentioned by Campbell 1977) also observed a drastic depletion in the glycogen content of *H. diminuta* following mebendazole treatment.

Benzimidazole derivatives have been found to uncouple oxidative phosphorylation (Jones and Watson 1967). Mebendazole also affects malate-induced phosphorylation in *Ascaris* mitochondria. However, a concentration of 9.2 mM mebendazole is needed for 50% inhibition (Van den Bossche 1972b). In *M. expansa* mebendazole was found to have a number of effects on energy metabolism (Rahman and Bryant 1977; Rahman et al. 1977). *In vitro* and *in vivo*, the drug diminished ATP synthesis and turnover of adenine nucleotides. These effects were observed within 30 min of exposure to the drug *in vitro* and 3 h after the treatment of sheep.

Recently, the progressive time-related micromorphological changes induced by mebendazole in adult *H. nana* have been reported (Verheyen et al. 1976). The cytoplasmic microtubules of the tegumental cells disappear in the early hours. They were almost totally lacking in the tegument of *H. nana* collected from mice medicated continuously for 6 hours with 500 ppm mebendazole in the food. After the disappearance of the microtubules, secretory vesicles accumulate in the Golgi areas and deterioration of the absorptive surface of the tapeworm occurs followed by degeneration of both nucleated and anucleated parts of the tegument.

Very similar changes were observed in the tegument of *C. fasciolaris* and in the intestinal cells of *A. suum* and *Syngamus trachea* (Borgers et al. 1975) after treatment of the hosts with mebendazole. Similar results were obtained with the mebendazole analogue, flubendazole (XXVIII) (Borgers et al. 1975).

The variety of effects observed renders it difficult to state which particular effect or sequence of effects is responsible for the eradication of worms.

Therefore, the author agrees with Rahman and Bryant (1977), who stated that it is safer to conclude that mebendazole and other benzimidazole derivatives are capable of exerting a number of effects which all together account for their anthelmintic activity.

Mebendazole is well tolerated by various animal species (Marsboom 1973) and even at high doses the drug has very low, if any, toxicity in man (Brugmans et al. 1971; Kale 1975; Shafei 1976).

7. Fenbendazole - Oxfendazole. Hoechst researchers replaced the benzoyl group of mebendazole by a phenylthio group (Loewe and Urbanietz 1977). The latter compound has the common name fenbendazole (XXIX).

Different studies have shown good efficacy in the treatment of naturally acquired and experimental infestations with nematodes (Enigk et al. 1974, 1975a, b; Duncan et al. 1976; Strasser and Tiefenbach 1977; Düwel 1977; Anderson 1977). Fenbendazole at 5-10 mg/kg body weight produced 91-100% elimination of *M. expansa* (Düwel 1977; McBeath et al. 1977; Townsend et al. 1977). Fenbendazole given orally at 25 mg/kg was effective against *H. diminuta* in rats (Düwel et al. 1975).

Preliminary results obtained with *A. suum* have shown that fenbendazole (Düwel 1977) like mebendazole, cambendazole and parbendazole (Van den Bossche 1972a) interferes with the absorption of glucose and especially with the incorporation of glucose into glycogen.

Like most benzimidazole derivatives, fenbendazole is well tolerated (Enigk et al. 1975b; Düwel 1977).

It is of interest to note that research workers of Syntex, Hoechst and Bayer (see Loewe and Urbanietz 1977) showed that fenbendazole is easily oxidized to the corresponding sulfoxide i.e. oxfendazole (XXX). A dose of 5 mg oxfendazole/kg body weight provides efficacy > 95% against *Moniezia* in sheep (Averkin et al. 1975). Effective removal of *H. nana* from mice was obtained when oxfendazole was administered in the feed at 125 ppm for 18 days (Averkin *et al.* 1975).

C. *Phenols and Derivatives*

1. Hexylresorcinol. Hexylresorcinol (XXXI), as administered in ascariasis, is frequently effective in eliminating light infections. According to Baldwin (1943) hexylresorcinol paralyses *Ascaris in vitro*.

Piringer *et al.* (1960) found this phenolic substance active *in vitro* on the eggs of *H. nana*. It appears to interfere with the protein of the hyaline membrane.

2. Dichlorophen. Dichlorophen (XXXII), has been described by Craige and Kleckner (1946) to be active against the tapeworms of dogs. Dichlorophen was found active against *H. nana* in mice (Krotov and Kuvchur 1971). It has been used by Seaton (1956, 1960) for taeniasis in man. Biagi *et al.* (1959) cured 40 out of 68 patients with hymenolepiasis; the dose used was 62 mg/kg body weight.

Mild side-effects of nausea, vomiting, abdominal pain and urticaria have been reported (Miller 1976). The drug should not be used in the presence of jaundice or overt liver disease (Davis 1973).

Dichlorophen, like desaspidin (I, A, 1) reduces the incorporation of ^{32}P into ATP by intact *H. diminuta in vitro* and there is evidence that this inhibition is due to an inhibitory effect on the ^{32}P-ATP exchange reactions in mitochondria prepared from the rat tapeworm (Scheibel *et al.* 1968). Furthermore Yorke and Turton (1974) demonstrated that dichlorophen and a great number of anti-cestodal and fasciolicidal agents can act as uncouplers of electron-transport-linked phosphorylation in isolated mitochondria of *H. diminuta*. In addition oxidative phosphorylation of rat liver mitochondria is uncoupled by dichlorophen (Strufe and Gönnert 1967). The low toxicity of dichlorophen probably can be ascribed to the fact that little is absorbed from the gastrointestinal tract (Bueding 1969).

3. *Bithionol*. The dichlorophenol compound, bithionol (XXXIII) is established as the drug of choice for treating paragonimiasis (Yokogawa et al. 1961a, b; Miller 1976) and has been used successfully in human fascioliasis (Yoshida et al. 1962). Bithionol has also been found active against mature *H. nana* (Krotov and Kovchur 1971) and Kovalenko, I. I. et al. (1976) found it active against *Hymenolepis* in geese when given in the diet at 0.9 g/kg.

There is some evidence that bithionol interferes with ATP production in *Paragonimus westermani* (Hamajima 1973) and *F. hepatica* (Panitz and Knapp 1970; Benediktov 1975).

D. *Benzanilides*

1. *Niclosamide*. A drug of special interest is the salicylanilide, niclosamide (XXXIV) of which numerous trials have demonstrated the curative efficacy in infestations with *H. nana*, *T. solium*, *T. saginata* and *D. latum*.

This cestocide was discovered in the course of studies on the experimental infection of rats with *H. diminuta* (Gönnert and Schraufstätter 1960). The latter authors found the anti-*Hymenolepis* activity independent of the magnitude of infection but dependent on the age of infection. In addition, the drug has no effect on the cysticercoids of *H. nana* in the jejunal villi of mice (Krotov et al. 1974a).

Addition of niclosamide (100 mg/kg) to the diet of infected rats for 2-3 weeks eliminated ova and adult parasites (*H. nana* and *H. diminuta*) from the intestinal tract (Hughes et al. 1973). Niclosamide at 2 g/kg/day for 6 days completely cured all mice infected with *H. nana* (Arakcheeva et al. 1975).

Treatment with the drug at a concentration of the 0.33% active ingredient in the feed for 7 days cleared all hamsters of infection with *H. nana* (Ronald and Wagner 1975).

However, niclosamide fails to result in the total removal of *H. microstoma* from the bile ducts of laboratory infected mice receiving doses ranging from 50 to 6000 mg/kg (McGavock 1968). As the drug was found very effective *in vitro* (McGavock 1968), the low activity *in vivo* may be due to the low rate of absorption from the gastrointestinal tract (Hecht and Gloxhuber 1960).

Substitution of male fern - and pumpkin seed extracts by niclosamide (phenasal) for treatment of *H. nana* infection reduced the rate of infection in the population of Tadzhik, S.S.R., from 68% (15,300 persons investigated) in 1961-'63 to 2.6% (12,200 persons investigated) in 1971-'73 (Shalabaev et *al.* 1974).

Although cure rates of *H. nana* infections have been variable, a 7-day course of 2.0 g niclosamide daily has cured 98% of patients (Nagaty *et al.* 1962). Excellent results against hymenolepiasis in man were also obtained by Perera *et al.* (1970), Kovalev and Daibova (1972), Grinenko *et al.* (1973, 1974) and Huggins (1973).

Oxygen uptake by homogenates of *H. diminuta* incubated in saline solutions containing glucose was inhibited by niclosamide proportionally to the amount of niclosamide added (Strufe 1964). It is of interest to note that in experiments with compounds in which the OH - or the NH - group of niclosamide was irreversibly blocked (as with 2-methoxy-2', 5-dichloro-4'-nitrobenzanilide or 2', 5-dichloro-4'-nitro-salicylic acid N-methylanilide) there was practically no effect on the oxygen uptake (Strufe 1964).

When intact *H. diminuta*, freshly isolated from the intestines of rats, was incubated anaerobically in the presence of glucose, a nearly constant utilization of glucose was observed (Strufe 1964). As little as 0.1 ppm niclosamide inhibited glucose utilization. In anaerobic conditions, the amount of lactate formed was proportional to the amount of niclosamide present. Such tapeworms showed a loss of glycogen after even short contact with niclosamide (Strufe 1964).

The anaerobic incorporation of ^{32}P into ATP by intact *H. diminuta* and the ^{32}P-ATP exchange in *H. diminuta* mitochondria were inhibited by this salicylanilide (Scheibel *et al.* 1968). Niclosamide elicited a stimulation of oxygen uptake by *H. diminuta* mitochondria at low concentrations (0.2µM) but about a 50% inhibition at 0.1 mM (Yorke and Turton 1974). Niclosamide has the same inhibitory effect upon the ^{32}P-ATP exchange reaction in *A. suum* mitochondria as demonstrated in *H. diminuta* mitochondria (Saz and Lescure 1968). It also inhibits the malate-induced ^{32}P incorporation into ATP by *Ascaris* mitochondria (Saz 1972a, b; Van den Bossche 1972b). These findings may indicate that *Ascaris* and *Hymenolepis* mitochondria are similar. The failure of niclosamide to affect intact nematodes may be due to a permeability barrier (Saz 1972b).

Oxidative phosphorylation in the rat liver (Gönnert *et al.* 1963; Williamson and Metcalf 1967; Strufe and Gönnert 1967) and in the house fly (Williamson and Metcalf 1967) mitochondria is also uncoupled by niclosamide. Although niclosamide and other anthelmintics, e.g. dichlorophen, oxyclozanide, uncouple phosphorylation in mammalian mitochondria *in vitro*, they have a low, if any toxicity *in vivo* (Hecht and Gloxhuber 1960; Hughes *et al.* 1973; Huggins 1973; Ronald and Wagner 1975). This low toxicity may be due to their inability to penetrate the host tissues (Hecht and Gloxhuber 1960; Gönnert *et al.* 1963).

2. *Resorantel*. The 2, 6-dihydroxybenzoic acid-anilides have marked cestocidal properties when a substitution by halogen atoms is made in the anilide portion of the molecule. The good anti-cestodal activity of the 4'-bromo-2, 6-dihydroxybenzanilide, resorantel (XXXV) has been observed by various authors (e.g. Düwel 1970; Behrens and Matschullat 1970; Ruschig *et al.* 1973). Experiments with 12,000 sheep showed the compound to be well tolerated (Becker *et al.* 1970).

Incubation of *H. diminuta* in the presence of this tapeworm remedy resulted in a decrease in ATP, ADP, and glycogen concentration as well as a concomitant increase in AMP, and pyruvate levels (Schacht *et al.* 1971). In addition, resorantel stimulates the oxygen consumption of isolated *H. diminuta* mitochondria at low concentrations (0.5 µM) and inhibits the oxygen uptake (66% at 0.177 mM) at high concentrations (Yorke and Turton 1974).

3. *Oxyclozanide.* Oxyclozanide (XXXVI) is another salicylanilide that has been extensively used in the treatment of *F. hepatica* infections. This 2, 2'-dihydroxy-3, 3', 5, 5', 6-pentachlorobenzanilide at doses of 4 mg/kg removed 13-day-old *H. diminuta* and caused no obvious harmful effect to the rat host up to 256 mg/kg (Hopkins *et al.* 1973).

Oxyclozanide is a potent uncoupler of oxidative phosphorylation and other energy-linked electron transfer reactions (Corbett and Goose 1971; Yorke and Turton 1974; Veenendaal and De Waal 1974). Using DL-isocitrate as substrate, oxyclozanide (0.217 µM) stimulated the rate of respiration of *H. diminuta* mitochondria and relieved oligomycin-induced inhibition of ADP-stimulated respiration (Yorke and Turton 1974).

E. *Isothiocyanates*

1. *Bitoscanate.* Bitoscanate (XXXVII) has proved to be effective against a variety of nematodes and cestodes in experimental animals and in man (Bunnag and Harinasuta 1968; Bhandari and Shrimali 1969; Bhandari and Singh 1969; Raghavan and Nagendra 1969; Lämmler and Saupe 1969; Botero and Perez 1970; Davis 1973; Ahmed and Vaishnava 1975; Biagi 1975; Samuel 1975; Mutalik *et al.* 1975). Bitoscanate has also been shown to be effective in infections with *H. nana*. A cure rate between 67 and 95% and a egg reduction rate between 86 and 96% were found when bitoscanate was administered in gelatin capsules at 200 or 300 mg in 2 or 3 divided doses of 100 mg each at 12-hourly intervals, after food (Mutalik *et al.* 1975).

2. *Other Isothiocyanates.* Nitroscanate (XXXVIII), a 4-nitro-4'-isothiocyano-diphenylether, is active against *E. granulosus* and *T. hydatigena* in dogs (Gemmell *et al.* 1977a). Recently, 4-isothiocyanato-4'-nitrodiphenylamine (XXXIX) has been found to be active against intestinal nematodes, filariae and schistosomes (Striebel 1976; Bueding *et al.* 1976; Saz *et al.* 1977; Doshi *et al.* 1977) and has been described as a new antihookworm compound (Vakil *et al.* 1977; Doshi *et al.* 1977; Vaidya *et al.* 1977). Further studies are needed to establish the anti-tapeworm

activity of isothiocyanates.

F.   *Naphthamidines*

1. *Bunamidine*. A series of naphthamidines has been tested by Baltzly et al. (1965) for activity against *H. nana* and *Oochoristica symmetrica* in mice and against *T. pisiformis* in dogs. Bunamidine (XL) proved to be the most effective. Good activity was also found against *T. hydatigena*, *E. granulosus* and *D. caninum* in dogs, *H. taeniaeformis* and *Spirometra mansonoides* in the cat and *M. expansa* in sheep (Baltzly et al. 1965; Forbes 1966; Burrows and Lillis 1966). Bunamidine at 1.8×10^{-5}M (20 nmoles/mg protein) stimulates and at 8.8×10^{-5}M (99.4 nmoles/mg protein) inhibits the oxygen uptake (substrate: succinate) of isolated rat liver mitochondria (Van den Bossche, unpublished results). At 1.8×10^{-4}M 100% inhibition of the oxygen uptake was observed. These results indicate that bunamidine uncouples oxidative phosphorylation from the electron transport chain in rat liver mitochondria.

In the presence of bunamidine *H. nana* shows a decrease in the rate of glucose uptake and an increase in the rate of glucose efflux (Hart et al. 1977). A bunamidine concentration of 3×10^{-5}M produced 88% inhibition of glucose uptake. The activity of the integumentary phosphatase (substrate p-nitrophenyl disodium phosphate, pH 7.4) of worms treated with bunamidine is much greater than that of the control worms and much of the enzyme activity is released into the incubation medium. At a bunamidine concentration of 3×10^{-5}M the activity is 15 times that of the controls. The biochemical indications of tegumental damage are confirmed by ultrastructural studies which show that there is complete loss of the surface tissue down to the level of the fibrous basal lamina (Hart et al. 1977).

Whether the morphological deteriorations are the result of interference with the phosphorylation system cannot be concluded from the just mentioned studies since the effects described were noted on different species. However, since similar effects on membranes are found with known uncouplers e.g. hexachlorophene, rafoxanide and nitroxynil (for review see Van den Bossche 1976) further studies are warranted.

G. *Quinolines and Isoquinolines*

1. *Quinolinehydrazones.* Pellerano *et al.* (1975) tested 107 4-quinoline hydrazones against *H. nana* in mice. Two of them i.e. 2, 6-dimethyl-4-[(3-pyridinylmethylene) hydrazino] quinoline (XLI) and 2, 6-dimethyl-4- (2-[(6-methyl)pyridinyl methylene] hydrazino) quinoline (XLII) at 200 mg/kg body weight were 100% effective against *H. nana* in mice.

2. *Praziquantel.* Praziquantel (LXIII) is an acylated heterocyclic compound which was developed by joint research of Bayer and E. Merck (Thomas and Andrews 1977). It is effective against all species of schistosomes pathogenic to man (Seubert *et al.* 1977). In addition praziquantel proves to be effective in a single oral dose against mature cestodes in man and animals, including *E. granulosus* and *E. multilocularis* in dogs (Thomas and Andrews 1977; Baldock *et al.* 1977; Bylund *et al.* 1977; Gemmell *et al.* 1977c).

The effects of praziquantel on *Hymenolepis* were studied by Thomas and Andrews (1977). An efficacy of 98% was obtained when mice infected with mature *H. nana* were treated orally with 10 mg/kg body weight. In rats praziquantel was 100% effective at 2.5 mg/kg against *H. diminuta*. The efficacy of praziquantel on cestodes in the bile duct was studied in mice on *H. microstoma*. A complete elimination was obtained after a single oral or subcutaneous administration of 5 or 10 mg/kg. However, against 24- and 48 h-old larvae of *H. nana* in mice only a 25-73% effect could be obtained with a dose of 500 mg/kg. At about 70 h after infection with eggs, i.e. at the onset of the last step of the differentiation of sucker and scolex, the larvae were almost as susceptible to praziquantel as 96 h-old larvae. They were killed by a single oral dose of 25 mg/kg host (Thomas and Andrews 1977).

Praziquantel affects *in vitro* the glucose uptake by *H. diminuta*. About 50% inhibition was obtained at 3.2×10^{-7}M (Thomas and Andrews 1977). At the same dose a significant increase in lactate excretion was observed. This effect was found when the worms were incubated in the presence or absence of glucose, indicating that the lactate excreted was formed from endogenous carbohydrates. There was a marked drop in the glycogen content of *H. diminuta* collected from the intestine of rats two hours after treating with 25 mg/kg. Praziquantel also rendered the tegument permeable to glucose, in fact glucose was leaking from *H. diminuta* incubated in glucose-free-praziquantel-containing media.

Praziquantel, at low concentrations ($3.2 \times 10^{-9} - 3.2 \times 10^{-8}$M) *in vitro* stimulated the motility of *H. diminuta* and impaired the proper functioning of the suckers. At higher doses (3.2×10^{-7}M) it caused a very strong contraction of the entire strobila (Thomas and Andrews 1977). Fetterer *et al.* (1977) stated that incubation of paired *S. mansoni* in the presence of 10^{-6}M praziquantel also resulted in a rapid and marked spastic paralysis.

Much more studies are needed to relate the effects upon carbohydrate metabolism, membranes and musculature.

It is of interest to note that *H. diminuta* incubated in the presence of praziquantel and subsequently placed into drug-free medium regained their motility. Glucose uptake also recovered (Thomas and Andrews 1977). This reversibility *in vitro* and the apparent irreversibility *in vivo* focuses the attention on the role the host-parasite relationship may play in the anthelmintic activities. Thomas and Andrews (1977) found that the tegument is readily attacked by proteolytic enzymes in the presence of praziquantel. *In vivo*, the tapeworm may be damaged by proteolytic enzymes and dislodged in the intestine before the effect of praziquantel is reversed.

VI. CONCLUSIONS

Herbal preparations have been used for centuries as taeniafuges. However, they are difficult to standardize and none of them are devoid of toxicity.

Several drugs with good activity against cestodiasis are now available. Nevertheless, there is still need for compounds which act against all cestode species of importance in veterinary and human medicine.

The antitapeworm screening carried out against *H. diminuta* in rats and especially that against *H. nana* in mice can be regarded as excellent models because both tapeworms are parasitic in man and the reactions to drugs of both *Hymenolepis* species in their rodent host can be compared with the reaction of cestodes in animals and man.

The lack of knowledge of the effects of anthelmintics on the physiology, metabolic processes, uptake, distribution and metabolism in the parasite and of their interference with the host-parasite relationship makes it almost impossible at present to understand the mechanisms which lie at the basis of their anthelmintic activity. Many more studies are needed to obtain more insight into the host-parasite-relationship and differences so that different and more specific targets can be selected to work on.

ACKNOWLEDGMENTS

The author is grateful to Dr. Paul A. J. Janssen for his constant interest. Grateful appreciation is expressed to Prof. L. Cañedo, Mexico, for sending the books of J. L. Díaz, Maximino Martinez and F. Guerra. The author gratefully acknowledges Dr. D. Thienpont and Dr. J. P. Tollenaere for a number of fruitful discussions, Dr. H. Vanhove for help in preparing the manuscript and Mrs. A. Nuyts for typing the text.

No	Name	Structure
I	Diacetylphloroglucinol	
II	Aspidin	
III	Aspidinol	
IV	Flavaspidic acid	

V	Desaspidin	
VI	Ortho-desaspidin	
VII	Nor-flavaspidic acid	
VIII	Desaspidinol	

IX	Rottlerin
X	Ascaridol
XI	Arecoline
XII	Pelletierine

XIII	Diospyrol	
XIV	3-amino-3-carboxy pyrrolidin	
XV	tris(1-quinolinyl)-$\underline{N}^1,\underline{O}$-antimonate	R = R' = H R = H, R' = CH$_3$
XVI	$\underline{O}$-(6-iodo-8-quinolinyl)-metaantimonate	

XVII	Stibophen	
XVIII	Paromomycin	

XIX	Mepacrine	
XX	Acranil	
XXI	Acriflavine	(a) R = CH$_3$ (b) R = H
XXII	Thiabendazole	

XXIII	Cambendazole	
XXIV	Parbendazole	
XXV	Oxibendazole	
XXVI	Albendazole	
XXVII	Mebendazole	

XXVIII	Flubendazole	4-fluorobenzoyl-benzimidazole-2-methylcarbamate structure
XXIX	Fenbendazole	phenylthio-benzimidazole-2-methylcarbamate structure
XXX	Oxfendazole	phenylsulfinyl-benzimidazole-2-methylcarbamate structure
XXXI	Hexylresorcinol	4-hexylresorcinol structure

Dichlorophen	XXXII
Bithionol	XXXIII
Niclosamide	XXXIV
Resorantel	XXXV

XXXVI	Oxyclozanide	
XXXVII	Bitoscanate	
XXXVIII	Nitroscanate	
XXXIX	4-isothiocyanato-4'-nitro-diphenylamine	

XL		Bunamidine
XLI		2,6-dimethyl-4-[(3-pyridinyl-methylene)hydrazino] quinoline
XLII		2,6-dimethyl-4-{2-[(6-methyl)pyridinyl methylene] hydrazino} quinoline
XLIII		Praziquantel

REFERENCES

1. Actor, P., Anderson, E. L., Di Cuollo, C. J., Ferlauto, R. J., Hoover, J. R. E., Pagano, J. F., Ravin, L. C., Scheidy, S. F., Stedman, R. J. and Theodorides, V. J., *Nature*, London *215*, 312-322 (1967).
2. Aebi, A., Büchi, J. and Kapoor, A., *Helv. Chim. Acta 40*, 266-274 (1957).
3. Aguilar, F. J., Cifuentos, C. E. and Samayoa, A., Abstract *4th Latin Am. Cong. Parasitol.* San José, Costa Rica. (1976).
4. Ahmed, S. H. and Vaishnava, S., *In* "Progress in Drug Research" (E. Jucker, ed.), pp. 2-6. Birkhäuser Verlag, Basel. (1975).
5. Aikman, L., *Nath. Geographic 146*, 420-440 (1974).
6. Al-Jeboori, T. I. and Shafio, M. A., *J. Fac. Med. Baghdad 18*, 161-170 (1976).
7. Allen, R. W., *Am. J. Vet. Res. 34*, 61-63 (1973).
8. Anderson, N., *Res. Vet. Sci. 23*, 298-302 (1977).
9. Arakcheeva, S. G., Isaeva, Kh. B. and Zubitskaya, M. A., *Med. Zh. Uzb.* (9), 14-17 (1975).
10. Averkin, E. A., Beard, C. C., Dvorak, C. A., Edwards, J. A. Fried, J. H., Kilian, J. G., Schiltz, R. A., Kistner, T. P., Drudge, J. H., Lyons, E. T., Sharp, M. L., and Corwin, R. M., *J. Med. Chem 18*, 1164-1166 (1975).
11. Baldock, F. C., Flucke, W. J. and Hopkins, T. J., *Res. Vet. Sci. 23*, 237-238 (1977).
12. Baldwin, E., *Parasitology 35*, 89-111 (1943).
13. Baltzly, R., Burrows, R. B., Harfenist, M., Fuller, K. A., Keeling, J. E. D., Standen, O. D., Hatton, C. J., Nunns, V. J., Rawes, D. A., Blood, B. D., Moya, V. and Lelyveld, J. L., *Nature*, London *206*, 408-409 (1965).
14. Banjerjee, D., Prakush, O. and Kaliyuaperumal, V., *Indian J. Med. Res. 60*, 562-566 (1972).
15. Barrett, J., *In* "The Organization of Nematodes" (N. A. Croll, ed.), pp. 11-70. Academic Press, New York. (1976a).
16. Barrett, J., *In* "Biochemistry of Parasites and Host-Parasite Relationships" (H. Van den Bossche, ed.), pp. 67-80. North-Holland Publishing Co., Amsterdam. (1976b).
17. Beaver, P. C. and Sodeman, W. A., *J. Trop. Med.*

Hyg. 55, 92-99 (1952).
18. Becker, W., Humke, R. and Tiefenbach, B., *Blaue Hefte Tierarzt 43*, 75-78 (1970).
19. Behrens, H. and Matschullat, G., *Dtsch. tierärztl. Wschr. 77*, 101-104 (1970).
20. Beier, A., *Z. Tropenmed. Parasit. 16*, 433-436 (1965).
21. Bekhti, A., *Acta Gastro-ent. Belg. 37*, 302-306 (1974).
22. Bekhti, A., Schaaps, J. P., Capron, M., Dessaint, J. P., Santoro F., Capron, A., *Brit. Med. J.*, 1047-1051 (1977).
23. Bello, T. R., Amborski, G. F., Torbert, B. J. and Greer, G. J., *Am. J. Vet. Res. 34*, 771-777 (1973).
24. Benediktov, I. I., *Med. Parazitol. Parazitarn. Bolez. 44*, 473-477 (1975).
25. Bennett, D. G., *Am. J. Vet. Res. 29*, 2325-2330 (1968).
26. Benz, G. W., *Am. J. Vet. Res. 32*, 399-403 (1971a).
27. Benz, G. W., *J. Parasitol. 57*, 286-288 (1971b).
28. Benz, G. W., *J. Parasitol. 59*, 166-168 (1973).
29. Benz, G. W. and Ernst, J. V., *Am. J. Vet. Res. 38*, 1425-1426 (1977).
30. Bhandari, B. and Shrimali, L. N., *J. Trop. Med. Hyg. 72*, 164-166 (1969).
31. Bhandari, B. and Singh, S. V., *Ann. Trop. Med. Parasitol. 63*, 177-180 (1969).
32. Biagi, F., *In* "Progress in Drug Research" (E. Jucker, ed.) pp. 23-27. Birkhäuser Verlag, Basel. (1975).
33. Biagi, F., Gomez-Orozco, L. and Robledo, E., *Bol. méd. hosp. infantil.* (Mex.) *16*, 113-116 (1959).
34. Biagi, F., López, R. and Viso, J., *In* "Progress in Drug Research" (E. Jucker, ed.), pp. 10-22. Birkhäuser Verlag, Basal. (1975).
35. Biagi, F., Smyth, J. and Gonzalez, C., *La Pressa Medica Mexicana 39*, 3-5 (1974).
36. Bianchi, M., Cotta, E., Ferni, G., Grein, A., Julita, P., Mazzoleni, R. and Spalla, C., *Arch. Microbiol. 98*, 289-299 (1974).
37. Blakemore, R. C., Bowden, K., Broadbent, J. L. and Drysdale, A. C., *J. Pharm. Pharmacol. 16*, 464-471 (1964).
38. Borgers, M., De Nollin, S., Verheyen, A., De Brabander, M. and Thienpont, D., *In* "Micro-

tubules and Microtubular Inhibitors" (M. Borgers and M. De Brabander, eds.), pp. 497-508. North-Holland Publish.Co., Amsterdam. (1975).
39. Botero, D. R., *Am. J. Trop. Med. Hyg. 19*, 234-237 (1970).
40. Botero, D. R. and Perez, A. C., *Am. J. Trop. Med. Hyg. 19*, 471-475 (1970).
41. Bowden, K., Broadbent, J. L., Ross, W. J., *Brit. J. Pharmacol. 24*, 714-724 (1965).
42. Brody, G. and Elward, T. E., *J. Parasitol. 57*, 1068-1077 (1971).
43. Brown, H. W., *Clin. Pharmacol. Therap. 10*, 5-21 (1969).
44. Brown, H. D., Matzuk, A. R., Ilves, I. R., Peterson, L. H., Harris, S. A., Sarrett, L. H., Egerton, J. R., Yakstis, J. J., Campbell, W. C. and Cuckler, A. C., *J. Am. Chem. Soc. 88*, 1764-1765 (1961).
45. Brugmans, J. P., Thienpont, D. C., Van Wijngaarden, I., Vanparijs, O. F., Schuermans, V. L. and Lauwers, H. L., *J. Am. Med. Assoc. 217*, 313-316 (1971).
46. Bryant, C., Cornish, R. A. and Rahman, M. S., *In* "Biochemistry of Parasites and Host-Parasite Relationships". (H. Van den Bossche, ed.) pp. 599-604. North-Holland Publishing Co., Amsterdam. (1976).
47. Bueding, E., *Biochem. Pharmacol. 18*, 1541-1547 (1969).
48. Bueding, E., *In* "Comparative Biochemistry of Parasites" (H. Van den Bossche, ed.) pp. 25-32. Academic Press, New York. (1972).
49. Bueding, E., Batzinger, R. and Petterson, G., *Experientia 32*, 604-606 (1976).
50. Bueding, E. and Fisher, J., *Biochem. Pharmacol. 15*, 1197-1211 (1966).
51. Bueding, E. and Mansour, J. M., *Br. J. Pharmacol. 12*, 159-165 (1957).
52. Bunnag, D. and Harinasuta, T., *Ann. trop. Med. Parasitol. 62*, 416-421 (1968).
53. Burrows, R. B. and Lillis, W. G., *Am. J. Vet. Res. 27*, 1381-1384 (1966).
54. Bylund, G., Bång, B. and Wikgren, K., *J. Helminthol. 51*, 115-119 (1977).
55. Campbell, W. C., *Proc. Helminthol. Soc. Wash. 44*, 17-28 (1977).
56. Campbell, W. C. and Blair, L. S., *J. Parasitol.*

60, 1043-1052 (1974).
57. Campbell, W. C., McCracken, R. O. and Blair, L. S., *J. Am. Med. Assoc. 230*, 825 (1974).
58. Campbell, W. C., McCracken, R. O. and Blair, L. S., *J. Parasitol. 61*, 844-852 (1975).
59. Cavier, R., *In* "Chemotherapy of Helminthiasis" (R. Cavier and F. Hawking, eds.) pp. 215-436. Pergamon Press, Oxford. (1973).
60. Cavier, R., Cenac, J., Loiseau, G., *Ann. Pharm. Franc. 32*, 623-628 (1974).
61. Červenka, J., Zajiček, D. and Nydl, J., *Veterinárstvi 25*, 263-264 (1975).
62. Chaia, G. and Sales da Cunha, A., *A. Fôlha Medica 63*, 67-76 (1971).
63. Chaia, G., Métene, F., Chiari, L., De Moura Araujo, S. and Barbosa de Abreu, I., *A. Fôlha Medica 64*, 155-161 (1972).
64. Chanco, P. P., Tulane, M.P.H.H., and Atienza, M. R., *Philipp. J. Microbiol. Inf. Dis. 2*, 27-38.
65. Chang, J. and Wescott, R. B., *Am. J. Vet. Res. 30*, 77-79 (1969).
66. Chavarria, A. P., Swartzwelder, J. C., Villarejos, V. M. and Zeledon, R., *Am. J. Trop. Med. Hyg. 22*, 592-595 (1973).
67. Chavarria, A. P., Villarejos, V. M., Zeledon, R., *Am. J. Trop. Med. Hyg. 26*, 118-120 (1977).
68. Coles, G. C., *Int. J. Biochem. 4*, 319-337 (1973).
69. Coles, G. C., *Pestic. Sci. 8*, 536-543 (1977).
70. Corbett, J. R. and Goose, J., *Pestic. Sci. 2*, 119-121 (1971).
71. Craige, A. H. and Kleckner, A. L., *N. Am. Vet. 27*, 26-30 (1946).
72. Culbertson, J. T., *J. Pharmacol. 70*, 309-314 (1940).
73. Dǎnek, J., Pavliček, J. and Zajiček, D., *Helminthologia 11*, 243-246 (1970).
74. Davis, A., "Drug Treatment in Intestinal Helminthiasis". WHO, Geneva. (1973).
75. Davis, M. J., Cilo, M., Plaitakis, A. and Yahr, M. D., *Neurology 26*, 37-40 (1976).
76. de Carneri, I. and Vita, G., *In* "Chemotherapy of Helminthiasis" (R. Cavier and F. Hawking, eds.), pp. 145-213, Pergamon Press, Oxford. (1973).
77. del Castillo, J., *In* "Chemical Zoology" (M. Florkin and B. T. Scheer, eds.) Vol. III, pp.

521-554. Academic Press, New York.
78. Della Bruna, C., Ricciardi, M. L. and Sanfilipo, A., *Antimicrob. Agents Chemother. 3*, 708-710 (1973).
79. De Nollin, S. and Van den Bossche, H., *J. Parasitol. 59*, 970-976 (1973).
80. Díaz, J. L., "Indice y Sinonimia de las Plantas Medicinales de Mexico". Monografias Cientificas I. Instituto Mexicano para el estudio de las plantas medicinales, A. C. (1976a).
81. Díaz, J. L., "Usos de las Plantas Medicinales de Mexico". Monografias Cientificas II. Instituto Mexicano para el estudio de las plantas medicinales, A. C. (1976b).
82. Dikshit, S. K. and Lalit, O. P., *Indian J. med. Res. 58*, 611-621 (1970).
83. Doshi, J. C., Vaidya, A. B., Sen, H. G., Mankodi, N. A., Nair, C. N. and Grewal, R. S., *Am. J. Trop. Med. Hyg. 26*, 636-639 (1977).
84. Douglas, J. R. and Baker, N. F., *Ann. Rev. Pharmacol. 8*, 213-228 (1968).
85. Duncan, J. L., Armour, J., Bairden, K., Jennings, F. W. and Urquhart, G. M., *Vet. Rec. 98*, 342 (1976).
86. Dunlop, R. H., *Fed. Proceed. 26*, 1227-1243 (1967).
87. Düwel, D., *Dtsch. tierärztl. Wschr. 77*, 97-101 (1970).
88. Düwel, D., *Pestic. Sci. 8*, 550-555 (1977).
89. Düwel, D., Kirsch, R. and Reisenleiter, R., *Vet. Rec. 97*, 371 (1975).
90. Eckert, J. and Pohlenz, J., *Tropenmed. Parasit. 27*, 247-262 (1976).
91. Egerton, J. R. and Campbell, W. C., *Res. Vet. Sci. 11*, 193-195 (1970).
92. Egerton, J. R., Di Netta, J., Neu, D. C., Walther, R. J. and Campbell, W. C., *Res. Vet. Sci. 11*, 590-592 (1970).
93. El-Masry, N. A., Farid, Z. and Bassily, S., *E. Afr. Med. J. 51*, 532-535 (1974).
94. Enigk, K., Dey-Hazra, A. and Batke, J., *Avian Pathol. 2*, 67-74 (1973).
95. Enigk, K., Dey-Hazra, A. and Batke, J., *Dtsch. tierärztl. Wschr. 81*, 177-200 (1974).
96. Enigk, K., Dey-Hazra, A. and Batke, J., *Tierärztliche Umschau 30*, 324-338 (1975a).
97. Enigk, K., Dey-Hazra, A. and Batke, J., *Dtsch. tierärztl. Wschr. 82*, 137-139 (1975b).

98. Evans, W. S. and Novak, M., *Can. J. Zool. 54*, 1079-1083 (1976).
99. Fernando, S. E. E. and Denham, D. A., *J. Parasitol. 62*, 874-876 (1976).
100. Fetterer, R., Pax, R. and Bennett, J., Prog. and Abst. American Society of Parasitology, Las Vegas, November. (1977).
101. Forbes, L. S., *Vet. Rec. 79*, 306-307 (1966).
102. Garin, J. P., Kalb, J. C., Despeignes, J. and Vincent, G., *J. Parasitol. 56*, (No. 4, Section II, part 1), 112 (1970).
103. Gemmell, M. A., Johnstone, P. D. and Oudemans, G., *Res. Vet. Sci. 22*, 391-392 (1977a).
104. Gemmell, M. A., Johnstone, P. D. and Oudemans, G., *Res. Vet. Sci. 23*, 115-116 (1977b).
105. Gemmell, M. A., Johnstone, P. D. and Oudemans, G., *Res. Vet. Sci. 23*, 121-123 (1977c).
106. Gibbs, H. C. and Gupta, R. P., *Can. J. Comp. Med. Vet. Sci. 36*, 108-115 (1972).
107. Gibson, T. E., *Parasitology 54*, 545-550 (1964).
108. Gibson, T. E. and Parfitt, J. W., *Brit. Vet. J. 127*, 201-206 (1971).
109. Gilles, H. M., *Brit. Med. J.*, 1314-1316 (1976).
110. Gilman, R. E. and Marion, L., *Bull. Soc. Chim. France*, 1993-1995 (1961).
111. Goldsmid, J. M., *S. Afr. Med. J. 48*, 2265-2266 (1974).
112. Gönnert, R. and Schraufstätter, E., *Arzneim. Forsch. 10*, 881-890 (1960).
113. Gönnert, R., Johannis, J., Schraufstätter, E. and Strufe, R., *Medizin und Chemie*, Bayer, Leverkusen, VII, 540-567 (1963).
114. Goodman, H. T., *Med. J. Australia 2*, 662 (1976).
115. Grevel, V. and Eckert, J., *Schweiz. Archiv für Tierheilkunde 115*, 559-577 (1973).
116. Grinenko, N. V., Bereslavich, T. N., Vishnivetskaya, M. B., Zhelezova, N. I. and Al' Van, A. K. H., *Med. Parazitol. Parazitarn. Bolez. 42*, 163-167 (1973).
117. Grinenko, N. V., Bereslabish, T. N., Nerodo, A. B., Arutyunyan, G. K. and Evtushik, Z. M. A., *Vrachebnoe Delo (4)*, 146-149 (1974).
118. Hart, R. J., Turner, R. and Wilson, R. G., *Int. J. Parasitol. 7*, 129-134 (1977).
119. Hamajima, F., *Exp. Parasitol. 34*, 1-11 (1973).
120. Hawking, F., *In* "Progress in Drug Research"

(E. Jucker, ed.), pp. 191-222. Birkhäuser Verlag, Basel (1966).
121. Haynes, W., "The Chemical Age", p. 90. Secker and Warburg, London. (1946).
122. Heath, D. D. and Chevis, R. A. F., *Lancet (2)*, 218-219 (1974).
123. Heath, D. D., Christie, M. J. and Chevis, R. A. F., *Parasitology 70*, 273-285 (1975).
124. Hecht, G. and Gloxhuber, Chr., *Arzneim. Forsch. 10*, 884-885 (1960).
125. Herlich, H., *Am. J. Vet. Res. 38*, 1247-1248 (1977).
126. Herzig, P. T., "Estudio de las propiedades anthelminticas de las semillas de calabaza". Tesis. Fac. de Ciencias Quimicas Mexico. (1946).
127. Hirte, W., *Deut. med. Wchnschr. 76*, 1083-1085 (1951).
128. Hoff, D. R., Fisher, M. H., Bochis, R. J., Lusi, A., Waksmunski, F., Egerton, J. R., Yakstis, J. J., Cuckler, A. C. and Campbell, W. C., *Experientia 26*, 550-551 (1970).
129. Hopkins, C. A., Grant, P. M. and Stallard, H., *Parasitology 66*, 355-365 (1973).
130. Huggins, D., *An. Instituto Hig. Med. Trop. 1*, 41-43 (1973).
131. Hughes, H. C. Jr., Barthel, C. H. and Lang, C. M., *Lab. Animal Sci. 23*, 72-73 (1973).
132. Janssen Pharmaceutica Report. The anthelmintic activity of mebendazole in rodents. Report V 1021. (1972).
133. Jones, O. T. H. and Watson, W. A., *Biochem. J. 102*, 564-573 (1967).
134. Junod, Ch., *Press. méd. 72*, 1243 (1964).
135. Kale, O. O., *Am. J. Trop. Med. Hyg. 24*, 600-605 (1975).
136. Kammerer, W. C. and Judge, D. M., *Am. J. Trop. Med. Hyg. 25*, 714-717 (1976).
137. Kates, K. C., Colglazier, M. L., Enzie, F. D., Lindahl, I. L. and Samuelson, G., *Parasitol. 57*, 356-362 (1971).
138. Kates, K. C., Colglazier, M. L., Enzie, F. D., Lindahl, I. L., and Samuelson, G., *Proc. Helminthol. Soc. Wash. 40*, 87-92 (1973).
139. Kates, K. C., Colglazier, M. L. and Enzie, F. D., *Vet. Rec. 97*, 442-444 (1975).
140. Katz, N., *In* "Advances in Pharmacology and Chemotherapy" (S. Garatini, F. Hawking, A. Goldin, I. J. Kopin and R. J. Schnitzer, eds.),

Vol. 14, pp. 1-70. Academic Press, New York. (1977).
141. Kean, B. H. and Hoskins, D. W., *In:* "Drugs of Choice 1976-1977" (W. Modell, ed.), pp. 356-369. The C. V. Mosby Company, Saint Louis. (1976).
142. Knight, R. A. and Colglazier, M. L., *Am. J. Vet. Res. 38*, 807-808 (1977).
143. Kovalenko, I. I., Kal'chenko, A. A., Sikachina, V. I. and Sikachina, S. F., *Veterinariya (9)*, 51-52 (1976).
144. Kovalenko, F. P., Krotov, A. I., Budanova, I. S. and Razakov, Sh. A., *Med. parazitol. parazitarn. Bolez. 45*, 546-551 (1976).
145. Kovalev, N. E. and Daibova, M. Z., *In:* "Problemy parazitologii. Trudy VII Nauchnoi Konferentsii Parazitologov U.S.S.R.", Part I, pp. 362-363. Kiev, U.S.S.R. (1972).
146. Krotov, A. I. and Kovchur, V. N., *Med. Parazitol. Bolez. 40*, 177-182 (1971).
147. Krotov, A. I., Nurtaeva, K. S. and Dovzhenko, V. A., *In:* "Problemy obschchei i prikladnoi gel' mihtologii", pp. 201-205. Moscow. (1973).
148. Krotov, A. I., Bajandina, D. G., Bechli, A. F., Braude, M. B., Kozyreva, N. P. and Kolosova, M. O., *Med. parazitol. parazitarn. Bolez. 43*, 697-700 (1974a).
149. Krotov, A. I., Chernyaeva, A. I., Kovalenko, F. P., Bayandina, D. G., Budanova, I. S., Kuznetsova, O. E. and Voskoloinik, L. V., *Med. parazitol. parazitarn. Bolez. 43*, 314-319 (1974b).
150. Krotov, A. I., Chernyaeva, A. I. and Budanova, I. S., *Med. parazitol. parazitarn. Bolez. 45*, 164-168 (1976).
151. Kuhls, R., *Med. Klin. 48*, 1511-1514 (1953).
152. Kumar, S. P., Shivnani, G. V. and Joshi, H. C., *Indian J. Poultry Sci. 9*, 7-13 (1974).
153. Kunkle, D. W. and Theodorides, V. J., *J. Parasitol. 57*, 319 (1971).
154. Lämmler, G. and Saupe, E., *Z. Tropenmed. Parasit. 20*, 346-350 (1969).
155. Loewe, H. and Urbanietz, J., *Pestic. Sci. 8*, 544-549 (1977).
156. Lüdin, C. E., Gyr, K. and Karoussos, K. *J. Int. Med. Res. 5*, 367-368 (1977).
157. Luney, F. W., *Can. Med. Assoc. J. 30*, 385-386 (1934).
158. Madsen, D. C., "Some effects of quinacrine on

the metabolism of *Hymenolepis diminuta*". Thesis. University of Massachusetts. (1972).
159. Malkin, M. F. and Camacho, R. M., *J. Parasitol.* 58, 845-846 (1972).
160. Manson-Bahr, P. E. C., *In* "Side Effects of Drugs", Vol. III, pp. 433-436. Excerpta Medica, Amsterdam. (1972).
161. Mansour, T. E. and Bueding, E., *Br. J. Pharmacol.* 9, 459-462 (1954).
162. Marinoni, V. and Sperzani, G. L., *Archs. ital. Sci. med. trop. Parassit.* 47, 327-330 (1966).
163. Marsboom, R., *Toxicol. Appl. Pharmacol.* 24, 371-377 (1973).
164. Martinez-Fernandez, A. R. and Rodriguez-Coabeiro, F., "4th Intern. Conference on Trichinellosis". Poznan, Poland, Abstract No. 8.4. (1976).
165. Maximino Martinez, "Las Plantas Medicinales de Mexico", pp. 127-130. Quinta Edicion - Andres - Ediciones Botas - Mexico. (1969).
166. McBeath, D. G., Best, J. M. J. and Preston, N. K., *Vet. Rec.* 101, 408-409 (1977).
167. McGavock, W. D., *Diss. Abst.* 29, 416B (1968).
168. McManus, E. C., Washko, F. V. and Tocco, K. J., *Am. J. Vet. Res.* 27, 849-855 (1966).
169. Merck Sharp & Dohme, *Clin. Pharmacol. Therapeutics* 9, 277-281 (1968).
170. Miller, M. J., *In* "Progress in Drug Research" (E. Jucker, ed.), pp. 433-464. Birkhäuser Verlag, Basel. (1976).
171. Mineev, V. V., *In* "Helminths and Helminthiasis of Poultry in Kazakhstan", pp. 109-114. Alma-Ata: Izdat. Akad. Nauk. Kazakhstanskoi, S. S. R. (1964).
172. Mutalik, G. S., Gulati, R. B. and Iqbal, A. K., *In* "Progress in Drug Research" (E. Jucker, ed.), pp. 81-85. Birkhäuser Verlag, Basel. (1975).
173. Nagalingam, I., Lam, L. E., Robinson, M. J. and Dissanaika, A. S., *Am. J. Trop. Med. Hyg.* 25, 568-572 (1976).
174. Nagaty, H. F., Rifaat, M. A. and Salem, S., *J. Trop. Med. Hyg.* 65, 128-129 (1962).
175. Náquira, C., Delgado, E., Tantaleán, M., Náquira, F. and Elliot, A., *Revta Peruana Med. Trop.* 2, 37-41 (1973).
176. Nawalinski, T. and Theodorides, V. J., *Am. J. Vet. Res.* 37, 469-471 (1976).

177. Neghme, R. A., *Rev. chilena hist. nat. 43*, 97-99 (1939).
178. Neghme, R. A. and Faigeunbaum, J., *Rev. méd. Chile 75*, 54-57 (1947).
179. Newton, B. A., In "Biochemistry of Parasites and Host-Parasite Relationships" (H. Van den Bossche, ed.), pp. 459-476. North-Holland Publish. Co., Amsterdam. (1976).
180. Nurtaeva, K. S., *Med. Parazitol. Parazitarn. Bolez. 41*, 741-745 (1972).
181. Nurtaeva, K. S., *Med. Parazitol. Parazitarn. Bolez. 42*, 560-565 (1973).
182. Pampiglione, S., *Parasitologia 4*, 49-58 (1962).
183. Panitz, E. and Knapp, S. E., *Am. J. Vet. Res. 31*, 763-770 (1970).
184. Partono, F., Purnomo and Tangkilisan A., *S. E. Asian J. Trop. Med. Publ. Hlth. 5*, 258-264 (1974).
185. Pawlowski, Z., *J. Parasitol. 56*, (No. 4, Sect. II, Pt. 1), 261 (1970).
186. Pawlowski, Z., Kozakiewicz, B., Zatonski, J., *Vet. Parasitol. 2*, 299-302 (1976).
187. Pellarno, C., Savini, L., Berkoff, C. E., Thomas, J. and Actor, P., *Farmaco Edizione Scientifica 30*, 965-973 (1975).
188. Pentillä, A. and Sundman, J., *Nordisk Medicin 67*, 439-443 (1962).
189. Pentilla, A. and Sundman, J., *Acta Chem. Scand. 17*, 2361-2369 (1963).
190. Perera, D. R., Western, K. A. and Schultz, M. G., *Am. J. Trop. Med. Hyg. 19*, 610-612 (1970).
191. Peters, W., "Chemotherapy and Drug Resistance in Malaria", p. 6, Academic Press, London (1970).
192. Pharmacopoeia of Japan, Part I, p. 443. Society of Japanese Pharmacopoeia Yankuji Nippo Ltd. (1971).
193. Piringer, W. A., Luque, J. M. and Mezcy, K. C., *Z. Tropenmed. Parasit. 11*, 51-56 (1960).
194. Podesta, R. B. and Mettrick, D. F., In "Biochemistry of Parasites and Host-Parasite Relationships" (H. Van den Bossche, ed.), pp. 373-377. North-Holland Publish Co., Amsterdam. (1976a).
195. Podesta, R. B. and Mettrick, D. F., *Comp. Biochem. Physiol. 57A*, 265-273 (1976b).
196. Prichard, R. K., *Nature*, London *228*, 684-685 (1970).

197. Prichard, R. K., *Int. J. Parasitol. 3*, 409-417 (1973).
198. Prichard, R. K., "Proceedings 3rd International Congress of Parasitology", München, Vol. III, pp. 1446-1447. Facta Publications, Vienna. (1974).
199. Raghaven, P. and Nagendra, A. S., *J. Postgrad. Med. 11*, 176-181 (1969).
200. Rahman, M. S. and Bryant, C., *Int. J. Parasitol. 7*, 403-409 (1977).
201. Rahman, M. S., Cornish, R. A., Chevis, R. A. F. and Bryant, C., *New Zealand Vet. J. 25*, 79-83 (1977).
202. Rollo, I. M., *In* "The Pharmacological Basis of Therapeutics" (L. S. Goodman and A. Gilman, eds.), pp. 1058-1086. The Macmillan Co., New York. (1965).
203. Romanowski, R. D., Rhoads, M. L., Colglazier, M. L. and Kates, K. C., *J. Parasitol. 61*, 777-778 (1975).
204. Ronald, N. C. and Wagner, J. E., *Lab. Animal Sci. 25*, 219-220 (1975).
205. Rosendahl, H., *Pharm. J. 87*, 35 (1911).
206. Runeberg, L., *Biochem. Pharmacol. 11*, 237-242 (1962).
207. Runeberg, L., "The effect of desaspidin and related phlorobutyrophenone derivatives from fern extract on oxidative phosphorylation and muscle adenosinetriphosphates". Societas Scientiarum Fennica. Commentationes Biologicae. XXVL (7) pp. 1-69 Helsinki, Helsingfors. (1963).
208. Ruschig, H. König, J., Düwel, D. and Loewe, H., *Arzneim. Forsch. 23*, 1745-1758 (1973).
209. Sadun, E. H. and Vajrathira, S., *J. Parasitol. 40*, 49-53 (1954).
210. Saikkonem, J. I. and Mustakallio, K. K., *Lancet (1)*, 335 (1963).
211. Salunkhe, D. S., *J. Trop. Med. Hyg. 69*, 165 (1966).
212. Samuel, M. R., *In* "Progress in Drug Research" (E. Jucker, ed.), pp. 96-107. Birkhäuser Verlag, Basel. (1975).
213. Saz, D. K., Bonner, T. P., Karlin, M. and Saz, H. J., *J. Parasitol. 57*, 1153-1162 (1971).
214. Saz, H. J., *In* "Comparative Biochemistry of Parasites" (H. Van den Bossche, ed.), pp. 33-47. Academic Press, New York. (1972a).
215. Saz, H. J., *In* "Comparative Biochemistry of

Parasites" (H. Van den Bossche, ed.), pp. 445-454. Academic Press, New York. (1972b).
216. Saz, H. J. and Dunbar, G. A., *J. Parasitol. 61*, 794-801 (1975).
217. Saz, H. J. and Lescure, O. L., *Molec. Pharmacol. 4*, 407-410 (1968).
218. Saz, H. J., Dunbar, G. A., Bueding, E., *Am. J. Trop. Med. Hyg. 26*, 574-575 (1977).
219. Schacht, U., Düwel, D. and Kirsch, R., *Z. Parasitenk. 37*, 278-287 (1971).
220. Scheibel, L. W., *J. Florida Med. Ass. 60*, 21-24 (1973).
221. Scheibel, L. W., Saz, H. J. and Bueding, E., *J. biol. Chem. 243*, 2229-2235 (1968).
222. Seaton, D. R., *Lancet (1)*, 808-809 (1956).
223. Seaton, D. R., *Ann. Trop. Med. Parasit. 54*, 338-340 (1960).
224. Sen, A. B. and Hawking, F., *Brit. J. Pharmacol. 15*, 436-439 (1960a).
225. Sen, A. B. and Hawking, F., *Ann. Biochem. Exptl. Med. (Calcutta) Supp. 20*, 547-550 (1960b).
226. Sen, H. G., Joshi, B. S., Parthasarathy, P. C. and Kamat, V. N., *Arzneim. Forsch. 24*, 2000-2003 (1974).
227. Seubert, J., Pohlke, R. and Loebich, F., *Experientia 33*, 1036-1037 (1977).
228. Shafei, A. Z., *J. Trop. Med. Hyg. 79*, 197-200 (1976).
229. Shalabaev, G. A., Gabunova, L. G. and Ostrovskii, M. S., *Helminthol. Abst. 45*, 5443 (1974).
230. Singson, C. N., Banzon, T. C. and Cross, J. H., *Am. J. trop. Med. Hyg. 24*, 932-934 (1975).
231. Sonnet, J. and Thienpont, D., *Acta Clin. Belgica 32*, 297-302 (1977).
232. Spaldonová, R., Corba, J. and Tomašovicová, O., 4th Internat. Conference on Trichinellosis, Poznan, Poland. Abstract No. 8.5. (1976).
233. Srivastava, M. C. and Singh, S. W., *Ind. J. Med. Res. 55*, 629-632 (1967).
234. Srivastava, M. C., Singh, S. W. and Tewari, J. P., *Ind. J. Med. Res. 55*, 746-748 (1967).
235. Strasser, H. and Tiefenbach, B., *Dtsch. Tierärztl. Wschr. 84*, 453-492 (1977).
236. Steck, E. A., "The Chemotherapy of Protozoan Diseases", Vol. II, Section III, pp. 15.10 - 15.11. Walter Reed Army Institute of Research,

Washington, D.C. (1971).
237. Stone, O., Stone, C. and Mallius, J., *J. Am. Med. Assoc. 187*, 536-538 (1964).
238. Stoye, M., Enigk, K. and Bürger, H. J., *Tierärztl. Umschau 26*, 108-110 (1971).
239. Striebel, H. P., *Experientia 32*, 457-458 (1976).
240. Strufe, R., "Proceed. 3rd Int. Congress Chemotherapy" 2, 1544-1547 (Congress 1963; Publ. 1964). (1964).
241. Strufe, R. and Gönnert, R., *Z. Tropenmed. Parasit. 18*, 193-202 (1967).
242. Taffs, L. F., *Vet. Rec. 89*, 165-168 (1971).
243. Taffs, L. F., *J. Helminthol. 49*, 173-177 (1975).
244. Taffs, L. F., *Vet. Rec. 99*, 143-144 (1976).
245. Theodorides, V. J., Laderman, M. and Pagano, J. F., *Vet. Med. Small Anim. Clin. 63*, 257-264 (1968a).
246. Theodorides, V. J., Laderman, M. and Pagano, J. F., *Vet. Med. Small Anim. Clin. 63*, 370-371 (1968b).
247. Theodorides, V. J., Chang, J., DiCuollo, C. J., Grass, G. M., Parish, R. C. and Scott, G. C., *Brit. Vet. J. 129*, XCVII-XCVIII. (1973).
248. Theodorides, V. J., Gyurik, R. J., Kingsbury, W. D. and Parish, R. C., *Experientia 32*, 702-703 (1976b).
249. Theodorides, V. J., Nawalinski, T. and Chang, T., *Am. J. Vet. Res. 37*, 1515-1516 (1976c).
250. Theodorides, V. J., Nawalinski, T., Freeman, J. F. and Murphy, J. R., *Am. J. Vet. Res. 37*, 1207-1209 (1976a).
251. Theodorides, V. J., Nawalinski, T., Murphy, J. and Freeman, J., *Am. J. Vet. Res. 37*, 1517-1518 (1976d).
252. Thienpont, D., Vanparijs, O. F. and Vandesteene, R., *In* "Trichinellosis" (C. W. Kim, ed.), pp. 515-527. Intext Educational Publishers, New York. (1974a).
253. Thienpont, D., Vanparijs, O. F. and Hermans, L., *In* "Proceed. 3rd Int. Congress Parasitology", München, p. 593. Facta Publications, Vienna. (1974b).
254. Thomas, H. and Andrews, P., *Pestic. Sci. 8*, 556-560 (1977).
255. Tocco, D. J., *J. Med. Chem. 7*, 399-405 (1964).
256 Tocco, D. J., Egerton, J. R., Bowers, W.,

Christensen, V. W. and Rosenblum, C., *J. Pharmacol. Exptl. Therapeut.* 149, 263-271 (1965).
257. Townsend, R. B., Kelly, J. D., James, R. and Weston, E., *Res. Vet. Sci.* 23, 385-386 (1977).
258. Turner, J. A., *In:* "Diseases Transmitted from Animals to Man" (W. T. Hubbert, W. F. McCulloch and P. R. Schnurrenberger, eds.), pp. 708-744. Chas. C., Springfield, Illinois. (1975).
259. Ulivelli, A., *Acta 30th Congr. ital. Pediat.* 2, 229-234 (1964).
260. Ulivelli, A., *Giorn. Mal. infett. parasit.* 19, 308-310 (1967).
261. Ulivelli, A., 8th Int. Congress Trop. Med. Teheran, pp. 1089-1091 (1968).
262. Vaidya, A. B., Sen, H. G., Mankodi, N. A., Paul, T. and Sheth, U. K., *Br. J. Clin. Pharmac.* 4, 463-467 (1977).
263. Vakil, B. J., Dalal, N. J., and Shah, P. N., *Trans. Roy. Soc. Trop. Med. Hyg.* 71, 247-250 (1977).
264. Van den Bossche, H., *In:* "Comparative Biochemistry of Parasites" (H. Van den Bossche, ed.), pp. 139-157. Academic Press, New York. (1972a).
265. Van den Bossche, H., *In:* "Comparative Biochemistry of Parasites" (H. Van den Bossche, ed.), pp. 455-468. Academic Press, New York. (1972b).
266. Van den Bossche, H., *In:* "Biochemistry of Parasites and Host-Parasite Relationships" (H. Van den Bossche, ed.), pp. 553-572. North-Holland Publish Co., Amsterdam. (1976).
267. Van den Bossche, H. and De Nollin, S., *Int. J. Parasitol.* 3, 401-407 (1973).
268. Vandepitte, J., Gatti, F., Lontie, M., Krubwa, F., Nguete-Kikhela and Thienpont, D., *Bull. Soc. Path. Exot.* 66, 165-178 (1973a).
269. Vandepitte, J., Gatti, F., Krubwa, F. and Thienpont, D., *S. Afr. Med. J.* 47, 2205 (1973b).
270. Van Noordwijk. J., Mellink, J. J., Visser, B. J. and Wisse, J. H., *Rec. Trav. Chim. Pays Bas* 82, 763-772 (1963).
271. Van Vugt, F., "On the energy metabolism of the adult liver fluke, *Fasciola heptica*" (Ne, en). Thesis. State University of Utrecht, The Netherlands. (1977).
272. Vargas-Mena, J., Villarreal, A. C. and Montes, E., *Revta lat.-am. Microbiol.* 12, 27-33 (1970a).
273. Vargas-Mena, J., Rodriguez, M. E. and Montes, E., *Revta lat.-am. Microbiol.* 12, 35-39 (1970b).

274. Veenendael, G. H. and De Waal, M. J., *Brit. J. Pharmacol. 50*, 435-437 (1974).
275. Verheyen, A., Borgers, M., Vanparijs, O. F. and Thienpont, D., *In:* "Biochemistry of Parasites and Host-Parasite Relationships" (H. Van den Bossche, ed.), pp. 605-618. North-Holland Publish. Co., Amsterdam. (1976).
276. von Brand, R., "Biochemistry of Parasites", 2nd edition, pp. 134-140. Academic Press, New York. (1973).
277. Waitz, J. A., McClay, P. and Thompson, P. E., *J. Parasitol. 52*, 830-831 (1966).
278. Walker, D. and Knight, D., *Vet. Rec. 90*, 58-65 (1972).
279. Watkins, T. I., *J. Pharm. Pharmacol. 10*, 209-227 (1958).
280. Williamson, R. L. and Metcalf. R. L., *Science 158*, 1694-1695 (1967).
281. Wilson, C. G., Parke, V. D. and Cawthorne, M. A., *Biochem. Soc. Trans. 1*, 195-196 (1973).
282. Wittner, M. and Tanowitz, H., *Am. J. Trop. Med. Hyg. 20*, 433-435 (1971).
283. Yokogawa, M., Yoshimura, H., Sano, M., Okura, T., Tsuji, M., Takizawa, A., Harada, Y., Kihata, M., Iswaski, M., Hirose, H., *Jap. J. Parasitol. 10*, 302-316 (1961a).
284. Yokogawa, M., Yoshimura, H., Okura, T., Sano, M., Tsuji, M., Twasaki, M., Hirose, H., *Jap. J. Parasitol. 10*, 317-327 (1961b).
285. Yorke, R. E. and Turton, J. A., *Z. Parasitenkde. 45*, 1-10 (1974).
286. Yoshida, Y., Miyake, T., Makanishi, Y., Nishida, K., Yamashiki, Y., Ishikawa, T., Fujisaka, A., Tanaka, A. and Ebara, S., *Jap. J. Parasit. 11*, 411-420 (1962).
287. Zakhryalov, Ya. N. and Gorodovich, N. M., Dal'nevotochnoe Knizhnoe Izdatel'stvo: 82-85. *Helminthol. Abst. 45 (1976)*, 446 (1971).

INDEX

A

Absorption,
  of amino acids, 285, 385
  capacity for amino acids, 324–325
  of carbohydrates, 285, 385, 389–398
  of Cl⁻, 302
  in excretory system, 211
  of fatty acids, 312
  functioning of tegument in, 180
  of galactose, 392–398, 509, 524, 529
  of glucose, 143, 309, 325, 381, 389, 392, 398, 509, 517, 521, 522, 523
  of HCO_3^-, 301, 302
  of hexose, 392, 520
  host intestinal surface area for, 286
  inhibition by sodium taurocholate of, 386
  of monosaccharides, 296
  of niclosamide, 660–661
  of nutrients, 167
  of paromomycin, 648
  of proteins, 307
  by surface of *Hymenolepis diminuta*, 506–507
  of thymidine, 405–406
  of water, 316, 317, 325, 326
Acanthobothrium coronatum, stretch receptor of, 223
Acanthocephala,
  anatomical specialization for enteric parasitism of, 263
  collagen-type proteins in, 201
Acetate,
  accumulation affected by O_2, 474
  effect on DNA synthesis of, 406, 407
  formation of, 472, 473, 475
  formation catalyzed by pyruvic dehydrogenase, 494
  uptake by *Hymenolepis diminuta,* 582
Acetic acid, as end product of energy metabolism, 406
Acetylcholine,
  accumulation in motor end plates, 193
  functioning as inhibitory neurotransmitter, 193
  in neurons of *Hymenolepis diminuta,* 224

Acetylcholine esterase (AChE), distribution along major nerve tracts of, 214
Acetyl-CoA-carboxylase, effect of high carbohydrate diets on, 314
AcPyAD⁺, in hydride transfer in mitochondria, 482, 486
AcPyADH, as hydride ion receptor in mitochondria, 482, 486
Acranil,
  effect on neuromuscular system of *Taenia saginata,* 650
  structural formula of, (673)
Acridine dyes (see: mepacrine, acranil, acriflavine)
Acriflavine, efficacy against *Hymenolepis nana* of, 650
Actidione, inhibition of growth by, 437
Actimycin A,
  insensitivity of succinate oxidation to, 467
  insensitivity of cytochrome o to, 469
Actin (see also: microfilaments),
  in cytoplasm of collecting duct cells, 211
  in microvilli of host lumen, 286
  in muscle cell, (187), 189
  in two-filament sliding model of muscle contraction, 189, 191
Actinomycin D, in study of preformed informational RNA, 365
Adenosine diphosphate,
  effect of oxyclozanide on ADP-stimulated respiration, 663
  effect of resorantel on level of, 662
  O_2 uptake measurements in presence of, 468
  role in inhibition of 'reverse NADH → NADP⁺' reaction, 484
  in stimulation of malate plus pyruvate oxidation, 490
Adenosine monophosphate,
  enhancement of O_2 uptake in plant mitochondria uncoupled by FCCP, 468, 491
  inhibitor of 'reverse NADH → NADP⁺' reaction in *Hymenolepis diminuta,* 484
Adenosine phosphatase, in musculature and circular fibers of capsular wall, 138

Adenosine triphosphatase,
  in activity related to excretory system, 211
  in association with inner mitochondrial membrane, 470, 479
  increased in activity by glycocholate and taurocholate, 296
  role in absorption of, 284, 517
Adenosine triphosphate,
  aerobic generation of, 466, 467, 489, 493
  content in *Hymenolepis diminuta*, 409, 644, 650
  desaspidin inhibition of ^{32}P incorporation into, 641
  electron transport dependent generation of, 481
  generation via fumarate reductase, 488, 495
  hydrolysis during myofilament contraction, 193
  inhibition of pyruvate kinase isozymes by, 477
  modification of NADPH → NAD$^+$ transhydrogenase activity by, 484
  reduction by cambendazole of synthesis of, 653
  reduction by mebendazole of synthesis of, 657
  Site I coupled generation of, 468
Age resistance,
  to *Cittotaenia* sp., 552
  to *Moniezia expansa*, 552
Alanine,
  accumulation during glucose dissimilation of, 473
  fluxes across brush border, 527, 528, 529
  formation by transamination of pyruvate, 493
  inhibition of α-aminoisobutyric acid by, 137
  uptake inhibited by ouabain, 509
Albendazole,
  efficacy in treatment of helminth infections of, 654–655
  structural formula of, (674)
Alkaline phosphatase,
  presence in bile of, 295
  release stimulated by CCK-PZ, 292
Amiloride,
  asymmetric inhibiton by, 513
  effect on Na$^+$ pools of *Hymenolepis diminuta*, 515
  inhibitor of Na$^+$ flux across brush border, 510
Amino acids (see also: specific amino acids),
  diurnal changes in host lumen of, 324
  effect on growth of *Hymenolepis diminuta* of, 382–385
  host luminal gradients of, 307–308
p-aminobenzoic acid (PABA),
  diet supplemented by, 375
  effect of deficiency on worm growth of, 377
3-amino-3-carboxy pyrrolidin,
  as anthelmintic component of *Cucurbita*, 645
  structural formula of, (671)
α-aminoisobutyric acid (AIB),
  transport locus of, 143
  uptake of, 137
Aminopeptidase,
  activity on polypeptides of, 289
  locus of activity in host villus of, 285
Ammonia,
  as component in test diet, 620
  effect on DNA synthesis of, 406
Amphotericin B, use in culture medium of, 437
Amylase,
  in autolysis of embryophore, 96, 100, 102
  from bacteria, 428
  in host digestion, 291, 293
  in host saliva and pancreatic juices, 290
α-amylase,
  alteration of embryophore by, 100
  digestion of outer oncospheral envelope to, 74
  insensitivity of DNA to, 453
  resistance of inner oncospheral envelope to, 74
Amylopectin, hydrolysis by host amylase of, 290
Amylose, hydrolysis by host amylase of, 290
Amylo-(1, 4-1, 6)-transglucosidase, in scolex of *Hymenolepis diminuta* metacestode, 143
Anaerobic energy generation,
  in *Ascaris lumbricoides*, 466
  in *Hymenolepis diminuta*, 494–495
Anaerobic phosphorylation,
  in *Ascaris lumbricoides*, 466
  in *Hymenolepis diminuta*, 479, 493–496
Ancylostoma, effect of chenopodium oil on, 644
Ancylostomiasis, use of diospyrol in treatment of, 645
Anlagen (see also: primordia),
  labeling of, 183
  in neck of *Hymenolepis diminuta*, 161, 229
  stem cell origin of, 360
Anthelmintics (see: specific anthelmintic)

Index

Anti-acetylcholine esterase compounds, in stimulation of muscle activity, 193
Antibodies (see also: specific antibody), induction and functions of, 571–573
Antihistamine, action of promethazine as, 575
Anti-5-hydroxytryptamine, action of methysergide as, 575
Anti-inflammatory drugs, in suppression of worm rejection, 575
Antilymphocyte serum (ALS),
  delay of rejection by, 595
  immunosuppressive action of, 566–567
Antimonials (see: specific antimonial)
Antimycin A,
  inhibition of succinate oxidation by, 490
  insensitivity of anaerobic generation of ATP in *Hymenolepis diminuta* mitochondria to, 489
Antithymocytic serum (ATS), immunosuppressive action of, 566–567
Apolysis,
  alteration of rostellar tegument with, 236
  carbohydrate requirement during, 374
  initiation of, 265, 365
  description of, 161, (163)
  effect on excretory system during, 206
  effect on nervous system during, 217
  of *Hymenolepis diminuta* in mice, 595
Areca catechu (betel-nut palm), source of arecoline, 643
Arecoline, anthelmintic activity of, 643–644
Arecoline hydrobromide, anthelmintic activity against hymenolepidids in ducks, 644
Arginine
  absence in cytoplasmic layer of *Hymenolepis diminuta* metacestodes, 69, 75
  absence in 48 h hydrolysates of *Hymenolepis diminuta* metacestodes, 135
  lack of inhibitory effect on α-aminoisobutyric acid by, 137
Aryl sulfatase, in intermediate cell layer and tail parenchyma of capsules of *Hymenolepis diminuta* and *H. nana*, 138
Ascaridol
  active constituent in chenopodium oil, 643
  structural formula of, (670)
Ascaris
  effect of mebendazole on malate-induced phosphorylation in mitochondria of, 657
  O_2 requiring oxidative phosphorylation in, 468

  paralytic effect of hexyresorcinal on, 659
  satellite DNA from, 455
  synthesis of C_4 through C_6 acids by, 466
  toxicity of chenopodium oil to, 643
  use of extracts of *Cucurbita pepo* seeds against, 645
Ascaris lumbricoides
  comparison of 'malic' enzymes from *Hymenolepis diminuta* and, 480
  cross reactivity of *Hymenolepis nana* and, 587
  dissimilation of glucose in muscle of, 493
  fumarate as acceptor in electron transport system of, 494
  ineffectiveness in vitro of kamala against, 642
  microaerophilic or anaerobic nature of, 464
  similarities in electron transport systems of *Hymenolepis diminuta* and, 488
  similarities in energy metabolism of *Hymenolepis diminuta* and, 472, 478, 479
  transhydrogenase activity in, 486
  use of ^{14}C-NADH for anaerobic phosphorylation by mitochondria of, 471
Ascaris suum
  effect of mebendazole on intestinal cells of, 657
  effect of phenols on incorporation of ^{32}P into ATP by, 642
  effect of phenols on ^{32}P-ATP exchange reaction of, 642
  inhibition of ^{32}P-ATP exchange reaction by niclosamide in, 662
  interference by fenbendazole on glycogenesis in, 658
  interference of glucose uptake by fenbendazole in, 658
Ascorbate
  in determination of cytochrome oxidase, 490
  role in fostering oxidative phosphorylation in *Ascaris lumbricoides* mitochondria, 468
  use in measurement of O_2 utilization in *Hymenolepis diminuta*, 474
Aspartic acid, as competitive inhibitor of α-aminoisobutyric acid, 137
Aspidin, anthelmintic activity against *Hymenolepis nana* of, 641
Aspidinol, ineffectiveness against *Hymenolepis nana*, 641
Aspidium, use as an anthelmintic, 640
Atabrine (see: mepacrine)

Atractyloside, inhibition of ADP-stimulated oxidation of malate plus pyruvate by, 491
Avitellina centripunctata
  effect of axenomycin D on, 649
  histogenesis of parenchymal muscle in, 199
Axenomycins, anthelmintic activity of, 648–649
Axons
  cable studies on, 535
  movement of fuchsinophilic material into, 367
Azide
  insensitivity of succinate oxidation to, 467
  sensitivity of cytochrome oxidase-like activity to, 491

B

Bacteroides sp., electron transport system with cytochrome b in, 469
Basal (basement) lamina
  bunamidine damage of tegument to level of, 664
  of distal cytoplasm, (91), (119), 120, 122, (128), 175, 180
  of oncospheral surface membrane, 82, 89, 113
  of vaginal epithelial lining, 254
Benzanilides, efficacy as anthelmintics of, 660–663
Benzimidazoles, anthelmintic efficacy of, 651–659
Bicarbonate ion
  fluxes in host small intestine of, 301–302
  from host pancreas, 288
  release from pancreas stimulated by secretin, 288, 321
Bicircum flux, in epithelial syncytium of *Hymenolepis diminuta*, 511–514
Bile
  activity of components of, 296–298
  composition in rat, 295
  effect on growth of, 386
  in excystment of cysticercoids, 434
  regulation of host secretion of, 295
  toxicity of, 440, 442
  use in culture medium of hamster, 438, 440
  use in culture medium of sheep, 440
Bile acids
  in activation and excystment of cysticercoids, 1, 385, 432, 434, 438, 440
  bacterial activity on, 317

facilation of absorption of fatty acids by, 386
inactivation of brush border by, 540
relation to CCK-PZ of, 292
role in release of enterokinase of, 293
role of, 296
Bilirubin
  bacterial action on, 317
  effect of aspidium on uptake into liver cells of, 640
  facilitation by bile salts in transport of, 296
Biotic potential
  of *Diphyllobothrium latum*, 240
  of *Hymenolepis diminuta*, 3, 357
  of *Taenia saginata*, 240
Biotin
  effect on establishment and growth dietary deficiency of, 377
  in host diet, 375
Bithionol, anthelmintic activity of, 660
Bitoscanate, anthelmintic activity of, 663
Blood
  of rabbit in culture medium, 434
  of rabbit in replacement of sheep's in culture medium, 436
  of man in culture medium, 442
Blood agar, as culture medium, 434, 435
Brugia pahangi, microaerophilic or anaerobic nature of, 464
Brunner's glands, in duodenal submucosa of rat gut, 292
Bunamidine, anthelmintic activity of, 664

C

Calliobothrium verticillatum
  effect of glucose and galactose on Na$^+$ efflux in, 522
  efflux of radiosodium in, 515
  Na$^+$ and glucose influx in, 520
  ultrastructure of tegument of, 171
Cambendazole
  anthelmintic activity of, 652–653
  effect on glucose absorption and glycogenesis of, 658
Capillaria hepatica, cross reactivity of *Hymenolepis nana* and, 587
Capillariasis, mebendazole in treatment of, 655
Capsule
  formation of, 66, 252
  role in viability of oncosphere of, 3

Index

Carbohydrate (see also: specific carbohydrate)
  competition for host dietary, 370, 371, 386, 403, 405
  effects on worm development of host dietary, 310, 371, 384, 593
  dissimilation in *Hymenolepis diminuta*, (465), 493–494
Carbon dioxide,
  concentration in rat intestine of, 535
  fixation of, 465, 475, 477, 479, 493, 494
Carbon tetrachloride, anthelmintic activity of, 552
Carbonyl cyanide m-chlorophenolhydrozone, malate dependent phosphorylation inhibited by, 479
Carboxypeptidase A, in hydrolysis of peptides, 291
Carboxypeptidase B, in hydrolysis of peptides, 291
β-carotene, facilitation by bile sales in absorption of, 296
Caryophyllaeus laticeps, ultrastructure of tegument of, 171
Casein, in host diet, 381, 388
Catalase, deficiency in *Ascaris lumbricoides* of, 467
Catenotaenia pusilla,
  hook formation in, 81
  myofilament formation in oncospheres of, 82
  persistence of capsule in, 61, 78
Cesium chloride,
  in characterization of nuclear DNA, 452–453
  in isolation procedure of mtDNA, 456
Cestodin, anthelmintic action of, 646
Chemodeoxycholic acid, role in absorption of fluid and electrolytes in rat intestine of, 296
Chenopodium ambrosioides, as source of chenopodium oil, 643
Chenopodium foetidum, as source of chenopodium oil, 643
Chenopodium graveolens, as source of chenopodium oil, 643
Chenopodium oil, anthelmintic action of, 643
Chlorella vulgaris, proton transport in, 521
Chloroblasts, nonelectrolyte transport in, 516
Chlorosalicylamide, as inhibitor of mitochondrial phosphorylation in adult *Hymenolepis diminuta*, 492
Choanotaenia infundibulum, unicellular glands in, 84

Cholate, in excystment of cysticercoids, 432
Cholecystokinin-pancreozymin (CCK-PZ),
  in control of bile flow in dogs, 295
  role in gastrointestinal secretion of, 321–322
  in stimulating release of host intestinal enzymes, 292
  synthesis by chromaffin cells of, 283
Cholesterol
  bacterial action on, 317
  distribution in *Hymenolepis diminuta*, 143
  metabolism of, 295–296
Cholesterol esterase, protection by bile salts from proteolytic attack of, 296
Cholic acid
  effect on ATPase by conjugates of, 296
  as precursor of bile acids, 295
Choline
  component of vitamin G complex in host diet, 375
  as replacement for cations in glucose uptake, 393
Cholinesterase, activity in larval tegument and nerves of scolex of, 138
Chorionic gonadotropin, effect on growth of, 376
Chromaffin cells
  in crypts of host intestinal mucosa, 283
  in synthesis of CCK-PZ, 283
Chyme, characteristics of, 288
Chymotrypsin
  activity in mid-gut of *Tenebrio molitor* larvae of, 101
  activity inhibited by intestinal mucosa, 294
  adsorption of, 92
  role in digestion of embryophore of, 102
Chymotrypsinogen, as precursor of chymotrypsin, 290
Cilia (see also: sensilla, flame cell)
  in lumen of capillary tubule of excretory system, 208
  as mis-identification of microvilli of vaginal wall, 254
  in terminal expansion of senory dendrite, 223
  on terminus of neurosensory processes, 179
Cirrus
  component of male copulatory apparatus, 250
  differentiation from somatic primordium, 246
  localization of AChE in, 218
  localization of 5-HT in sphincter musculature of, 193

Cittotaenia sp., age resistance of, 552
Cleavage, in *Hymenolepis diminuta*, 62–64
Clostridium formicoaceticum, electron transport system with cytochrome b linked with fumarate reduction, 469
Clostridium thermoaceticum, electron transport system with cytochrome c linked with fumarate reduction, 469
Colchicine, in arrest of mitotic activity in *Hymenolepis diminuta*, 362
Collagen (see also: connective tissue)
  role of smooth muscle in synthesis of, 204
  structure, function and origin of, 200–202
Commissures, in nervous system of *Hymenolepis diminuta*, 161, 215
Complement, activation by IgA of, 576
Concanavalin A, crypt cell agglutination by, 286
Concretions, as source of carbonate and phosphate buffer components, 535
Connective tissue
  in association with rostellar suckers, 230
  in binding of myofibrils, 186
  in capsule of rostellum, 234
  in forming basement membrane of tegument, 171, 175
  general characteristics of, 199–200
  in intercellular space of *Hymenolepis diminuta*, 164, 197, 206
  myocytons in elaboration of, 198, 265
  role in body movement of, 189
  ultrastructure, histogenesis and function in *Hymenolepis diminuta*, 201–204
Contracircum flux, in epithelial syncytium of *Hymenolepis diminuta*, 511–514, 537
Coprophagy, role in vitamin B_6 deficiency of, 377–379, 403
Corpuscles, calcareous, 511
Cortisone
  effect on methionine and sodium acetate transport in immunosuppressed rats and mice by, 582
  immunosuppressive action in mice, 561–563
  suppression of rejection by, 557, 558, 590, 593
C. P. Read principle, 505
Crowding effect
  on cysticercoids in beetles, 145
  in definitive host, 354–365
  mechanism of, 401–410
  of *Moniliformis dubius* on *Hymenolepis diminuta*, 387, 388
  nutrients as a factor in, 312, 593
  premunition and, 368, 551, 591
Crypts of Lieberkühn, in host intestine, 292
Cucurbita, anthelmintic action of ground seeds of, 645
Cucurbita maxima, anthelmintic activity of ground seeds of, 645
Cucurbita moschata, anthelmintic action of ground seeds of, 645
Cucurbita pepo, anthelmintic action of ground seeds of, 645
Cuticle (see also: tegument)
  O_2 requirement for synthesis of *Ascaris lumbricoides*, 464
  term erroneously used in reference to tapeworm surfaces, 161, 172
Cyanide
  inhibition of *Hymenolepis diminuta* succinate oxidation by, 490
  insensitivity of cytochrome o in *Ascaris lumbriocoides* to, 469
  insensitivity of succinate dependent O_2 consumption in *Hymenolepis diminuta* to, 489
  insensitivity of succinate oxidation in *Ascaris lumbricoides* muscle to, 467
Cyanobalamin (see: vitamin B_{12})
Cyclohexamide, inhibition of in vitro growth of *Hymenolepis diminuta* by, 437
Cyclophosphamide (Cy), immunosuppressant activity of, 563–566
Cyst
  activity of scolex in, 432
  development of, 431
  wall structure of, 117, (118)
Cystacanth, of *Moniliformis dubius* in concurrent infections with *Hymenolepis diminuta*, 387, 618
Cysteine,
  in culture medium, 430, 431
  effect in host diet of, 382
Cysticercoid (metacestode),
  development of, 3, 4, 59–60, 108, 110–111, 116, 431, 432, 433
  effect of mebendazole on development of *Hymenolepis diminuta*, 655
  efficacy of kamala on, 643
  efficacy of mepacrine on *Hymenolepis nana*, 649
  efficacy of paromomycin on *Hymenolepis nana*, 648
  excystment in vitro of, 432
  excystment of, 1, 357, 440

Index 701

immunogenic effect of *Hymenolepis nana*, 586
immunogenic effect of irradiated *Hymenolepis diminuta*, 598
informational RNA in, 365
in vitro cultivation of, 426–427, 434
in vitro cultivation of *Hymenolepis nana*, 437
in vitro gas phase requirements of, 474–475
isozyme of lactic dehydrogenase in, 478
motility of, 432
stem cells in, 358

Cysticercus fasciolaris,
efficacy of mebendazole on, 656
mebendazole in reduction of glycogen content in, 657

Cystine, in capsule of mature larvae of *Hymenolepis diminuta*, 69, 75
Cytochromes (see: specific cytochrome)
Cytochrome a, in ascarid system, 469
Cytochrome a_3, in ascarid system, 469
Cytochrome b,
in ascarid system, 469
in *Ascaris lumbricoides* muscle, 469
Cytochrome b_{550}, in *Ascaris lumbricoides* muscle, 469
Cytochrome o, roles of, 469–470
Cytochrome oxidase,
activity in *Hymenolepis diminuta*, 490–491
activity in mitochondria from *Ascaris lumbricoides*, 464
involvement in ascarid electron transport system by, 467
levels in *Ascaris lumbricoides* of, 464
Cytoplasm, resistance of, 533

D

Dendrites (see: nervous system, sensilla, neurons)
Dense bodies,
attachment to actin filaments, 189
in distal cytoplasmic layer of cysticercoids, 87–88
function of, 189
as site of interaction between muscle and connective tissues, 202
Deoxypyridine, inhibition of in vitro growth of *Hymenolepis diminuta* by, 379
Deoxycholate, inhibition of ATPase activity in rat intestine by, 296
Deoxycholic acid, role in absorption of fluid and electrolytes in rat intestine of, 296

Deoxyribonuclease,
in treatment of worm conditioned saline, 410
sensitivity of satellite DNAs to, 453
Deoxyribonucleic acid,
AT/GC content of, 453, 454
buoyant density of nuclear, 452, 453
buoyant density of satellite, 453, 454, 455, 456, 457
changes during development in concentrations of, 371
content in *Hymenolepis diminuta*, 451
effect of worm conditioned saline on incorporation of ^{3}H-thymidine into, 405–406, (407), 409
functions of, 456, 457
genome size, 455
isolation and characterization of, 452–456
kinetic complexity of, 455
lacking in embryonic envelopes and capsule of *Hymenolepis diminuta*, 69, 74
in mitochondria of *Ascaris lumbricoides* muscle, 466
in mitochondria of *Hymenolepis diminuta*, 479
mitochondrial (mtDNA), 456
radioactivity from tritiation of, 362, 405, 406, 407, 409, 455
relationship of crowding effect to replication of, 365
roles of satellites of, 456–457
satellites of, 453, 455, 456, 457
in species of hymenolepidids, 455, 456
synthesis of, 402, 405, 406–409, 458
T_m of, 453
yield from *Hymenolepis diminuta* of, 450
Dermestes vulpinus, 'emergence' medium from saline extracts of, 96
Desaspidin,
anthelmintic of choice for *Diphyllobothrium latum* in Finland, 641
inhibition of ^{32}P-ATP exchange reaction in *Hymenolepis diminuta* by, 641–642, 659
inhibitor of phosphorylation in *Hymenolepis diminuta* mitochondria, 492
Desaspidinol,
structural formula of, (669)
uncoupler of oxidative phosphorylation in rat liver mitochondria, 641
Desmosomes (see also: dense bodies),
attachment to blade of hook, 81, (92)
at attachment of sensory dendrites and tegument, 169, 179, (221), 223

junctional complexes mis-interpreted as, 89
in planarians, 207
Destrobilation,
as criterion in worm development, 554–555
in *Hymenolepis* with increase in intensity of infection, 369
as reaction to host immune response, 581–582
as result of host dietary restriction, 372, 631
Desulfovibrio gigas, electron transport system with cytochrome b linked to fumarate reduction in, 469
Development,
of adult, 2
chemical changes during, 371–372
of cysticercoid, 3, 4, 60, 116, 431, 432, 433, 655
in definitive host, 310, 357–423, 616, 631
effect of in vitro temperature on, 4
of scolex, 231, 431
Dextrin,
absorption of, 389
effect on growth of, 372
effect on host intestinal pH of, 299
as product of starch hydrolysis, 290
relative incorporation of ^{14}C-glucose into limit, 399, (400)
Diacetylphloroglucinol,
activity in vitro against *Hymenolepis nana* of, 641
structural formula of, (668)
3,3′-diaminobenzidine (DAB),
detection of cytochrome oxidase-like activity in *Hymenolepis diminuta* based on oxidation of, 490
detection of peroxidase activity using, 492
2′,5-dichloro-4′-nitrosalicylic acid, effect on O_2 uptake of *Hymenolepis diminuta* homogenates of, 661
Dichlorophen,
effect on ^{32}P-ATP exchange reaction of, 659
effect on ^{32}P incorporation into ATP by *Hymenolepis diminuta* in vitro of, 659
efficacy in treatment of cestodes of mammals of, 659
uncoupler of electron transport linked phosphorylation in mitochondria of *Hymenolepis diminuta*, 659, 662
structural formulas of, (676)
Dictol, in vaccination against *Dictyocaulus viviparus*, 553

Dictyocaulus,
efficacy of albendazole in treatment of sheep and cattle against, 654
succinate production in, (473)
Dictyocaulus viviparus, use of Dictol as vaccine against, 553
Diets,
carbohydrate components of, 310–314
effects of deprivation of, 620
effects on migration of, 620–621, 627
as external factors, 371–385
isocaloric, 310
Differentiation,
of gonads, 541
lack of cellular, 265–266
lack of regional, 170
rapid and/or sustained growth without, 168
of somatic and reproductive tissues, 161
Diffusion,
ionic, 534
molecular, 137, 534
Dihydrofolate reductase, in reduction of dihydrofolate, 566
Dihydrolipoyl dehydrogenase, in inner mitochondrial membrane of *Ascaris lumbricoides*, 471
2,6-dimethyl-4-[2-([6-methyl] pyrindinyl methylene) hydrazino] quinoline,
efficacy against *Hymenolepis nana* in mice of, 665
structural formula of, (678)
2,6-dimethyl-4-(3-pyridinyl methylene) hydrazino quinoline,
efficacy against *Hymenolepis nana* in mice of, 665
structural formula of, (678)
2,4-dinitrophenol, inhibitor of electron transport associated phosphorylation, 479
Diospyrol,
efficacy against *Hymenolepis nana* in mice of, 645
structural formula of, (671)
Diospyros mollis, as source of diospyrol, 645
Dipeptidases, in host intestinal epithelium, 284
Dipetalonema viteae, energy generating metabolism in, 464
Diphyllobothrium dendriticum,
cell cycle of stem cells in, 362
histogenesis of nervous tissue in, 218
plerocercoids of, 362
stem cell origin of all cell types in, 359
stem cells in plerocercoids of, 358

Diphyllobothrium latum,
  biotic potential of, 340
  plerocercoids of, 358
  tegument development in, 184
  use of desaspidin against, 641
  use of mepacrine against, 649
  use of niclosamide against, 660
  use of oleoresin of aspidium against, 660
Diphyllobothrium spp., use of axenomycin D in dogs against, 649
Dipylidium caninum,
  efficacy of bunamidine in dogs against, 664
  fine structure of tegument of, 171
  hook structure of, 81
  use of axenomycin D in dogs against, 649
Disaccharidases,
  in host intestinal epithelium, 284
  secretion in mammals of, 291
Distal cytoplasm (see: tegument, syncytium)
Distribution,
  geographical, 9–28
  of host of *Hymenolepis diminuta*, 9–28
  intraintestinal, 617, 618, 619, 627
Dixon plot, for glucose absorption by *Hymenolepis diminuta*, 393
Drepan otaenia, efficacy of arecoline in geese against, 644
Drosophila, gap junctions in epithelium of salivary glands of, 533
Dryopteris austrica, as source of desaspidin, 641
Dryopteris dilatata, as source of aspidin, phloropyrone and aspidinol, 641
Dryopteris filix-mas, as source of flavaspidic acid, aspidinol and oleoresin of aspidium, 640–641
Dugesia tigrina, genome size of, 455

E

Eagle's basal medium, use in in vitro culture of *Hymenolepis microstoma*, 442
Eagle's medium (modified),
  use in in vitro culture of *Hymenolepis nana*, 438, (441)
  use in in vitro culture of *Hymenolepis microstoma*, 442
Earle's saline, use in collection of eggs of *Hymenolepis nana*, *H. diminuta*, *H. microstoma* and *H. citelli*, 428, 429
Echinococcus granulosus,
  efficacy of bunamidine in dogs infected with, 664

  efficacy of mebendazole against cysts of, 656
  efficacy of nitroscanate in dogs infected with, 663
  efficacy of praziquantel in dogs infected with, 665
  immunity to, 552
  rostellar glands of, 569
  stem cells in adults of, 358
  vaccination against, 598
Echinococcus multilocularis,
  efficacy of mebendazole against larval stages of, 656
  efficacy of praziquantel in dogs against, 665
  stem cells in cysts of, 358
ED_{92}, of kamala in mice infected with *Hymenolepis nana*, 644
Eggs (see also: capsule),
  capsule of, 4
  collection and sterilization of, 428
  effect of bitoscanate on *Hymenolepis nana* production of, 663
  effect of hexyresorcinol on hyaline membrane of *Hymenolepis nana*, 659
  in host feces, 365
  host sex hormonal effect on production of, 3, 375, 376
  immunological challenge by infection with, 587
  in vitro emergence of oncospheres from, 426
  in vitro production of, 436
  isozyme of lactic dehydrogenase in, 478
  lipid transfer to, 198
  loss as reaction to immune response, 562
  PAS positive material on outer coat of, 263
  production affected by dietary deficiencies, 372, 376
  production depressed in bileless hosts, 386
  production of *Taenia saginata* and *Diphyllobothrium latum*, 442
  rDNA in, 452
  in reference to capsule, 59
  sequence in development of, 253
  'shell' of, 69
Elastase,
  resistance of oxytalan to, 200
  in succus entericus, 290
Elastin, in vertebrate elastic tissue, 200
Electron transport,
  bunamidine uncoupling of oxidative phosphorylation reaction involving, 664

effect of oxyclozanide on reactions involving, 663
fumarate as terminal acceptor in ascarid, 466, 488
Electrotonic coupling, in *Hymenolepis diminuta,* 533–536, 537
Embryophore,
  atypical nature of *Hymenolepis diminuta,* 3
  disruption during emergence of oncosphere of, 96
  structure of, 71–77
Embryo,
  morphogenesis of, 77, 183
  release of, 3
Emergence (see also: hatching), of *Hymenolepis diminuta* oncosphere, 94–102
Emigration,
  definition of, 615
  of helminths, 616
Emptying time, of host stomach, 619
Endocircum flux, in *Hymenolepis diminuta,* 511–514
Endopeptidase, in pancreatic juices of host, 289, 290
Endoplasmic reticulum
  absence in stem cells, 358
  in cells of lacunar wall of cysticercoid, 113
  in connective tissue-forming cells, 202
  in cytoplasmic layer of cyst wall formed by type II cells, 122
  of cytoplasm of myoblasts of oncospheres, 82
  of cytoplasm of outer envelope of embryo, 66
  in endocrine cells, (225)
  ion transport in frog skin via, 533
  in mammalian columnar epithelial cells, (181)
  in mucous glands of ootype, 262
  in muscle cells, (187), 187, 189, 191, 194, 203
  of penetration glands of oncospheres, 84
  in pericanicular cytons, 207
  in perikarya, 220
  in rostellar tegumentary cyton, (237)
  in secretory cells in wall of cysticdrcoid, 120
  in serous glands of ootype, 261, (261)
  of surface epithelium, 87, 88, 178
  in Type A spermatogonia, 243
  in Type B spermatogonia, 244
  in vertebrate fibroblasts, 201
  in vitelline cells, 61, 257, (257), 258

Enterohepatic circulation, role in resorption of bile acids of, 295
Enterokinase
  action on trypsinogen of, 290
  activation of protelytic enzymes by, 293
  release of, 290, 291
  in succus entericus, 290
Enteropeptidase, site of activity of, 285
Entobdella soleae, endogenous circadian rhythm in, 631
Envelope,
  inner embryonic, 4, 71
  outer embryonic, 3, 4, 64
Enzymes (see also: specific enzymes),
  inhibitors of proteolytic, 293
  lytic, 563
  proteolytic, 290
Epazote del zorillo (see: *Chenopodium graveolens*)
Epithelial syncytium,
  adaptation to host enzymes by, 538
  adaptation to host immunological attack by, 538
  adaptation to parasitism by, 540
  evolutionary aspects of, 530–538
  of *Hymenolepis diminuta,* 507–515, 539–541
  information transfer by, 536
  ion and sugar fluxes across, 539
  response to detergent action by, 538
  role in inactivation of bile acids of, 538
  water transport across, 526–538
Escherichia coli, tissue equivalency to *Hymenolepis diminuta,* 450
Estrone, inability to reverse effect of host castration on worm growth by, 375
Ethylenediamine tetraacetate (EDTA), inhibition of NADH $\rightarrow$ NADP$_E$ reaction by, 484
Excretory system,
  elements in cortex of proglottid, 163, (164), (168), (254)
  elements in rostellum, 235
  elements in scolex, 239–240
  of metacestode, 127, (132)
  of strobilate stage, 204–214
  structure of, 165–166
Exocircum flux, in *Hymenolepis diminuta,* 511–514
Exocrino-enteric circulation,
  amino acids and lipids in, 381
  increase in flow during pregnancy and lactation of host of, 558

influence on worm survival of, 599
in meeting requirements for growth of
Hymenolepis diminuta, 631
External factors,
influencing development, 144
influencing migratory response, 631

F

Farnesol (farnesal methyl ether), effect on in vitro development of *Hymenolepis diminuta* by, 436
Fasciola, structure of glycocalyx of, 596
Fasciola hepatica,
collagen-type proteins in, 201
in concurrent infections with *Hymenolepis diminuta,* 625
cytochrome o in, 469
effect of bithionol on ATP production in, 660
effect of thiabendazole on fumarate reductase system of, 651, 652
efficacy of albendazole in sheep infected with, 654
efficacy of oxyclozanide in treatment of, 663
succinate formation in, (473)
Fasciolopsis buski, ineffectiveness of kamala on, 642
Fenbendazole,
in treatment of *Moniezia expansa,* 658
structural formula of, (675)
Ferricyanide, mitochondrial succinate dependent reduction of, 470
Fertilization, in *Hymenolepis diminuta,* 60
Ficin, dispersal of cytoplasmic layer of oncosphere by, 102
Filaria,
activity of nitroscanate on, 663
stibophen in chemotherapy of, 647
Flagellum, of spermatozoa, 244, (246)
Flame cells (see also: excretory system),
absence in scolex of adult, 240
in excretory system of cysticercoid, 127
structure and function of, 206, 207–213
Flavaspidic acid,
effect on respiration in rat liver mitochondria of, 641
structural formula of, (668)
Flavin,
involvement in succinoxidase activity of, 467
succinate dehydrogenase in, 489

Flubendazole,
effect on tegument of *Hymenolepis nana* and *Cysticercus fasciolaris* and intestinal cells of *Ascaris suum* and *Syngamus tracheae* of, 657
structural formula of, (675)
Fluoride, stimulation of mitochondrial phosphorylation by, 479
Folic acid,
effect on jejunal glycolytic enzymes of, 313
effect on worm growth with dietary deficiency of, 375, 377
Fructosans, hydrolysis of, 290
Fructose,
adaptive response of glycolytic enzymes to increase in dietary, 313
competitive inhibition of glucose uptake in metacestode of *Hymenolepis diminuta* by, 143
deleterious effect of dietary, 372
from hydrolysis of dietary disaccharides, 312
Fructose-1, 6-diphosphate, in activation of isozymes of pyruvate kinase, 137, 477
Fumarase,
activity in cell-free preparations and mitochondria of *Hymenolepis diminuta,* 480
in intermembrane space of mitochondria of *Ascaris,* 470
mitochondrial fumarate formation by, 466
in removal of H_2O from malate, 493
Fumarate,
formation by dehydration of malate by mitochondrial fumarase, 466, 493
in generation of ATP, 495
reduction of, 489
termination of electron transport activities with reduction of, 482, 494
utilization of NADH stimulated by, 482
Fumarate reductase,
inhibition of activity by cambendazole, 653
in mitochondrial malate dismutation, 479–484
in NADH coupled activity, 481–483, (485), 489, 493–494
in reduction of fumarate in *Ascaris lumbricoides,* 466
similarity in function of *Ascaris* succinate to, 467, 489
in Site I anaerobic phosphorylation, 492
system in *Haemonchus contortus, Fasciola hepatica* and *Hymenolepis diminuta* affected by thiabendazole, 651, 652

G

Galactose,
absorption of, 389–392, (394)
asymmetry of epithelial syncytium in transport of, 510
effect on host intestinal pH by, 310
effect on worm growth by dietary, 310
inhibitor of glucose uptake in metacestodes of *Hymenolepis diminuta*, 143
product of hydrolysis of dietary disaccharides, 312
role in Na^+ flux of, 522
role of Na^+ in transport of, 525–528, (527), 529
in test diet to assess migratory response in *Hymenolepis diminuta*, 620
as test solute in brush border fluxes, 513, 518, (519), (524)
transport in rabbit ileum in diffusive-convective model, 523
uptake inhibited by ouabain, 509
Galactosyl transferase, distribution in host crypt cell of, 286
Ganglia,
bilateral, 239
cerebral, 215–217, (216), (219), (221), (222)
Hymenolepis microstoma, metacestode cephalic, 221–222
nerve cell bodies in cephalic, 218
of transverse commissures and major nerve cords, 218
Gap junctions (see also: nexus),
between adjacent muscle cells, 194
of cestode parenchymal and tegumental cells, 220
effect of Ca^{++} concentration on cell communication via, 535
in *Hymenolepis diminuta*, 534
in lateral nerve cords, 111
in salivary glands of *Drosophila*, 533
Gas phase,
air as, 431, 438, 444, 474, 475
carbon dioxide and nitrogen as, 429, 431, 434, 438, 440, 474, 475
of in vitro incubation system, 306–307
oxygen with nitrogen as, 435, 440, 475
Gastric inhibitory peptide, in host gastrointestinal tract, 321
Gastrins,
control of host secretion by, 322
as factor in bile flow control in dogs, 295
in host gastrointestinal tract, 321
from pyloric gland area of host stomach and duodenum, 322
Genitalia (see: reproductive system, specific organs)
Germinative area (see also: neck, stem cells), cytology and histogenesis in, 358–362, (359), (360), (361)
effect of carbohydrate deficiency on cell division in, 404
Glands, endocrine,
gap junction between muscle and, 189, (190)
in neck region, (225)
response to variation in blood plasma components of, 320
role in modulation of muscle activity of, 192–193
in suckers, (232), 233
Glands, Mehlis',
mucous-type element of, (261)
proximity of ootype to, 260
role of, 262–263
serous-type element of, 262–263
as source of lipoprotein in oocyte membrane formation, 61
Glands, penetration,
in *Hymenolepis* metacestode, 84–86, (109)
use by oncosphere in penetration through gut wall of intermediate host, 3
Glands, rostellar,
as origin of antigens, 569
secretion of, (234), 235–238, (236), (237), (238), (239)
Glands, vitelline,
differentiation of, 241, 257
innervation of duct of, 218
as origin of vitelline cell, 253
position and ultrastructure of, (254)
Globule leucocyte,
in gut epithelium at time of worm rejection, 580
response to *Hymenolepis diminuta* of, 574
Glucagon,
biological action of, 321
insulin release affected by, 320
secretion of α-cells of pancreas, 291
secretion inhibited by hypoglycaemia, 320
in stimulation of hepatic glycogenolysis and gluconeogenesis, 321
Gluconeogenesis,
effect of high carbohydrate diets on concentration of enzymes controlling, 314
stimulation by glucagon of, 321

Glucose,
  absorption as a function of development, 392, (393), (394), 397, 398–399, (402)
  absorption impaired in riboflavin-deficient diets, 380
  adaptive enzyme response to, 313
  anaerobic path of metabolism of, 140
  bile salt inhibition of anaerobic fermentation of, 386
  competitive inhibition of transport of, 143
  concentration in excretory canals, 209–210
  effect of blood plasma levels of, 320
  effect of cations on absorption of, 393–396
  effect of *Hymenolepis diminuta* on host absorption of, 325–326
  effect of Na^+ concentration on transport of, 516, 520–521
  effect of Na^+ influx across brush border of, 510, 521
  effect of Na^+ pools of, 515, 522–523
  effect of parasitism on intestinal pH of rats fed, 298, 299
  effect of pH on mucosal, 301
  effect on worm growth of dietary, 2, 310, 372, 373, 374
  efflux from host mucosa of, 312
  gradients in host intestine of, 311
  -independent Na^+ uptake, 522
  incorporation of, 62, 650, 658
  incorporation into glycogen of, 399–401
  in increased solute/water flux ratios, 526
  influence on crowding effect of, 404–405
  inhibition by ouabain of transport of, 509
  pathway for catabolism of, (465), 472–478, 493–494
  as primary dietary source of carbohydrate, 310
  requirement in in vitro culture for, 435
  starch as optimal source of dietary, 372, 389
  in test diets to assess migratory response of *Hymenolepis diminuta*, 620, 621
  uptake by cysticercoids of, 143
^{14}C-glucose, incorporation into glycogen of, 62
D-glucose, uptake unaffected in cortisone-treated hosts, 582
Glucocorticosteroids, effects on host blood cell elements of, 563
Glucose-6-phosphate, activity of glycogen synthase with, 401
Glucose phosphorylase, pyridoxal phosphate as cofactor of, 379
Glutamate,
  as source of excretory nitrogen in cysticercoids, 140
  uptake of O_2 by mitochondria in presence of malate and, 491
Glutamic pyruvic transaminase, pyridoxal phosphate requirement of, 379
Glutathione reductase, coupled with $NADPH \rightarrow NADP^+$ reaction, 483
Glycerol, dependency on Na^+ concentration for transport of, 516
α-glycerol phosphate,
  generation of ATP by oxidation of, 492
  role in mitochondrial oxidative phosphorylation in *Ascaris lumbricoides* of, 468
α-glycerophosphate dehydrogenase, activity in cell-free preparation in presence of cytochrome c, 490
  role in ATP generation in *Hymenolepis diminuta*, mitochondria of, 492
Glycine,
  absorption as peptide by intestinal mucosa of, 309
  conjugates affecting activity of ATPase, 296
  in formation of bile acids, 295, 297
Glycocalyx,
  adsorption of IgA on, 572
  antigenic materials from breakdown of, 570, 596
  enzymes associated with microvillar, 284
  protecitive nature of, 538
  response to immune mediated attack of, 582
  as surface layer of tegument, 175
Glycocholate,
  in in vitro excystment of *Hymenolepis diminuta*, 432
  inhibition of glycolysis by, 386
  inhibition of intestinal ATPase by, 296
Glycogen,
  in cercomer, scolex musculature and tegument of cysticercoid, (76), 140
  changes during development in content of, 370–371, 451
  in cortical region of immature proglottid, (165), (172)
  in cytoplasm of inner envelope of oncosphere, 74
  in cytoplasmic bodies of medullary parenchyma, 195
  depletion in worms during host starvation, 374
  effect of cambendazole on *Moniezia expansa* utilization of, 653
  effect of mebendazole on *Cysticercus fasciolaris* utilization of, 656–657

effect of mebendazole on *Hymenolepis diminuta* and *H. nana* utilization of, 657
effect of mepacrine on *Hymenolepis diminuta* synthesis and catabolism of, 650
effect of niclosamide on *Hymenolepis diminuta* utilization of, 661
effect of praziquantel on *Hymenolepis diminuta* utilization of, 666
effect of resorantel on *Hymenolepis diminuta* utilization of, 662
in epithelial cells of oviductal lining, (260)
interference by fenbendazole in *Ascaris suum* of glucose incorporation into, 658
loss during fixation, 196
in medullary muscles of neck region, (185)
molecular weight species of, 399
in myocytons, 194
in myocytons surrounding mucous-type element of Mehlis' gland, (261)
in myocytons surrounding terminal organ of excretory system, (213)
in non-contractile elements of muscle cells, 164, 178, 194
requirement for CO_2 for anaerobic synthesis of, 475
as source of energy for penetration of oncosphere, (87), 106
in spermatozoa, 245
storage in parenchymal myocyton, 198, 199
synthesis of, 398–401
synthesis in musculature, 198
synthesis stimulated by CO_2, 476
in tegument, (179)
in vitelline cells, 62, 258
α-glycogen,
in cells lining lacuna of *Hymenolepis citelli* cysticercoid, 140
in perinuclear cytoplasm of myoblast, 82
in peripheral cytoplasm of medullary myocyton, (197)
β-glycogen,
in cells lining lacuna of cysticercoids of *Hymenolepis citelli*, 140
in cytoplasm of inner envelope of preoncosphere, 71, 74
in cytoplasm of penetration cells of oncospheres, 84–85
in fibrillar portion of muscle cell, (187), (188)
in myofibers of cyticercoids of *Hymenolepis citelli*, 112, 140
in perikarya, 222
in terminal expansion of sensory dendrite, 223

Desmo-glycogen, measurement of, 371
Lyo-glycogen, measurement of, 371
Glycogen phosphorylase, reduction in activity in pyridoxine deficient and limited hosts of, 379
Glycogen synthase, activities in developing worms of I and D forms of, 401
Glycogen synthetase, activity in scolex, inner envelope, cercomer, and wall musculature of cysticercoids, 143
Glycogenesis, requirement of CO_2 in, 476
Glycogenolysis, effect of glucagon on, 291, 321
Glucoproteins, of differentiated host villus cell, 286
Golgi apparatus,
in binucleate cell forming surface epithelium of oncosphere, 87, 88
in cerebral ganglion, (219)
in columnar epithelium of mammalian intestine, (181)
in cytoplasm of inner envelope, 71
in cytoplasm of Type A cell of fibrous region of wall of cysticercoid, 120
in cytoplasm of vitelline cells of preoncosphere, 61
in endocrine cell, (225)
in macromere during early cleavage, 62
in maturing vitelline cells, 257, (257)
in mucous cells of Mehlis' gland, 261, (261)
in oncoblasts of *Catenotaenia pusilla* oncospheres, 81
in perikarya, 220, (222), 223, 226, (227), 233
in perinuclear cytoplasm of tegumentary cytons, 178, (179)
in rostellar tegumentary cytons, 236, (237)
in serous cells of Mehlis' gland, 262, (262)
in syncytial epithelium of oviduct, 259, (260)
Glycolysis
in *Ascaris lumbricoides,* (465)
effect of high carbohydrate diets on, 314
in *Hymenolepis diminuta,* 471–474, 493–494, (494)
stimulation by 5-hydroxytryptamine of, 227
Glycosyltransferase, distribution in host crypt walls, 286
Gradients
chemical, 508
electrical potential, 508
electrochemical potential, 516, 517, 530
in intestine and migratory behavior, 630
Na^+, 516, 517
Growth
curve, 2, 362–364

of cysticercoids, 4, 427, 554
effect of host nutrients on, 307, 310, 311, 371–385, 386, 388, 403, 431
exponential, 2, 265, 363
in definitive host, 2, 287, 310, 357–423, 557
rate of, 2, 265, 310, 362–363, 365, 440
zone, 360
Gyrocotyle, satellite DNA of, 455

H

Haemonchus contortus, effect of thiabendazole on fumarate reductase system in, 651
Hank's balanced salt solution
use in collection of cysticercoids, 437, 440, (441)
use in in vitro culture, 434
Hatching (see also: emergence)
laboratory procedures for, 428–429
of oncospheres in vitro, 427
Hemin, as requirement for in vitro strobilation of *Hymenolepis microstoma*, 442, 443
Hemocytes, in encapsulation of cysticercoids, 127
Hemidesmosomes (see: desmosomes, dense bodies)
Heterakis gallinae, succinate production by, (473)
Hexacanth larva (see also: oncosphere)
effect of PAS reaction of host connective tissue of, 108
emergence of, 95–102
hooks of, 95
polarity of, 228
production of, 3
Hexachlorophene, in uncoupling of phosphorylation system, 664
Hexose
absorption dependent on Na^+, 392
asymmetry in permeability of membranes in transport of, 510
brush border transport of, 507
effect of ouabain on transport of, 507
ion-gradient hypothesis for transport of, 518, 520, 522
transport accelerated by Na^+, 395
Hexyresorcinal
effect on protein of hyaline membrane of *Hymenolepis nana* eggs of, 659
structural formula of, 675
Histamine
effect on worm survival by introduction of exogenous, 580
release by mast cells of, 575

Histidine
in inner envelope of oncosphere, 75
in oncosphere, 69
Histogenesis
of connective tissue, 202–204
of cysticercoid, 116
of muscle, 198–199
of nervous system, 218–222
of reproductive organs, 241–263
of scolex, 229–230
of tegument, 182–185
Holdfast (see also: scolex, suckers)
alternative term for scolex, 229
in reversal of polarity, 110
Homeostasis, in host lumen, 323–325
Hook, formation of, 78
Hookworm, use of nitroscanate against, 663
Hormones, of host gastrointestinal tract, 321, 558
Hosts
definitive, 1, 2, 9–23, 59, 304, 384, 385, 386, 404, 553, 557, 616, 621, 625, 627, 642, 644, 646, 647, 648, 649, 651, 652, 653, 654, 655, 656
human, 1, 20–23, 364, 367, 369, 373, 374, 381, 639, 643, 646
intermediate, 3, 24–28, 59, 95, 96, 97, 99, 102, 105, 106, 108, 110, 217, 131, 134, 144–145, 146
Host diet, effects on development of, 311, 371–385, 619
Humatin (see: paromomycin)
Hyaluronic acid, in association with protein forming ground substance of cells, 137
Hydatidosis, mebendazole in treatment of, 656
Hydatigera taeniaeformis
bunamidine in treatment of cats infected with, 664
paromomycin in treatment of cats infected with, 648
Hydrocortisone acetate, monocytopaenia in response to, 563
Hydroxyproline, requirement for O_2 by *Ascaris lumbricoides* for formation of, 464
5-hydroxytryptamine (serotonin, 5-HT)
chromaffin cells in synthesis of, 283
in cirrus sphincter musculature, 193, 218
for determining pattern of nervous system, 214
function as metabolic regulator, 227–228
influence on worm growth of exogenous, 580
lacking in majority of neurons in *Hymenolepis diminuta*, 224

mast cell production of, 575
role in neurotransmission of, 193
in vesicles in neuron of neck region, 226
Hymenolepis cantaniana, development of scolex of cysticeroid of, 4
Hymenolepis carioca, efficacy of tin compounds in treatment of fowl infected with, 646
Hymenolepis citelli
collection and sterilization of eggs of, 428
cross reactivity of *Hymenolepis diminuta* and, 586, 587, 588, 589
culture medium for, 429–430
culture temperature requirements of, 431
development of cysticercoid scolex in, 4
diel migration in hamsters of, 625, 627
duration of immunological protection against, 560
effect of sucrose diet on, 372
encapsulation by *Tribolium confusum* hemocytes of cysticercoids of, 131
glycogen in myofibers of metacestodes, 112, 140
hatching medium for, 428–429
immune response in mice to, 599
immunity to, 553
intestinal distribution of, (626)
in vitro development of cysticercoids of, 431, 433
in vitro excystment of cysticercoids of, 432
in vitro gas phase for culture of cysticercoids of, 431
in vitro hatching of eggs of, 428
in vitro maintenance of cysticercoids of, 431
lamella-like folds on surface cytoplasm of oncosphere of, 127
motility in cysticercoids of, 432
myoblast and 'parenchymal' cell precursors in embryo of, 199
nuclear types associated with musculature of, (79)
in *Peromyscus maniculatus*, 553
rate of in vitro development of, (433)
rejection threshold in numbers of, 556, 598
satellite DNA of, (91)
surface structure of metacestode scolex of, 134
taxonomic position of, 8
ultrastructure of hooks of, 81, (92)
Hymenolepis diminuta
active transport in, 582–583
antibodies against, 571–578

antigenic threshold for, 593–595
collection and sterilization of eggs of, 3, 4, 428
cross reactivity of *Hymenolepis citelli* and, 586, 589
cross reactivity of *Hymenolepis microstoma* and, 588–589
cross reactivity of *Hymenolepis nana* and, 586–588
cross reactivity of *Moniliformis dubius* and, 387–388, 586
cross reactivity of *Nematospiroides dubius* and, 590
cross reactivity of *Nippostrongylus brasiliensis* and, 388–389, 589
cross reactivity of *Trichinella spiralis* and, 589–590
darkened areas of, 581–582
development of strobilate stage of, 2
effect of age on immune response in mice infected with, 556–557
effect of anti-inflammatory drugs on immune response in mice infected with, 575, 580
effect of antithymocyte serum and antilymphocyte serum on immune response of mice infected with, 566–567
effect on CO_2 concentration in rat intestine of, 537
effect of cortisone on immune response of mice infected with, 562–563, 590, 593
effect of crowding on, 145, 311, 364–365, 366, 368, 387, 388, 401–410, 551, 591, 593
effect of cyclophosphamide on immune response of mice infected with, 563–566
effect of lactation on immune response of mice infected with, 558
effect of mast cells on immune response of mice infected with, 574–575
effect of methotrexate on immune response of mice infected with, 566
effect of numbers of worms on immune response of mice infected with, 556
effect of passive protection on immune response of mice infected with, 577
effect of pregnancy on immune response of mice infected with, 558
effect of prostaglandins on immune response of mice infected with, 580
effect of sex of host on immune response of mice infected with, 558
effect of strain of host on immune response of mice infected with, 557

Index

effect of thymectomy on immune response of mice infected with, 578
effect of X-irradiation on immune response of mice infected with, 567–568, 578
eggs of, 376, 426
immune response in rats to, 318, 591–595
intestinal migration of, 2, 103, 298–299, 313, 387, 585, 615–638
in vitro culture of cysticercoids of, 430
in vitro culture of mouse fibroblasts and cysticercoids of, 426
in vitro culture of strobilate stage of, 426, 434–437
in vitro development of cysticercoids of, 431, 433, 474, 475
in vitro effect of antibiotics on strobilate stage of, 437
in vitro effect of vitamin B_6 on strobilate stage of, 438, 445
in vitro excystment of cysticercoids of, 432, 434
in vitro gas phase requirements of cysticercoids of, 307, 431, 474, 475
in vitro hatching of eggs of, 428
in vitro maintenance of cysticercoids of, 431
in vitro surface sterilization of strobilate stage of, 436
longevity of, 3, 554, 591–592
measurement of immune response of mice infected with, 554–555
memory of immune response in mice infected with, 559, 561
'nude mice' as hosts of, 578–579
'nude rats' as host of, 595
source of antigens of, 569–570
T cells in rejection of, 578–579
vaccination against, 596–598
Hymenolepis exigua, scolex development in cysticercoids of, 4
Hymenolepis flavopunctata, synonym of *Hymenolepis diminuta*, 157–159
Hymenolepis lanceolata, efficacy of mebendazole in treatment of geese infected with, 655
Hymenolepis microstoma
   antibodies against, 573
   binding of mouse immunoglobulin to tegument of, 318
   collection and sterilization of eggs of, 428
   cross reactivity of, 588–589
   cross reactivity of *Hymenolepis nana* and, 587
   effect of crowding on, 401

effect of *Fasciola hepatica* on site selection in, 625
effect of IgA on, 573
effect of IgM on, 576
efficacy of parbendazole in treatment of mice infected with, 653
efficacy of praziquantel in treatment of mice infected with, 665
efficacy of niclosamide in treatment of mice infected with, 660
immune responses to, 318, 553
immunological studies on mice infected with, 553, 599
in vitro culture of cysticercoids of, 427
in vitro culture in media of various freezing point depressions of strobilate stage of, 445
in vitro culture medium for cysticercoids of, 430
in vitro culture of strobilate stage of, 438–444
in vitro development of cysticercoids of, 433
in vitro effects of antibiotics on strobilate stage of, 437
in vitro effect of horse serum on strobilate stage of, 440
in vitro effect of sheep bile on strobilate stage of, 440
in vitro excystment of cysticercoids of, 434
in vitro gas phase requirements of cysticercoids of, 431
in vitro hatching of eggs of, 429
in vitro maintenance of cysticercoids of, 431
musculature of metacestode of, (117)
neurosecretory cells in, 226
nonspecific acid phosphatase activity in intermediate cell layer and tail parenchyma of capsules of, 138
reciprocity in immune response of *Hymenolepis diminuta* with, 588, 589
rejection threshold in numbers of, 556
response of *Tribolium confusum* to metacestodes of, 131
satellite DNA of, 455
scolex retraction in metacestode of, 113, (116)
sensory perikarya in rostellar and cerebral ganglia of, 223
site selection in, 623–624
synaptic junctions in metacestodes of, 218
vesicle types in cephalic ganglia of, 221–222
Hymenolepis nana,
   activity of acranil and acriflavine against, 650

activity of bithionol against, 660
activity of dichlorophen in mice against, 659
anthelmintic action of thiabendazole in mice against, 651
characteristics of eggs of, 3
collection and sterilization of eggs of, 428
complement fixation by 'cell sap' antigens of, 591
cross reactivity of *Ascaris lumbricoides* with, 587
cross reactivity of *Capillaria hepatica* with, 587
cross reactivity of *Hymenolepis diminuta* with, 586–588
cross reactivity of *Trichinella spiralis* with, 587, 590
development of, 4, 432, 586
effect of bunamidine on glucose uptake and efflux in, 664
effect of crowding on, 401
effect of sucrose diet of host on, 372
effectiveness of oxfendazole in ridding mice of, 658–659
efficacy of antimony complexes of 8-oxyquinolines in mouse infections of, 647
efficacy of aspidin in mouse infections of, 641
efficacy of aspidinol in mouse infections of, 641
efficacy of axenomycin D in dog infections of, 649
efficacy of bitoscanate in human infections of, 663
efficacy of diospyrol in mice with concurrent infections of *Nematospiroides dubius* and, 645
efficacy of flavaspidic acid in mouse infections of, 641
efficacy of kamala in human infections of, 643
efficacy of kamala in mouse infections of, 642
efficacy of mepacrine in human infections of, 649
efficacy of niclosamide in human infections of, 661
efficacy of niclosamide in rat and mouse infections of, 660
efficacy of parbendazole in mouse infections of, 653
efficacy of paromomycin in human infections of, 648

efficacy of praziquantel in mouse infections of, 665
efficacy of oxibendazole in mouse infections of, 654
efficacy of 4-quinoline hydrazones in mouse infections of, 665
efficacy of thiabendazole in human infections of, 651
hook formation in, 78
immune response of mice to, 552, 586
ineffectiveness of pelletierine against, 644
induction by mebendazole of time-related micro-morphological changes of tegument of, 657
influence of *Trichinella spiralis* on infections of, 590
intercurrent infections of *Hymenolepis diminuta* and, 586–588
in vitro culture of, 430–435, 475
in vitro culture of strobilate stage of, 426, 437
in vitro effect of diacetylphloroglucinol on, 641
in vitro effect of horse serum on strobilate stage of, 444
in vitro hatching of eggs of, 429, 475
in vitro motility of cysticercoids of, 432
β-phospholipase increase in mouse intestine infected with, 580
scolex development in cysticercoids of, 4
toxicity of chenopodium oil to, 643
vaccination against, 596
Hymenolepis peromysci, diel migration in, 625, 627, (628)
Hymenolepis setigera, efficacy of mebendazole in geese infected with, 655
Hymenolepis spp.
efficacy of arecoline in geese infected with, 644
efficacy of bithionol in geese infected with, 660
efficacy of mebendazole in geese infected with, 655
production of temporary paralysis by extracts of *Cucurbita* seeds in, 645
Hymenolepis tenuirostris, scolex development in cysticercoids of, 4
Hyperglycaemia, role of glucagon in host, 321
Hypoglycaemia, role of glucagon in host, 291

I

I cells, in production of CCK-PZ, 322
Immunity
against *Hymenolepis diminuta*, 368–369
and *Hymenolepis diminuta*, 551–614

Immunoglobulin
  antigen uptake inhibited by, 569
  effects on transport across brush border surface of, 541
  induction and activity of IgM, 576
  induction and function of IgA, 572–574
  presence in serum of rats infected with *Hymenolepis diminuta* of IgE, 576–577
  presence in serum of rats infected with *Hymenolepis diminuta* of IgG_a, 576
  presence on surface of *Hymenolepis diminuta* in mice of IgG_1, 577
  presence on surface of *Hymenolepis diminuta* in mice of IgG_2, 577
  presence on surface of *Hymenolepis diminuta* of IgM, 577
  rejection of *Hymenolepis diminuta* by IgE, 576
  role of epithelial syncytium against, 540
Inermicapsifer madagascarensis, ultrastructure of mature hooks of, 81
Inhibitors (see also specific inhibitors), secretion of growth, 405–410
Inositol, as dietary replacement, 375, 377
Insulin
  indirect inhibition of hypoglycaemia by, 320
  secretion by host pancreatic β-cells, 291
  secretion stimulated by secretin-glucagon group of hormones, 321
Intestine
  analogy of *Hymenolepis diminuta* to, 166, 180, (181)
  changes effected by methotrexate in, 566
  changes with age in lymphoid tissue of, 556–557
  characteristics of host, 282–326
  distribution of *Hymenolepis citelli* in hamster, (626)
  distribution of *Hymenolepis diminuta* in hamster, (629)
  distribution of *Hymenolepis peromysci* in hamster, (628)
  effect of amines on, 575
  effect of amino acid imbalance in, 384
  effect of challenge infections of *Hymenolepis diminuta* on, 584–585
  effect of cortisone on permeability of, 562
  effect of host diet on microflora of, 317
  effect of *Hymenolepis diminuta* infection on microflora of, 315–317
  effect of *Hymenolepis nana* infections on α-phospholipase in wall of mouse, 580
  effect of infection on luminal gases of, 304–306
  effect of microflora on luminal gases of, 306
  fluctuations in characteristics of host, 529, 534
  equivalent concentrations of succinate in worm conditioned saline and, 407
  gradients of amino acids in lumen of, 307–310, 324
  gradients of carbohydrates in lumen of, 310–314
  gradients of lipids in lumen of, 314
  gradients of lumen of, 307–314
  helminth-host interactions in, 631
  host digestion in, 319–320
  of intermediate host, 103–104, (104), 105
  immunological rejection of worms from lumen of, 553
  macromolecular uptake by, 573, 597
  migratory activity of *Hymenolepis diminuta* in rat, 618–623
  numbers and kinds of microflora in host, 314–315
  production of protective antigens by *Hymenolepis diminuta* in, 596
  response to migratory hexacanth in tissue of intermediate host, 108
  role in nutrition of microflora in host, 296, 297, 314, 325
  site of oncospheral penetration in, 103
  site selection by *Hymenolepis diminuta* in rat, 616–618
  transplanting of worms in, 560, 584
  of vertebrates as a habitat for parasites, 263
In vitro cultivation, of species of *Hymenolepis*, 435–448
Intrafamilial relationships of *Hymenolepis diminuta*, 5–8
Isocaloric diets
  in determination of carbohydrate requirements for worm growth, 310
  growth retardation in glucose-containing, 373, 374
  in studies on B vitamin deficiencies, 377, 379
Isocitrate, as substrate for oxyclozanide stimulation of mitochondrial respiration in *Hymenolepis diminuta*, 663
Isocitrate dehydrogenase, coupled with exogenous $NADP^+ \to NAD^+$ reaction in *Hymenolepis diminuta* mitochondria, 483
Isopelletierine
  from bark of *Punica granatum*, 644
  efficacy against *Taenia* spp. and *Hymenolepis nana* of, 644

Isoquinolines (see: praziquantel)
Isorotterlin, active component of kamala, 642
Isothiocyanates (see: bitoscanate and nitroscanate)
4-isothiocyanato-4'-nitro-diphenylamine (see also: nitroscanate)
  structural formula of, (677)

J

Junctions (see also: dense bodies, desmosomes)
  electrical potential difference and, 530–533
  electrotonic, 536
  electrotonic coupling and, 533–536
  gap, 178, 181, (190), 220, 233, 533, 534, 535
  leaky, 506, 531, 532
  of muscle cells, 189, (190), 194, 196
  of muscle and tegument, 189, (190)
  neuromuscular, 192, 193, 220, 251
  of neurons, (195)
  of parenchymal cell and excretory ducts, 206, 213
  of parenchymal and tegumentary cells, 220
  permeability of gap, 535
  synaptic, 218
  tight, 506, 508, 509, 530, 531, 532
  transepithelial resistance and, 530–533
  transport across epithelial syncytium without, 539–540
  vertebrate cholinergic myoneural, 193
  variety of, 169

K

K_t (apparent transport constant)
  for galactose, 392, 394–398, 404
  for glucose, 392, 394–398, 404
  for glucose in metacestodes, 143
Kamala
  anthelmintic action against hymenolepidids in ducks of, 642
  anthelmintic action in rats and in vitro against *Hymenolepis* nana and *H. diminuta* of, 642
  anthelmintic action in human cases of *Hymenolepis nana* of, 643
  effect on smooth muscles of host and parasite of, 643
  efficacy in treatment of *Drepanotaenia* in geese and *Hymenolepis nana* in mice of, 644
  from *Mallotus philippinensis*

Keimzone (see: neck, germinative area)
Keratin
  in cytoplasmic layer of oncosphere, 75
  lacking in capsule of oncosphere, 69
  similarity of fibers in hooks to, 81–82
  α-ketoglutarate, effect on O_2 uptake by *Hymenolepis diminuta* mitochondria of, 491
Kinetics
  of efflux, 513
  of influx, 513
  initial rate, 515, 516
  steady state, 515
Krebs' phosphate solution, use in collection of adult worms, 435
Krebs' Ringer's phosphate solution, in excystment medium, 432

L

Lacistorhynchus tenuis, ultrastructure of, 171
Lactase
  activity during starch degradation, 291, 293
  distribution of villar, 285
Lactate
  accumulation in *Hymenolepis diminuta* unaffected by O_2, 474
  change with worm age in concentration of, 475
  effect of cambendazole on production of, 653
  effect of niclosamide on production of, 661
  effect of praziquantel on production of, 665
  effect on DNA synthesis of, 406, 407
  excretion of, 302
  in excretory canal fluid of *Hymenolepis diminuta*, 209, 211
  formation via glycolysis in cell-free preparations of *Hymenolepis diminuta*, 472–473
  in worm conditioned saline, 406, (407), (408)
Lactate dehydrogenase
  isozymes of, 478
  in larvae and cysticercoids of *Hymenolepis diminuta*, 137–138
  in metabolism of PEP, 493
Lactation, effect on *Hymenolepis diminuta*, during host, 558
Lactose, in host diet, 373
Lanthanum, penetration of tight junctions by, 531
LD_{50}, of kamala in *Hymenolepis diminuta* infections in mice, 643

'Leak lesions', result of inflammatory response of intestine to amines, 575
Lecithin, role of bile salts in transport of, 296
Length
  of worm in relation to host species, 2
  of worms in relation to intensity of infection, 2, 145, 313, 364–365
Leptotriches, as extensions into parenchyma from tubule of flame cell, 209, (209), (210)
Leucine aminopeptidase, site of activity of, 285
Life history
  of *Hymenolepis diminuta*, 1–4
  of *Diphyllobothrium latum*, 240
Lipase
  activity enhanced by bile acids, 295
  in hydrolysis of fats, 289
  inhibitors of, 293
Lipid
  bile salts and digestion of, 296
  changes during development in concentrations of, 370, 371, (372)
  concentration in crowded worms, 403–404
  concentration in worms of, 371, 404
  concentration in worms of hosts with glucose as sole carbohydrate source, 373
  distribution in cysticercoids, 143
  effects on development of dietary, 372, 381
  effect of host dietary modification of, 381
  effect of parasitism on intestinal content of, 314
  homeostatic regulation of luminal, 323
  host intestinal gradient of, 314
  in inner envelope and embryophore of mature larvae, 74, 75, 97
  in mature larvae of *Hymenolepis diminuta*, 69, (72)
  in medullary parenchyma, 195, (197)
  in myocytons of rostellum, (237)
  in non-contractile region of myocyton, 164, (166), (179)
  site of transport of, 507
  storage in musculo-parenchyma, 198
Lipoprotein, in membrane surrounding oocyte and vitelline cell, 61
Litomosoides carinii, requirement for aerobic component in energy generating metabolism of, 464
Liver extract
  in culture medium, 436
  of hamsters in culture medium, 438
  of lambs in culture medium, 437
  preparation of, 437
  of rats in culture medium, 437
  of sheep in culture medium, 438
Location specificity (see: site selection)
Logistic equation, specific growth pattern fitted to, 364
Longevity
  of *Hymenolepis diminuta* in mice, 554
  of *Hymenolepis diminuta* in rats, 3, 591–592
Lysine, effect in host diet of, 382

M

Macromere, role in early ontogeny of *Hymenolepis diminuta* of, 62–65
Malate,
  accumulation via CO_2 fixation and malate dehydrogenase of, 476, 478
  anaerobic dismutation in *Ascaris lumbricoides* of, 466–471, (472)
  dismutation in *Hymenolepis diminuta* of, 494
  in phosphorylation leading to succinate accumulation, 479, 488, 489
Malate dehydrogenase,
  malate accumulation via CO_2 fixation by, 485
  oxidation to pyruvate and CO_2 by, 466
  reduction of oxalacetate to malate by, 465, 477, 493
  as source of reducing equivalents, 480
Malate dependent phosphorylarion,
  in *Ascaris lumbricoides*, 466, 467, 468
  in *Hymenolepis diminuta*, 479
Malate dismutation,
  in *Ascaris lumbricoides*, 466
  in *Hymenolepis diminuta*, 480, 493
Maleate,
  in inhibition of proteolytic enzymes, 294
  in stimulation of pancreatic lipase, 294
'Malic' enzyme,
  absolute specificity for $NADP^+$ in *Hymenolepis diminuta* of, 480
  of ascarids, 470
  in dismutation of malate, 466, 494
  in *Hymenolepis diminuta*, 476
  localization in *Hymenolepis diminuta* mitochondria of, 480, 486–488, (487)
  requirement for hydride ion transfer generated by, 482
Mallotus philippinensis, as source of kamala, 642
Malonate
  inhibition of ascarid phosphorylation by, 467, 479

inhibition of succinate dependent O$_2$ consumption by, 489
Maltase
    activity regulated by specific dietary sugars, 312
    distribution of activity in villi of, 285
    fructose in production of adaptive response of, 313
    reinforcement of pancreatic disaccharidase activity by, 293
    secretion of mammals of, 291
Maltose
    effect of reducing conditions on absorption of, 389–392
    inability of *Hymenolepis diminuta* to utilize, 372, 373, 402
    lack of worm growth with dietary, 310
    as product of starch hydrolysis, 290
    relative rate of host absorption of, 284, 289
Maltotriose, inability of *Hymenolepis diminuta* to absorb, 389
Mast cells, induction and role of, 574–576
Mebendazole
    in affecting tegument of *Hymenolepis nana* and *Cysticercus fasciolaris* and intestinal cells of *Ascaris suum* and *Syngamus tracheae*, 657
    effect on glucose uptake by nematodes, *Cysticercus fasciolaris*, *Moniezia expansa*, *Hymenolepis nana* and *H. diminuta* of, 656–657
    effect on metacestodes of, 146, 655
    efficacy in treatment of *Hymenolepis* sp. in geese of, 655
    efficacy in treatment of *Hymenolepis nana* infections in mice and man of, 656
    efficacy in treatment of hydatidosis of, 656
    efficacy in treatment of human cases of *Taenia solium* of, 656
    in uncoupling of oxidative phosphorylation, 657
    structural formula of, (674)
Membranes
    of ascarid mitochondria, 470, 471
    association of enzymes with microvillar, 284, 286
    asymmetry in function of, 509, 510
    of dense bodies, 71
    derivation of larval envelopes from vitelline cell, 258
    digestion by pancreatic amylase, 291, 570
    distance between, 187
    electrical potential across, 508
    of embryos, 6, 61, 95
    hyaline, 659
    of *Hymenolepis diminuta*, 505–550
    of inner envelope, 71
    inward-facing, 508, 509, 510, 511, 513, 518
    of larvae, 59
    of myofibril, 187, (188), 189
    in myoneural junction, 192, (221)
    of nucleus during mitosis, 361
    ouabain inhibition of inward-facing, 517
    ouabain-sensitive site of hexose transport of, 508
    ouabain-sensitive site of Na$^+$ transport of, 508
    outward-facing, 508, 509, 510, 511, 513, 518
    potentials of, 533
    protective functions of, 507
    protective role of brush border, 294
    in reference to generic name of *Hymenolepis diminuta*, 157
    resistance pathways in, 509
    of tegument, 171, 175, (177), (179), 182
    transport across, 506–507
    unstirred layers and, 287, 306
    untake of antigens across, 592
Mepacrine
    concentration in radial musculature in scolex of *Taenia saginata*, 649
    inhibition of glucose uptake and glycogenesis and stimulation of glycogenolysis in *Hymenolepis diminuta* by, 650
    structural formula of, (673)
    in treatment of *Taenia saginata*, *T. solium* and *Hymenolepis nana* in man, 649
Mesocestoides corti, effect of mebendazole on tetrathyridia of, 656
Mesophore, cellular composition of, 78
Metabolism,
    anaerobic, 197–198, 653
    anaerobic mitochondrial, 478–492
    of carbohydrates, 389–401
    of cholesterol, 295
    effect of H$^+$ concentration on cellular, 301
    effect of imbalance in amino acid uptake on protein, 324
    effect of sodium taurocholate on glucose, 386
    hormonal effect on, 320
    incomplete catabolism of glucose in helminth, 463

Index

of rapidly dividing cells affected by antilymphocytic serum, 566
stimulation by 5-HT of trematode, 227
Methionine,
  effect on *Hymenolepis diminuta* from cortisone-treated hosts of, 582
  in protein-free diets, 385
  as source of excretory nitrogen in cysticercoids, 140
  in 36 h hydrolysates of cysticercoids, 135
Methotrexate, effect on cell division of, 566
2-methoxy-2', 5-dichloro-4'-dinitrobenzanilide, as blocking agent of OH- or
Methylene blue, stimulation of succinate dependent O_2 consumption in cell-free homogenates of *Hymenolepis diminuta* by, 489
  NH-groups of niclosamide, 661
Methylpelletierine, as alkaloid component of bark of *Punica granatum*, 644
Michaelis' constant (K_t), effect of external Na^+ on, 520
Microfilaments (see also: actin),
  in cytoplasm of excretory duct epithelium, 206, 211
  of microtriches, 173, (173), (174)
Microtriches (see: microvilli)
Microtubules
  in cilium of flame cell, 208, (212)
  effect of mebendazole on tegumental cytoplasmic, 657
  in flagellar axoneme of spermatozoa, 244–245, (246)
  in internuncial process of tegumentary cyton, 178
  in relation to oncospheral membrane, (76)
  synthesis in cysticercoids, 120
Microvilli (microtriches)
  chronology of formation of, 134
  dispersion of exogenous and endogenous products of lumen by pulsation of, 286
  of distal cytoplasm of metacestode, (124)
  enzymes associated with plasma membrane of, 284
  formation of, 131–134
  on lining of vagina and seminal vesicle, 253–254, (255)
  of lumenal surface of excretory canals, 206, (207), (208), 211
  on lumenal surface of oviduct, 259, (260)
  on lumenal surface of sperm ducts, 248, (249)
  on lumenal surface of uterus, 263, (264)

maintenance of integrity after worm conditioned saline treatment of, 409
  of mammalian small intestine, (181), 283
  origin from lamellar folds of surface of metacestode, 127
  on outer margin of metacestode, (119)
  protective function of, 131, 538
  relationship to absorptive surface area of host gut of, 286, 287
  of rostellar tegument, 233, (235), 238, (238)
  of tegument, (165), (166), 171–173, (1974), (176), (177), (179)
Mitochondria
  anaerobic metabolism of adult *Hymenolepis diminuta*, 478–492
  in areas of *Hymenolepis diminuta* attacked by immune response, 581
  in cells surrounding primitive lacuna of cysticercoid, 113
  in cytoplasm of inner envelope, 71, (72), 74
  in cytoplasm of outer envelope, 66, (76)
  in dendritic processes of tegument, 179, (179)
  DNA from, 451, 452
  in ductal cytoplasm of excretory system, 206
  effects of desaspidin on oxidative phosphorylation in *Ascaris suum*, 642
  effect of mebendazole on malate-induced phosphorylation in *Ascaris*, 657
  electrochemical potential gradients of ions in, 516
  in embryophore, 72–73, (76)
  enzymatic activity of ascarid, 466–471
  in epithelium of mammalian small intestine, (181)
  in fertilzed oocyte, (259)
  inhibition of O_2 uptake by bunamidine in rat liver, 664
  inhibition of ^{32}P-ATP exchange by desaspidin in *Hymenolepis diminuta*, 641
  inhibition of ^{32}P-ATP exchange reaction by dichlorophen in *Hymenolepis diminuta* and *Ascaris suum*, 659, 662
  inhibition of ^{32}P-ATP exchange reaction by niclosamide in *Hymenolepis diminuta* and *Ascaris suum*, 661–662
  isolation and characterization of DNA from, 456
  in macromere of preoncosphere, 62
  malic dismutation in, 493
  in maturing vitelline cells, 257, (257)
  in musculature of scolex, 138
  in myofibrilar cytoplasm, (188), 189

in oncoblast of *Catenotaenia pusilla* oncosphere, 81
in penetration glands of oncosphere, 84
in perikarya, 220, (222)
in oocyte, 256, (259)
in primary spermatocytes, 244, (245)
in scolex tegument, (177), 178
in spermatids, 244
in surface epithelium of oncosphere, 88, 122, 133, (133)
in stem cells, 358
stimulation of respiratory rate by oxyclozanide in *Hymenolepis diminuta*, 663
in Type A spermatogonia, 243
in Type B spermatogonia, 244
uncoupling effect of dichlorophen on elecoron transport linked phosphorylation in *Hymenolepis diminuta* and rat liver, 659
uncoupling by niclosamide of oxidative phosphorylation in rat liver, housefly and mammalian, 662
Migration
of *Hymenolepis citelli* in hamsters, 625–626
of *Hymenolepis diminuta* in hamsters, 622
of *Hymenolepis diminuta* in rats, 191, 623
of *Hymenolepis diminuta* in relation to intestinal gradients, 311
of *Hymenolepis diminuta* in response to intestinal pH and other physicochemical characteristics of host intestine, 298
of *Hymenolepis diminuta* in single and multiple worm infections, 622–623
of *Hymenolepis microstoma* in hamsters, 623
of *Hymenolepis microstoma* in mice, 623–624
of *Hymenolepis microstoma* with *Fasciola hepatic* in mice, 625
of *Hymenolepis peromysci* in hamsters, 627–628
of intestinal worms, 618–632
as pattern of circadian rhythm, 615
Mitosis (cell division)
effect of methotrexate on, 566
as index of limits of neck, 358
influence of crowding on, 401–402, 404
in spermatozoa, 243
in stem cells, (361), 362
Moniezia benedeni
efficacy of axenomycin D in lambs infected with, 649
vitamin B_6 content in, 379

Moniezia expansa
activity of axenomycin D on, 649
activity of kamala on, 642
age resistance to, 552
effect of cambendazole on carbohydrate metabolism in, 652–653
effect of mebendazole on energy metabolism in, 656, 657
efficacy of albendazole in treatment of sheep infected with, 654
efficacy of bunamidine in treatment of, 664
efficacy of fenbendazole in treatment of, 658
immunological protection in sheep from, 597
keratin in, 68
role of cytochrome o in reduction of fumarate in, 469–470
succinate production in, (473)
Moniliformis dubius
cross reactivity of *Hymenolepis diminuta* and, 586
effect of *Hymenolepis diminuta* of concurrent infections with 387–388, 586, 618
effect on site selection by *Hymenolepis diminuta* of, 618
succinate formation in, 473 (473)
Motor end plates (see also: neuromuscular junctions), in longitudinal musculature of *Hymenolepis diminuta*, 192, 193, 217
Mucosal transport pool, in *Hymenolepis diminuta*, 511, (512), 514
Musculature (see also: muscle, myocyton)
of adult *Hymenolepis diminuta*, 186–191
of cysticercoid scolex, 113
of cysticercoid wall, 117, (117), 122
fluid flow in excretory system controlled by body, 206
of oncosphere, 82–83
of *Tenebrio molitor* intestine, 102–104, 108
Muscle (see also, myocyton, myofibril, musculature)
activity of particulate fraction from *Ascaris lumbricoides*, 467
carbohydrate dissimilation in *Ascaris lumbricoides*, 465, (465)
CO_2 stimulation of, 537
characterization of, 265
of copulatory organ, 250, (250)
effect of mepacrine on scolex and body, 649–650
electrical coupling of epithelial syncytium and, 540
histogenesis of, 198–199, 359
5-hydroxytryptamine as modulator of, 226

innervation of, 165, 192–194, 215–217, (216), 218, (219), 220
interference by aspidium of activity of, 643
interference by kamala of activity of, 643
malate dismutation in *Ascaris lumbricoides*, 466
in medullary zone of proglottid, 163, 164, (164), (166), (172)
mitochondria in *Ascaris lumbricoides*, 466
of neck region, (185)
of oncospheral hooks, (83), (84), (85), 106
of oviduct, 260
propagation of action potentials to, 536
of rostellum, 233–235, (237)
of scolex, (177), 230–233, (231), (234)
sites of connective tissue interaction with, 202, (204)
of sperm duct, 249, (249)
of vaginal complex, 254, (255)
Myoblast
origin in Class II cells of oncosphere, 82
as precursor to all muscle units, 198–199
in preoncosphere, 89
staining reaction to Golgi procedures, 214
Myocyton (see also: muscle)
component of muscle cell, 186
in connective tissue protein synthesis, 202, (203), 203–204
cortical, (172)
fibrillar vesicles in parenchymal, 202
fine structure of, 194–199
medullary, (179), (185), (190), (261)
in musculature of rostellum, 235, (237)
in radial musculature of suckers, 231, (232)
for storage of carbohydrate in cells of excretory ducts, (207)
terminal organ of excretory system surrounded by glycogen-rich, (213)
Myofibril (see also: myosin, actin)
composition of, 186
dense body associated with sarcolemma of, 202
elaboration by myoblast in *Avitellina centripunctata*, 199
fine structure of, 186–191
in glycogen-rich extensions of musculoparenchyma cells of superficial body musculature, 178, (179), (185)
in preoncosphere, 89
in radial musculature of suckers, 231, (232)
in somatic musculature of oncosphere, 82
Myosin
comparison to vertebrate myosin filaments to worm, 188–189
in contractile myofibril, 186, (187)
in two-filament sliding model of muscle contraction, 189, 191
Mystatin, in control of fungal contaminants in culture media, 435, 537

N

NAD$^+$
control of lactic dehydrogenase by cytoplasmic, 478
-linked malate dehydrogenase, 480
-linked 'malic' enzyme, 466, 470
malate dehydrogenase regeneration of, 465, 477, 493
in mitochondrial electron transport, 470, 471, 482–488
in Site I coupled generation of ATP, 468
NAD$^+$ transhydrogenase, in mitochondria of *Hymenolepis diminuta*, 483–488, (487)
NADH
aerobic utilization of, 467
-coupled fumarate reductase activity in *Hymenolepis diminuta*, 481–482
generation of intramitochondrial, 466, 470, 480
reducing equivalents from malate dismutation in form of, 470, 493
-stimulated O$_2$ uptake sensitive to rotenone, 489
in transhydrogenase reaction, 471, 483–488, (487)
NADH dehydrogenase
in *Ascaris lumbricoides* muscle, 467
mitochondrial location of, 470
NADH:NADP transhydrogenase
inhibition by 2' AMP, AMP, ADP, and ATP of, 484
in mitochondrial membranes of *Hymenolepis diminuta*, 483
NADH oxidase
in *Ascaris lumbricoides* muscle, 467
in mitochondria of adult *Hymenolepis diminuta*, 481, 485, 489
role in ATP generation of, 492
NADH-tetrazolium reductase, activity in inner envelope of, 74
NADPH:NAD transhydrogenase
activity stimulated by bacterial 2' AMP and ATP, 484
in cysticercoids of *Hymenolepis diminuta*, (141)

in electron transport with fumarate reductase, 484–486
in mitochondria of *Hymenolepis diminuta*, 482, (487)
unaffected by EDTA, 484
Naphthamimidines (see: bunamidine)
Neck
  as body component of adult tapeworm, 160
  germinal anlagen in, 229
  interconnection of longitudinal nerve trunks in, 217
  lateral nerve cords in, (195), (227)
  multipolar perikarya in, 233
  muscle innervation in, 192
  neurosecretory release sites in, 226
  as region of proglottid formation, 182, (1982), 241
Nematospiroides dubius
  cross reactivity of *Hymenolepis diminuta* and, 590
  efficacy of diospyrol on mouse infections of, 645
  immunosuppresive effect on, 590
Nerve cells (neurons)
  cytology of, 220–224, (221), (222)
  histology of, 218, (219)
  junctions of, 218–220
  in myoneural junctions, 169
  in relation to 'neuron doctrine', 169
  secretions of, 224–228, (227)
  stem cell origin of, 359
Nervous system
  neuromuscular interactions of, 192–194, 251
  position of major nerve trunks of, 163–164, 164–165
  role in site selection and migration of *Hymenolepis diminuta* of, 631
  structure and functions of, 214–228
Neuromuscular tissue
  effect of acranil on *Taenia saginata*, 650
  ionic and membrane events accompanying excitability in, 541
Neuropile
  in cephalic ganglion, 218, (218)
  neuromuscular junction in, 220
  in relation to lateral nerve cord, (227)
Neurosecretion
  in *Hymenolepis diminuta*, 224–228, (225), (227)
  in *Hymenolepis microstoma*, 222, 367
  influence on endocrine glands by, 233

Neurosecretory cells
  in *Hymenolepis diminuta*, 630
  in *Hymenolepis microstoma*, 367
Nexus (see: junctions)
Niacin
  absorption of, 381
  as dietary supplement, 375
  inhibition of worm growth with deficiency of, 377
Niche (see: site)
Niclosamide
  anthelmintic action of, 660–662
  structural formula of, (676)
Nippostrongylus brasiliensis
  anthelmintic action of thiabendazole on, 652
  concentration of thiabendazole by, 651
  concurrent infections of *Hymenolepis diminuta* and, 382, (383), 388–389, (390), (391)
  cross reactivity of *Hymenolepis diminuta* and, 589
  energy metabolism of, 464
  globule leucocytes and mast cells in rejection of, 573–574
  immunological threshold in numbers of, 594
  intestinal migration of, 596
  modification of intraintestinal environment by, 387
  passive protection against, 577
  prostaglandins in rejection of, 580
Nitroscanate
  anthelmintic activity of, 664
  structural formula of, (677)
Nitroxynil, tegumentary damage by, 664
Nor-flavaspidic acid
  in uncoupling of oxidative phosphorylation in rat liver mitochondria, 641
  structural formula of, (669)
Nucleic acids
  isolation of, 451
  role of acriflavine in studies on structure and functions of, 650
Nucleosidases, intracellular enzymes from mucosal cells, 293
Nucleotidases, extracellular secretion from mucosal cells, 293
Nucleotides, permeability of gap junctions to, 534
Nucleases
  extracellular secretion of, 293
  in *Hymenolepis diminuta*, 458
Nucleus
  chromosomes in, 78

Index

of Class I embryonic cells, (94)
of cortical myocyton, (196)
of endocrine cell, (225)
^{3}H-thymidine labeling of, 183, (184)
of medullary myocyton, (197)
of oocyte, 258, (259)
of penetration glands, 84
in plasmodium formation, 168
in spermatozoa, (255)
in spermiogenesis, 243–244, (247), (248)
of stem cells, 358, (359)
of syncytium surrounding embryo, 64–65
of tegumental cell, (124), 178, (179)
types of, (79)
of vitelline cell, 61, 257, (257), (258)
'Nude' mice, role of T-cells in, 578–579
'Nude' rats, inability to reject infections of *Hymenolepis diminuta* by, 595
Nutrient agar, in culture medium, 442
Nutrition, parenteral, 631

O

Oesophagostomum columbianum, immunological threshold in sheep of, 594
Oleoresin of aspidium
  from rhizomes of *Dryopteris filix-mas*, 640
  in treatment of *Diphyllobothrium latum*, 640
Oligomycin
  inhibition of mitochondrial malate dependent phosphorylation by, 480
  oxyclozanide in relief of inhibition of ADP-stimulated respiration induced by, 663
Oligosaccharide, secretion by mammals, 291
Olive oil, in test diet to assess effect on migratory response of *Hymenolepis diminuta*, 620–621
Oncoblast, in hook formation, 78
Oncophore, in hook differentiation, 78
Oncosphere
  description of, 89
  diagram of, (93)
  emergence of, 4, 428–429
  hooks of, 3, 81
  in vitro culture of 426, 427, 474
  in vitro development of, 431–432
  membranes of, 76
  penetration of, 94, 102
  tegumentary epithelium of, 86, 183
Oochoristica symmetrica, activity of bunamidine in mice infected with, 664

Oocyte (see also: eggs)
  description of, 256, (259)
  in process of oogenesis, 60–62
  rDNA of, 457
Oogenesis, in *Hymenolepis diminuta*, 60
Ootype, secretory glands of, 253, 260–263
Ortho-desapidin
  in uncoupling of oxidative phosphorylation in rat liver mitochondria, 641
  structural formula of, (669)
Osmoregulation
  in *Hymenolepis diminuta*, 165–166
  by epithelial syncytium of *Hymenolepis diminuta*, 532
Ouabain
  asymmetric inhibition of transport across membranes by, 508, 510, 514, 518, (519), 520
  effect on cellular Na$^+$ concentration by, 523, (524)
  effect on size and t½ of intracellular pool of tissue Na$^+$ of, 515
  inhibition of Na$^+$-pump of inward-facing membrane by, 517
  sensitivity of membranes of epithelial syncytium to, 509–510
Ova (see: eggs, oocytes)
Ovary
  differentiation of, 256
  differentiation of oocyte in, 253
  histogenesis of, 241
  in mature proglottid, (168), (254), 365
  in production of oocytes, 60
Oviduct
  course of oocyte through, 253
  histogenesis of, 256
  in mature proglottid, (254)
  microanatomy of, 259–260, (260)
Oxalacetate
  formation by PEPCK, 476, 493
  malate dehydrogenase in reduction of, 477
  decarboxylation of, 480
Oxfendazole
  efficacy against *Moniezia* in sheep of, 658
  structural formula of, (675)
Oxibendazole
  activity against *Dictyocaulus* in sheep and cattle, 654
  structural formula of, (674)
Oxidation-reduction potential
  effect of H$^+$ concentration in host intestine of, 303

effect of *Hymenolepis diminuta* infections on, 303–304
effect on microflora of intestine of, 303
of host intestine, 302–304
Oxyclozanide
in uncoupling of phosphorylation in mammalian mitochondria, 662
in treatment of *Fasciola hepatica* and *Hymenolepis diminuta* infections, 663
structural formula of, (677)
Oxygen
inhibitory effect during development of *Hymenolepis diminuta* of, 405, 464, 468, 488
uptake in *Hymenolepis diminuta*, 464, 468, 472, 488, 489, 661, 662, 664
8-oxyquinoline
antimonial complexes of, 647
O-(6-ido-8-quinolinyl)-meta-antimonate as antimonial complex of, (671)
tris (1-quinolinyl)-N′-, O-antimonate as antimonial complex of, (671)
Oxytalan (see also: connective tissue)
similarity of elements in *Hymenolepis diminuta* connective tissue to, 201, 204

P

Pancreatic amylase
reduction of starch digestion in absence of, 293
role in carbohydrate hydrolysis of, 290–291
Pancreatic islet cells, glucagon and insulin production by, 291
Pancreatic juices
buffering role of, 289
composition of, 290–292
Pancreatic lipase
inhibition of, 294
stimulation by bile salts of, 296
Pancreatic proteases
activation by enterokinase of, 293
influence of high protein diets on secretion of, 291
involvement in release of macromolecules from brush border of, 292
Paneth cells
distribution in intestinal crypts of, 283
in recruitment of endogenous amino acids, 324
in secretion of zymogens, 283
Pantothenate, inhibition of worm growth with deficiency of, 377

Pantothenic acid
as dietary supplement, 375
inhibition of worm growth with deficiency of, 377
Papain, in dispersal of cytoplasmic layer of inner envelope of oncosphere, 102
Paragonimus westermani
interference by bithionol of ATP production in, 660
succinate formation in, (473)
Parbendazole
destrobilation effect on *Moniezia expansa* of, 653
efficacy against *Hymenolepis diminuta* and *H. nana* in mice of, 653
interference of glucose absorption and glycogenesis by, 658
structural formula of, (674)
Parenchyma
in capsular tail of metacestode, 138
cells in, 541
collecting tubules in cortical, 206
medullary, 359
membrane transport properties of, 514
myocytons of, 202
organization of, 196–197
relationship of muscle and, 164, 199, 359
Parenchymal transport pool, of *Hymenolepis diminuta*, 511, (512)
Parietal cells, in secretion of hydrochloric acid, 288
Paromomycin (humatin)
efficacy against *Hymenolepis nana* in mice, *H. diminuta* in rats, and *Hydatigera taeniaeformis* in cats of, 647–648
structural formula of, (672)
Pelletierine,
efficacy against *Taenia* spp. and *Hymenolepis nana* of, 644
side effects of, 645
structural formula of, 645
Penicillin
as antibacterial agent in culture media, 430, 434, 435, 437
in excystment medium, 437–438
as sterilizing agent in egg collection, 428
Pepsin
in dispersal of cytoplasmic layer of inner envelope of oncosphere, 102
in excystment medium, 432, 434, 438, 440
optimum pH for activity of gastric, 288
Peptidase, in digestion of oncospheral embryophore, 101, 102

Peptone, stimulation of CCK-PZ secretion by, 322
Perikarya (see also: cytons), effect of worm conditioned saline on, 409
Permeability coefficients, effect of unstirred water layer on, 287
Peromyscus maniculatus, immunological studies on *Hymenolepis citelli* in, 553
Peroxidase
  in mitochondria of *Hymenolepis diminuta*, 492
  in *Trichinella spiralis*, 580
Peyer's patches, sensitization of β-cells by specific antigens in, 571
pH
  changes with diet, 298–301
  changes with infection, 298–301
  effect on transport of, 301
  of host intestine, 298–301
Phenol oxidase, in tanning of *Schistosoma mansoni* eggs, 464
Phenol red, in culture medium, (441)
Phenolase, absent in mature larvae and adults of *Hymenolepis diminuta*, 69
Phenylalanine, in shell protein of *Hymenolepis diminuta*, 69
Phisophex, in sterilization of adult tapeworm tegument, 436
Phlorizin
  in inhibition of glucose uptake, 522
  in inhibition of Na_E efflux, 522
Phloroglucinol compounds (see: aspidin, aspindinol, desapidin, desapidinol, flavaspidic acid, kamala, nor-flavaspidic acid, oleoresin of aspidium, ortho-desapidin, phloropyrone)
Phloropyrone, activity against *Hymenolepis nana*, 641
Phosphatase
  activity in collecting ducts, 211
  activity in host villus of, 285, 293
  effect of bunamidine on *Hymenolepis nana* tegumentary, 664
  in intermediate cell layer and tail parenchyma of capsules, 138
  in oncospheres and cysticercoids, 138–140, 143
  in synthesis of microtubules by secretory cells, 120
Phosphoenolpyruvate (PEP)
  formation by PEPCK in *Hymenolepis diminuta*, 476
  in glucose catabolism of *Ascaris lumbricoides* muscle, 465, 476

malate formation and regeneration of NAD_E by CO_K fixation of, 477, 478
Phosphoenolpyruvate carboxykinase (PEPCK)
  in formation of oxalacetate and PEP, 476
  inhibition in *Moniezia expansa* by cambendazole of, 653
  metabolic activities of, 476, 472–478
  in CO_K fixation, 465, 493
Phosphofructokinase, effect of antimonials on schistosome, 647
β-phospholipase, in *Hymenolepis nana*, 580
Phospholipids
  concentration changes during development, 370, (370), 371
  concentration in worms, 371
  in cytoplasmic region of outer envelope, 97
  in mature hooks of oncosphere, 82
  in mature larvae, 74
Phosphorus
  incorporation of, 641, 659, 661
  in $_{xx}$P-ATP exchange reaction, 479, 642, 659, 661–662
Phosphorus/malate ratio, for *Ascaris lumbricoides*, 466
Phosphorylase
  effect of glucagon on cellular concentration of, 291
  in scolex, inner envelope and cercomer of metacestode, 143
Phosphorylase b kinase, in control of ratio of α- to β-phosphorylases, 143
Phosphorylation
  Ascaris lumbricoides Site I, 492, 493–494
  benzimidazole derivatives in uncoupling of oxidative, 657
  bunamidine uncoupling of rat liver mitochondrial oxidative, 663
  dichlorophen uncoupling of *Hymenolepis diminuta* electron transport-linked, 659
  dichlorophen uncoupling of rat liver mitochondrial oxidative, 659, 662
  effect of desaspidin on *Hymenolepis diminuta* mitochondrial, 642
  enhancement by fluoride of mitochondrial, 479
  fumarate reductase coupled Site I, 492, 493–494
  malate dependent, 479–480
  O_K requirement of *Ascaris* oxidative, 468
  oxyclozanide uncoupling of oxidative, 663
  phlorobutyrophene derivatives in uncoupling of oxidative, 641

p-trifluromethyoxyphenylhydrazone uncoupling of artichoke mitochondrial, 468–469
Phytohemagglutinin (PHA), in stimulation of T-cells, 579
Plasmodia (see also: spermatogenesis)
 formation of, 168
 formation in spermatogenesis, 169, 243, (245)
Polyembryony, in Digenea, 266
Potassium, effect on glucose transport of ionic, 392, 393, 395, 396
Praziquantel
 effect on glucose uptake in *Hymenolepis diminuta* in vitro of, 665–666
 effect on *Echinococcus granulosus* and *E. multilocularis* in dogs of, 665
 effect on human species of schistosomes of, 665
 effect on musculature of *Hymenolepis diminuta* in vitro of, 666
 efficacy against *Hymenolepis diminuta* in rats of, 665
 efficacy against *Hymenolepis nana* and *H. diminuta* in mice of, 665
Pregnancy, of host affecting in vivo growth of *Hymenolepis diminuta*, 375, 558
Premunition, in superinfections of *Hymenolepis diminuta*, 367, 368
Preoncosphere, ontogeny of, 77–78
Primitive lacuna, development of, 111–112
Primordia
 development of peripheral and central, 241
 differentiation of male genitalia from somatic, 245–246
 differentiation of ovary and vitelline glands from central, 256, 257
 differentiation of terminal genitalia from somatic, 253
 differentiation of testes from germinative and germinative-somatic cells of peripheral, 242–243
 early primary, 241
 role in chronology of histogenesis of proglottid of, 365
Proflavine
 effect on *Hymenolepis nana* of, 650
 structural formula of, (673)
Progesterone
 effect on egg production in castrated hosts of, 376

 in support of worm growth in castrated hosts, 375
 unsupportive of worm growth in spayed hosts, 375
Proglottid (proglottis)
 development of, 2, 365–367, 404
 diagram of mature, (254)
 differences in absorption related to maturity of, 397–398
 early development of, 241, 358
 effect of crowding on production of, 403–404
 effect of host diet on production of, 372–374, 377
 general structure of, 161–170
 immune mediated attack dependent on age of, 582
 micrograph of teminal, (163)
 of *Moniezia expansa* as source of antigen, 597
 number in *Hymenolepis diminuta* of, 163, 357, (366)
 rate of development of, 265
 role in reproductive potential of, 266
 zones of, 163
Proline
 absorbed as peptides by host intestine, 309
 in shell protein, 69
Promethazine, effect on rejection of *Hymenolepis diminuta* in mice of, 575
Propionyl-Co A carboxylase, absent in *Hymenolepis diminuta*, 476
Prostaglandins
 in rejection of *Nippostrongylus* from rats, 580
 synthesis by chromaffin cells of, 283
Protease
 in digestion of inner envelope, 98, 100
 effect on growth inhibiting substances of, 410
Protein
 cell-free synthesis of, 458
 content of *Hymenolepis diminuta*, 451
 effects on worm development of host dietary, 307, 309, 372, 381, 383
Protein kinase, in control of ratio of α- to β-phosphorylase in metacestodes, 143
Protein synthesis
 amino acid requirement from endogenous protein for, 312
 in connective tissue cells, 202, 204
 effect of crowding on, 409

informational RNA and, 365
inhibition of, 313
in vitro cell-free system for, 457
in tegumentary cytons, 180, 182
Protonephridia
applicability of term to cestode system of, 204–205
canals of, 536
flame cells as terminal organs of, 206
in H_E secretion, 300
in metacestodes, (132)
Pseudopelletierine, from bark of *Punica granatum*, 644
Ptyalin (salivary amylase), in starch hydrolysis, 290
Punica granatum (pomegranate tree), as source of pelletierine, 644
Pyridoxine (and pyridoxal, pyridoxamine, vitamin B_K),
as dietary requirement, 375, 403
effects of dietary deficiency of, 377–381, (378)
Pyruvate,
acetate formed via pyruvate dehydrogenase from, 480, 494
alanine accumulation via transamination of, 473, 493
formation during malate dismutation, 466
increase during *Hymenolepis diminuta* incubation with resorantel, 662
oxalacetate decarboxylation in formation of, 480
in oxidative phosphorylation, 468
oxidation in presence of malate stimulated by ADP and cytochrome c, 490
Pyruvate carboxylase, absent in *Hymenolepis diminuta*, 476
Pyruvate dehydrogenase, formation of acetate from pyruvate via, 480, 494
Pyruvate kinase,
activity in ascarid muscle of, 465
activity in *Hymenolepis diminuta* of, 477–478, 493
in oncospheres and cysticercoids of *Hymenolepis diminuta*, 137

Q

Quinacrine (see: mepacrine)
Quinolinehydrazones, in tests against *Hymenolepis nana*, 665

Quinone, in color change and hardening of shells, 69
Quinolines, anthelmintic activity of, 665–666

R

Rafoxanide, in uncoupling of phosphorylation systems, 664
Raillietina cesticillus,
effect of crowding on, 401
effect of host starvation on, 593
immune response of fowl to, 599
immunity to, 553
mast cell increase in response to infection with, 575
protein distribution in, 135
Receptors,
chemoreceptors, 536, 630
mechanoreceptors, 536
sensory, 536, 541
Regeneration,
of scolex, 229
of strobila, 229
Reproductive system (see also: specific organs), general structure and functions of, 240–263
Resorantel,
effect on ATP, ADP and glycogen concentrations in *Hymenolepis diminuta* of, 662
effect of O_K consumption of isolated *Hymenolepis diminuta* mitochondria of, 662
structural formula of, (676)
Rhabditis macrocerca, in vitro activity of axenomycin A, B, and D against, 648
Rhodoquinone, coupling of ascarid electron transport system to, 467
Rhythms,
circadian, 615
diel, 615
diurnal,
periodic activity as, 615
Riboflavin, requirement in host diet of, 375, 377, 379–381
Ribonuclease,
effect on satellite DNAs of, 453
effect on worm conditioned saline of, 410
Ribonucleic acid,
absent in mature larvae, 69, 74
in binucleate medullary center for hook formation, 86

changes during development in concentrations of, 370, 371
content in *Hymenolepis diminuta,* 451
effect of crowding on synthesis of, 409, (410)
in *Hymenolepis diminuta,* 449–459
messenger (mRNA), 365, 458, 459
mitochondrial (mtRNA), 457, 458
synthesis of, 135, 402, 409, 410, 458
synthesis in germinative region of informational, 365
synthesis in wall of cysticercoid, 135
transfer (tRNA), 457
Ribosomes
in binucleate cell of oncosphere, 87
in connective tissue forming inner fibrous region of wall of cysticercoid, 120
in cortical myocyton, (196)
in cytons of surface epithelium, 134, 178, 195
in cytoplasm of cells forming wall of cyst, 112
in cytoplasm of flame cells, 209
in cytoplasm of outer envelope, 66
in endocrine cell, (225)
in epithelial squamous cells lining primitive lacuna, 113
in fibrogenic cell, 202, (203)
in intermediate layer of distal cytoplasmic layer of oncosphere, 88
in macromeres, 62
in mucous cells of Mehlis' gland, 261, (261)
in oocytes, 256
in perikarya, 220
purification of, 457
in rostellar tegumentary cyton, (237)
in secondary spermatocytes, 244
in serous cells of Mehlis' gland, 262, (262)
in stem cells, 358
in syncytial epithelium of oviduct, 259
in Type A and B spermatogonia, 243–244
in vitelline cells, 61
Ringer's phosphate solution, use in harvesting adult tapeworms, 435
Roller tubes, use in in vitro cultivation, 437, 438, 440
Rostellum (see also: scolex)
bipolar fuchsinophilic cells in, 367
excretory system in, 205–206
functions of, 229
general features of, 161, (162), (230), (231), 233–240, (234), (235), (237)
innervation of, 215, (216)
in members of the genus *Hymenolepis,* 8
sensory perikarya in, 223, (227)
tegument of, (177), (238), (239)
Rotenone
effect on mitochondrial fumarate reductase activity of, (483)
inhibition of electron transport associated$n$phosphorylation by, 479–480
inhibition of malate dependent mitochondrial phosphorylation by, 480
inhibition of Site I phosphorylation by, 482, 489
Rotterlin
as component of kamala, 642
structural formula of, (670)
Roughage, in host diet, 373

S

Salicylanilide (see: niclosamide)
Schistocephalus solidus, cultivation of fragments of, 570
Scolex (see also: holdfast)
adenosine phosphatase in musculature of cysticercoid, 138
alkaline phosphatase in tegument of, 140
amylo-(1, 4-1, 6)-transglucosidase in, 143
attachment as index of intestinal distribution of worms, 617, 622
cholinesterase activity in nerves of, 138
cultivation of, 426
development of, 4, (135)
effect of temperature on withdrawal of, 144
glycogen in musculature of, 140
longevity of destrobilated, 581, 582
microtrich formation on, 120, 131, 431, 432
mitotic activity in, 358
NADH → NBT reductase in tegument and parenchyma of cysticercoid, 138
phosphatase activity in metacestode, 138
phosphorylase system in cysticercoid, 143
as primary source of antigens, 561, 569, 570
retraction of, 112–114, (116), 131, 431, 432
succinic dehydrogenase activity in cysticercoid, 137
Schistosoma mansoni
activity of axenomycin A, B, and D against, 648
collection of DNA from, 452
energy metabolism in, 464
O_2 requirement for normal egg development in, 464

Index

oxytalan-type connective tissue in, 201
spastic paralysis caused by praziquantel in, 666
Schistosoma spp.
  4-isothiocyanato-4′-nitrodiphenylamine activity against, 663
  praziquantel activity against all human, 665
  stibophen in chemotherapy of, 647
Secretin
  control of bile flow in dogs by, 295
  control of water and bicarbonate secretion from pancreas by, 288
  distribution and concentration in host of, 321–322
  inhibition of acid secretion and stimulation of insulin release by, 321
  synthesis by chromaffin cells of, 283
Secretion (see also: neurosecretion)
  of CCK-PZ, 322
  by cells in wall of cysticercoid, 120, (121)
  diurnal periodicity of intestinal hormone, 309
  of endocrine cells, 309
  of gastrin I and II, 322
  of glucagon, 322
  of growth hormone, 322
  of H^+, 300–301
  of HCO_3^-, 301–302
  of insulin, 320
  of lipoprotein from Mehlis' gland, 61
  from Paneth cells, 324
  of penetration glands, 84–85, (87), 104, 106–108
  of proteins, 307
  by specialized cells in host intestinal epithelium, 283
  by uterus, 68
  of vitelline cells, 61
Seminal receptacle
  formation from vagina, 253
  microvilli on lining of, 254, (255)
  storage of spermatozoa in, 253, (255)
Seminal vesicle
  differentiation from somatic primordium of, 246
  expansion of sperm duct as, 242, 247–248, (250)
  location in proglottid of, (164), (168), (251), (254)
  in rats as index of sex hormonal status, 372
  storage of spermatozoa in, 242
Sensilla
  of *Acanthobothrium coronatum*, 223

chemo- and/or tacto-sensory nature of, 179, 223
in rostellar tegument, 215
in scolex tegument, 216, (221), 239
structure of, (179), 223
in tegument, 179, 223
Serine, in inner layer of inner envelope, 75
Serine dehydrogenase, influence of high carbohydrate diets on concentrations of, 314
Serotonin (see: 5-hydroxytryptamine)
Serum
  of calf in culture medium, 430
  of horse in culture medium, 426, 436, 437, 438, 442, 444
Sex hormones, of host affecting worm growth, 3, 145, 375–377
Sialytransferase, on villus of host intestine, 286
Site
  definition of, 615
  -finding behavior, 616
  selection, 616, 617–618, 627, 632
Sodium
  effect on glucose transport of ionic, 392, 393, 395, 396, 517, 520–521, 523–524
  -pump, 517
Sodium acetate
  absorption by metacestodes of, 143
  effect of cortisone on transport of, 582
Sodium butyrate, inhibition of sodium acetate absorption by, 143
Sodium cholate, inhibition of anaerobic fermentation of glucose by, 386
Sodium propionate, inhibition of sodium acetate uptake by, 143
Sodium stearate, uptake of sodium acetate not affected by, 143
Sodium taurocholate, in excystment medium, 434, 438, 440
Sodium tauroglycocholate, in excystment medium, 434, 438, 440
Somatophore (see also: oncophore)
  cellular composition of, 78
Sperm duct
  differentiation from somatic primordium of, 246
  passage of spermatozoa in, 242
  structure and functions of, 245–249, (249)
Spermatogenesis, in *Hymenolepis diminuta*, 60, 242–245
Spermatozoa
  development from single primary spermatogonium, 243

fertilization by, 253
formation of capsule over, 66
storage of, 248, (249), (255)
storage in external seminal vesicle of, (164)
ultrastructure of, 244–245, (246), (247)
Spirometra mansonoides
  activity of bunamidine in cats against, 664
  in vitro cultivation of, 426
  mechanism of microtrich formation in, 134
  succinate formation in, (473)
Starch, in host diet, 293, 310–311, 372, 373, 384, 403, 404, 620, 623
Stem cells
  cell cycle of, 362
  characterization of, 358–361, (359), (360), (361)
Stereospecificity
  of carrier-mediated transport systems, 516
  of inward- and outward-facing membranes of epithelial syncytium, 510
Steroids, variation in mammals in susceptibility to, 563
Stibophen
  in chemotherapy of schistosomes, 647
  structural formula of, (672)
Stilbesterol, effect on worm growth with deficiency of, 375
Streptomyces, protease from, 410
Streptomyces lisandri, axenomycin A, B, and D from, 648–649
Streptomyces rimosus, paromomycin from, 647
Streptomycin
  sterilization of adult worms with, 435, 437
  sterilization of eggs with, 428
  use in culture medium of, 430, 434
Strobila (see also: proglottids)
  cell proliferation in, 358
  as component of tapeworm body, 160–161
  contraction of longitudinal muscles of, 194
  difference in glucose absorption along the length of, 397–398
  effect of praziquantel on, 666
  effect of rejection on, 582
  formation of, 3, 168, 183, 241, 444
  growth of, 229–230
  immunogenic role of, 569–570
  production and maturation of proglottids of, 365–367
  segmentation of, 163, (163)
  stem cells in formation of, 359
Succinic acid, as end product of energy metabolism, 406

Succinic dehydrogenase
  activity in intermediate cell layer of capsule of metacestode, 138
  in *Ascaris lumbricoides* muscle, 467
  in fumarate reduction in *Hymenolepis diminuta*, 489
  in inner envelope of mature larvae, 74
  in matrix side of inner membrane of mitochondria of *Ascaris lumbricoides*, 470
  presence in several species of *Hymenolepis*, 137
Succinate
  accumulation from dissimilation of carbohydrate in *Ascaris lumbricoides*, 464, 465, 473, 494, 495
  $^{14}CO_2$ incorporation into, 476–478
  dependency of O_2 uptake on, 489, 491
  effect on DNA synthesis of, 410
  fermentation ratios of, 475
  in fluid of excretory canal, 209, 211
  formation by helminths, (473)
  formation from malate dismutation of, 466, 467, 470, (472), 479, 482
  oxidation inhibited by antimycin A and KCN, 490
  secretion of, 406
  in worm conditioned saline, 406–408
Succinoxidase
  in mitochondria of *Hymenolepis diminuta*, 489, 492
  in particulate fraction of *Ascaris lumbricoides* muscle, 467
Succus entericus
  characterization of, 292–294
  enterokinase in, 290
Suckers (see also: scolex)
  in attachment to host intestine, 161, 231
  development in metacestode, 113, (114), 131
  function impaired by praziquantel, 666
  innervation of, 215–217
  modulation of muscle activity in, 192
  myofibrils in musculature of, 186
  in relationship to rostellum, (162)
  structure of, 230–233, (232)
  as taxonomic character, 6, 8
Sucrase
  in mammals, 291
  regulation by dietary sucrose in man, 312–313
  in reinforcing action of pancreatic disaccharidases, 293
  secretion stimulated by CCK-PZ, 292

Index 729

Sucrose
  adaptive enzymatic activity in response to, 313
  gradients in host gut, 311
  parallel to crowding effect of dietary, 403
  rate of absorption of, 284
  worm growth not supported by dietary, 310
Superinfections
  in crowding effect, 591
  in premunition, 367–368, 552
Synapse (see also: junctions), as distinguished from junctions, 226
Syncytiotrophoblast, of mammals, 168
Syncytium
  of acetabular tegument, (232)
  of collecting ducts, 206, (207)
  of excretory canals of scolex, (236)
  in mammalian development, 184
  musculo-parenchymal tissue as, 196
  of outer envelope, 64, 66
  of oviduct, 259, (260)
  of preoncospheral surface, 97
  prevalence of, 167–168
  of sperm ducts, 248, (249)
  of surfaces, 265
  ultrastructure of, (177)
  of uterus, 263
  of vagina and seminal receptacle, 253, (255)
Syngamus tracheae, effect of mebendazole on intestinal cells of, 657
Synonymy, of *Hymenolepis diminuta*, 5
Syphacia muris, succinate formation in, (473)
Systematic position, of *Hymenolepis diminuta*, 4–5, 157–158

T

Taenia
  occurrence of premunition in human infections of, 591
  tapeworm adults all formerly assigned to, 157
  vaccination against, 598
Taenia crassiceps
  activity of cambendazole in mice on metacestodes of, 652
  activity of oxibendazole in mice against, 654
  effectiveness of mebendazole against cysticercus of, 656
  gas phase in in vitro culture of, 475
  growth of tegument of, 183–184
  plasma membrane of tegument of, 175

Taenia diminuta
  synonym of *Hymenolepis diminuta*, 5, 6, 157
  synonym of *Hymenolepis flavopunctata* with, 157–158
Taenia hydatigena,
  activity of bunamidine in dogs against, 664
  activity of cambendazole in dogs against, 652
  activity of nitroscanate in dogs against, 663
Taenia pisiformis,
  effectiveness of axenomycin D in dogs against, 649
  efficacy of mebendazole against cysticercoid of, 656
  polysaccharide complexes in penetration glands of, 106
Taenia saginata,
  effect of acranil on neuromuscular system of, 650
  effect of cambendazole on viability of cysticercoid of, 652
  effectiveness of acranil in treatment of, 650
  efficacy of extracts of *Cucurbita* seed in human infections of, 646
  efficacy of niclosamide against, 660
  efficacy of paromomycin in human cases of, 648
  egg production of, 240
  polysaccharide complexes in penetration glands of, 106
  use of infusion of bark of pomegranate tree against, 644
  use of mepacrine in treatment of, 649
Taenia solium,
  action of mebendazole against, 656
  efficacy of niclosamide against, 660
  efficacy of paromomycin in infections of, 648
  use of mepacrine in treatment of, 649
Taenia spp.
  effectiveness of pelletierine against, 644
  role of paromomycin in changing tegumental ultrastruce of, 648
  use of minced seed of *Cucurbita pepo* in treatment of, 645
Taenia taeniaeformis,
  succinate production by larvae and adults of, (473)
  ultrastructure of hooks of, 81
Taeniasis, effectiveness of thiabendazole in treatment of, 651
Taurine
  conjugation in duodenun of, 297

formation of bile acids from, 295
stimulation of ATPase activity by conjugates of, 296
Taurocholate
in excystment medium, 432, 434
inhibition of glycolysis by, 386
Tauroglycocholate, in excystment medium, 434
Taxonomy, of *Hymenolepis diminuta*, 4–5, 157–158
Tegument
alkaline phosphatase in scolex, 140
alteration by paromomycin of *Taenia*, 648
alteration in staining characteristics of rostellar, 235–236, (236), (237), (238)
antigens from 569, 570
binding of immunoglobulins to, 318
effect of bunamidine on *Hymenolepis nana*, 664
effect of immune attack on, 580, 581–582
effect of mebendazole on *Hymenolepis nana*, 664
effect of praziquantel on *Hymenolepis nana*, 666
effect of worm conditioned saline treatment on, 408–409
formation during cysticercoid development, 4
functional correlates of, 180–185
gap junctions between muscles and, 189, (190)
immunological damage of transport agencies of, 582–583
membranes of, 318, 648
phosphatase activity of scolex, 140
position of unstriated muscle of metacestode in relation to, 113
production of proteolytic enzyme inhibitor by, 294
protective role of, 131
relative efficiency in nutrient uptake by host mucosa and tapeworm, 287–288
of scolex during reorganization of oncosphere, 110
sensilla in distal cytoplasm of, 223, 239
sensilla in rostellar, 215
unstirred water layer as source of error in calculating uptake rates of, 287
Tenebrio molitor
glycogen levels in oncosphere during penetration of gut of larval, 106
growth of metacestodes in gnotobiotic, 108

histology of midgut in larval and adult, 102, (103), (104
as intermediate host of *Hymenolepis diminuta*, 95
saline preparations and midgut contents of, 96, 98, (99), (100)
sequence of events during emergence of *Hymenolepis diminuta* in, (97)
tryptic activity of larval midgut extracts from, 101
Terpenic peroxide (see: ascaridol)
Testes
differentiation from peripheral primordium of, 241, 242–243
glycogen in, 62
position in proglottid of, 164, 168
in spermatogenesis, 242, (245)
use as taxonomic character of, 6
Testosterone
effect on egg production of worms in castrated and diet-deficient female hosts of, 376
effect of worm growth in normal or spayed hosts on deficient diets of, 375
Tetrahydrofolate, role in purine and thymine synthesis, 566
N, N, N', N'-tetramethyl-p-phenylene diamine (TMPD)
assay of cytochrome oxidase with ascorbate and, 474, 490
in oxidative phosphorylation in *Ascaris lumbricoides* mitochondria, 468
Theelin (see: estrone)
Thiabendazole
effect on fumarate reductase in *Haemonchus contortus, Fasciola hepatica* and *Hymenolepis diminuta*, 651
efficacy in treatment of hyman cases of *Hymenolepis nana*, 651
efficacy in treatment of taeniasis of, 651
in vitro concentration by *Nippostrongylus brasiliensis, Fasciola hepatica* and *Hymenolepis diminuta* of, 651–652
Thiamine
absorption of, 381
requirement in diet for, 375, 376, 377
Threonine, lacking in 48 h hydrolysates of cysticercoids, 135
T lymphocytes
in rejection of *Hymenolepis diminuta*, 578–579
in rejection of *Trichinella spiralis*, 578

Thymidine
  cell cycle chronology estimated by labelling with, 362
  DNA incorporation of, 405
  effect of worm conditioned saline on DNA incorporation of, 406
  transport dependent on Na$^+$ concentration, 516
Thymidine kinase, role in synthesis of DNA of, 458
Thymine, role of dihydrofolate dehydrogenase in synthesis of, 566
Thysanosoma actinoides, action of cambendazole on, 652
Tin compounds, anthelmintic activity of, 646–647
Toluidine blue positive cells, histochemical evidence of intestinal mast cells and globule leucocytes from, 574
Total transport pool, in *Hymenolepis diminuta*, 511, (512)
Transplantation (implanting)
  in assessment of site selection in *Hymenolepis diminuta*, 617–618
  in determining duration of memory to immunizing infections, 560–561
Transhydrogenase
  activity in *Ascaris* mitochondria, 470–471, 482
  activity in *Hymenolepis diminuta* mitochondria, 482–488
Transport
  of alanine, 509
  of amino acids, 507
  competitive inhibition of glucose, 395
  via convective coupling, 516, 520–526, 529
  via coupling mechanisms and volume regulation, 516, 526–532
  in coupled systems, 516–532
  effect of Na$^+$ concentration on, 521
  effect on Na$^+$ concentration on glucose, 520–521, 523
  of galactose, 509, 510, 523–525
  of glucose, 509, 520–523
  of hexose, 507, 513, 518
  of ions, 507, 513
  ion-gradient hypothesis of, 516–520
  of lipids, 507
  by microvilli of glucose, 286
  Na$^+$-coupled nonelectrolyte, 509, 521, 529
  of Na$^+$-sensitive amino acids, 509
  of nucleosides, 507
  of nutrients, 506, 539
  of purines, 507
  of pyrimidines, 507
  transepithelial, 507, 509
  of vitamins, 507
Triaenophorus nodulosus, plerocercoids of, 358
Tribolium, development of larval *Hymenolepis diminuta* in, 4
Tribolium castaneum, intensity of infection and development of *Hymenolepis diminuta* in, 145
Tribolium confusum
  comparison of developmental rates of cysticercoids in vitro and in, (433)
  cysticercoids for in vitro culture taken from 437, 440
  intensity of infection of *Hymenolepis diminuta* in, 145
  intensity of infection and size of metacestodes of *Hymenolepis diminuta* affected by age of, 146
  response to infections of *Hymenolepis citelli*, *H. microstoma* and *H. diminuta* by, 131
Tricarboxylic acid cycle
  inoperative as energy generating sequence in *Ascaris lumbricoides*, 464–465
  lacking in *Hymenolepis diminuta*, 474, 495
Trichinella spiralis
  cross reactivity of *Hymenolepis diminuta* and, 589–590
  cross reactivity of *Hymenolepis nana* and, 587, 590
  effect of mebendazole on encysted stages of, 655
  in vitro cultivation of, 426
  peroxidase in, 580
  stichosome as antigenic source in, 570
  succinate production in, (473)
  T cells in rejection of, 578
  vaccination against, 596
Trichinosis, use of thiabendazole in, 651
Trichuris muris
  antigenic threshold of, 595
  source of antigens of, 570
  vaccination against, 596
Trichuris vulpis, succinate production in, (473)
p-trifluromethyoxyphenylhydrozone (FCCP), uncoupling of mitochondrial phosphorylation system in Jerusalem artichokes by, 469

Triglycerides, resynthesis of, 296
Triple Eagle's medium, use in cultivation of
    Hymenolepis microstoma of, 444
Trivalent antimonials (see: stibophen)
Trypanosomes, action of acriflavine on, 650
Trypsin
    activation by enterokinase, 291, 293
    adsorption to intestinal mucosal cells by, 292
    alteration of outer envelope by, 68, 74
    dispersal of cytoplasmic region of inner envelope, 96
    in excystment medium, 432, 434, 438, 440
    influence of diet on secretion of, 291
    inhibition of activity of, 294
    in pancreatic juice, 290
    requirement in hatching of oncospheres, 428
    use in defined medium for digestion of embryophore of, 102
Trypsinogen
    activation by enterokinase of, 293
    in pancreatic juice, 290
Tryptar, in hatching medium of *Hymenolepis citelli* and *H. nana*, 428, 429
Tryptophan
    in capsule of *Hymenolepis diminuta*, 68
    in capsule of *Raillietina cesticillus*, 135
    in embryophore of *Hymenolepis diminuta*, 75
    in 'shell' of *Hymenolepis diminuta*, 68
Two-membrane hypothesis
    asymmetry of function in, 517, 518, 520
    model for, 507–509, 539
Tyrode's solution, in excystment medium, 434
Tyrosine
    distribution in tissues of cysticdrcoid, 135, 137
    in inner envelope and embryophore, 74, 75
    in layers of capsule, 68, 69, (70)

U

Ubiquinone, coupling in mammalian electron transport system, 467
Uridine
    labelling of DNA with radioactive, 458
    Na^+ requirement for membrane transport of, 516
    periodicity in uptake of, 309, 631, 633
    uptake inhibited by worm conditioned saline, 409, (412)
Urea
    action of intestinal bacteria on, 317
    effect on DNA synthesis of, 406

Uterus
    development of, 263
    initiation of cleavage of oocyte in, 62
    location in proglottid of, (254)
    maturation of larvae in, 253, (264)
    microanatomy of, 263
    role in 'shell' formation of, 68

V

V_{max} (maximum transport velocity), of glucose and galactose, 394, 398
Vagina
    differentiation from somatic primordium of, 241
    histology of, 253–256
    position in proglottid of, 253
Vasoactive intestinal peptide (VIP), activity in gastrointestinal tract of, 321
Vibrio succinogenes, electron transport system linked to reduction of fumarate in, 469
Vitamins (see also: specific vitamins)
    requirements of *Hymenolepis diminuta* for, 374–381
    transport across brush border of, 507
Vitamin A, requirement for, 375
Vitamin B_1 (see: thiamine)
Vitamin B_6 (see: pyridoxine)
Vitamin B_{12} (cyanocobalamin)
    effect of egg production by *Hymenolepis diminuta* of, 376
    effect on establishment and growth with deficiency of, 377
    effect of H^+ concentration on binding of, 301
    requirement for, 376
Vitamin D
    requirement for, 375
    requirement for bile salts in absorption of, 296
Vitamin E
    requirement for, 375
    requirement for bile salts in absorption of, 296
'Vitamin G complex', requirement for, 375
Vitamin K, requirement for bile salts in absorption of, 296
Vitelline cells
    differentiation from central primordium of, 242, 257
    in embryonic development, 61–62
    in envelope formation, 253
    fusion with oocyte by, 253

Index 733

Vitelline ducts
 in female reproductive system, 253, 258
 innervation of, 218

W

Worm conditioned saline (WCS), characterization and activities of, 405–410

X

X-irradiation
 destruction of T-cells by, 578
 immunosuppressive effects of, 567–568

Y

Yeast extract, use in culture medium of, 436, 437, 438, 442

Z

'Zanil', activity as a vermifuge of, 588, 593
Z-disc, lacking in myofibrils of *Hymenolepis diminuta,* 186
Zein, in test diets, 381
Zygote, development of membranes of, 253
Zymogens, enzymes secreted as, 293
Zymogen cells, similarity in structure of Paneth cells and, 283

ARY OF DAV